Mav 04

Surgical Care at the District Hospital

World Health Organization

WHO Library Cataloguing-in-Publication Data

Surgical care at the district hospital.

1. Surgery – methods 2. Surgical procedures, Operative – methods 3. Anesthesia – methods 4. Wounds and injuries – surgery 5. Hospitals, District – organization and administration 6. Pregnancy complications – surgery 7. Manuals I. World Health Organization.

Incorporates: Primary trauma care manual.

ISBN 92 4 154575 5 (NLM classification: WO 39)

Typeset in London

Printed in Malta by Interprint Limited

Contents

PART 6: TRAUMATOLOGY AND ORTHOPAEDICS

Preface

Many patients who present to district (first-referral) level hospitals require surgical treatment for trauma, obstetric, abdominal and orthopaedic emergencies. Often surgery cannot be safely postponed to allow their transfer to a secondary or tertiary-level hospital, but many district hospitals in developing countries have no specialist surgical teams and are staffed by medical, nursing and paramedical personnel who perform a wide range of surgical procedures, often with inadequate training. The quality of surgical and acute care is often further constrained by poor facilities, inadequate low-technology apparatus and limited supplies of drugs, materials and other essentials.

All these factors contribute to unacceptable rates of mortality resulting from trauma, obstetric complications and non-traumatic surgical disorders as well as disability resulting from injury.

District hospitals should be able to manage all common surgical and obstetric procedures. However, the establishment and maintenance of effective district surgical services requires:

- Personnel with appropriate education and training
- Practical continuing education programmes in clinical management to maintain quality in care
- Appropriate physical facilities
- Suitable equipment and instruments
- A reliable system for the supply of drugs and medications, surgical materials and other consumables
- A quality system, including standards, clinical guidelines, standard operating procedures, records and audit.

The mission of the team responsible for Devices and Clinical Technology in the World Health Organization Department of Blood Safety and Clinical Technology (WHO/BCT) is to promote the quality of clinical care through the identification, promotion and standardization of appropriate procedures, equipment and materials, particularly at district hospital level.

WHO/BCT has identified education and training as a particular priority, especially for non-specialist practitioners who practise surgery and anaesthesia. It has therefore developed *Surgical Care at the District Hospital* as a practical resource for individual practitioners and for use in undergraduate and postgraduate programmes, in-service training and continuing medical education programmes. The manual is a successor of three earlier publications that are widely used throughout the world and that remain important reference texts:

- *General Surgery at the District Hospital* (WHO, 1988)
- *Surgery at the District Hospital: Obstetrics Gynaecology, Orthopaedics and Traumatology* (WHO, 1991)
- *Anaesthesia at the District Hospital* (WHO, 1988; second edition 2000).

This new manual draws together material from these three publications into a single volume which includes new and updated material, as well as material from *Managing Complications in Pregnancy and Childbirth: A guide for midwives and doctors* (WHO, 2000).

It also incorporates the *Primary Trauma Care Manual: Trauma Management in District and Remote Locations* which has been developed to help teach Primary Trauma Care (PTC), a system designed specifically for hospitals with limited resources. This edition of the *Primary Trauma Care Manual* has been adapted for WHO and is reproduced by permission of the Primary Trauma Care Foundation.

Surgical Care at the District Hospital has been written by an international team of specialist surgeons, anaesthetists and a medical educator. The authors and clinical editors acknowledge the important contributions made to this work by the previous authors. The manual has been reviewed by clinical specialists from all parts of the world and by the WHO Departments of Child and Adolescent Health and Development, Reproductive Health and Research, Organization and Service Delivery, and Injuries and Violence Prevention.

WHO recognizes the important contributions of practitioners who care for the surgical patients at the district hospital and hopes that this manual will assist them to provide consistently high standards of care for their patients.

Dr Jean C. Emmanuel
Director
Department of Blood Safety and Clinical Technology
World Health Organization

Acknowledgements

The World Health Organization acknowledges with special thanks the clinical specialists who have contributed to the development of *Surgical Care at the District Hospital*.

Project Director

Dr Jean C. Emmanuel, Director, Department of Blood Safety and Clinical Technology, WHO

Project Manager

Ms Jan Fordham, Director, Open Learning Associates, London, United Kingdom

Project Co-worker

Dr Meena Nathan Cherian, Medical Officer, Devices and Clinical Technology, Department of Blood Safety and Clinical Technology, WHO

Clinical Editors

Dr Michael Dobson, Consultant Anaesthetist, John Radcliffe Hospital, Oxford, United Kingdom

Dr Richard Fisher, Associate Professor, Department of Orthopaedics, University of Colorado Health Science Centre, Denver, Colorado, USA

Authors

Dr Michael Dobson, Consultant Anaesthetist, John Radcliffe Hospital, Oxford, United Kingdom

Dr Paul Fenton, formerly Associate Professor, College of Medicine, Blantyre, Malawi

Dr Richard Fisher, Associate Professor, Department of Orthopaedics, University of Colorado Health Science Centre, Denver, Colorado, USA

Dr Ronald Lett, President and International Director, Canadian Network for International Surgery, Vancouver, Canada

Dr Matthews Mathai, Professor and Head of Department of Obstetrics and Gynaecology, Christian Medical College and Hospital, Vellore, India

Dr Ambrose Wasunna, Professor of Surgery, Kenyatta Memorial Hospital, Nairobi, Kenya

Dr Shayna Watson, Assistant Professor, Department of Family Medicine, Queen's University, Ontario, Canada

Dr Douglas Wilkinson, Clinical Director, Nuffield Department of Anaesthetics, John Radcliffe Hospital, Oxford, United Kingdom

Part 1 **Organizing the District Surgical Service**
Dr Shayna Watson

Part 2 **Fundamentals of Surgical Practice**
Dr Ronald Lett and Dr Shayna Watson

Part 3 **The Abdomen**
Dr Ambrose Wasunna and Dr Ronald Lett

Part 4 **Emergency Obstetric Care**
Dr Matthews Mathai

Part 5 **Resuscitation and Anaesthesia**
Dr Paul Fenton and Dr Michael Dobson

Part 6 **Traumatology and Orthopaedics**
Dr Richard Fisher and Dr Douglas Wilkinson

Annex **Primary Trauma Care Manual: Trauma Management in District and Remote Locations**
Dr Douglas Wilkinson and Dr Marcus F. Skinner

Contributors

Dr Stephen Bickler, Assistant Clinical Professor of Surgery and Paediatrics, University Hospital of San Diego, California, USA

Dr Marcus F. Skinner, Consultant, Intensive Care Unit, Hobart Hospital, Tasmania, Australia

Dr Harald Ostensen, Coordinator, Diagnostic Imaging and Laboratory Services, Department of Blood Safety and Clinical Technology, WHO

Dr Martin Weber, Medical Officer, Department of Child and Adolescent Health and Development, WHO

Dr Luc de Bernis, Medical Officer, Making Pregnancy Safer, Department of Reproductive Health and Research, WHO

Dr Pierre Bwale, Medical Officer, Department of Injuries and Violence Prevention, WHO

Dr Naeema Al-Gasseer, Medical Officer, Department of Health Service Provision, WHO

Illustration and design

Derek Atherton

Dominique Autier

Richard Fisher

Pat Thorne

Introduction

Surgical Care at the District Hospital provides a comprehensive guide to surgical procedures that are commonly performed at the district hospital. It is intentionally limited to emergency and very common problems and is not designed as a major textbook of surgery.

The manual is presented in seven parts with an initial section on organizing the district surgical service followed by clinical sections which include basic surgical procedures, the abdomen, emergency obstetrics, resuscitation and anaesthesia, acute trauma management and orthopaedics. It concludes with a course manual for teaching primary trauma care.

Using the manual

The manual is designed particularly for use by non-specialist clinicians, including:

- District medical officers and other general practitioners working in isolation
- Postgraduate medical officers (registrars)
- Junior doctors
- Medical students
- Senior paramedical staff, including clinical officers and nurse anaesthetists
- Medical and paramedical staff responsible for supervising the care and maintenance of equipment.

It should also be a valuable resource for:

- Medical and paramedical personnel at secondary and tertiary levels, particularly those working in specialist areas, such as trauma care
- Trainers in:
  - Medical schools and university teaching hospitals
  - Nursing schools
  - Paramedical training institutions
  - Continuing medical education programmes.

The evidence base for clinical practice

The interventions described in this manual are based on the latest available scientific evidence. It is planned to update it as new information becomes available but, since the evidence base for effective clinical practice is constantly evolving, you are encouraged to consult up-to-date sources of information such as the Cochrane Library, the National Library of Medicine database and the WHO Reproductive Health Library (see following page).

WHO would be pleased to receive comments and suggestions regarding the manual and experience in its use. This will be of considerable value in the preparation of future editions.

Sources for the evidence base for clinical practice

The Cochrane Library. Systematic reviews of the effects of health care interventions, available on diskette, CD-ROM and via the Internet. There are Cochrane Centres in Africa, Asia, Australasia, Europe, North America and South America. For information, contact: UK Cochrane Centre, NHS Research and Development Programme, Summertown Pavilion, Middle Way, Oxford OX2 7LG, UK. Tel: +44 1865 516300. Fax: +44 1865 516311. www.cochrane.org

National Library of Medicine: An online biomedical library, including Medline which contains references and abstracts from 4300 biomedical journals and Clinical Trials which provides information on clinical research studies. National Library of Medicine, 8600 Rockville Pike, Bethesda, MD 20894, USA. www.nlm.nih.gov

WHO Reproductive Health Library: An electronic review journal focusing on evidence-based solutions to reproductive health problems in developing countries. Available on CD-ROM from Reproductive Health and Research, World Health Organization, 1211 Geneva 27, Switzerland. www.who.int

Part 1

Organizing the District Hospital Surgical Service

Organization and management of the district hospital surgical service

1

1.1 THE DISTRICT HOSPITAL

You, your staff, systems and site

The hospital plays a unique role in any community:

- It is the focus of many health care services
- It can provide a significant amount of local employment
- It is a point of intersection for members of different communities
- It may be a community in its own right
- It must be involved in community public health education and political solutions to common health problems.

Organizations grow and change; hospitals are no different.

As a doctor or senior health care provider, you may be the most highly trained person in a district hospital. In this capacity, other hospital staff will expect leadership to be a part of your job.

As a leader (especially if you are newly arrived), other members of the health care team or the community may turn to you with frustrations or with hopes for solutions to problems. These tasks may not be directly related to your work on the wards or in the operating room, but they will become part of your job.

When assuming a new role or advanced leadership responsibilities, one of the challenges is to see what is familiar as if you were seeing it for the first time. It is difficult but important to avoid bringing old ideas or grudges to a new position. Use your past experiences, but also begin a new role with a broader view and an attitude unbiased by prejudgements. When you arrive in a new place or take on a new job or role at a familiar place, be alert to the physical and human resources and try to learn as much as possible about the work and culture of the place.

Familiarize yourself with the people, hospital and its resources. Try to get an overview of the organizational and communications systems that are used (not just those that are *supposed* to be used, but what is *really* happening).

Approach a new work environment or job as you would approach a patient by taking a full history and examination. Be observant and attentive to all aspects of the encounter. Asking questions is important; be a good listener.

KEY POINTS

- Leadership is a part of your job
- Apply the medical skills of evaluation and planning to your work as a manager
- Respect the knowledge and expertise of senior hospital staff
- Every institution has a history and the legacy of what has happened and why things have worked or not worked is held in the memory of the employees
- The pride people feel in their workplace and the services they offer is a valuable commodity and is the greatest resource of any health care facility.

1

Hear what people have to say. Try to understand what works well, where the problems lie and what the hopes of your co-workers are.

It will not be possible to understand everything at once or to fix all problems, but a full history and examination of the site provides the starting point for understanding and improvement. Any efforts to change practices or introduce new ones should include consultation with representatives of all interested parties; this is part of taking the "history" of the place and is equivalent to talking to the family members of a patient. As with patients, any management plan needs to be worked out with the people involved and carried out as a partnership.

As a health care provider, you will be entering into the lives of others who will have worked hard to create and maintain the place in which they work. Being sensitive to this will help you to fit in. The pride people feel in their workplace and the services they offer is a valuable commodity and is the greatest resource of any health care facility.

Community partners

The district hospital is part of a wider community of people and agencies, all of whom are working to improve the health of individuals, communities and society. Remember that these people and groups are your friends and allies. In discouraging times you can help one another and, by working together, can make things better. Find out who the other individuals and groups are and reach out and work with them – you have much to teach and learn from each other.

> In addition to identifying the opinion leaders, you must be sensitive to any groups or subgroups whose voices are unlikely to be heard. You must find ways of reaching out and listening to them.

Health is a concern for all people and can provide an opportunity to bring people together across divisions. In areas of conflict, when the district hospital and other parts of the health care system are accessible to all members of society without prejudice, it can provide an example of cooperation and develop the feeling of belonging to a broader and more inclusive group which respects and meets common needs.

KEY POINTS

- The leader is not expected to make all the decisions or do all the work, but must encourage others and co-ordinate efforts; the final responsibility for any endeavour rests with the leader
- Leadership requires a set of skills that can be learned and developed over time.

1.2 LEADERSHIP, TEAM SKILLS AND MANAGEMENT

A leader is best when people barely know he exists.
Not so good when people obey and acclaim him.
Worse when they despise him.
Fail to honour people, they fail to honour you.
But of a good leader, who talks little
When his work is done, his aim fulfilled,
The people will say "We did this ourselves".

Lao-tse

ROLE OF THE LEADER WITHIN A HEALTH CARE TEAM

Health care providers are only a part of the health team which includes support staff, administrative staff and those at satellite locations. The team consists of a group of people who share a common health goal and common objectives, as determined by community needs. Each member contributes according to his or her competence and skills and in coordination with the others.

The health care team exists to serve the community. Even if working for a manager or other employer, you are ultimately responsible to the people you serve clinically: the community and users of your service. It is from these people and groups that you must seek direction. Observing, listening and learning, discussing and deciding, organizing, participating and informing are the foundation of the relationship between the community and the team.

The leader is not expected to make all the decisions or do all the work, but must encourage others and coordinate efforts. Final responsibility for any endeavour rests with the leader.

Responsibility is the essence of leadership.

Leaders can be *given* authority by the group or by an outside power, they can *assume* authority or *earn* authority and responsibility. They can be appointed, elected or chosen by a group. Leadership can be shared by two or more people or rotated within a group. In an informal situation, different members of a group may take leadership roles with respect to different issues or tasks. It is important that all members of a group share the same idea of what the leader's role will be.

Some people adopt leadership roles with greater ease than others, but there are no born leaders. Leadership requires a set of skills that can be learned and developed over time. They include:

- Listening
- Observing
- Organizing
- Making decisions
- Communicating effectively and working well with others
- Encouraging and facilitating others
- Fostering enthusiasm and vision
- Goal setting and evaluation
- Giving and receiving feedback
- Coordinating the efforts of others
- Chairing a meeting
- Being willing to accept responsibility.

1

LEADERSHIP STYLES

There are many different leadership styles.

Democratic
The leader is chosen by the group and is expected to act with the wishes of the group in mind. The leader follows a course of action that represents the will of the group. Not everyone may agree, but most people mostly agree.

Autocratic
The decisions are made by the leader and the other members of the group are expected to follow. In this situation, one person makes the decisions and tells the others what to do.

Laissez-faire
The laissez-faire leader allows the members of the group unconstrained freedoms.

Anarchic
No leadership is shown and individuals or groups of people do what they want and resist efforts to organize or coordinate.

Consensus
Members of the group attempt to find a mutually agreeable solution or course of action. This is not so much a leadership style as a group style where all members agree on a course of action

Situational
No single style of leadership will work in all situations; different situations will demand different styles of leadership. A leader who is responsive to the group and the situation is practising situational leadership.

In times of crisis, an autocratic leader can make sure that things get done quickly and efficiently. When time and situation permit, democratic and consensus based leadership can be very effective and make people feel more involved and can even increase satisfaction and morale within groups.

COMMUNICATION

An effective communicator:

- Listens
- Speaks clearly so that others will understand
- Confirms understanding and asks others to do the same
- Does not use jargon
- Asks for questions and encourages others to speak
- Is patient
- Presents information in small amounts
- Does not overwhelm others.

Think about how people communicate in your hospital:

- What works and what does not work?
- How could you do more of what works and less of what does not?

Listening

Listening is a culturally based activity and skill. In some situations, eye contact is appropriate and avoiding eye contact can be seen to be evasive whereas, in others, eye contact is seen as being very aggressive and diverting one's eyes is a sign of respect. No matter what the cultural norms, effective listening is active, not passive. Active listeners are attentive – they communicate interest and concern with their words and body language. Effective listeners summarize what they have heard and how they understand what has been said. This allows for clarification and early correction of misunderstandings. Everyone likes to be heard and listening is a way of showing respect and concern.

KEY POINTS

- Active listeners are attentive – they communicate interest and concern with their words and body language
- Effective listeners summarize – what they have heard and how they understand what has been said.

WORKING WITH OTHERS

A skilled leader recognizes the expertise and input of others. Different things motivate different people, but everyone likes to do work of value, to do it well and to be recognized for it.

The effective leader can help people stay motivated and interested:

- **Achievement**: help people achieve work related and personal goals
- **Recognition**: give praise when it is due
- **Responsibility**: help others take responsibility
- **Advancement**: help others train for promotion and learn new skills
- **Self-improvement**: provide opportunities for personal development
- **The work itself**: explain the value of work, make work meaningful; if possible, allow people to do work which appeals to them, or allow people to pursue special projects or ideas they may have
- **Involvement**: when people work hard for an organization or cause they are investing in it, not financially but personally and emotionally; this leads to feelings of pride and responsibility – a sense of ownership.

KEY POINTS

- Help people and groups find common ground in times of difference and conflict
- Be a role model: in the way you work, demonstrate the behaviours you value.

Just as there are ways of motivating people, recognize the factors that may discourage them and create dissatisfaction:

- Poor personal relations
- Poor leadership
- Low pay
- Unsafe or unpleasant working conditions
- Inefficient administration
- Incompetent supervision.

Remember that healthy organizations:

- Orient new members to the group and the ways the group works
- Have ways of dealing with challenges, questions, discussions and disagreements

- Encourage new ideas and efforts
- Are places that people want to join and to stay.

The staff may have representation from groups in society which may have a history of conflict or be actively engaged in conflict. In a situation like this, the ability to develop and maintain healthy working relationships and a work environment of respect and peace can be an important community health initiative of its own.

Meetings

When groups of people get together for discussion, a formal meeting structure is sometimes adopted. The goal of formalizing communication in this way is to ensure that everyone has a fair opportunity to contribute and that there is sufficient time for discussion and decisions. Having a structure can be especially important if difficult or complex issues are being dealt with. Do your homework before the meeting, anticipate questions and have answers and information available. Be prepared.

Effective meetings:

- Have clear objectives and expected outcomes: people need to know what the meeting is about
- Have an agenda or a plan of how things will proceed; this can be created by the group but, at the very least, must be agreed on by those attending the meeting
- Have a chairperson: the role of the chairperson is to run the meeting, not to voice his or her own opinions; in a difficult situation, it may be appropriate for an uninvolved person to chair the meeting
- Stick to schedule and end on time, proceeding according to the agreed agenda or plan: it can be changed, if necessary, but should not be ignored
- Are comfortable physically: the space must be neither too hot nor too cold and have enough room for all the people in attendance to participate
- Are conducted in a way that makes all participants feel welcome and comfortable: use names, encourage input and recognize the work and contribution of others
- Allow everyone the opportunity to speak: before people speak a second time, make sure everyone who wants to has had a turn to speak once.

Be clear about what you are doing and why: confirm the plan at the beginning of the meeting, allow people to express feelings and suggestions about the meeting at the end, evaluate the meeting and try to think of ways of making the next meeting better: meetings are an expression of how a group works.

Feedback

Feedback is most helpful if comments are constructive in nature and suggest changes in a way that is encouraging rather than threatening. Comments should be very specific and deal with a person's behaviour rather than expressing an opinion about them as a person. "All your patients get infections; you must be a bad surgeon" is hurtful and not constructive. "You have very good technical skills; perhaps if you would scrub for longer before coming to the operating room, we could decrease our infection rates" is much more helpful. This example is also specific; it gives the other person an idea of what she or he can do to be a better surgeon.

Comments are most helpful when they occur close to the time of an event. While it is important not to speak in haste or anger, it is also important not to leave things so long that they are difficult to remember or are no longer relevant. It is important that comments are given in private in order to respect the privacy of patients and staff and allow for discussion.

Seek out feedback from people who will be honest with you and may be outside your usual circle of friends.

Feedback should be specific, timely, constructive and given in a respectful manner. A culture of communication can grow if those in positions of responsibility seek and gracefully receive feedback from others. This will help everyone feel more comfortable with the ongoing process of improvement. It is not always easy to do, but is well worth the effort.

1.3 ETHICS

As health care providers, we adhere to the dictates of our profession and the expectations of society. In our professional roles, we are acting not just as individuals but also as representatives of our profession.

Work within the limits of your training.

PATIENT CONSENT

Before performing a procedure, it is important to receive consent from the patient:

- Ask permission to make an examination
- Explain what you intend to do before doing it
- Ask the patient if he or she has questions and answer them
- Check that the patient has understood
- Obtain permission to proceed
- Be mindful of the comfort and privacy of others.

With invasive and surgical procedures, it is particularly important to give a full explanation of what you are proposing, your reasons for wishing to undertake the procedure and what you hope to find or accomplish. Ensure that you use language that can be understood; draw pictures and use an interpreter, if necessary. Allow the patient and family members to ask questions and to think about what you have said. In some situations, it may be necessary to consult with a family member or community elder who may not be present; allow for this if the patient's condition permits. If a person is too ill to give consent (for example, if they are unconscious) and their condition will not allow further delay, you should proceed, without formal consent, acting in the best interest of the patient. Record your reasoning and plan.

KEY POINT

- Informed consent means that the patient and the patient's family understand what is to take place, including the potential risks and complications of both proceeding and not proceeding, and have given permission for a course of action.

1

> Be attentive to legal, religious, cultural, linguistic and family norms and differences.

Some hospitals require patients to sign a document indicating that the surgical procedure and potential complications have been explained and that permission to proceed has been granted. This paper is then included in the patient's record. If this is not a formal requirement in your hospital, document the conversation in which consent was given and include the names of people present at the discussion.

Informed consent means that the patient and the patient's family understand what is to take place, including the potential risks and complications of both proceeding and not proceeding, and have given permission for a course of action. It should be a choice made free from coercion.

In our jobs as health care providers, we sometimes experience situations which demand things with which we, as individuals, may feel uncomfortable. Our duty as professionals to provide service and care can come into conflict with our personal opinions. It is important to be aware of these feelings when they occur and to understand where they are coming from. If we are asked to care for someone who is alleged to have committed a crime, it is not our responsibility to administer justice. However, it *is* our responsibility to provide care. This can be difficult, but it is important to recognize that:

> Our job is not to judge, but to provide care to all without regard to social status or any other considerations.

By acting in this way, we will be seen to be fair and equitable by the community we serve.

DISCLOSURE

Any information gained about the patient's condition belongs to the patient, and must be communicated. The delivery of bad news is very difficult and one can become more skilled at it over time; it is never easy. Arrange to talk to the patient in the company of family, preferably away from other patients. In some cultures, it is not common to give difficult news directly to the patient. We must be aware of the norms and customs of our patients as well as our own culture and the evolving culture of medicine. Navigating the different needs and expectations of these groups can be a challenge at times.

Be clear and direct with what you mean, and what you are saying. Do not say growth or neoplasm if what you mean, and what will be understood, is cancer. Often we try to soften the delivery of bad news by saying too much and confusing the matter, or by saying too little and leaving people with unanswered questions. Be clear, allow people to understand and feel some of the impact of the news and then to ask questions. It is often necessary to repeat the information to other members of the family, or to the same family and patient, the next day.

CARING FOR CARE GIVERS

At times, systems and individuals can be overwhelmed. When this occurs, be as kind to yourself as you would be to someone else. Tend to your own needs, whether they are physical, emotional or spiritual. Take the time you need and return refreshed. Being chronically overwhelmed can lead to "burn-out" and increases the risk of physical and mental ill health and use of destructive coping mechanisms such as drugs and alcohol.

Some factors will be beyond your control, such as a shortage of supplies, whether from a lack of resources, theft or corruption. The balance between advocating for improvement and driving yourself crazy with an unfixable problem can be difficult. Trying too hard to fix a problem can lead to frustration and eventually to cynicism; too little effort will ensure that things will never change. Be realistic about what you can accomplish as an individual and as part of an organization. You did not create the situation, but you can speak the truth about it and work for improvement.

Working in leadership and management roles means you will be dealing with your colleagues and co-workers and be faced with many of their problems. You will have to deal with absenteeism, poor job performance and the results of illness and disease. These are problems that you did not create and may not be able to fix. Be clear about your expectations and put systems for reporting, evaluation and remedy in place. This will help to make expectations clear and avoid the problem of dealing with things on a person by person basis.

Do not tie your sense of self worth or job performance to the resolution of systemic or long-standing problems. Set reasonable goals in areas that are within your control.

KEY POINTS

- Some factors are beyond your control
- Be realistic about what you can accomplish
- You did not create the situation, but you can speak the truth and work for improvement.

1.4 EDUCATION

Education is a key part of providing health care – we educate ourselves, our patients, our colleagues and the wider community. Education is the mainstay of our work and the key to positive change, whether it is health based patient education, community education or planning a community health centre. Like leadership, education is a core surgical skill.

KEY POINTS

- Leadership and education are essential surgical skills
- Planning, implementation and evaluation are the keys to successful educational initiatives.

PLANNING

Everyone in the hospital needs to have access to teaching and learning opportunities. Health care is constantly changing and developing and it is no longer possible to learn in a few short years all that will be needed over the course of a career. Medical or nursing school is just the beginning of a career-long education. Continuing medical education and professional development are important ways of investing in hospital staff and improving patient care as well as challenging and stimulating the interest of staff.

Planning, implementation and evaluation are the keys to successful educational initiatives. In addition to organizing structured in-service training on new technology, medications or treatment regimens, education can also take place alongside and during the active provision of patient care through:

1

- Morning report
- Bedside teaching to review and improve clinical skills and the care and management of specific patient groups
- Formal educational rounds
- Morbidity and mortality meetings
- Team training in critical care.

Poor performance can be related to knowledge, skills or attitudes.

You can plan an educational programme with learning outcomes and activities to teach knowledge, skills or attitudes. In-service training should be directly related to the work people do and the care they provide; this will help people to do their job better and improve patient care as well as boosting staff morale and motivation. Educational efforts are more effective if they are clearly applicable and relevant.

It is helpful to use clinical problems as a basis for learning. Learning outcomes are a useful way of stating what you expect people to be able to do as a result of training. For example:

- Problem: there is an increasing number of postoperative wound infections
- Teaching aim: to review the factors that affect postoperative wound infections
- Learning outcome: all staff working with surgical patients will be more aware of the factors contributing to postoperative wound infection rates.

In a teaching session, you could discuss some patients who have had post-operative wound infections and review possible causes of these infections. This could involve reviewing the course of the patient's illness and care in hospital and highlighting all the opportunities for infection to be introduced. Involve the participants in developing this list of possibilities. Review procedures for each of these situations (e.g. hand washing, dressing changes, the role of antibiotics for prophylaxis and treatment and how to recognize infection early). Rather than simply giving a lecture, try to include activities and time to practise skills being reviewed. Give everyone a chance to present information and ask questions.

KEY POINTS

- People may forget what they are told but will remember what they do
- When learning:
  - Ask questions
  - Be involved in your own learning
  - Try to understand new information in relation to what you already know – how do your new ideas change your old ideas?

Learning can occur in many ways and individuals differ in the ways they learn best. For example, some people can learn by reading, while others need to hear an explanation or be shown something before they can understand it. These different ways of learning can be called learning styles:

- How do you learn best?
- How do others in your organization learn best?

It is important to provide information in a variety of ways to take into account different learning styles and different educational levels.

People can learn by watching others and benefit from seeing and discussing how others have managed a specific situation. By discussing cases and problems, everyone can learn from everyone else. Design and organize learning experiences that involve the participants. Allow people to practise new skills under supervision, until they are able to apply them. People tend to forget what they are *told*, but remember what they *do*. Providing supportive supervision reinforces learning and enables the teacher to evaluate the effectiveness of his or her teaching.

In addition to clinical skills, staff also need to learn information that relates to specific tasks. For example, while learning how to start an intravenous infusion, it is equally important to understand the indications for an intravenous drip and to know what to do if the attempt does not work and how to manage complications.

Do not neglect your own professional education. Take part in educational activities at your hospital and in your region. Get together with colleagues and form a journal club to read and review articles published in the medical literature. If you are the sole medical officer, start an independent study programme to explore questions arising from your practice and then present your findings to other members of your staff. Spend time with visiting colleagues or make time to go to another hospital for some further instruction. Take advantage of any educational opportunity available to you; there will always be too much work to do and it will never be completed so you must make your own education a priority when opportunities present themselves. Make an educational plan and stick to it.

There are many educational programmes and initiatives which are called "distance learning". In this way, people can use printed materials, video, audiotapes or even computer networks to learn together, even though they may be geographically separated. If programmes of this kind are available, consider making use of them yourself or offering them to others in your organization.

If you are the most senior person in the hospital, who will help you learn? You can learn a great deal from your patients, colleagues in other fields and co-workers, but it may also be necessary to find someone to act as your mentor and help you think through problems or develop new skills. This person need not necessarily be close at hand, but should be available to you when needed through the post, by telephone or in person. We all need colleagues and support. It is an important part of your job to find and maintain these connections.

ROUNDS

Morning report

Morning report is a review of the night's activities, of admissions and a hand-over of patients to the day staff. This meeting can be used for education as well as information sharing by reviewing patient assessment and management and highlighting points about the presenting illness. It provides an opportunity for members of the health care team to share ideas and help one another. If there is sufficient time, patient cases can be presented in a more formal manner with broader discussion of medical and patient care issues.

1

Bedside teaching rounds

Bedside teaching rounds provide an opportunity for the people involved in the care of patients to meet with patients and discuss their illnesses and their management. This approach to teaching uses specific patients to illustrate particular illnesses, surgical procedures or interventions. Individual patients provide a starting point for a broader discussion which does not have to occur at the bedside and could continue later away from the wards. The bedside is also a good place to review clinical skills and specific physical findings.

Traditionally, these rounds have been used for the instruction of junior doctors, but they can also be used for interdisciplinary teaching involving nursing, midwifery and pharmacy staff as well as medical officers. They also give patients and their families an opportunity to ask questions of all the people involved in their care.

Any discussion of a patient on a bedside teaching round must be with the consent of the patient and should actively involve the patient.

Formal educational rounds

Unlike hand-over rounds or bedside teaching rounds, formal educational rounds are a clearly educational event and are separate from the service work of running the wards. They can be organized on a regular basis or when guests with unique experience or expertise are on site.

Morbidity and mortality meetings

Morbidity and mortality meetings are a periodic review of illness and deaths in the population served by the hospital. A systematic review of morbidity and mortality can assist practitioners in reviewing the management of cases and discussing ways of managing similar cases in the future. It is essential that discussions of this kind are used as a learning activity and *not* as a way of assigning blame.

Team training in critical care practice

If your hospital has a dedicated area to receive emergency patients, it can be helpful to designate time each week for staff to practise managing different scenarios. Have one person pretend to be the patient and work through all the actions and procedures that should take place when that patient arrives at the hospital. Rehearsing scenarios gives people a chance to practise their skills and working together as a team. It also provides an opportunity to identify any further training needs. As a group, decide what roles are needed and what tasks are required of each person. Once this has been decided, post this information for easy reference during a real emergency.

The Annex: *Primary Trauma Care Manual* provides a structured outline for a short course in primary trauma care that can be used for staff, including medical, nursing and paramedical staff.

Hospital library

Store educational and resource materials together in a central place to which staff seeking information have easy access. If the hospital has a visitor who offers teaching on a specific topic, or if people present useful information at educational rounds, designate someone to make notes and include them in the library. If possible, keep interesting X-rays and notes on unusual cases.

Designate a specific person to be responsible for the care and organization of the collection, including making a list of materials and keeping a record of items that are borrowed in order to ensure their return. Make known your interest in developing a library of learning materials to any external organizations or donor agencies with whom your hospital has contact and make specific requests and suggestions for books, journals and other resources.

1.5 RECORD KEEPING

KEY POINTS

- Even if your hospital maintains records, it is essential that patients receive a written note of any diagnosis or procedure performed
- All records should be clear, accurate, complete and signed.

Medical records exist for the benefit of the patient and for reference by future health care providers. If your hospital's policy is for records to stay at the hospital rather than being kept by patients, it is essential that they are well maintained and organized for future reference. This requires well trained staff as well as secure and dedicated space.

Records are confidential and should be available only to people involved directly in the care of the patient.

Even if your hospital maintains records, each patient should receive a written note of any diagnosis or procedure performed. If a woman has had a ruptured uterus, for example, it is essential that she knows this so that she can communicate this information to health care providers in the future.

Clinical notes are an important means of communication for the team involved in a patient's care by documenting the management plan and the care offered; they can also be used to improve patient care when reviewed as part of an audit. Notes may also be requested for insurance and medico-legal purposes.

All members of the health care team are responsible for ensuring that records are:

- Complete
- Accurate
- Legible and easily understood
- Current, written at the time of patient contact, whenever possible
- Signed, with the date, time, name and position of the person making the entry.

Once written, notes must not be changed; a subsequent entry can be made if there is a change in the patient's condition or management.

1

Admission note/preoperative note

The preoperative assessment should be documented, including a full history and physical examination, as well as the management plan and patient consent.

Operating room records

Operating room records can be kept in a book or can be kept as separate notes on each procedure. Standardized forms save time and encourage staff to record all required information.

A theatre record usually includes:

- Patient identity
- Procedure performed
- Persons involved
- Complications.

By looking at records of all procedures, a hospital can evaluate occurrences such as complications and postoperative wound infections or review the type and number of procedures being performed. Such evaluation, which should be the regular duty of one member of the hospital team, permits assessment of the application of aseptic routine within the hospital and allows for future planning.

Delivery book

The delivery book should contain a chronological list of deliveries and procedures, including interventions, complications and outcomes. It may contain some of the same information that would be included in a theatre record.

The operative note

After a surgical procedure, an "operative note" must be written in the patient's clinical notes. Include orders for postoperative care with your operative note.

Postoperative note

All patients should be assessed at least once a day, even those who are not seriously ill. Vital signs should be taken as dictated by the patient's condition and recorded; this can be done on a standard form or graph and can also include the fluid balance record. Progress notes need not be long, but must comment on the patient's condition and note any changes in the management plan. They should be signed by the person writing the note.

Notes can be organized in the "SOAP" format:

Subjective	How the patient feels
Objective	Findings on physical examination, vital signs and laboratory results
Assessment	What the practitioner thinks
Plan	Management plan; this may also include directives which can be written in a specific location as "orders".

A consistent approach such as this ensures that all areas are included and that it is easy for other members of the team to find information.

See Unit 3: *The Surgical Patient* for more detailed guidance on preoperative, operative and postoperative notes.

Discharge note

On discharging the patient from the ward, record:

- Admitting and definitive diagnoses
- Summary of patient's course in hospital
- Instructions about further management as an outpatient, including any medication and the length of administration and planned follow-up.

Standard operating procedures

Create and record standard operating procedures for the hospital. These should be followed by all staff at all times. Keep copies of these procedures in a central location as well as the place where each procedure is performed so they are available for easy reference.

Interhospital communication

Each patient who is transferred to another hospital should be accompanied by a letter of referral which includes:

- Patient identity
- Name and position of the practitioner making the referral
- Patient history, findings and management plan to date
- Reason for referral.

1.6 EVALUATION

To evaluate means to judge the value, quality or outcome of something against a predetermined standard.

At a district hospital, the act of evaluation will generate information that will enable a judgement to be made on whether the hospital is providing high standards of care and is making the best possible use of resources, including:

- Performance of staff, equipment or a particular intervention
- Clinical effectiveness of a type of treatment
- Efficiency in relation to the use of resource (cost-effectiveness).

Evaluation is part of a continuous loop of information gathering, analysis, planning, intervention and further evaluation and involves the following steps.

1 Set goals and targets.

2 Define indicators (previously stated standards, intended results or norms) that can be used to assess whether these goals and targets are being met.

3 Collect information to measure observed achievements.

KEY POINTS

- Evaluation is an essential part of ensuring high quality care
- With any change:
  - Plan (observe, consult and set goals)
  - Implement the change
  - Evaluate the outcome.

4 Compare achievements with goals and targets.
5 Identify any deficiencies or failures and analyse the causes.
6 Identify, plan and implement any interventions required for improvement, such as training.
7 Re-evaluate and identify any further interventions required.

Evaluation may be as simple as asking the question "Are all babies weighed in the outpatients department?" If the answer is "No", the next step is to ask the question "Why not?" and to use the answer to identify possible steps to resolve the problem.

Evaluation will often be more complex, however. For example, a hospital recognizes that it has very high postoperative wound infection rates. All potential sources and causes of postoperative infection are studied and, after careful review and consultation, a plan is developed and implemented. After a defined period of time, a review of postoperative wound infections is again undertaken as a measurement of observed achievement. This is then compared with both previous results and expected outcomes.

If there has been a drop in the infection rate, the team can decide whether the desired outcome has been achieved and whether the measures taken should be adopted as regular practice. By changing only one thing at a time, it is possible to determine whether any improvement is related to the intervention. If the intervention does not result in the desired change, it is important to identify why it has been unsuccessful before trying another intervention.

Chart audit

Patient charts contain important information about individuals, their illnesses and course in hospital. This is valuable information for evaluation. If records are kept after patients have been discharged, a chart audit can assist in monitoring the services provided by a hospital, diagnosing areas of concern and identifying areas for improvement, including:

- Consistency of approach
- Infection rates
- Length of patient stay
- Transfusion rates
- Complication rates.

A chart audit involves the following steps.

1 Ask a specific question, such as "What is our postoperative wound infection rate?"
2 Define the period of time for which the charts to be monitored will be selected.
3 Define the size of the sample of charts to be reviewed.
4 Develop a system for tabulating the data.
5 Make a systematic review of the charts of patients who had surgery during the defined time period.
6 Collate, analyse and interpret the results.

Once the wound infection rate has been documented, it is possible to assess whether it is acceptable. If it could be lowered, an improvement strategy can be devised and implemented. After a period of time, a second chart review can be undertaken, the change evaluated and adjustments made to practice.

Evaluation takes time and effort, but is a necessary part of a commitment to quality care.

1.7 DISASTER AND TRAUMA PLANNING

DISASTERS

A disaster is any situation that threatens to overwhelm the ability of local resources to cope, including:

- Trauma disasters, such as major road traffic accidents
- Natural disasters, such as hurricanes, earthquakes and floods
- Public health disasters, such as water contamination or the outbreak of a virulent disease
- War and civil disorder.

Each country should have a national disaster plan, but it is the responsibility of the district hospital to plan and prepare for disaster situations at the local level. Disaster planning requires consultation and discussion to develop a realistic plan, made in advance, that anticipates a time when it will be too late to plan.

Disaster planning involves the following steps.

1 Identify situations that could potentially overwhelm a district hospital.

2 Identify the staff and resources required to cope with each kind of disaster situation, including equipment, materials, drugs and blood.

3 Meet with representatives of all hospital departments and staff groups who would be involved, including medical, nursing, paramedical, laboratory and blood bank staff, ambulance attendants and support staff to discuss their role in managing a major emergency.

4 Liaise with other services and authorities, such as the Ministry of Health, local government, fire service, police, army, non-governmental organizations and aid and relief agencies.

5 Develop a disaster plan to cope with each situation and communicate this to all members of staff.

It is impossible to anticipate every situation, but a disaster plan should include:

- Designating a senior person to be team leader
- Defining the roles and responsibilities of each member of staff
- Establishing disaster management protocols
- Setting up systems for:
  - Identification of key personnel
  - Communication within the hospital
  - Calling in extra staff, if required
  - Obtaining additional supplies, if required
  - Triage

  - Communicating patients' triage level and medical need
  - Transportation of patients to other hospitals, if possible
- Mapping evacuation priorities and designating evacuation facilities
- Identifying training needs, including disaster management and trauma triage, and training staff
- Practising the management of disaster scenarios, including handling the arrival of a large number of patients at the same time
- Establishing a system for communication with other services, authorities and agencies and the media.

In the event of a local disaster, such as a major road traffic accident involving many persons, systems will then be in place. These will help the staff on duty to deal with a sudden and dramatic increase in need for services and to summon help to deal with such a situation.

It is vital to develop a written disaster plan if your hospital does not yet have one. Inform staff about the plan and keep copies of it in busy areas of the hospital. Ensure that it is reviewed regularly and that staff practise implementing it using different scenarios so that any problems can be identified and resolved before a real disaster occurs.

Triage

Triage is a system of making a rapid assessment of each patient and assigning a priority rating on the basis of clinical need and urgency. The goal of triage is to do the greatest good for the greatest number. People who are in greatest need should therefore be treated first. It is not helpful to spend huge amounts of time and resources on individuals whose needs exceed the services available, especially if this is at the expense of other patients who could be helped with the skills and resources available locally.

TRAUMA TEAM

Just as every district hospital needs to be prepared for a situation where there are many patients with competing needs, the staff also need to be skilled at dealing with multiply injured or critically ill patients requiring the care of many people at the same time. A "trauma team" that is experienced in working together in times of stress and urgency is also an important part of the disaster plan.

Identify the different jobs to be undertaken in an emergency and ensure that all members of the team know what those roles are and are trained to perform their own role. The area in which emergency patients are received should be organized so that equipment and materials are easy to find. It is helpful to make a map showing where in the room/area people need to be stationed and the jobs that are associated with the different positions.

Team leader

A team leader should be designated to take charge in a disaster or trauma situation. Ensure that all members of the team know who the leader is.

In the event of a major disaster, the leader should oversee the implementation of the disaster plan and delegate specific tasks.

In the case of an individual trauma case, the team leader is usually responsible for the following activities:

- Perform the primary survey and coordinate the management of airway, breathing and circulation
- Ensure that a good history has been taken from the patient, family and/or bystanders
- Perform the secondary survey to assess the extent of other injuries
- Consider tetanus prophylaxis and the use of prophylactic or treatment doses of antibiotics
- Reassess the patient and the efforts of the team
- Ensure patient documentation is completed, including diagnosis, procedure, medications, allergies, last meal and events leading up to the injury
- Communicate with other areas of the hospital and staff members
- Communicate with other people and institutions outside the hospital
- Prepare the patient for transfer
- Liaise with relatives.

Information should flow to and through the leader:

- Know and use the names of the other members of the team and ensure that they have heard and understood directions
- Check back with members of the team to make sure designated tasks have been completed: for example, "How is the airway?", "Are you having any trouble bagging?", "Have you had to suction much?", "Is the second IV started?"
- Ask for input from the team, but ensure that all directions come from only one person.

If only a small number of people are available, each team member will have to assume a number of roles. If there is only one person with airway management skills, for example, that person must manage the airway as well as acting as the leader. If there is more than one person with airway skills, one can be assigned to manage the airway and the other to act as the leader. It is difficult to perform emergency tasks while at the same time keeping an eye on the overall situation, so recruit as much help as you can. Practise often and communicate clearly.

> In an emergency, stay calm and speak clearly.

Members of the trauma team

Members of the team are responsible for:

- Accepting the authority of the leader: this is not a time for consensus decision making
- Speaking to and through the team leader

- Clearly and concisely reporting back to the leader once a task is completed: for example, "IV line established in the right antecubital fossa using a 14 gauge cannula".

If teams are involved in planning disaster and trauma management and regularly practise implementing the plan, they will be more effective and less stressed when a real event happens. Taking turns in acting out different roles within the trauma team will help each person to have a greater understanding of the roles of other team members and the demands of each role.

Trauma management is covered in depth in Unit 16: *Acute Trauma Management* and in the Annex: *Primary Trauma Care Manual.*

The surgical domain:

Creating the environment for surgery

2

2.1 INFECTION CONTROL AND ASEPSIS

KEY POINTS

- Hand washing is the single most important measure for the prevention of infection
- Treat all body substances of all people as potentially infectious
- Asepsis depends on standard procedures, staff training, personal discipline and careful attention to detail.

INFECTION PREVENTION AND UNIVERSAL PRECAUTIONS

Infection control measures are intended to protect patients, health care providers, hospital workers and other people in the health care setting. While infection prevention is most commonly associated with the prevention of HIV transmission, these procedures also guard against other blood borne pathogens, such as hepatitis B and C, syphilis and Chagas disease and should be considered standard practice. It is very easy for an outbreak of enteric illness to occur in a crowded hospital, especially without proper precautions and hand washing.

Infection prevention depends upon a system of practices in which all blood and body fluids, including cerebrospinal fluid, sputum and semen, are considered to be infectious. *All blood and body fluids from all people* are treated with the same degree of caution so no judgement is required about the potential infectivity of a particular specimen.

Hand washing, the use of barrier protection such as gloves and aprons, the safe handling and disposal of "sharps" and medical waste and proper disinfection, cleaning and sterilization are all part of creating a safe hospital.

HAND WASHING

Hand washing is intended to remove contamination and to decrease the natural bacterial load. Plain soap and water is effective for the removal of visible contaminants. There are special circumstances when it will be necessary to further cleanse hands by using an antimicrobial soap, such as in an intensive care unit or neonatal unit, or when caring for immunocompromized patients. Even when using these antimicrobial soaps and scrubs, it is impossible to completely eliminate microorganisms from our hands.

Wash your hands with a vigorous mechanical action on all surfaces of the hands to remove visible soiling and contaminants. Continue for at least 15 seconds. Wash above the wrists and remove jewellery, if possible. The nails are the area of greatest contamination and need to be specially cleaned at the beginning of each day. Shorter nails are easier to clean and are less likely to tear gloves. Rinse under running or poured water. Be sure to dry your hands thoroughly as moisture on the hands provides a breeding ground for bacteria. Disposable towels decrease the potential for contamination. If the sink does not have foot controls or long handles to operate with your elbow, have someone else to turn off the tap, or use the towel to turn off the tap, to avoid re-contaminating your hands.

2

Ensure the skin on your hands does not become dry and damaged. In these conditions, the hands show a higher bacterial load which is more difficult to remove than with healthy, intact skin.

Some organisms can grow on bars of soap, in the water that collects around soap dishes and on reusable nailbrushes. Keep the areas around bar soap clean and dry and store the soap in a container that drains water. Wash and sterilize reusable brushes. Store these items dry.

Set a good example and encourage hand washing by your co-workers, patients, relatives and other visitors. Make it easy for people to wash their hands by ensuring that soap and water are always available.

Although gloves provide some protection, they cannot provide 100% protection; they may have small defects that are not visible and it is easy to contaminate hands during the removal of gloves. The warm, moist environment inside gloves allows microorganisms to multiply.

Always wash your hands after removing your gloves.

KEY POINTS

- A safe injection does not harm the recipient, does not expose the provider to any avoidable risk and does not result in any waste that is dangerous for other people
- Use a sterile syringe and needle for each injection and to reconstitute each unit of medication
- Ideally, use new, quality controlled disposable syringes and needles
- If single-use syringes and needles are unavailable, use equipment designed for steam sterilization
- Prepare each injection in a clean, designated area where blood or body fluid contamination is unlikely
- Use single-dose vials rather than multi-dose vials
- If multi-dose vials must be used, always pierce the septum with a sterile needle; avoid leaving a needle in place in the stopper of the vial
- Once opened, store multi-dose vials in a refrigerator.

PREVENTION OF TRANSMISSION OF THE HUMAN IMMUNODEFICIENCY VIRUS (HIV)

In the clinical setting, HIV may be transmitted by:

- Injury with needles or sharp instruments contaminated with blood or body fluids
- The use of equipment that has not been properly disinfected, cleaned and sterilized
- Contact between open wounds, broken skin (for example, caused by dermatitis) or mucous membranes and contaminated blood or body fluids
- Transfusion of infected blood or blood products
- "Vertical" transmission between mother and child during pregnancy, delivery and breast feeding.

Most of the small number of reported infections of health workers with HIV have resulted from injuries caused by needles (for example, during recapping) and other sharp instruments. After use, always put disposable needles and scalpel blades ("sharps") into a puncture- and tamper-proof container that has been labelled clearly. The risk of transmission in the case of any given exposure is related to the prevalence of the disease in the area, the portal of entry (cutaneous, percutaneous or transfusion) and the inoculum dose from the exposure.

Take care of your patients, your co-workers and yourself:

- Do not recap needles
- Set up sharps containers in the places where you use sharps; the further you have to move to dispose of a sharp the greater the chance of an accident
- Do not use the same injection set on more than one patient
- Dispose of your own sharps
- Pass needles, scalpels and scissors with care and consideration.

Several points of aseptic routine applicable to members of the surgical team are also particularly relevant to the prevention of transmission of HIV:

- Protect areas of broken skin and open wounds with watertight dressings
- Wear gloves during exposure to blood or body fluids and wash your hands with soap and water afterwards
- Wash immediately in the case of skin exposure or contamination, whether from a splash, glove puncture or non-gloved contact
- Wear protective glasses where blood splashes may occur, such as during major surgery; wash out your eyes as soon as possible if they are inadvertently splashed
- Wear a protective gown or apron if splash potential exists
- Clean blood spills immediately and safely.

The purpose of infection precautions and aseptic technique is to prevent the transmission of infection. The best protection against HIV and other transmissible infection is attention to every detail of asepsis, with special care to avoid injury during operation. In some places, prophylactic medications are offered after needlestick injury or other potentially infectious contact. Each hospital should have clear guidelines for the management of injury or exposure to infectious materials.

Latex allergy

Increased exposure to latex has resulted in reactions by some people to certain proteins in latex rubber. Reactions range from mild irritation to anaphylaxis. When caring for a patient with latex allergy, always check the composition of tape, tubes, catheters, gloves and anaesthetic equipment. Even the stoppers at the top of medication vials may contain latex. All health care workers should be aware of this possibility and, if sensitized, consider the composition of gloves and using non-latex gloves.

Aseptic technique

> Infection is the most important and preventable cause of impaired wound healing.

Microorganisms can reach the tissues during an operation or manipulation of the surgical wound. They are carried and transmitted by:

- People, including the patient
- Inanimate objects, including instruments, sutures, linen, swabs, solutions, mattresses and blankets
- Air around a wound, which can be contaminated by dust and droplets of moisture from anyone assisting at the operation or caring for the wound.

The aseptic treatment of a wound is an attempt to prevent contamination by bacteria from all these sources, during the operation and throughout the initial phase of healing. Bacteria can never be absolutely eliminated from the operating field, but aseptic measures can reduce the risk of contamination.

Aseptic technique includes attention to innumerable details of operating technique and behaviour. Anyone entering the operating room, for whatever reason, should first put on:

2

- Clean clothes
- An impermeable mask to cover the mouth and nose
- A cap or hood to cover all the hair on the head and face
- A clean pair of shoes or clean shoe-covers.

Caps, gowns and masks are worn to decrease the risk of patient exposure to contamination or infection from the surgical team. Sterile instruments, gloves and drapes are also key elements in the fight against contamination.

Operative procedure list

An operative procedure list is needed whenever the surgical team will perform several operations in succession. The list is a planned ordering of the cases on a given day. Elements such as urgency, the age of the patient, diabetes, infection and the length of the procedure should all be considered when drawing up the list.

Operate on "clean" cases before infected cases since the potential for wound infection increases as the list proceeds. Also consider other factors when making up the operative list: children and diabetic patients should be operated on early in the day to avoid being subjected to prolonged periods without food.

Ensure that between operations:

- The operating theatre is cleaned
- Instruments are re-sterilized
- Fresh linen is provided.

It is essential to have clear standard procedures for cleaning and the storage of operating room equipment; these must be followed by all staff at all times. The probability of wound infection increases in proportion to the number of breaches of aseptic technique and the length of the procedure.

2.2 EQUIPMENT

Anaesthesia and life support equipment, monitoring devices, lights, the operating table and the operating room itself are all essential to surgical care and need to be cared for and maintained. Equipment should be kept strictly for use in the operating room, treatment room or emergency department in order to ensure that it will be available, in good repair and sterilized or cleaned ready for use.

Equipment and instruments

Care and repair

Surgical instruments and equipment used in the operating room should be dedicated to this use and should not be removed; the surgeon, nurse and anaesthetist will expect them to be available during the next case. It is essential that all personnel check the medications and equipment they will be using prior to beginning a case or procedure.

You must have resuscitation equipment, such as oxygen and suction, available wherever critically ill patients are cared for and where medications which can cause apnoea (such as narcotics and sedatives) are administered. The treatment room, emergency department, case room and operating room are obvious examples of such areas.

Medical equipment is expensive and can be quite delicate. Have a regular plan of maintenance for equipment and plan in advance for the repair and replacement of equipment. Create a list (inventory) of the equipment you have, then work out when the various items will need to be serviced and ultimately replaced.

Use

Many types of surgical instruments are available. There are broad groupings within this range:

- Forceps and instruments for holding tissue
- Needle holders
- Scissors
- Retractors.

The decision about which instrument to use sometimes has to be made on the basis of what is available. When you have a choice between instruments:

- Choose the shortest instrument that will comfortably reach the operative site
- If cutting suture or other non-tissue material, avoid using fine scissors that are designed to cut tissue or dissect tissue planes; use larger and blunter scissors for non-tissue materials
- Choose instruments in good repair; forceps that cross at the tip, scissors that do not cut easily and needle drivers that do not grip the needle securely can be frustrating and dangerous.

When holding instruments:

- Use three-point control: have three points of contact between your hand and the instrument to stabilize the instruments and increase the precision of use (Figure 2.1)
- When using instruments that open and close, extend your index finger along the instrument to provide extra control and stability
- Place only the tips of your fingers and thumb through the handles on instruments that open and close. In this way, rotation of the instrument can come from your wrist and forearm and provide a greater arc of control. It is also quicker and less cumbersome to pick up and put down the instrument.

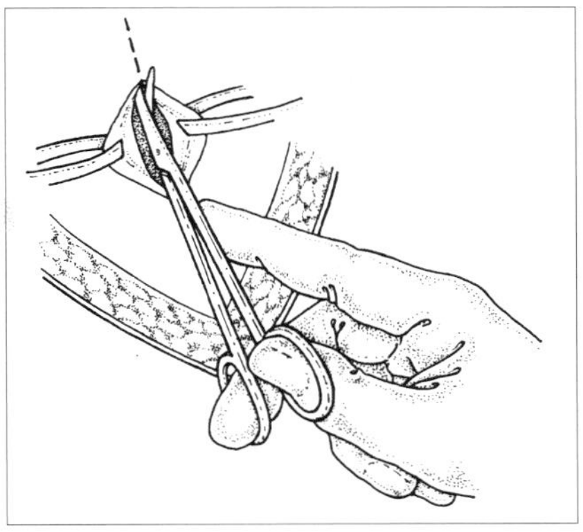

Figure 2.1

Scalpel

The way in which the scalpel is held depends on its size and the procedure being performed. Most procedures are performed with a #3 handle and either a #10, 11 or 15 blade. Use a #10 blade for large incisions, #11 for stab incision and #15 for fine precision work (Figure 2.2). If a larger #4 handle is used, use a #20 or #22 blade.

When incising the skin or abdominal wall, use the larger scalpel and blade. Hold the knife parallel to the surface with your third to fifth finger, thumb and index finger; this provides the three-point control. Your index finger will guide the blade and determine the degree of pressure applied.

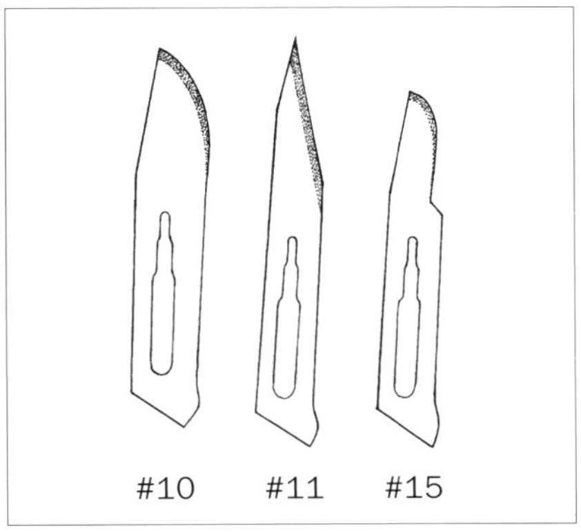

Figure 2.2

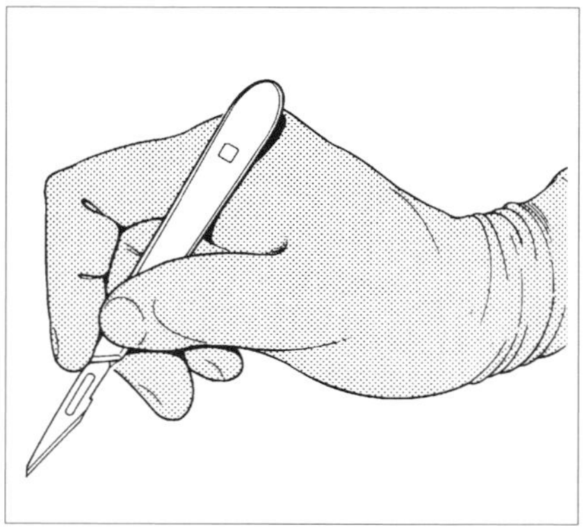

Figure 2.3

When using the scalpel for dissection, use a smaller knife and hold the instrument like a pen with your thumb, third finger and index finger holding the knife and your index finger controlling the dissection (Figure 2.3).

Forceps

Forceps are either toothed or non-toothed. Toothed forceps are also referred to as "atraumatic" as they are less likely to crush tissue. Hold these forceps like the small scalpel or a pen.

Artery forceps come in many sizes and shapes. Place your thumb and fingers through the handles just enough to sufficiently control the instrument. Place your index finger on the shaft of the instrument to provide three-point control. Hold curved dissection scissors in the same way.

Using your left hand

Scissors are designed so that the blades come together when used in the right hand. When right handed scissors are used in the left hand, the motion of cutting actually separates the tips of the scissors and widens the space between the blades; this makes cutting difficult, if not impossible. In order to use them with your left hand, it is necessary to hold them and apply pressure in a way that brings the blades closer together.

2.3 OPERATING ROOM

The operating theatre is a room specifically for use by the anaesthesia and surgical teams and must not be used for other purposes. A treatment room has equipment similar to an operating theatre, but on a smaller scale. Both rooms require:

- Good lighting and ventilation
- Dedicated equipment for procedures
- Equipment to monitor patients, as required for the procedure
- Drugs and other consumables, such as sutures, for routine and emergency use.

Ensure that procedures are established for the correct use of the operating room and that all staff are trained to follow them:

- Keep all doors to the operating room closed, except as needed for the passage of equipment, personnel and the patient
- Store some sutures and extra instruments in the operating room to decrease the need for people to enter and leave the operating room during a case
- Keep to a minimum the number of people allowed to enter the operating room, especially after an operation has started
- Keep the operating room uncluttered and easy to clean
- Between cases, clean and disinfect the table and instrument surfaces
- At the end of each day, clean the operating room: start at the top and continue to the floor, including all furniture, overhead equipment and lights; use a liquid disinfectant at a dilution recommended by the manufacturer

- Sterilize all surgical instruments and supplies after use and store them protected and ready for the next use
- Leave the operating room ready for use in case of an emergency.

SPONGE AND INSTRUMENT COUNTS

It is essential to keep track of the materials being used in the operating room and during any complicated procedure in order to avoid inadvertent disposal or the potentially disastrous loss of sponges and instruments in the wound.

It is standard practice to count supplies (instruments, needles and sponges):

- Before beginning a case
- Before final closure
- On completing the procedure.

The aim is to ensure that materials are not left behind or lost. Pay special attention to small items and sponges.

Create and make copies of a standard list of equipment for use as a checklist to check equipment as it is set up for the case and then as counts are completed during the case. Include space for suture material and other consumables added during the case.

When trays are created with the instruments for a specific case, such as a Caesarean section, also make a checklist of the instruments included in that tray for future reference.

SCRUBBING AND GOWNING

Before each operation, all members of the surgical team – that is, those who will touch the sterile surgical field, surgical instruments or the wound – should scrub their hands and arms to the elbows. Scrubbing cannot completely sterilize the skin, but will decrease the bacterial load and risk of wound contamination from the hands.

Every hospital should develop a written procedure for scrubbing that specifies the length and type of scrub to be undertaken. It is usual that the first scrub of the day is longer (minimum 5 minutes) than any subsequent scrubs between consecutive clean operations (minimum 3 minutes).

When scrubbing (Figure 2.4 on page 2 – 8):

- Remove all jewellery and trim the nails
- Use soap, a brush (on the nails and finger tips) and running water to clean thoroughly around and underneath the nails
- Scrub your hands and arms up to the elbows
- After scrubbing, hold up your arms to allow water to drip off your elbows
- Turn off the tap with your elbow.

After scrubbing your hands:

- Dry them with a sterile towel and make sure the towel does not become contaminated

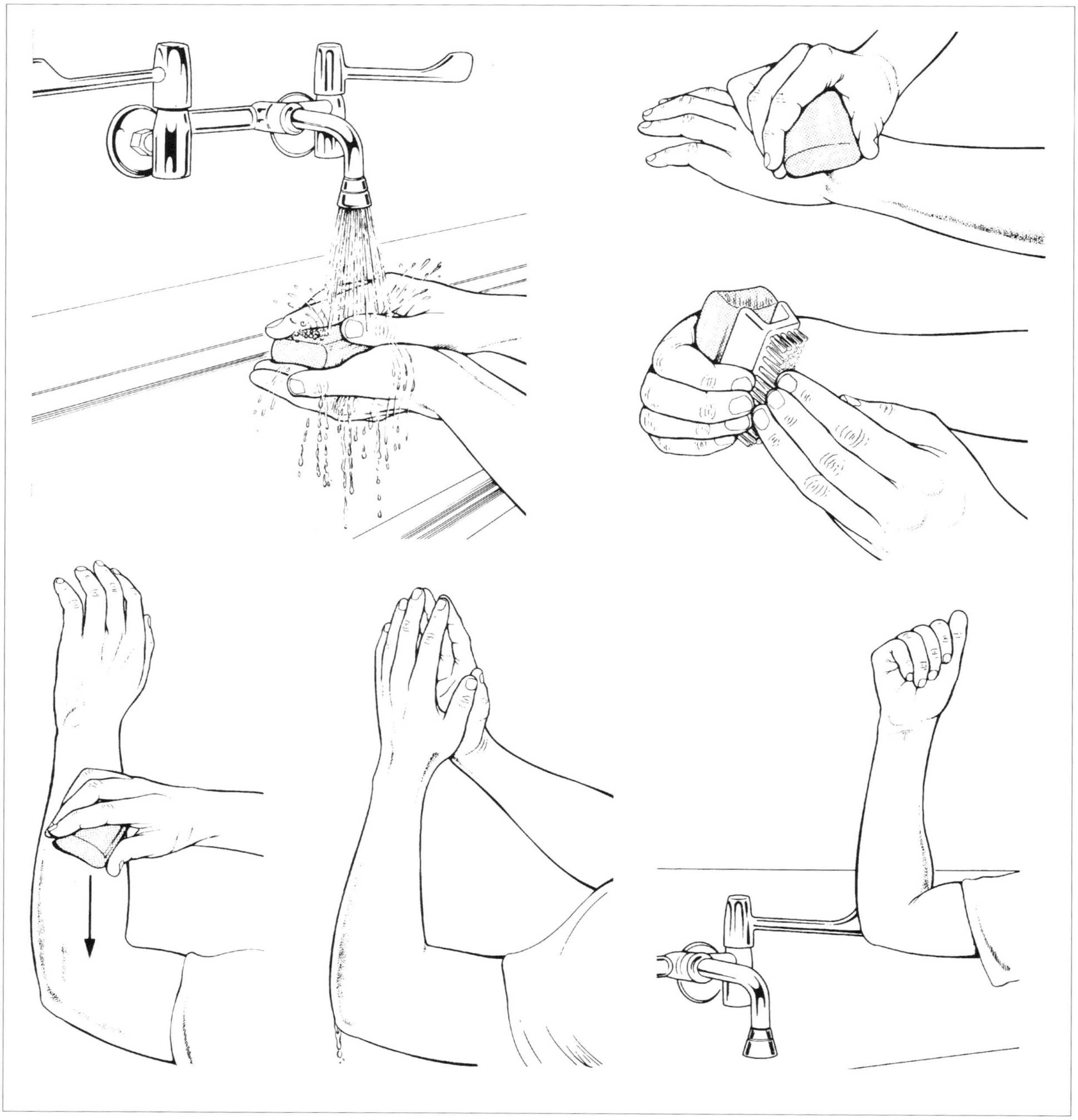

Figure 2.4

- Hold your hands and forearms away from your body and higher than your elbows until you put on a sterile gown and sterile gloves (Figures 2.5 and 2.6).

Surgical gloves prevent transmission of HIV through contact with blood, but there is always the possibility of accidental injury and of a glove being punctured. Promptly change a glove punctured during an operation and rinse your hand with antiseptic or re-scrub if the glove has leaked during the puncture. Patient safety is of primary concern; do not compromise it. Change your gloves only when it is safe for the patient.

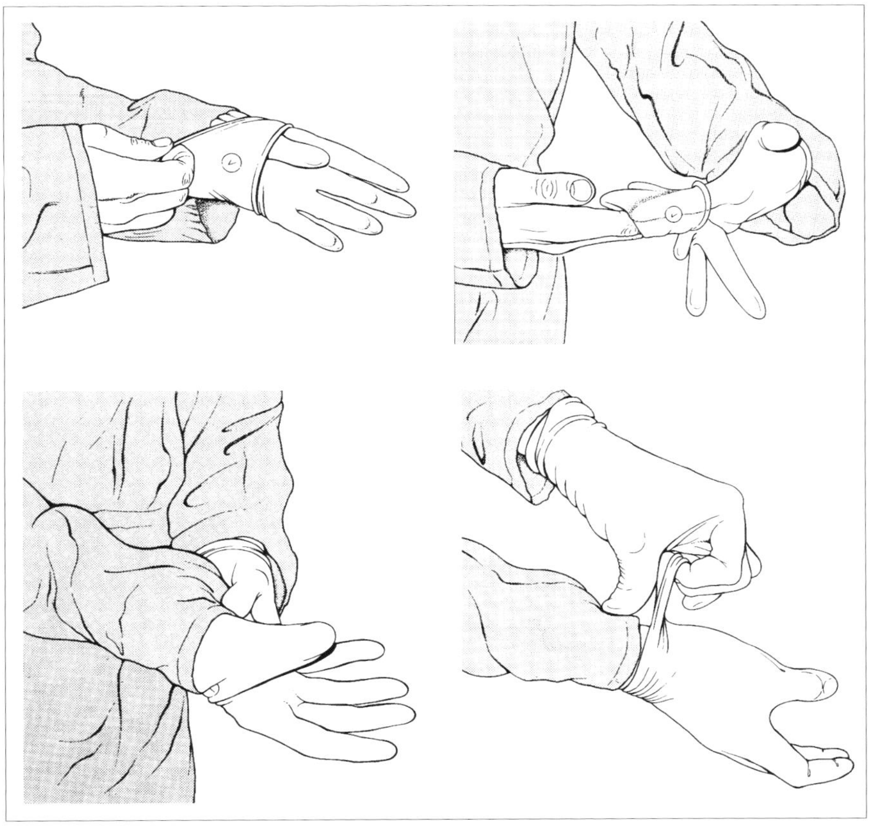

Figure 2.5

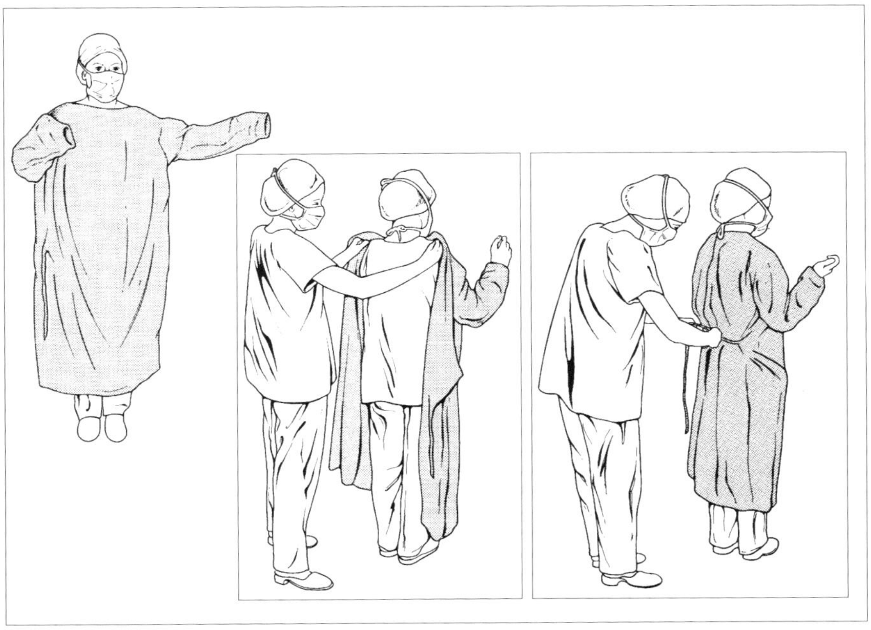

Figure 2.6

2

SKIN PREPARATION

The patient should bathe the night before an elective operation. Hair in the operative site should not be removed unless it will interfere with the surgical procedure. Shaving can damage the skin so clipping is better if hair removal is required; it should be done in the operating room.

Just before the operation, wash the operation site and the area surrounding it with soap and water. Prepare the skin with antiseptic solution, starting in the centre and moving out to the periphery (Figure 2.7). This area should be large enough to include the entire incision and an adjacent working area, so that you can manoeuvre during the operation without touching unprepared skin. Chlorhexidine gluconate and iodine are preferable to alcohol and are less irritating to the skin. The solution should remain wet on the skin for at least two minutes.

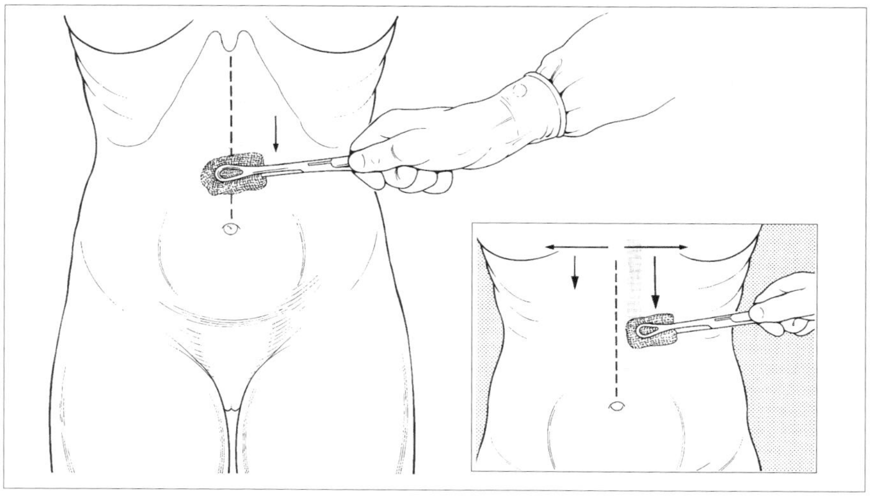

Figure 2.7

DRAPING

Scrub, gown and glove before covering the patient with sterile drapes. Leave uncovered only the operative field and those areas necessary for the maintenance of anaesthesia. Secure the drapes with towel clips at each corner (Figure 2.8).

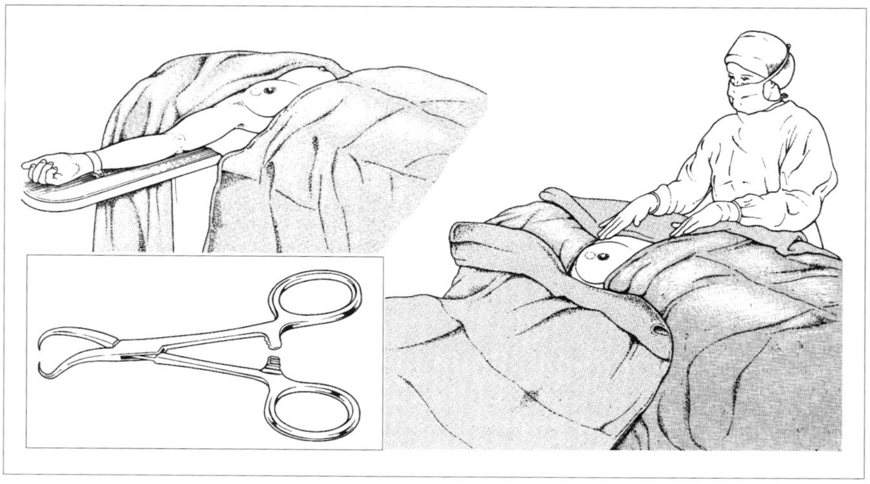

Figure 2.8

2

Draping exposes the area of the operative field and provides a sterile field for the operative staff to work. This is designed to maximize surgical exposure and limit potential for contamination. There are many approaches to draping, some of which depend on the kind of drapes being used. Do not place drapes until you are gowned and gloved, so as to maintain the sterility of the drapes. It is important to secure good exposure and a large sterile area. When laying out the drapes, the edges and folds (which hang below the operating table) are considered to be non-sterile.

2.4 CLEANING, STERILIZATION AND DISINFECTION

DISINFECTION

Disinfectant solutions are used to inactivate any infectious agents that may be present in blood or other body fluids. They must always be available for cleaning working surfaces, equipment that cannot be autoclaved and non-disposable items and for dealing with any spillages involving pathological specimens or other known infectious material.

Needles and instruments should routinely be soaked in a chemical disinfectant for 30 minutes before cleaning. Disinfection decreases the viral and bacterial burden of an instrument, but does *not* clean debris from the instrument or confer sterility. The purpose of disinfection is to reduce the risk to those who have to handle the instruments during further cleaning.

Reusable needles must always be used with great care. After use, they should be placed in a special container of disinfectant before being cleaned and sterilized. Thick gloves should be worn when needles and sharp instruments are being cleaned.

There are many disinfectant solutions, with varying degrees of effectiveness. In most countries, the most widely available disinfectant is sodium hypochlorite solution (commonly known as bleach or *chloros*), which is a particularly effective antiviral disinfectant solution.

To ensure effective disinfection, follow the manufacturer's instructions or any other specific guidelines that have been given and dilute the concentrated solution to the correct working strength. It is important to use all disinfectant solutions within their expiry date as some solutions, such as hypochlorite, lose their activity very quickly.

Disinfection must be performed before cleaning with detergent. There are many different disinfectants available and these act in different ways, so it is important to use the appropriate one in order to ensure effective disinfection. All disinfectants have what is known as a "contact time", which means that they must be left in contact with an infectious agent for a certain period of time to ensure that it is completely inactivated. However, some disinfectants are themselves inactivated by the presence of organic material and so higher concentrations of disinfectant and longer contact times must be used in certain situations, such as a large spill of infected blood.

After disinfection, you can clean with normal detergent and water to remove the inactivated material and the used disinfectant. Even if disinfection is performed correctly, all the waste material generated should be disposed of safely.

KEY POINTS

- Cleaning removes debris
- Disinfection decreases the viral and bacterial burden of an instrument, but does not clean debris or confer sterility
- Sterilization kills microbes.

Take great care when using any disinfectants containing chlorine. In the presence of some chemicals, it is very easy to liberate poisonous chlorine gas from some chlorine-containing solutions (when bleach and acid are mixed, for example). If you have any doubts about the exact composition of a spilt mixture containing infectious agents, you can neutralize any acid present by adding a small amount of saturated sodium bicarbonate before adding bleach or hypochlorite solution.

Linen soiled with blood should be handled with gloves and should be collected and transported in leak-proof bags. Wash the linen first in cool water and then disinfect with a dilute chlorine solution. Then wash it with detergent for 25 minutes at a temperature of at least 71°C.

Before sterilization, all equipment must be disinfected and then cleaned to remove debris. Sterilization is intended to kill living organisms, but is not a method of cleaning.

STERILIZATION

The methods of sterilization in common use are:

- Autoclaving or steam sterilization
- Exposure to dry heat
- Treatment with chemical antiseptics.

Autoclaving should be the main form of sterilization at the district hospital.

Autoclaving

Before sterilizing medical items, they must first be disinfected and vigorously cleaned to remove all organic material. Proper disinfection decreases the risk for the person who will be cleaning the instruments. Sterilization of all surgical instruments and supplies is crucial in preventing HIV transmission. All viruses, including HIV, are inactivated by steam sterilization (autoclaving) for 20 minutes at 121°C–132°C or for 30 minutes if the instruments are in wrapped packs.

For efficient use, an autoclave requires a trained operator and depends on regular maintenance. The selection of a suitable autoclave requires serious consideration not only of the cost, but also:

- Anticipated use
- Workload
- Size
- Complexity
- Power source.

In general, the smaller the capacity, the shorter the whole process and the less damage to soft materials. It is often more practical to use a small autoclave several times a day than to use a large machine once.

Appropriate indicators must be used each time to show that sterilization has been accomplished. At the end of the procedure, the outsides of the packs of instruments should not have wet spots, which may indicate that sterilization has not occurred.

Dry heat

If items cannot be autoclaved, they can be sterilized by dry heat for 1–2 hours at 170 °C. Instruments must be clean and free of grease or oil. However, sterilizing by hot air is a poor alternative to autoclaving since it is suitable only for metal instruments and a few natural suture materials.

> Boiling instruments is now regarded as an unreliable means of sterilization and is not recommended as a routine in hospital practice.

Antiseptics

In general, instruments are no longer stored in liquid antiseptic. However, sharp instruments, other delicate equipment and certain catheters and tubes can be sterilized by exposure to formaldehyde, glutaral (glutaraldehyde) or chlorhexidine.

If you are using formaldehyde, carefully clean the equipment and then expose it to vapour from paraformaldehyde tablets in a closed container for 48 hours. Ensure that this process is carried out correctly.

Glutaral is a disinfectant that is extremely effective against bacteria, fungi and a wide range of viruses. Always follow the manufacturer's instructions for use.

Failure of normal methods of sterilization

Failure of an autoclave or a power supply may suddenly interrupt normal sterilization procedures. If an extra set of sterile equipment and drapes are not available, the following "antiseptic technique" will allow some surgery to continue.

1 Immerse towels and drapes for 1 hour in a reliable antiseptic such as aqueous chlorhexidine, wring them out and lay them moist on the skin of the patient.

2 Treat gauze packs and swabs similarly, but rinse them in diluted (1: 1000) chlorhexidine solution before using them in the wound. From time to time during the operation, rinse gauze in use in this solution.

3 Immerse instruments, needles, and natural suture materials in strong antiseptic for 1 hour and rinse them in weak antiseptic just before use.

2.5 WASTE DISPOSAL

All biological waste must be carefully stored and disposed of safely. Contaminated materials such as blood bags, dirty dressings and disposable needles are also potentially hazardous and must be treated accordingly. If biological waste and contaminated materials are not disposed of properly, staff and members of the community could be exposed to infectious material

2

and become infected. It is essential for the hospital to have protocols for dealing with biological waste and contaminated materials. All staff must be familiar with them and follow them.

The disposal of biohazardous materials is time consuming and expensive, so it is important to separate non-contaminated material such as waste paper, packaging and non-sterile but not biologically contaminated materials. Make separate disposal containers available where waste is created so that staff can sort the waste as it is being discarded. Organize things in a way to discourage the need for people to be in contact with contaminated waste.

All infected waste should then be disposed of by incineration. Incinerators must be operated in accordance with local regulations and the approval of the public health department.

Incineration is the ideal method for the final disposal of waste but, if this is not possible, other suitable methods must be used. These should also be regulated and approved by the public health department.

Burying waste is the only option in some areas. If this is the case, you should do as much as possible before burying it to minimize the risk of infection. Small amounts of infected waste should be soaked in a hypochlorite solution for at least 12 hours, put into a pit and then covered. Larger quantities should be put into a pit with a final concentration of 10% sodium hypochlorite, before covering immediately.

Do not mix waste chemicals, unless you are certain that a chemical reaction will not take place. This is essential to prevent any unwanted or even dangerous reactions occurring between the chemicals, which could endanger laboratory staff. Always follow local guidelines on the disposal of waste chemicals to ensure that chemical contamination of the surrounding land or water supply does not occur.

Provide a safe system for getting rid of disposable items such as scalpel blades or needles. The risk of injury with sharp objects increases with the distance they are carried and the amount they are manipulated. A container for the safe disposal of sharp objects should be:

- Well labelled
- Puncture proof
- Watertight
- Break resistant (a glass container could break and provide a serious hazard to the person cleaning up the mess)
- Opening large enough to pass needles and scalpel blades, but never large enough for someone to reach into
- Secured to a surface, such as a wall or counter, to ensure stability during use
- Removable for disposal.

These containers must then be disposed of safely.

Part 2

Fundamentals of Surgical Practice

The surgical patient

3

3.1 APPROACH TO THE SURGICAL PATIENT

A skilled surgeon can make diagnosis appear very easy, almost intuitive. The process of problem analysis and decision making may be faster, but it is the same for every practitioner, whatever his or her experience. It consists of:

- History
- Physical examination
- Differential diagnosis
- Investigations, if required, to confirm your diagnosis
- Treatment
- Observation of the effects of treatment
- Re-evaluation of the situation, the diagnosis and the treatment.

Skilled practitioners go through the same process for both a puzzling case and one that, at the outset, seems to have an obvious diagnosis. If you make the diagnosis too early, you may miss the opportunity to collect important information. Do not jump to conclusions. A diagnostic algorithm can be helpful, but cannot replace active thinking about the case. Talk to, examine and think about the patient.

KEY POINTS

- Talk to, examine and think about the patient
- The patient's history and physical examination are key parts of surgical decision making
- The history and physical examination should not delay resuscitation of the acutely ill surgical patient.

History and physical examination

The patient's history and physical examination are key parts of surgical decision making. It is not enough simply to examine the abdomen when the presentation is abdominal pain. Examine the whole patient, assess his/her general health, nutrition and volume status and look for anaemia. Remember to ask about chronic or intercurrent illnesses.

A full medical history includes the following:

- Patient identification: name, sex, address and date of birth
- Presenting complaint
- History of the present symptoms/illness
- Past medical history, especially previous surgery and any complications, including:
  - Allergies
  - Medications, including non-prescription and locally obtained drugs
  - Immunizations
  - Use of tobacco and alcohol
- Family history
- Social history
- Functional inquiry which reviews all systems.

Investigations: general principles

Use laboratory and diagnostic imaging investigations to confirm a clinical hypothesis; they will not make the diagnosis in isolation.

3

Remember to inform the patient of the results of any tests. Take time and care if the results are unexpected or are likely to cause emotional trauma.

Do not delay an urgent procedure if laboratory services or diagnostic imaging are not available. The decision to operate must often be made on purely clinical grounds, even though investigations provide additional information and further support for the diagnosis and management plan.

Only ask for an investigation if:

- You know why you want it and can interpret the result
- Your management plan depends on the result.

If the patient's condition changes, return to the beginning of the process and re-evaluate everything. Gather information and communicate the assessment and plan to everyone who needs to know.

Remember that the surgical practitioner does *not* exist in isolation, but is part of an operative team. The surgical practitioner's primary colleagues in the operating room are the anaesthetist and nurses; communication and coordinated efforts are essential between these people. Technical staff and porters are valuable members of the team. The instruments, equipment, drugs and the operating room itself are also essential components that require your active attention.

Before undertaking a procedure, contact other members of the surgical team and enlist their involvement and cooperation. Assess the surgical and anaesthetic risk and explain it to the patient (and the patient's family, if appropriate). See the sections on consent on pages 1–7 to 1–8 and 13–23.

The ability to provide consistent postoperative care can limit the surgical capabilities of a hospital. In this situation, the whole surgical team needs to work together to improve it. The surgical team is ultimately responsible for all aspects of surgical care and must be involved in its ongoing evaluation and development.

Decision making

Your clinical assessment of the patient may indicate that surgery is required. If so, consider the following important issues.

Can we do the procedure here?

- Is the operating room safe and fit for use?
- Are the necessary equipment and drugs available?
- Are all members of the team available?
- Do I have the knowledge and skill to perform the necessary procedure?

Can we manage this patient?

- Is there back up or extra support available, if required?
- Can we manage the potential complications if problems arise?
- Do we have nursing facilities for good postoperative care?

If the answer to any of these questions is "No", it is inadvisable to proceed with surgery. If transfer is not possible or the patient could not withstand such a stress, then be aware of, and communicate, the increased risk of the procedure and proceed with great caution.

Is this patient stable enough to be transferred elsewhere?

At times it will be necessary to transfer an ill patient. Make contact with the centre to which you wish to send the patient; make sure they agree to the transfer and are expecting the patient. If you are finding it difficult to manage a patient in your hospital, be aware that it will be even more difficult to manage that patient in transport. Whether transport is by land, air or water, the environment will be noisier, bumpier and more crowded than where you are when you make the decision to transport the patient. Preparation and planning are essential for a successful transport.

1 Make a diagnosis and treatment plan. Do not simply refer the patient without thinking about what is going on. Manage and care for the patient while awaiting transfer and while in transit.
2 Do not refer the patient unless the referral centre can provide a higher level of expertise and care and the patient can tolerate the transfer.
3 When possible, talk to the person to whom you are sending the patient. Make sure they are aware of and willing to accept the patient.
4 Identify the transportation options that are available and decide which is best for the patient.
5 Stabilize the patient before transportation; the highest priorities are airway, breathing and circulation (ABC). Immobilize fractures, control pain and prevent further injury. Place a nasogastric tube if gastrointestinal obstruction is suspected.
6 Assess the need for care and intervention during transport. Send the patient with the equipment and staffing required.
7 Try to anticipate and prepare for any changes that may occur on the way.
8 Send a referral or transfer letter with the patient's notes and the results of any investigations. The letter should contain the same information as in the preoperative note (see below).

If it is usual for your hospital to transport patients, make a list of the equipment commonly required, use this as a checklist and consider having a kit with this equipment, ready for use. Make it someone's job to restock the kit after each use. Devise a sealing system to ensure that nothing is taken from the kit and that it is possible to see, simply by looking, that it is stocked and ready for use.

Preoperative note

The preoperative note should:

- Document:
  - The history and physical examination
  - Results of laboratory and other investigations
  - Diagnosis
  - Proposed surgery
- Document your discussion with the patient and family and their consent to proceed

- Demonstrate:
  - The thought process leading to the decision to operate
  - That you have considered possible alternatives and the risks and benefits of each.

Preparation for surgery

The patient must be seen by the surgical and anaesthetic practitioners preoperatively. This can range from days or weeks in advance in the case of an elective procedure to minutes before in an emergency. If there is a long time between initial assessment and surgical procedure, it is essential to ensure that there have been no changes in the patient's condition in the intervening period.

The patient's stay in hospital before an operation should be as short as possible. Complete as much preoperative investigation and treatment as possible on an outpatient basis. Before the operation, correct gross malnutrition, treat serious bacterial infection, investigate and correct gross anaemia, and control diabetes.

On the day of surgery

Always see the patient on the day of surgery. Make sure that the patient has fasted for an appropriate time before the operation.

It is the surgical practitioner's responsibility to ensure that the side to be operated on is clearly marked just before the operation. Recheck this immediately before the patient is anaesthetized. The patient's notes, laboratory reports and X-rays must accompany the patient to the operating room.

Intraoperative care

It is the anaesthetic practitioner's responsibility to provide safe and effective anaesthesia for the patient. The anaesthetic of choice for any given procedure will depend on his or her training and experience, the range of equipment and drugs available and the clinical situation. It is important for the surgical and anaesthetic practitioners to communicate any changes or findings to one another during the procedure.

The operative note

After an operation, an "operative note" must be written in the patient's clinical notes. It should include at least:

- Names of persons in attendance during the procedure
- Pre- and postoperative diagnoses
- Procedure carried out
- Findings and unusual occurrences
- Length of procedure
- Estimated blood loss
- Anaesthesia record (normally a separate sheet)
- Fluids administered (may also be on anaesthesia record)
- Specimens removed or taken
- Complications, including contamination or potential for infection

- Method of closure or other information that will be important to know before operating again (for example, the type of incision on the uterus after Caesarean section)
- Postoperative expectations and management plan
- Presence of any tubes or drains.

Postoperative note and orders

The patient should be discharged to the ward with comprehensive orders for the following:

- Vital signs
- Pain control
- Rate and type of intravenous fluid
- Urine and gastrointestinal fluid output
- Other medications
- Laboratory investigations.

The patient's progress should be monitored and should include at least:

- A comment on medical and nursing observations
- A specific comment on the wound or operation site
- Any complications
- Any changes made in treatment.

Aftercare

Prevention of complications

- Encourage early mobilization:
  - Deep breathing and coughing
  - Active daily exercise
  - Joint range of motion
  - Muscular strengthening
  - Make walking aids such as canes, crutches and walkers available and provide instructions for their use
- Ensure adequate nutrition
- Prevent skin breakdown and pressure sores:
  - Turn the patient frequently
  - Keep urine and faeces off skin
- Provide adequate pain control.

Pain management

Pain is often the patient's presenting symptom. It can provide useful clinical information and it is your responsibility to use this information to help the patient and alleviate suffering. Manage pain wherever you see patients (emergency, operating room and on the ward) and anticipate their needs for pain management after surgery and discharge. Do not unnecessarily delay the treatment of pain; for example, do not transport a patient without analgesia simply so that the next practitioner can appreciate how much pain the person is experiencing.

Pain management is our job.

3

Discharge note

On discharging the patient from the ward, record in the notes:

- Diagnosis on admission and discharge
- Summary of course in hospital
- Instructions about further management, including drugs prescribed.

Ensure that a copy of this information is given to the patient, together with details of any follow-up appointment.

KEY POINTS

- Infants and children differ from adults in significant physiological and anatomical ways
- Infants and small children have much smaller physiological reserves than adults and minor deviations from normal levels require early attention
- Infants and children are at special risk of becoming dehydrated and hypoglycaemic
- Monitor fluid status, electrolytes and haemoglobin diligently and correct any abnormalities promptly
- Maintenance fluid requirements must be supplemented to compensate for all losses.

3.2 THE PAEDIATRIC PATIENT

Infants and children under 10 years of age have important physiological differences that influence the way in which they should be cared for before, during and after surgery. The pattern of surgical disease is also different; congenital disorders must be considered in all children, but especially in neonates.

Children are not just little adults.

PHYSIOLOGICAL CONSIDERATIONS

Vital signs

Infants and children have a more rapid metabolic rate than adults. This is reflected in their normal vital signs.

Vital signs (normal and at rest)

Age (years)	Heart rate Beats/minute	Systolic blood pressure mmHg	Respiratory rate Breaths/minute
<1	120–160	70–90	30–40
1–5	100–120	80–90	25–30
5–12	80–100	90–110	20–25
>12	60–100	100–120	15–20

KEY POINT

- Infants and young children, especially those with little subcutaneous fat, are unable to maintain a normal body temperature when there are wide variations in the ambient temperature or when they have been anaesthetized.

Temperature regulation

Children lose heat more rapidly than adults because they have a greater relative surface area and are poorly insulated. Hypothermia can affect drug metabolism, anaesthesia and blood coagulation. Children are especially prone to hypothermia in the operating room.

Prevent hypothermia by:

- Turning off any air conditioning in the operating room (aim for a room temperature of >28 °C)
- Using warmed intravenous fluids
- Avoiding long procedures

- Monitoring the child's temperature at least every 30 minutes and at the completion of the case.

It is easier to keep children warm than to warm them up when cold. Encourage the mother to keep the child warm.

Compensatory mechanisms for shock

Children compensate for shock differently from adults, mainly by increasing their heart rate. A rapid heart rate in a child may be a sign of impending circulatory collapse. Do not ignore a decreased blood pressure. A slow heart rate in a child is hypoxia until proven otherwise.

Blood volume

Children have smaller blood volumes than adults:

- Even small amounts of blood loss can be life threatening
- Intravenous fluid replacement is needed when blood loss exceeds 10% of the total blood volume
- Chronic anaemia should be slowly corrected before elective operations with iron, folic acid or other supplements, as appropriate
- Make sure that safe blood will be available in the operating room if blood loss is anticipated during surgical procedures.

See *The Clinical Use of Blood* (WHO, 2000) for additional information on the use of blood in paediatrics and neonatology.

Paediatric blood volumes

Blood volume	**ml/kg body weight**
Neonates	85–90
Children	80
Adults	70

Nutrition and hypoglycaemia

Infants and children are at special risk for nutritional problems because of their higher caloric needs for growth. Poor nutrition affects response to injury and ability to heal wounds. Many surgical conditions, such as burns, increase caloric needs or prevent adequate intake of needed nutrition.

Good nutrition helps healing. Poor nutrition prevents it.

Infants are at risk for developing hypoglycaemia because of a limited ability to utilize fat and protein to synthesize glucose. If prolonged periods of fasting are anticipated (>6 hours), give intravenous fluids that contain glucose.

KEY POINTS

- Malnutrition can impair the response of children to injury and their ability to heal and recover
- When completing a preoperative assessment on a child, consider nutritional status and anaemia; treat chronic anaemia as part of the preparation for surgery.

Fluid and electrolytes

Baseline fluid and electrolyte requirements are related to the child's weight. However, the actual fluid requirements may vary markedly, depending on the surgical condition (see page 13 – 17).

KEY POINTS

- Whenever possible, give fluids by mouth
- Use the intravenous route for rapid resuscitation (20 ml/kg bolus of normal saline) and for cases where the oral route is not available or inadequate
- Intraosseous puncture can provide the quickest access to the circulation in a shocked child in whom venous cannulation is impossible (see pages 13–14 to 13–15).

Total daily maintenance fluid requirements

Body weight	**Fluid (ml/day)**
<10 kg	100–120
10–19 kg	90–120
>20 kg	50–90

Example

Body weight	**Fluid (ml/day)**
2	220
4	440
6	660
8	900
10	1100
15	1500
20	1800

Hourly maintenance fluid requirements can be calculated using the 4:2:1 rule.

Hourly maintenance fluid requirements

Body weight (kg)	**Fluid (ml/hour)**
First 10 kg	4
Plus	
Second 10 kg	2
Plus	
Thereafter	1

Example: Hourly maintenance fluid requirements for a 22 kg child

	Fluid (ml/hour)
10 x 4	40
Plus	
10 x 2 ml	20
Plus	
2 x 1 ml	2
Total	**62**

Fluid requirements in surgical patients commonly exceed maintenance requirements. Children with abdominal operations typically require up to 50% more than baseline requirements and even larger amounts if peritonitis is present. Special care is needed with fluid therapy in children; pay close attention to ongoing losses (e.g. nasogastric drainage) and monitor urine output. In the case of fever, add 12% to total maintenance requirements per 1 °C rise above 37.5 °C temperature measured rectally.

The most sensitive indicator of fluid status in a child is urine output. If urinary retention is suspected, pass a Foley catheter. A catheter also allows hourly measurements of urine output that can prove invaluable in the severely ill patient.

Normal urine output: Infants 1–2 ml/kg/hour
Children 1 ml/kg/hour

Infants are unable to concentrate urine as well as adults, making them more susceptible to electrolyte abnormalities.

Establishing intravenous access in paediatric patients can be challenging. See pages 13–11 to 13–15 for IV access techniques.

Anaesthesia and pain control

Anaesthesia in children poses special problems. The smaller diameter airway makes children especially susceptible to airway obstruction. Children often need intubation to protect their airway during surgical procedures. Ketamine anaesthesia is widely used for children in rural centres (see pages 14–14 to 14–21), but is also good for pain control.

Children suffer from pain as much as adults, but may show it in different ways. Make surgical procedures as painless as possible:

- Oral paracetamol can be given several hours prior to operation
- Local anaesthetics (bupivacaine 0.25%, not to exceed 1 ml/kg) administered in the operating room can decrease incisional pain
- Paracetamol (10–15 mg/kg every 4–6 hours) administered by mouth or rectally is a safe and effective method for controlling postoperative pain
- For more severe pain, use intravenous narcotics (morphine sulfate 0.05–0.1 mg/kg IV) every 2–4 hours
- Ibuprofen 10 mg/kg can be administered by mouth every 6–8 hours
- Codeine suspension 0.5–1 mg/kg can be administered by mouth every 6 hours, as needed.

Pre- and postoperative care

The pre- and postoperative care of children with surgical problems is often as important as the procedure itself. For this reason, surgical care of children does not begin or end in the operating room. Good care requires teamwork, with doctors, nurses and parents all having important roles to play:

- Prepare the patient and family for the procedure
- Ensure that the needed paediatric supplies (such as intravenous catheters, endotracheal tubes and Foley catheters) are available in the operating room to complete the procedure
- Monitor the patient's vital signs during the critical period of recovery
- Encourage a parent to stay with the child in the hospital and to be involved in his/her care.

SURGICAL PROBLEMS IN NEONATES

While there are many types of congenital anomalies, only a few of them are common. Some require urgent surgical attention while others should be left alone until the child is older. However, resuscitation cannot await referral and you may need to perform essential life-saving interventions prior to referral of the child for definitive surgery.

KEY POINTS

- By recognizing common congenital conditions you can identify when urgent referral is required
- Jaundice in the newborn is usually physiological or due to ABO incompatibility; if it is progressive, however, consider a congenital abnormality of the biliary tree.

3

Intestinal obstruction

Any newborn with abdominal distension, vomiting or no stool output, has a bowel obstruction until proven otherwise.

Bile stained (green) vomiting can be a sign of a life threatening condition. A peristaltic wave across the abdomen can sometimes be seen just before the child vomits:

- Place a nasogastric tube
- Start intravenous fluids
- Keep the child warm
- Transfer the child, if possible.

If transfer is not possible, perform a laparotomy (see pages 6–1 to 6–4) to rule out midgut volvulus which can result in gangrene of the entire small intestine. Under ketamine anaesthesia, untwist the bowel. Close the abdomen and, when the child is stable, refer for definitive management.

Hypertrophic pyloric stenosis

Non-bilious (not green) vomiting can be caused by hypertrophic pyloric stenosis. This condition is caused by enlargement of the muscle that controls stomach emptying (pylorus). In a relaxed infant, a mass is palpable in the upper abdomen at the midline or slightly to the right of the midline.

The condition most commonly occurs in male infants 2–5 weeks of age. It is treated with pyloromyotomy. Infants with pyloric stenosis commonly present with dehydration and electrolyte imbalances. Intravenous fluid resuscitation is required urgently:

- Use normal saline (20 ml/kg bolus) and insert a nasogastric tube
- Repeat the fluid boluses until the infant is urinating and vital signs have corrected to normal (2 or 3 boluses may be required).

Once the fluid and electrolyte abnormalities have been corrected, provide for maintenance for ongoing losses and transfer the patient for urgent management by a qualified surgeon.

Oesophageal atresia

Failure of oesophageal development is often associated with a fistula from the oesophagus to the trachea. The newborn presents with drooling or regurgitation of the first and subsequent feeds. Choking or coughing on feeding is frequent. An X-ray with a nasogastric tube coiled up in an air filled pouch is diagnostic.

Keep the infant warm and nurse in the 30° head up position. Place a sump drain in the oesophageal pouch and administer intravenous fluids calculated according to weight. The child will inevitably get pneumonia, so give antibiotics. Refer the stable infant to a paediatric surgeon.

Abdominal wall defects

Defects of the abdominal wall occur at or beside the umbilicus:

- In omphalocoele, there is a transparent covering over the extruding bowel

- In gastroschisis, the bowel is exposed:
  - If the bowel is strangulated in a gastroschisis, make an incision in the full thickness of the abdominal wall to increase the size of the opening and relieve the obstruction
  - Apply a sterile dressing and then cover with a plastic bag to prevent fluid loss; exposed bowel can lead to rapid fluid loss and hypothermia
  - Transfer the baby urgently to a qualified surgeon.

Anorectal anomalies

Imperforate anus can occur in a variety of forms. The diagnosis should be made at birth by examining the anus. There may be no opening at all. In other instances, a tiny opening discharging a little meconium may be seen at the base of the penis or just inside the vagina.

Delay in diagnosis may cause severe abdominal distension, leading to bowel perforation. Place a nasogastric tube, start intravenous fluids and transfer the child to a surgeon. A transverse loop colostomy is the emergency treatment of anorectal obstruction. Arrange for repair of the anomaly by a qualified surgeon on an elective basis.

Meningomyelocele (spina bifida)

Meningomyelocele is the name given to a small sac that protrudes through a bony defect in the skull or vertebrae. The most common site is the lumbar region. It may be associated with neurological problems (bowel, bladder and motor deficits in the lower extremities) and hydrocephalus. These patients should always be referred:

- Hydrocephalus will progress without a shunt being placed
- Meningitis occurs if the spinal defect is open.

The defect should be covered with sterile dressings and treated with strict aseptic technique until closure.

Cleft lip and palate

Cleft lip and palate may occur together or separately. A baby with a cleft palate may have difficulty sucking, leading to malnutrition. An infant with cleft lip or palate who is not growing normally should be fed with a spoon. The operation for a cleft lip is best done at 6 months of age and cleft palate at 1 year. Urgent referral is not required.

Congenital orthopaedic disorders

Disability can be avoided with early treatment of two of the most common congenital orthopedic disorders:

- Talipes equinovarus (club foot)
- Congenital hip dislocation.

Talipes equinovarus (club foot)

Club foot is a deformity that may be bilateral. It can often be corrected by early treatment (see pages 19–3 to 19–4).

3

Dislocation of the hip

All children should be screened for this problem at birth. The diagnosis is suggested by clinical examination:

- When the dislocation is unilateral:
  - The limb is short
  - There is limited abduction when the hip is flexed
  - The skin crease at the back of the hip appears asymmetrical
- When the flexed hip is abducted, a click can often be felt as the dislocated femoral head enters the acetabulum (Ortolani's sign).

In some regions of the world, this problem is uncommon because infants are carried on the mother's back.

See pages 19–1 to 19–2 for treatment.

Other common problems seen in neonates

Condition	Finding	Cause	Treatment
Clavicle fracture	Swelling and tenderness over clavicle	Birth trauma	None
Humerus or femur fracture	Deformity of limb	Birth trauma	Elastic bandage
Arm weakness (Erbs palsy)	No arm movement	Birth trauma	Physical therapy
Large breast	Large breast	Effects of maternal oestrogen	None

KEY POINTS

- Injuries, including burns and surgical infections, are common problems in children; the calculation of doses, based on weight, for fluids, transfusions and drugs is crucial to correct management
- The principles of priority apply to children with injuries
- Burns, especially scald injuries, are very common in children; children with burns are at increased risk for infection.
- Underlying malnutrition and immunosuppression from chronic parasitic infections greatly affect wound healing and the risk of infection.

SURGICAL PROBLEMS IN YOUNG CHILDREN

The differences in physiology between adults and children must always be considered and careful calculation of doses for fluids, blood transfusions and drugs based on body weight is crucial to the correct management of injuries, including burns, in children. Underlying malnutrition and immunosuppression from chronic parasitic infections greatly affect wound healing and the risk of infection.

Injuries

Most of the principles of adult trauma also apply to children, but there are important differences. See Unit 16: *Acute Trauma Management* and the Annex: *Primary Trauma Care Manual.* The initial assessment and priorities apply to children.

Burns

Burns, especially scald injuries, are very common in children. Children with burns are at increased risk for infection. See pages 5–13 to 5–16 and pages 34–37 in the Annex: *Primary Trauma Care Manual.*

Surgical infections

The treatment of abscess, pyomyositis, osteomyelitis, and septic arthritis in children is similar to that of adults, although the diagnosis may depend more on physical examination as the history is often limited or unavailable. Systemic illness and fever may overshadow localizing symptoms. Avoid the pitfall of identifying all childhood fever as malaria or other infectious disease.

In the diagnosis of surgical infections, pain is the most important symptom and tenderness the most important sign that differentiates them from infectious diseases. Use the specific sections on abscess in Unit 5: *Basic Surgical Procedures* and Unit 19: *General Orthopaedics* for information on management.

KEY POINTS

- Abscess, pyomyositis, osteomyelitis and septic arthritis have similar presentations and treatment in children as in adults
- The systemic illness and fever may overshadow localizing symptoms; careful history and physical examination is necessary to avoid the pitfall of idenfifying all childhood fever as malaria
- Pain is the most important symptom and tenderness the most important sign suggesting infection.

Acute abdominal conditions

Abdominal pain

Children commonly complain of abdominal pain. Serial observations are important in making a decision on whether there is an indication to operate. Be concerned about a child with:

- Unrelenting abdominal pain (>6 hours)
- Marked tenderness with guarding
- Pain that is associated with persistent nausea and vomiting.

The goal in assessing a child with abdominal pain is to determine if peritonitis (inflammation of the lining of the abdominal cavity) is present. The most common causes of peritonitis in children are:

- Appendicitis
- Other causes of bowel perforations:
  - Bowel obstructions
  - Typhoid fever.

Peritonitis may be difficult to diagnose in young children. The signs of peritonitis are:

- Tenderness
- Guarding (spasm of abdominal musculature following palpation)
- Pain with movement.

Simple methods for assessing the presence of peritonitis include:

- Asking the child to jump up and down, shaking the pelvis or pounding on the bottom of the foot
- Pressing down on the abdomen then quickly removing the hand; if there is exaggerated pain, peritonitis is present.

Most causes of peritonitis require laparotomy.

Appendicitis

The most common cause of peritonitis in children is appendicitis. The most important physical finding in appendicitis is steady abdominal pain that is localized in the right lower quadrant of the abdomen. There is usually vomiting. If appendicitis is not recognized early and treated, perforation may result. In children under two years of age, most cases of appendicitis are diagnosed after perforation. See pages 7–10 to 7–13 for clinical management.

3

Bowel obstruction

The clinical signs of a bowel obstruction are the same as in adults and include:

- Vomiting
- Constipation
- Abdominal pain
- Distension.

Children swallow air that can increase the amount of distension. The bowel can rupture if it becomes too dilated. The most common causes of bowel obstruction in children are:

- Incarcerated hernia: can be reduced if it presents early and is then referred for surgery
- Intussusception: can be reduced with barium enema if it presents early
- Adhesions (scarring): small bowel obstruction due to adhesions is initially treated non-operatively with nasogastric suction and intravenous fluids.

Reduction of the intussusception and lysis of adhesions both at laparotomy and herniotomy are the surgical treatments when non-operative management is unsuccessful or in late presentations.

See pages 7–2 to 7–5 for the clinical management of intestinal obstruction and pages 7–13 to 7–14 for the management of intussusception.

If the bowel is blocked with large numbers of Ascaris worms, treat with antihelminthics. If blockage is found at laparotomy, do not open the small intestine, but milk the worms into the large intestine and give antihelminthics postoperatively.

Hernias

The most common hernias in children are:

- Umbilical
- Inguinal.

Umbilical hernias are common in newborns. They are usually asymptomatic. Repair if the hernia has ever been incarcerated, otherwise avoid surgery as spontaneous resolution can occur up to 10 years of age (see pages 8–9 to 8–10 for a description of umbilical herniorraphy).

Inguinal hernias occur where the spermatic cord exits the abdomen. The clinical sign of an inguinal hernia is swelling in the groin. Distinguish hernias from hydrocoeles. Hydrocoeles are collections of fluid around the testicle that often resolve during the first year of life and do not require surgical repair. Hydrocoeles that fluctuate in size, called communicating hydrocoeles, are a form of hernia. These are an exception and require surgery. Refer possible communicating hydrocoeles for definitive diagnosis and treatment.

Surgery in paediatric inguinal hernia is indicated to prevent incarceration. The procedure is high ligation of the sac, but repair is only rarely required. See pages 8–2 to 8–6 for the description of inguinal and umbilical hernia.

Surgical techniques 4

4.1 TISSUE HANDLING

Technique

When making an incision:

1 Plan the incision to give adequate exposure.

2 Stabilize the skin with one hand and, using the belly of the scalpel blade, open the skin in a continuous motion (Figure 4.1).

3 Deepen the wound to reach the target organ, using the whole length of the incision. Do not shorten the incision with each layer. If time permits, ensure that haemostasis is achieved as the operation proceeds. In an emergency situation, this can be done once the situation and the patient are stabilized.

4 Close the operation wound in layers with non-absorbable sutures. Braided materials may provide a focus for infection and should not be used in potentially contaminated wounds. Bring the wound edges together loosely, but without gaps, taking a "bite" of about 1 cm of tissue on either side, and leaving an interval of 1 cm between each stitch (Figure 4.2).

A potentially contaminated wound is best left open lightly packed with damp saline soaked gauze and the suture closed as delayed primary closure after 2–5 days (Figure 4.3).

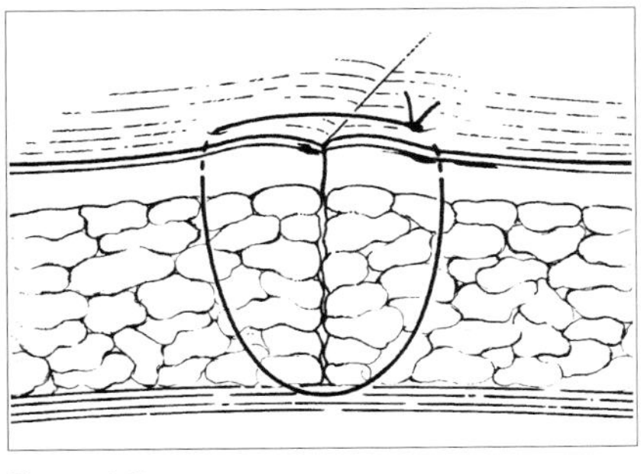

Figure 4.2

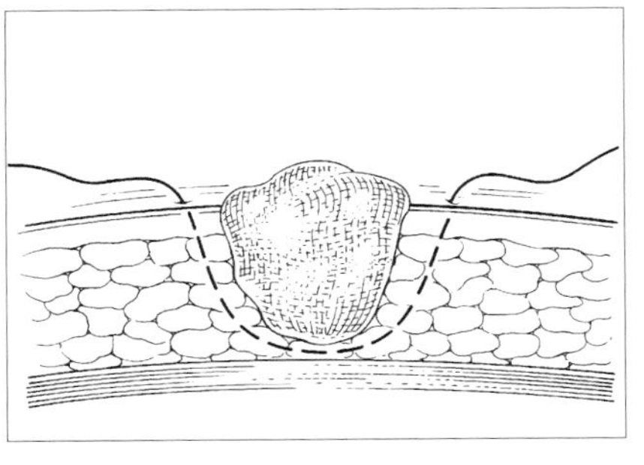

Figure 4.3

KEY POINTS

- Handle tissues gently
- Prevent bleeding. Minimizing blood loss minimizes the need for blood replacement or transfusion. This is especially important in areas where a safe and consistent blood supply is in doubt.

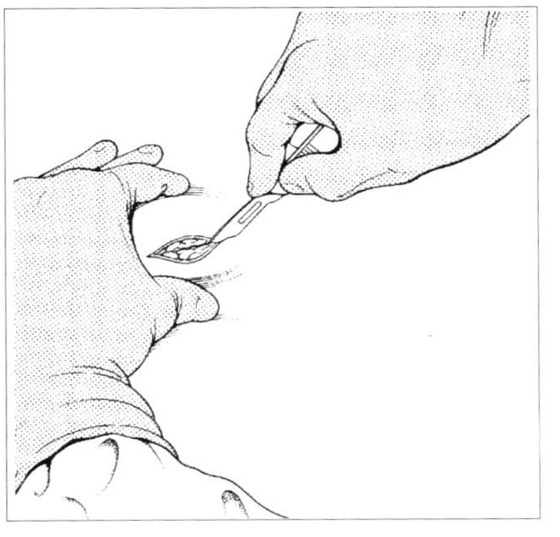

Figure 4.1

HAEMOSTASIS

Minimizing blood loss is essential and is of the highest priority in patients who are medically compromised by anaemia or chronic illness.

As the risks of transfusion (from infections such as malaria, Chagas, hepatitis and HIV) have increased, the challenge of establishing a safe and consistent blood supply has been highlighted. Minimizing blood loss is part of excellent surgical technique and safe medical practice. Meticulous haemostasis at all stages of operative procedures, decreased operative times and improved surgical skill and knowledge will all help to decrease blood loss and minimize the need for blood replacement or transfusion.

4

Technique

- Control initial oozing of blood from the cut surfaces by pressure over gauze
- Control individual bleeding vessels with cautery or suture ligation using fine suture; when tying off bleeders, cut the ligature short
- Avoid diathermy near the skin where it may cause damage and devitalize tissue
- When tying off a large vessel, or to ensure that the suture will not come off the end of a vessel, use a suture ligature. This involves passing the needle through the vessel before securing the tie around the vessel (Figure 4.4). Place a second free tie below the suture ligature.

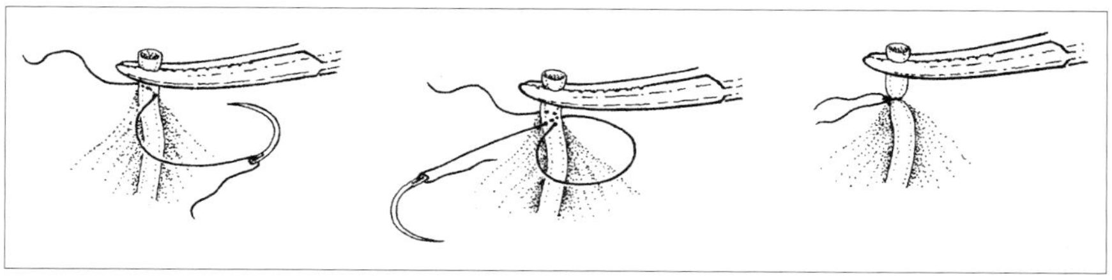

Figure 4.4

KEY POINTS

- Suture is made of a variety of materials with a variety of properties
- There are many types of suture and a variety of materials; learn the properties of each, become confident using a few and regularly use those you are most comfortable with
- Suturing is the most versatile, least expensive and most widely used technique of securing tissue during an operative procedure.

4.2 SUTURE AND SUTURE TECHNIQUE

Suture is made of a variety of materials with a variety of properties. It may be synthetic or biological, absorbable or non-absorbable and constructed with a single or multiple filaments.

Nylon is an example of a synthetic suture. Biological suture, such as gut, increases physiological response and is not good for use in the skin. Silk is a braided biological suture, which should not be used in dirty wounds. The multiple filaments create space, allowing bacterial trapping, and silk is absorbed slowly.

Choice among these materials depends on:

- Availability
- Individual preference in handling
- Security of knots
- Behaviour of the material in the presence of infection
- Cost.

If you want a suture to last, for example when closing the abdominal wall or ligating a major vessel, use one made of non-absorbable material. Use absorbable material in the urinary tract to avoid the encrustation and stone formation associated with non-absorbable suture.

All varieties of suture material may be used in the skin, but a reactive suture such as silk should be removed within a few days. In skin wounds, remove sutures early to reduce visible markings.

Because of the ease of tying, braided suture may be easier to use for interrupted stitches. Absorbable and non-absorbable monofilament suture is convenient for continuous running stitches.

The commercial suture package is marked with the needle shape and size, the suture material and the suture thickness. Suture is graded according to size. The most popular grading system rates the suture material downward from a very heavy 2 to a very fine ophthalmic suture of 10/0. Most common operations can be completed with suture material between sizes 4/0 and 1.

Different materials have different strength characteristics. The strength of all sutures increases with their size.

Suture can be purchased in reels and packaged and sterilized on site as a less expensive alternative to packages from the manufacturer.

ABSORBABLE SUTURE

A suture that degrades and loses its tensile strength within 60 days is generally considered to be absorbable.

Polyglycolic acid is the most popular suture material because it is absorbable and has long lasting tensile strength. It is an appropriate suture for abdominal closure. The absorption time for this suture is considered to be 60 – 90 days.

Catgut is pliable, is easy to handle and inexpensive. Chromic catgut lasts for 2–3 weeks and is used for ligatures and tissue suture. Do not use it for closing fascial layers of abdominal wounds, or in situations where prolonged support is needed. Plain catgut is absorbed in 5–7 days, and is therefore useful when healing is expected within this period. It is also useful for suturing mucous membranes or when it is not possible for the patient to return for skin suture removal.

NON-ABSORBABLE SUTURE

Braided suture is usually made of natural products (silk, linen or cotton). It is acceptable in many situations, but is contraindicated in a wound that is, or may be, contaminated.

Synthetic monofilament suture, such as nylon polypropamide, may be left in the deeper layers, and is not contraindicated in situations of contamination. It is often used as continuous suture. The knots are less secure than those in braided suture or in polyglycolic acid suture and more throws are used for a secure knot.

Use non-absorbable suture material when possible. Sterilized polyester thread and nylon line produced for non-surgical purposes are acceptable compromises when commercial suture is unavailable.

NEEDLES

Surgical needles are classified in three categories:

- Round bodied
- Cutting
- Trochar.

4

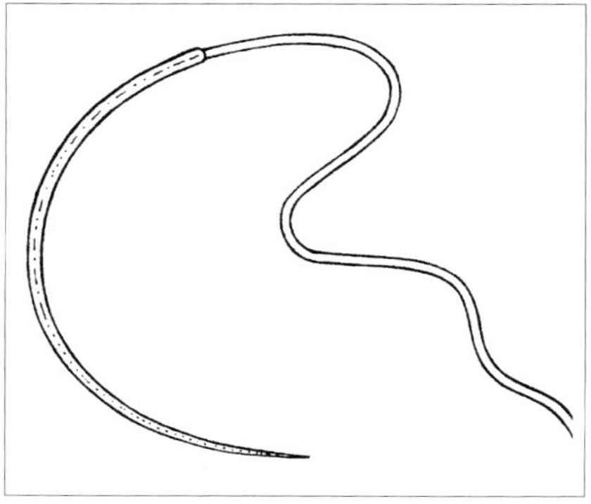

Figure 4.5

Within these categories, there are hundreds of different types.

Use cutting needles on the skin, and for securing structures like drains. Use round bodied needles in fragile tissue, for example when performing an intestinal anastomosis. Do not use a cutting needle in this situation.

Trochar needles have a sharp tip but a round body. They are useful when it is necessary to perforate tough tissue, but when cutting the tissue would be undesirable, as in the linea alba when closing the abdominal wall.

Needles are attached to the suture commercially (sweged on: see Figure 4.5) or have eyes to pass the suture through (free needles). Sweged on needles are preferable, but every centre should have free needles available as an alternative when more expensive suture is unavailable or when a needle breaks off the suture before the task has been completed.

Techniques

There are many ways to secure tissue during an operative procedure and to repair discontinuity in the skin: tape, glue, staples and suture. The aim of all these techniques is to approximate the wound edges without gaps and without tension. Staples are an expensive alternative and glue may not be widely available. Suturing is the most versatile, least expensive and most widely used technique.

Suturing techniques include:

- Interrupted simple
- Continuous simple
- Vertical mattress
- Horizontal mattress
- Subcuticular
- Purse string
- Retention/tension.

The size of the bite, and the interval between bites, should be consistent and will depend on the thickness of the tissue being approximated.

Use the minimal size and amount of suture material required to close the wound.

Leave skin sutures in place for an average of 7 days. In locations where healing is slow and cosmesis is less important (the back and legs), leave sutures for 10–14 days. In locations where cosmesis is important (the face), sutures can be removed after 3 days but the wound should be reinforced with skin tapes.

1 Use the needle driver to hold the needle, grasping the needle with the tip of the driver, between half and two thirds of the way along the needle. If the needle is held less than half way along, it will be difficult to take proper bites and to use the angle of the needle. Holding the needle too close to the end where the suture is attached may result in a flattening of the needle and a lack of control. Hold the needle driver so that your fingers are free of the rings and so that you can rotate your wrist and/or the driver.
2 Pass the needle tip through the skin at 90 degrees.

3 Use the curve of the needle by turning the needle through the tissue; do not try to push it as you would a straight needle.

4 Close deep wounds in layers with either absorbable or monofilament non-absorbable sutures (Figure 4.6).

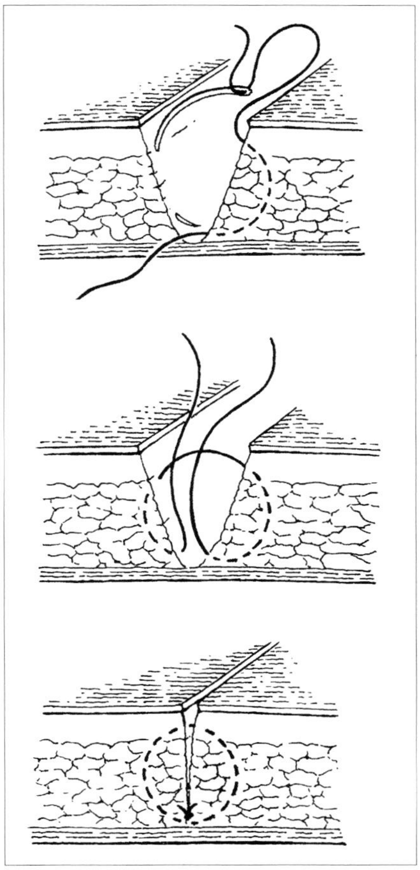

Figure 4.6

Interrupted sutures

- Most commonly used to repair lacerations
- Permit good eversion of the wound edges, as well as apposition; entering the tissue close to the wound edge will increase control over the position of the edge
- Use only when there is minimal skin tension
- Ensure that bites are of equal volume
- If the wound is unequal, bring the thicker side to meet the thinner to avoid putting extra tension on the thinner side
- The needle should pass through tissue at 90 degrees and exit at the same angle
- Use non-absorbable suture and remove it at an appropriate time.

Continuous/running sutures

- Less time-consuming than interrupted sutures; fewer knots are tied and less suture is used
- Less precision in approximating edges of the wound
- Poorer cosmetic result than other options
- Inclusion cysts and epithelialization of the suture track are potential complications
- Suture passes at 90 degrees to the line of the incision and crosses internally under the top of the incision at 45–60 degrees.

Mattress sutures

- Provide a relief of wound tension and precise apposition of the wound edges
- More complex and therefore more time-consuming to put in.

Vertical mattress technique

Vertical mattress sutures are best for allowing eversion of wound edges and perfect apposition and to relieve tension from the skin edges (Figures 4.7 and 4.8).

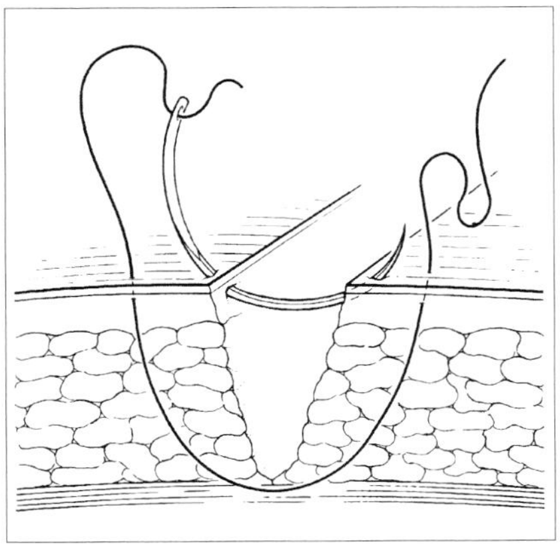

Figure 4.7

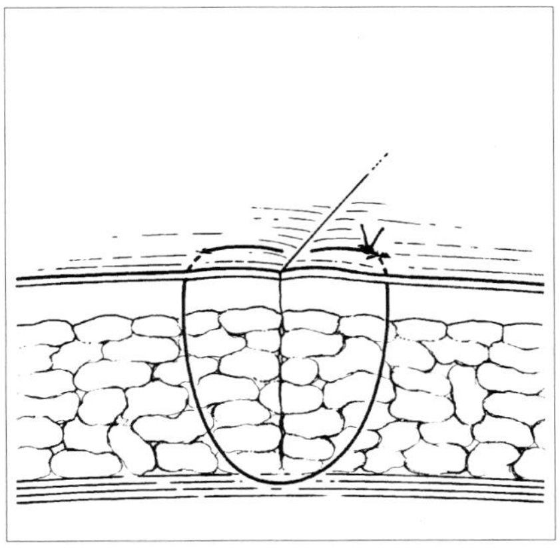

Figure 4.8

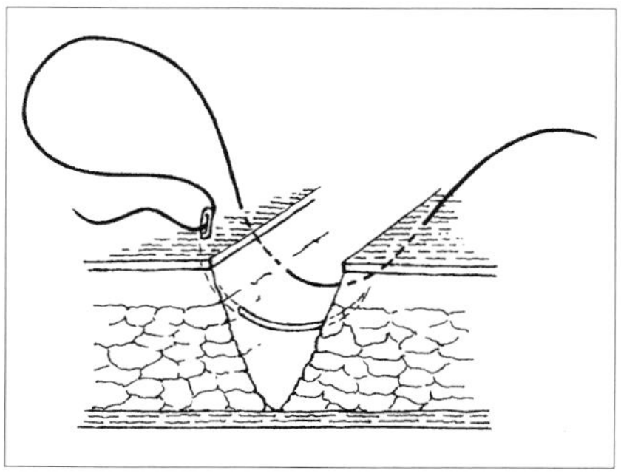

Figure 4.9

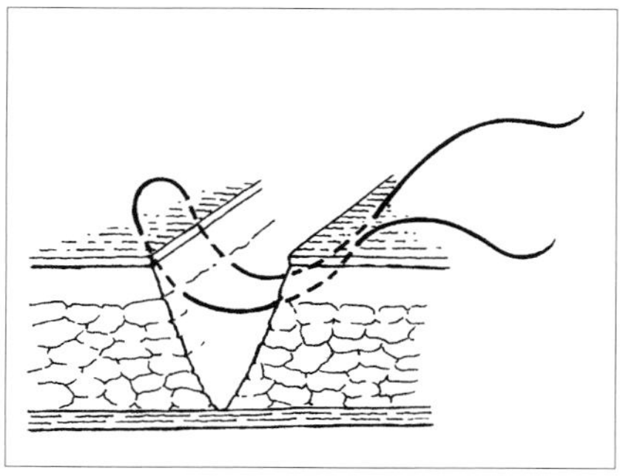

Figure 4.10

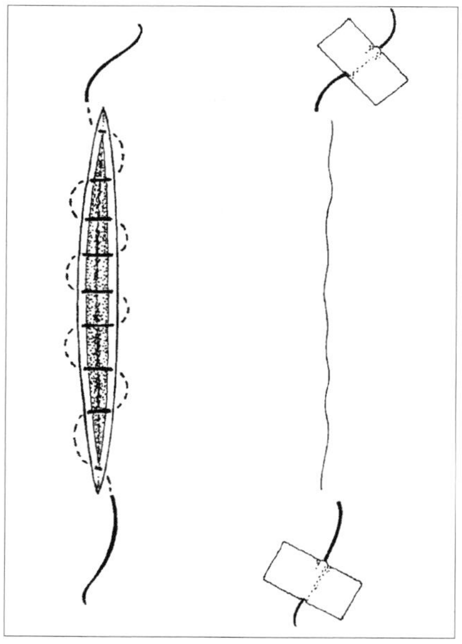

Figure 4.11

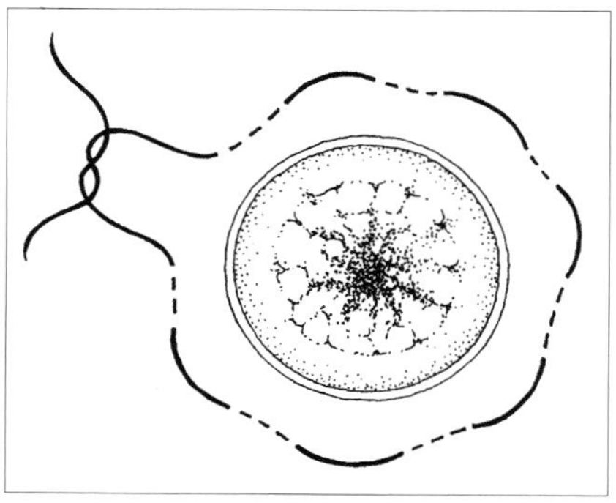

Figure 4.12

1 Start the first bite wide of the incision and pass to the same position on the other side of the wound.

2 The second step is a similar bite which starts on the side of the incision where the needle has just exited the skin. Pass the needle through the skin between the exit point and the wound edge, in line with the original entry point. From this point, take a small bite; the final exit point is in a similar position on the other side of the wound.

3 Tie the knot so that it does not lie over the incision line. This suture approximates the subcutaneous tissue and the skin edge.

Horizontal mattress technique

Horizontal mattress sutures reinforce the subcutaneous tissue and provide more strength and support along the length of the wound; this keeps tension off the scar (Figures 4.9 and 4.10).

1 The two sutures are aligned beside one another. The first stitch is aligned across the wound; the second begins on the side that the first ends.

2 Tie the knot on the side of the original entry point.

Continuous subcuticular sutures

- Excellent cosmetic result
- Use fine, absorbable braided or monofilament suture
- Do not require removal if absorbable sutures are used
- Useful in wounds with strong skin tension, especially for patients who are prone to keloid formation
- Anchor the suture in the wound and, from the apex, take bites below the dermal-epidermal border
- Start the next stitch directly opposite the one that precedes it (Figure 4.11).

Purse string sutures

- A circular pattern that draws together the tissue in the path of the suture when the ends are brought together and tied (Figure 4.12).

Retention sutures

- All abdominal layers are held together without tension; the sutures take the tension off the wound edges
- Use for patients debilitated as a result of malnutrition, old age, immune deficiency or advanced cancer; those with impaired healing and patients suffering from conditions associated with increased intra-abdominal pressure, such as obesity, asthma or chronic cough
- Also use in cases of abdominal wound dehiscence
- Monofilament nylon is a suitable material.

Retention sutures technique

1 Insert retention sutures through the entire thickness of the abdominal wall leaving them untied at first. Sutures may be simple (through-and-through) or mattress in type.

2 Insert a continuous peritoneal suture and continue to close the wound in layers.
3 When skin closure is complete, tie each suture after threading it through a short length of plastic or rubber tubing (Figures 4.13–4.16). Do not tie the sutures under tension to avoid compromising blood supply to the healing tissues.
4 Leave the sutures in place for at least 14 days.

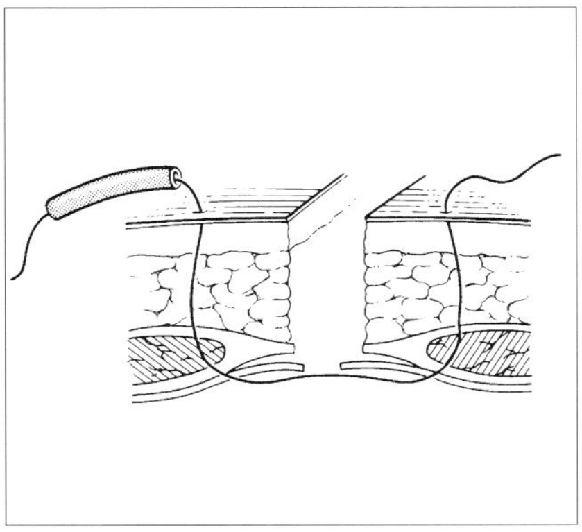
Figure 4.13

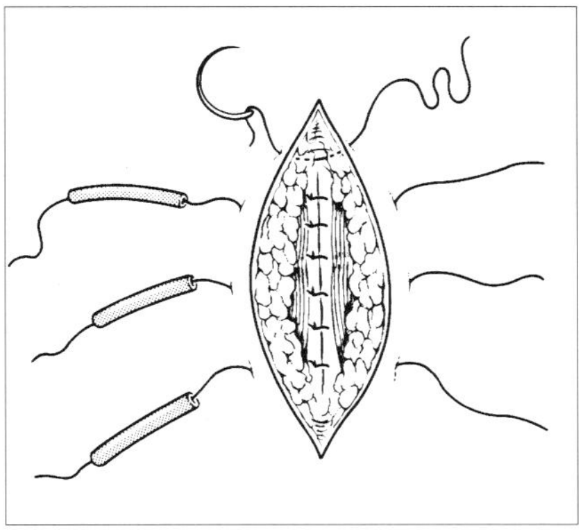
Figure 4.14

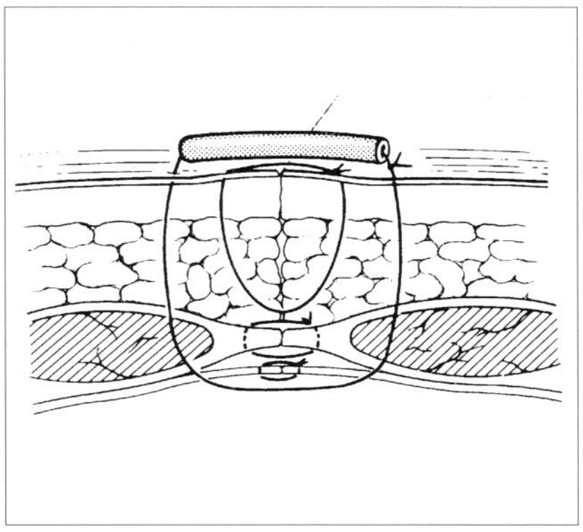
Figure 4.15

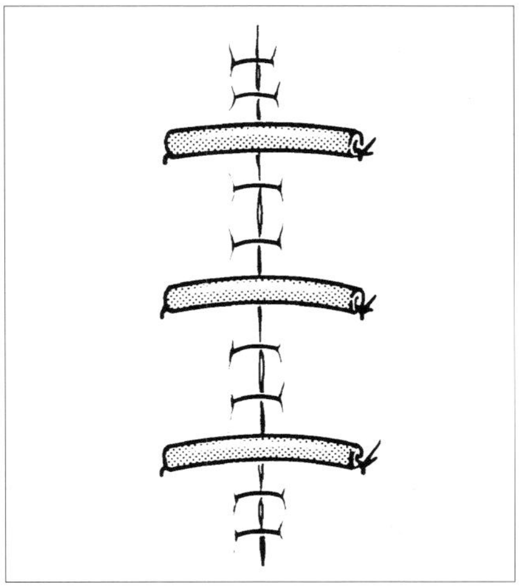
Figure 4.16

KNOT TYING

There are many knot tying variations and techniques, all with the intention of completing a secure, square knot. A complete square knot consists of two sequential throws that lie in opposite directions. This is necessary to create a knot that will not slip (Figure 4.17).

A surgeon's knot is a variation in which a double throw is followed by a single throw to increase the friction on the suture material and to decrease the initial slip until a full square knot has been completed (Figure 4.18).

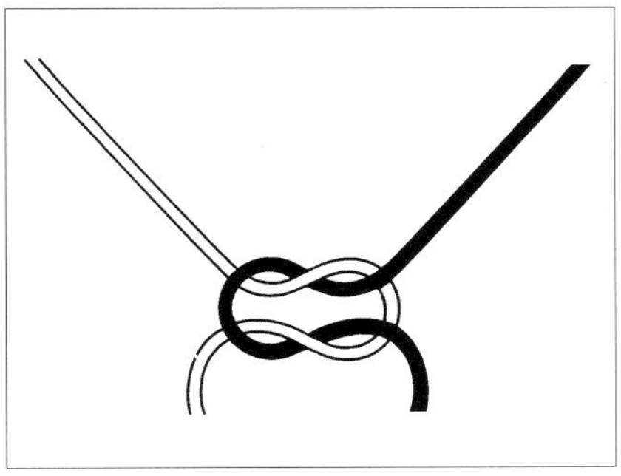
Figure 4.17

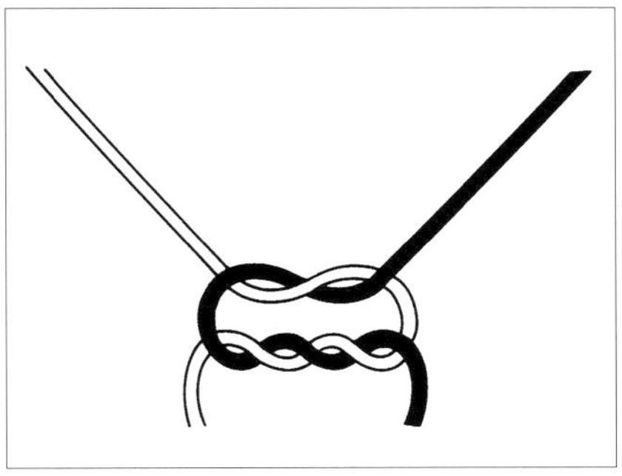
Figure 4.18

Use a minimum of two complete square knots on any substantive vessel and more when using monofilament suture. If the suture material is slippery, more knot throws will be required to ensure that the suture does not come undone or slip. When using a relatively "non-slippery" material such as silk, as few as three throws may be sufficient to ensure a secure knot.

Cut sutures of slippery materials longer than those of "non-slippery" materials. There is a balance between the need for security of the knot and the desire to leave as little foreign material in the wound as possible.

Techniques

There are three basic techniques of knot tying.

1 Instrument tie

- This is the most straightforward and the most commonly used technique; take care to ensure that the knots are tied correctly
- You must cross your hands to produce a square knot; to prevent slipping, use a surgeon's knot on the first throw only
- Do not use instrument ties if the patient's life depends on the security of the knot (Figure 4.19).

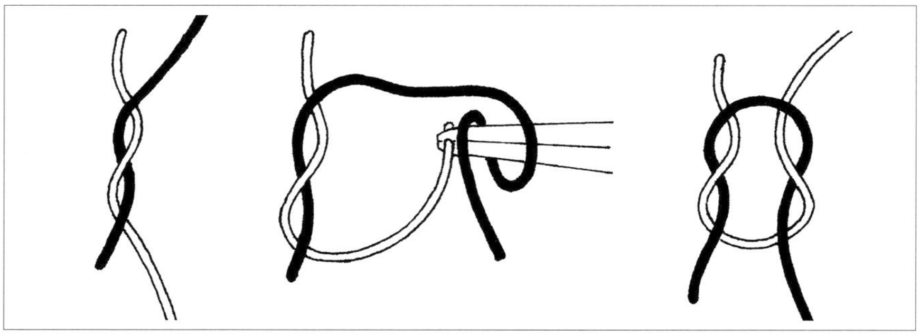

Figure 4.19

2 One handed knot

- Use the one handed technique to place deep seated knots and when one limb of the suture is immobilized by a needle or instrument
- Hand tying has the advantage of tactile sensations lost when using instruments; if you place the first throw of the knot twice, it will slide into place, but will have enough friction to hold while the next throw is placed
- This is an alternative to the surgeon's knot, but must be followed with a square knot
- To attain a square knot, the limbs of the suture must be crossed even when the knot is placed deeply (Figure 4.20).

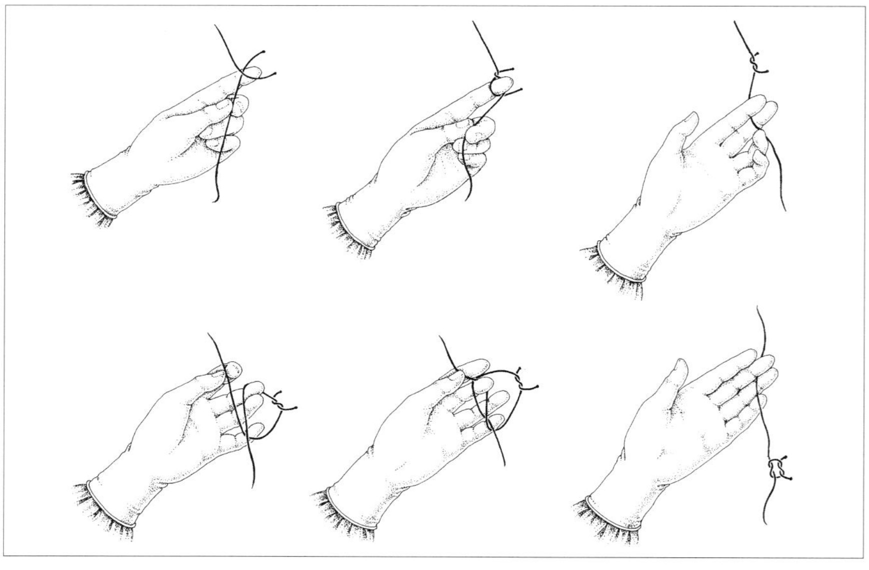

Figure 4.20

3 Two handed knot

- The two handed knot is the most secure. Both limbs of the suture are moved during its placement. A surgeon's knot is easily formed using a two handed technique (Figure 4.21).

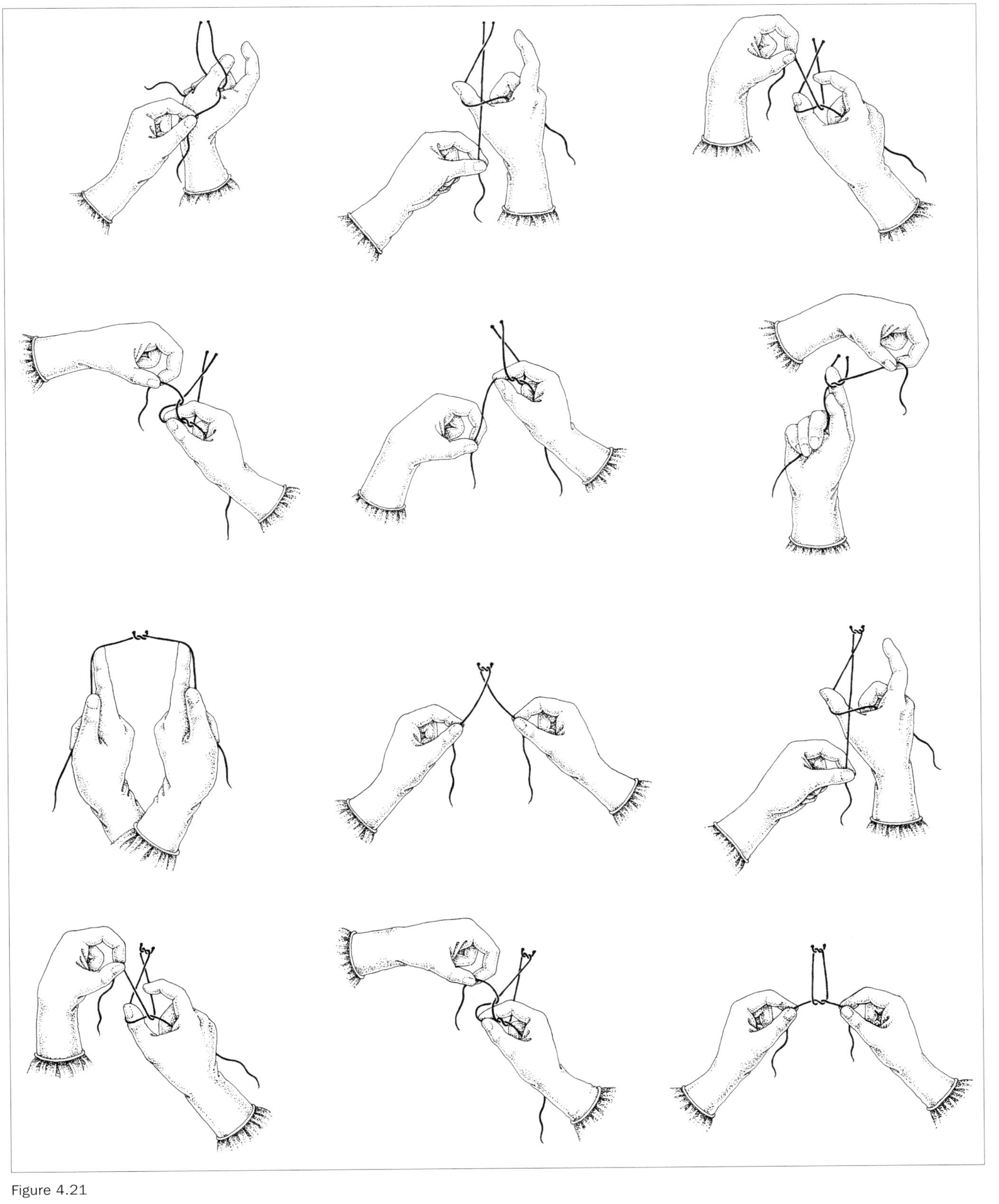

Figure 4.21

4

With practice, the feel of knot tying will begin to seem automatic. As with learning any motor skill, we develop "muscle memory". Our brain teaches our hands how to tie the knots, and eventually our hands tie knots so well, we are no longer consciously completing each step.

To teach knot tying (or any other skill) to someone else, remember the discrete steps involved. Demonstrate the whole skill of tying a knot; then demonstrate each step. Let the learner practice each step. Watch carefully and reinforce the correct actions, while making suggestions to correct problems. Once each step is mastered, the learner should put them together to tie a complete knot on his/her own. The learner must then practice tying knots over and over again, until the steps become a more fluid action requiring less conscious thought.

KEY POINTS

- Give prophylactic antibiotics in cases of wound contamination
- Immunize the non-immune patient against tetanus with tetanus toxoid and give immune globulin if the wound is tetanus prone.

4.3 PROPHYLAXIS

ANTIBIOTIC PROPHYLAXIS

Antibiotic prophylaxis is different from antibiotic treatment. Prophylaxis is intended to prevent infection or to decrease the potential for infection. It is not intended to prevent infection in situations of gross contamination. Use therapeutic doses if infection is present or likely:

- Administer antibiotics prior to surgery, within the 2 hours before the skin is cut, so that tissue levels are adequate during the surgery
- More than one dose may be given if the procedure is long (>6 hours) or if there is significant blood loss.

The use of topical antibiotics and washing wounds with antibiotic solutions are not recommended.

Use antibiotic prophylaxis in cases where there are:

- Biomechanical considerations that increase the risk of infection:
  - Implantation of a foreign body
  - Known valvular heart disease
  - Indwelling prosthesis
- Medical considerations that compromise the healing capacity or increase the infection risk:
  - Diabetes
  - Peripheral vascular disease
  - Possibility of gangrene or tetanus
  - Immunocompromise
- High-risk wounds or situations:
  - Penetrating wounds
  - Abdominal trauma
  - Compound fractures
  - Wounds with devitalized tissue
  - Lacerations greater than 5 cm or stellate lacerations
  - Contaminated wounds

- High risk anatomical sites such as hand or foot
- Biliary and bowel surgery.

Consider using prophylaxis:
- For traumatic wounds which may not require surgical intervention
- When surgical intervention will be delayed for more than 6 hours.

Use intravenous (IV) antibiotics for prophylaxis in clean surgical situations to reduce the risk of postoperative infection, since skin and instruments are never completely sterile.

For the prophylaxis of endocarditis in patients with known valvular heart disease:
- Oral and upper respiratory procedures: give amoxycillin 3 g orally, 1 hour before surgery and 1.5 g, 6 hours after first dose
- Gastrointestinal and genitourinary procedures: give ampicillin 3 g, 1 hour before surgery *and* gentamicin 1.5 mg/kg intramuscularly (IM) or IV (maximum dose 80 mg), 30 minutes before surgery.

ANTIBIOTIC TREATMENT

When a wound is extensive and more than 6 hours old, you should consider it to be colonized with bacteria, and use therapeutic doses and regimens. Penicillin and metronidazole provide good coverage and are widely available.

Monitor wound healing and infection regularly. Make use of culture and sensitivity findings if they are available. Continue therapeutic doses of antibiotics for 5–7 days.

TETANUS PROPHYLAXIS

Active immunization with tetanus toxoid (TT) prevents tetanus and is given together with diphtheria vaccine (TD). Women should be immunized during pregnancy to prevent neonatal tetanus. Childhood immunization regimes include diphtheria, pertussis and tetanus. Individuals who have not received three doses of tetanus toxoid are not considered immune and require immunization.

A non-immune person with a minor wound can be immunized if the wound is tetanus prone; give both TT or TD and tetanus immune globulin (TIG). A non-immunized person will require repeat immunization at six weeks and at six months to complete the immunization series.

Examples of tetanus prone wounds include:
- Wounds contaminated with dirt or faeces
- Puncture wounds
- Burns
- Frostbite
- High velocity missile injuries.

4

Tetanus prophylaxis regime

	Clean wounds	**Moderate risk**	**High risk**
Immunized and booster within 5 years	Nil	Nil	Nil
Immunized and 5–10 years since booster	Nil	TT or TD	TT or TD
Immunized and >10 years since booster	TT or TD	TT or TD	TT or TD
Incomplete immunization or unknown	TT or TD	TT or TD and TIG	TT or TD and TIG

Do not give TIG if the person is known to have had two primary doses of TT or TD

Basic surgical procedures

5

5.1 WOUND MANAGEMENT

SURGICAL WOUND CLASSIFICATION

Surgical wounds can be classified as follows:

- Clean
- Clean contaminated: a wound involving normal but colonized tissue
- Contaminated: a wound containing foreign or infected material
- Infected: a wound with pus present.

Factors that affect wound healing and the potential for infection

- Patient:
  - Age
  - Underlying illnesses or disease: consider anaemia, diabetes or immunocompromise
  - Effect of the injury on healing (e.g. devascularization)
- Wound:
  - Organ or tissue injured
  - Extent of injury
  - Nature of injury (for example, a laceration will be a less complicated wound than a crush injury)
  - Contamination or infection
  - Time between injury and treatment (sooner is better)
- Local factors:
  - Haemostasis and debridement
  - Timing of closure

- Close clean wounds immediately to allow healing by primary intention
- Do not close contaminated and infected wounds, but leave them open to heal by secondary intention
- In treating clean contaminated wounds and clean wounds that are more than six hours old, manage with surgical toilet, leave open and then close 48 hours later. This is delayed primary closure.

KEY POINTS

- Many important procedures can be performed under local anaesthesia and do not require a surgical specialist
- In most outpatient procedures, local or field block anaesthesia will be sufficient but general anaesthesia, including ketamine, may be necessary in children and should be available
- Irrespective of the seriousness of a wound, give initial management priority to the airway, breathing and circulation
- Good lighting and basic instruments are important for adequate wound examination and management
- Work efficiently to avoid prolonging the operation unnecessarily; *the risk of infection increases with time*
- Universal precautions are necessary to avoid the transmission of the HIV, hepatitis, Ebola and other viruses
- Clear the operative field of devitalized tissue and foreign material
- While not a substitute for appropriate haemostasis, placement of a drain is an option if a wound is oozing; the collection of fluid and blood leads to increased risk of infection and delayed healing
- Minimize dead space when closing a wound.

WOUND

Primary repair

Primary closure requires that clean tissue is approximated without tension. Injudicious closure of a contaminated wound will promote infection and delay healing.

Essential suturing techniques (see Unit 4) include:

- Interrupted simple
- Continuous simple

- Vertical mattress
- Horizontal mattress
- Intradermal.

Staples are an expensive, but rapid, alternative to sutures for skin closure. The aim with all techniques is to approximate the wound edges without gaps or tension. The size of the suture "bite" and the interval between bites should be equal in length and proportional to the thickness of tissue being approximated (see pages 4–4 to 4–7):

- As suture is a foreign body, use the minimal size and amount of suture material required to close the wound
- Leave skin sutures in place for 5 days; leave the sutures in longer if healing is expected to be slow due to the blood supply of a particular location or the patient's condition
- If appearance is important and suture marks unacceptable, as in the face, remove sutures as early as 3 days. In this case, re-enforce the wound with skin tapes
- Close deep wounds in layers, using absorbable sutures for the deep layers. Place a latex drain in deep oozing wounds to prevent haematoma formation.

Delayed primary closure

Irrigate clean contaminated wounds; then pack them open with damp saline gauze. Close the wounds with sutures at 2 days. These sutures can be placed at the time of wound irrigation or at the time of wound closure (see pages 4–4 to 4–7).

Secondary healing

To promote healing by secondary intention, perform wound toilet and surgical debridement. Surgical wound toilet involves:

- Cleaning the skin with antiseptics
- Irrigation of wounds with saline
- Surgical debridement of all dead tissue and foreign matter. Dead tissue does not bleed when cut.

During wound debridement, gentle handling of tissues minimizes bleeding. Control residual bleeding with compression, ligation or cautery.

Dead or devitalized muscle is dark in colour, soft, easily damaged and does not contract when pinched. During debridement, excise only a very thin margin of skin from the wound edge (Figure 5.1).

1 Systematically perform wound toilet and surgical debridement, initially to the superficial layers of tissues and subsequently to the deeper layers (Figures 5.2, 5.3). After scrubbing the skin with soap and irrigating the wound with saline, prep the skin with antiseptic. Do *not* use antiseptics within the wound.

2 Debride the wound meticulously to remove any loose foreign material such as dirt, grass, wood, glass or clothing. With a scalpel or dissecting

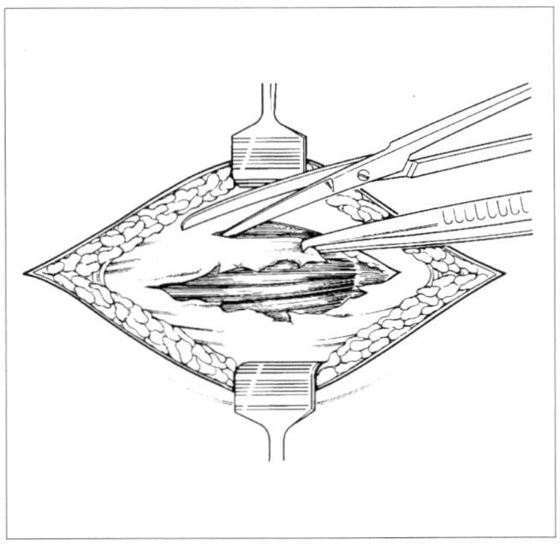

Figure 5.1

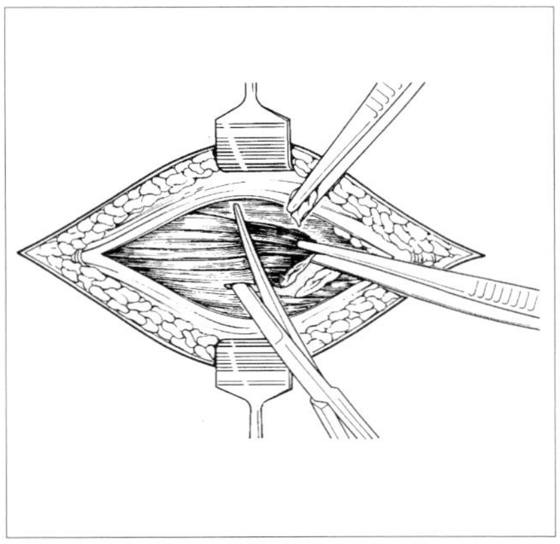

Figure 5.2

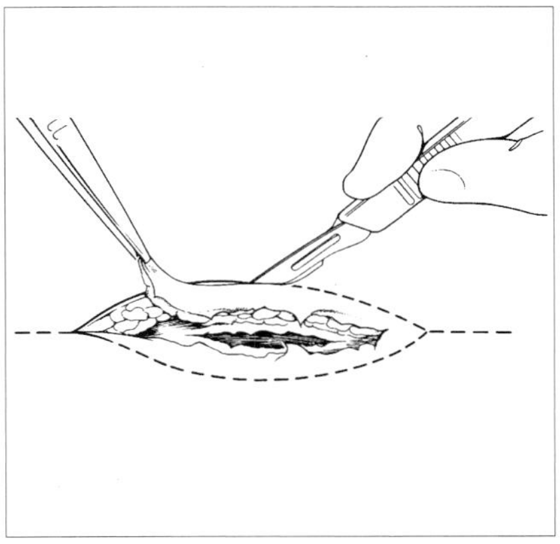

Figure 5.3

scissors, remove all adherent foreign material along with a thin margin of underlying tissue and then irrigate the wound again. Continue the cycle of surgical debridement and saline irrigation until the wound is completely clean.

3 Leave the wound open after debridement to allow healing by secondary intention. Pack it lightly with damp saline gauze and cover the packed wound with a dry dressing. Change the packing and dressing daily or more often if the outer dressing becomes damp with blood or other body fluids. Large defects will require closure with flaps or skin grafts but may be initially managed with saline packing.

Drains

Drainage of a wound or body cavity is indicated when there is risk of blood or serous fluid collection or when there is pus or gross wound contamination. The type of drain used depends on both indication and availability.

Drains are classified as open or closed and active or passive:

- Closed drains do not allow the entry of atmospheric air and require either suction or differential pressure to function
- Open drains allow atmospheric air access to the wound or body cavity
- Continuous suction drains with air vents are open but active drains.

Drains are not a substitute for good haemostasis or for good surgical technique and should not be left in place too long. They are usually left in place only until the situation which indicated insertion is resolved, there is no longer any fluid drainage or the drain is not functioning. Leaving a non-functioning drain in place unnecessarily exposes the patient to an increased risk of infection.

KEY POINTS

- Suction drains are active and closed
- Differential pressure drains are closed and passive
- Latex drains, which function by capillary action, are passive and open.

SPLIT-SKIN GRAFTING

Skin is the best cover for a wound. If a wound cannot be closed primarily, close it with a skin graft. Closure of a large defect with a skin graft requires a qualified practitioner who has received specific training.

- The recipient site should be healthy with no evidence of infection: a fresh clean wound or a wound with healthy granulation tissue

- The donor site is usually the anterolateral or posterolateral surface of the thigh
- Local anaesthetics are appropriate for small grafts; spinal or general anaesthesia is necessary for large grafts.

Technique

1 To perform a skin graft, prepare the donor site with antiseptic, isolate with drapes and lubricate with mineral oil.

2 Take small grafts with a razor blade held with an artery forcep or an adapted shaving instrument. Start by applying the cutting edge of the blade at an angle to the skin; after the first incision lay the blade flat.

For large grafts, use a skin-grafting knife or electric dermatome (Figure 5.4) in one hand and apply traction to the grafting board on the donor site. Instruct an assistant to apply counter-traction to keep the skin taut by holding a second board in the same manner. Cut the skin with regular back-and-forth movements while progressively sliding the first board ahead of the knife (Figure 5.5).

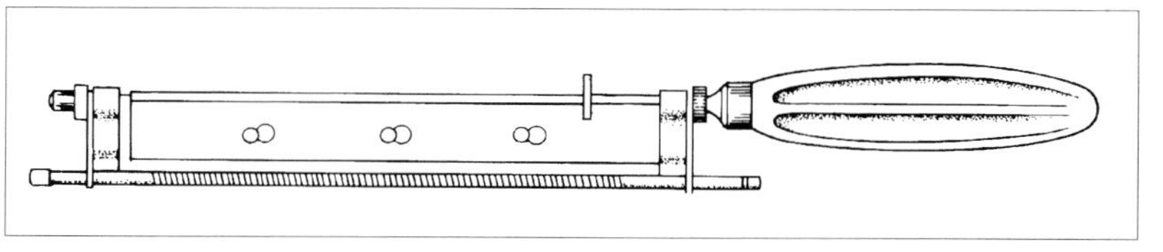

Figure 5.4

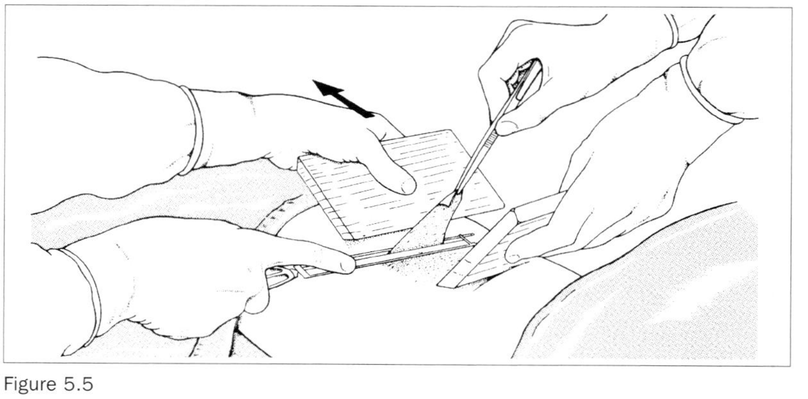

Figure 5.5

3 If the donor area has a homogeneous bleeding surface after the graft has been taken, it is split-skin thickness; exposed fat on the donor site indicates that the graft is too deep and full thickness skin has been removed. Adjust the blade and your technique to make the cut closer to the surface.

As the cut skin appears over the blade, instruct an assistant to lift it gently out of the way with non-toothed dissecting forceps.

4 Place the new graft in saline and cover the donor area with petroleum gauze. Spread the skin graft, with the raw surface upwards, on saline gauze (Figure 5.6).

5 Clean the recipient area with saline. Suture the graft in place at a few points and then secure it with sutures around all edges of the wound. During the procedure, keep the graft moist with saline and do not pinch it with instruments.

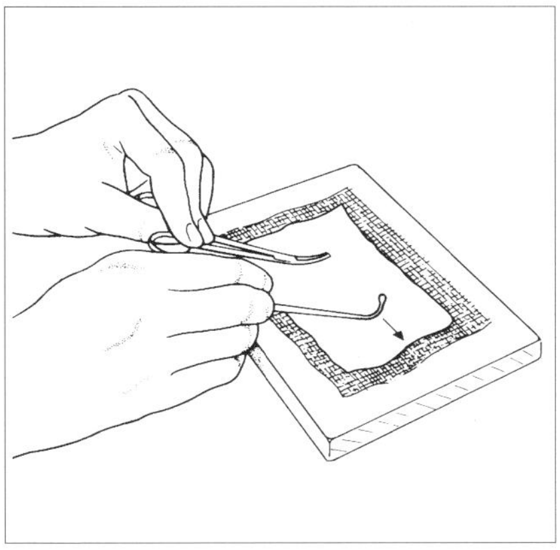

Figure 5.6

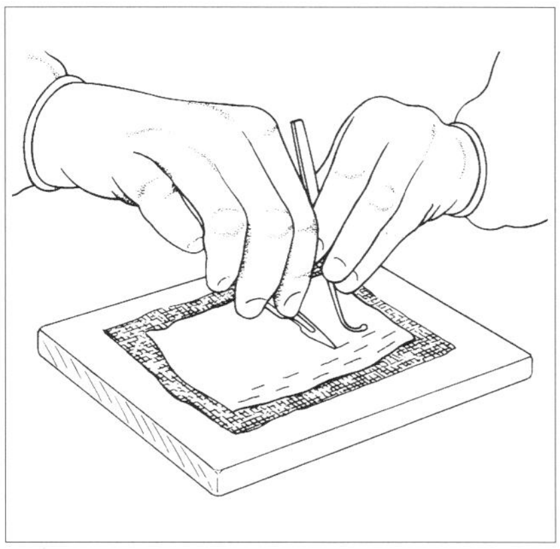

Figure 5.7

Haematoma formation under the graft is the most common reason for failure. To prevent it, apply petroleum gauze dressing moulded over the graft. Secure it with a simple dressing or tie in place with sutures over a bolus dressing. Small perforations in the graft (Figure 5.7) allow blood to escape and help prevent the formation of a haematoma.

6 Apply additional layers of gauze and cotton wool and, finally, a firm, even bandage. Leave the graft undisturbed for 5 days unless infection or haematoma is suspected. After that, change the dressing daily or every other day. After the initial dressing change, inspect the graft at least every 48 hours. If the graft is raised with serum, release the collection by aspirating with a hypodermic syringe or puncture the graft with a knife.

7 After 7 to 10 days, remove any sutures, gently wash the grafted area, and lubricate it with mineral oil. The second week after grafting, instruct the patient in regular massage and exercise of the grafted area, especially if it is located on the hand, the neck or extremities.

5.2 SPECIFIC LACERATIONS AND WOUNDS

BLOOD VESSELS, NERVES AND TENDONS

Assess the function of tendons, nerves and blood vessels distal to the laceration. Ligate lacerated vessels whether or not they are bleeding, as the vessels which are not bleeding may do so at a later time. Large damaged vessels may need to be divided between ligatures. Before dividing these larger vessels or an end artery, test the effect on the distal circulation by temporary occlusion of the vessel.

Loosely oppose the ends of divided nerves by inserting one or two sutures through the nerve sheath. Similarly fix tendon ends to prevent retraction. These sutures should be long enough to assist in tendon or nerve identification at a subsequent procedure. Formal repair of nerves and flexor tendons is not urgent and is best undertaken later by a qualified surgeon.

KEY POINTS

- Lacerations may be associated with neurovascular or other serious injury; a complete examination is required to identify injuries that are not immediately obvious
- Minor problems are important because mismanagement can lead to major detrimental consequences.

FACIAL LACERATIONS

It is appropriate to manage most facial wounds in the outpatient department. Clean the skin with soap and water, while protecting the patient's eyes. Irrigate

5

the wound with saline. Preserve tissue, especially skin, but remove all foreign material and all obviously devitalized tissue. Close with simple monofilament non-absorbable sutures of 4/0 or 5/0. Reinforce the skin closure with skin tapes. To avoid skin marking, remove sutures at 3 to 5 days. If the wound is contaminated, give prophylactic antibiotics to prevent cellulitis.

Large facial wounds or wounds associated with tissue loss require referral for specialized care after primary management. Arrest obvious bleeding, clean wounds and remove all foreign material. Tack the wound edges in place with a few monofilament sutures after the wound is packed with a sterile saline dressing.

LIP LACERATIONS

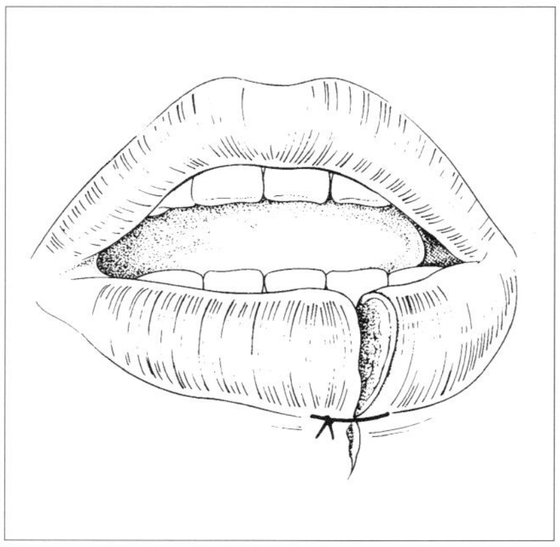

Figure 5.8

Small lacerations of the buccal mucosa do not require suturing. Advise the patient to rinse the mouth frequently, particularly after meals. Local anaesthesia is adequate for lacerations that do require suturing. For good cosmesis, proper anatomical alignment of the vermillion border is essential. To achieve this alignment, place the first stitch at the border (Figure 5.8). This region may be distorted by the swelling caused by local anaesthetic or blanched by adrenaline, so to assure accuracy, premark the vermillion border with a pen.

After the initial suture is inserted, repair the rest of the wound in layers, starting with the mucosa and progressing to the muscles and finally the skin (Figures 5.9, 5.10). Use interrupted 4/0 or 3/0 absorbable suture for the inner layers and 4/0 or 5/0 monofilament non-absorbable suture in the skin.

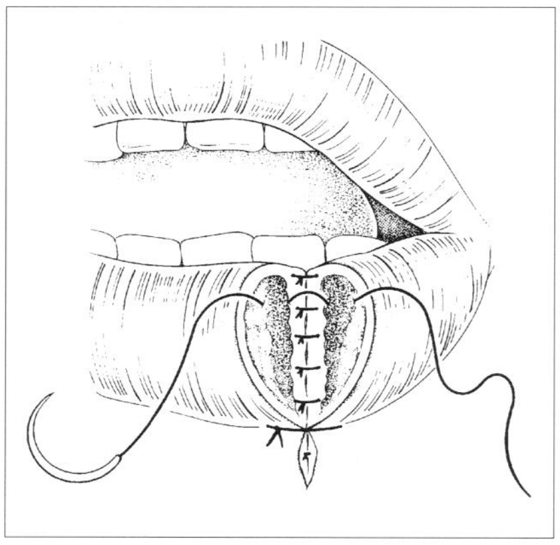

Figure 5.9

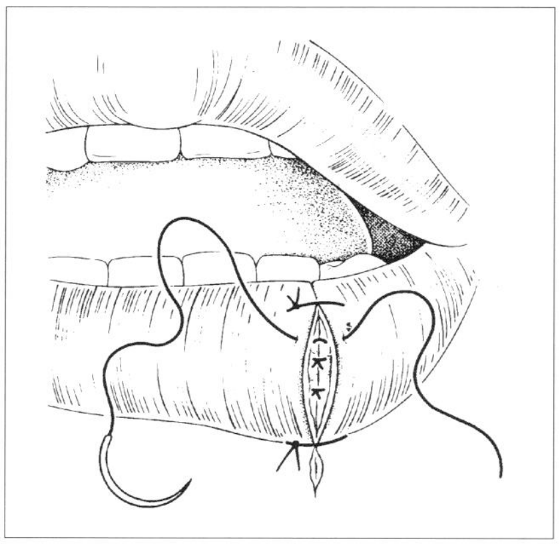

Figure 5.10

WOUNDS OF THE TONGUE

Most wounds of the tongue heal rapidly without suturing. Lacerations with a raised flap on the lateral border or the dorsum of the tongue need to be sutured (Figure 5.11). Suture the flap to its bed with 4/0 or 3/0 buried, absorbable stitches (Figure 5.12). Local anaesthesia is sufficient. Instruct the patient to rinse the mouth regularly until healing is complete.

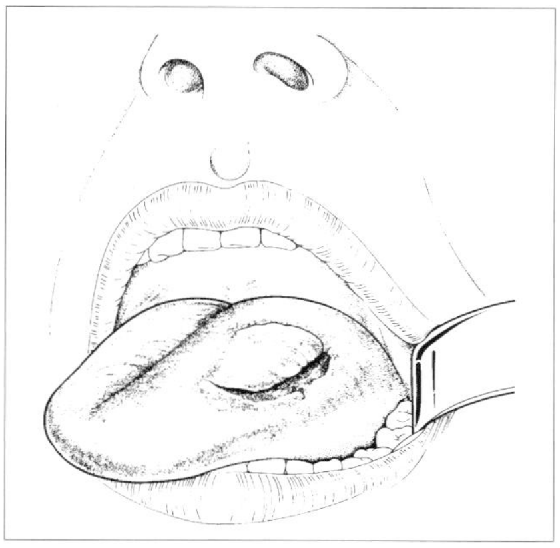

Figure 5.11

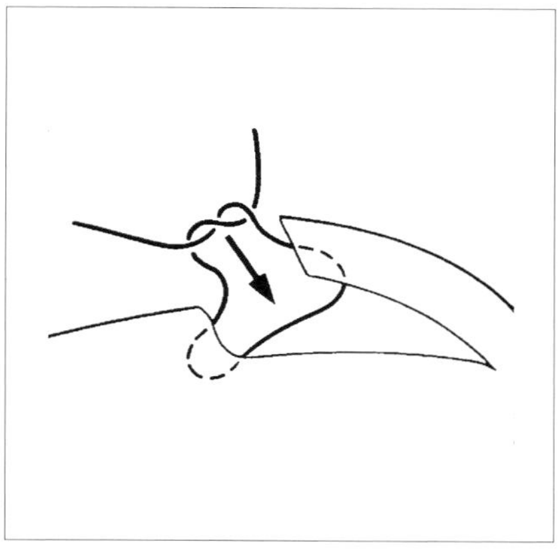

Figure 5.12

EAR AND NOSE LACERATIONS

The three-dimensional curves of the pinna and nares and the presence of cartilage present difficulties when injured. Wounds are commonly irregular, with cartilage exposed by loss of skin.

Use the folds of the ear or nose as landmarks to help restore anatomical alignment. Close the wound in layers with fine sutures, using absorbable sutures for the cartilage (Figures 5.13, 5.14).

The dressings are important. Support the pinna on both sides with moist cotton pads and firmly bandage to reduce haematoma formation (Figure 5.15). Cover exposed cartilage either by wound closure or split thickness skin grafts. Wounds of the ear and nose may result in deformities or necrosis of the cartilage.

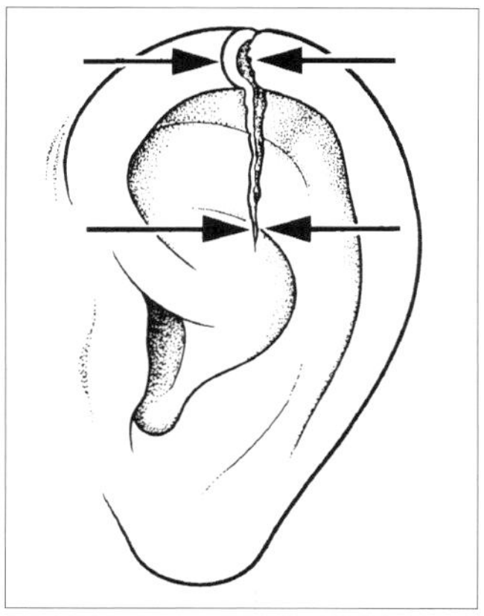

Figure 5.13

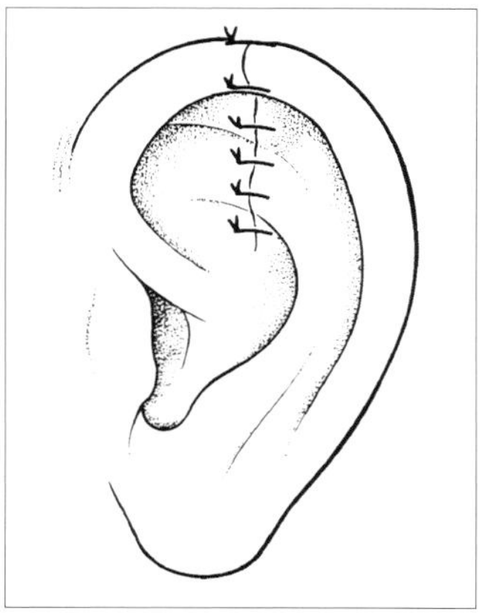

Figure 5.14

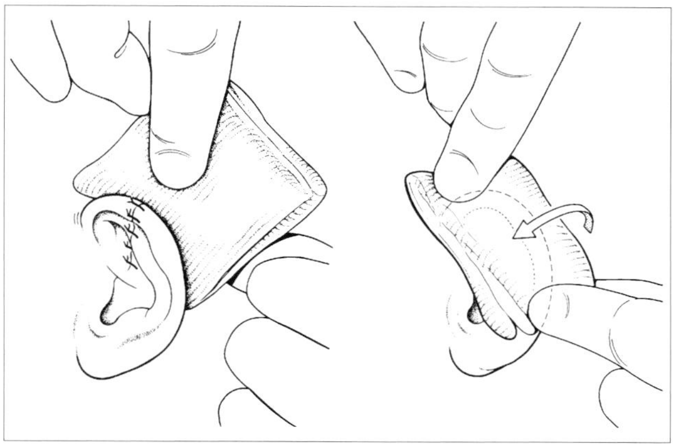

Figure 5.15

NOSE BLEED (EPISTAXIS)

Epistaxis often occurs from the plexus of veins in the anterior part of the nasal septum (Figure 5.16). In children it is often due to nose picking; other

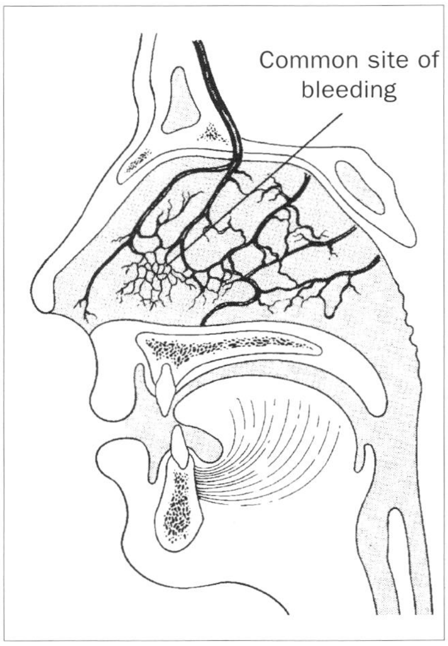

Figure 5.16

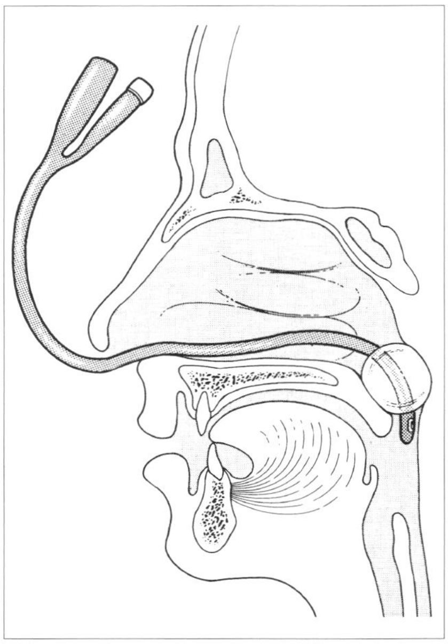

Figure 5.17

causes include trauma, a foreign body, Burkitt's lymphoma and nasopharyngeal carcinoma.

Manage epistaxis with the patient in a sitting position. Remove blood clots from the nose and throat to visualize the site of bleeding and confirm the diagnosis. Pinch the nose between your fingers and thumb while applying icepacks to the nose and forehead. Continue to apply pressure. Bleeding will usually stop within 10 minutes. If bleeding continues, pack the anterior nares with petroleum impregnated ribbon gauze.

If bleeding continues after packing, the posterior nasopharynx may be the source of bleeding. Apply pressure using the balloon of a Foley catheter. Lubricate the catheter, and pass it through the nose until the tip reaches the oropharynx. Withdraw it a short distance to bring the balloon into the nasopharynx. Inflate the balloon with water, enough to exert pressure but not to cause discomfort (5–10 ml of water is usually adequate for an adult, but use no more than 5 ml for a child). Gently pull the catheter forward until the balloon is held in the posterior choana (Figure 5.17).

Tape the catheter to the forehead or cheek in the same manner as a nasogastric tube. With the catheter in place, pack the anterior nares with petroleum gauze. Deflate the Foley catheter after 48 hours and, if bleeding does not recur, remove it.

OCULAR TRAUMA

Eye injuries are common and are an important cause of blindness. Early diagnosis and proper treatment are imperative to prevent blindness.

Superficial injuries

Superficial lacerations of the conjunctiva or cornea do not require surgical intervention. If a foreign body is not present, copiously irrigate the eyelid and eye with sterile saline, apply tetracycline 1% eye ointment and apply an eye pad with the eyelids closed. Leave the dressing in place for 24 hours, and then re-examine the eye and eyelids. If the injury has resolved or is improving, continue applying antibiotic eye ointment 3 times daily for 3 days.

Eyelid lacerations

Carry out wound toilet and minimal debridement, preserving as much tissue as possible. Never shave the brow or invert hair-bearing skin into the wound. If the laceration involves the lid margin, place an intermarginal suture behind the eyelashes to assure precise alignment of the wound (Figure 5.18). Carry out the repair in layers: the conjunctiva and tarsus with 6/0 absorbable suture, the skin with 6/0 non-absorbable suture and muscle (orbicularis oculi) with 6/0 absorbable suture (Figure 5.19). Tie suture knots away from the orbit.

Lacerations involving the inferior lacrimal canaliculus require canalicular repair. Refer the patient for specialized surgical management of the duct but, prior to referral, repair the lid laceration.

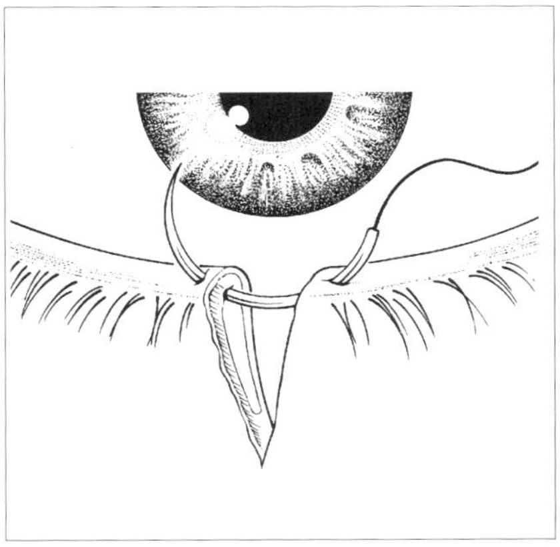

Figure 5.18

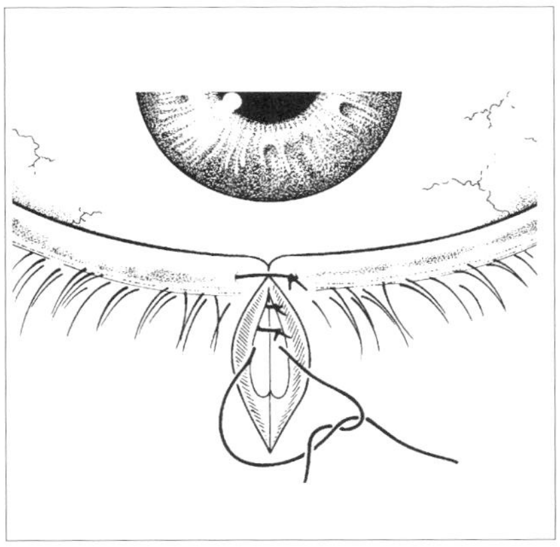

Figure 5.19

Eye

The first objective in the management of eye injuries is to save sight and to prevent the progression of conditions that could produce further damage.

Blunt trauma

Hyphaema (blood in the anterior chamber) is caused by blunt trauma. Check for raised intraocular pressure. If intraocular pressure is elevated or indicated by a total hyphaema or pain, administer acetazolamide 250 mg orally every 6 hours. If a patient has hyphaema, admit to hospital, put on complete bed rest, sedate, and patch both eyes. Examine and dress the eye daily. If the hyphaema is not resolving in 5 days, refer the patient.

Lacerations and penetrating trauma

Manage perforations of the cornea without iris prolapse and with a deep intact anterior chamber with local atropine (1% drops or ointment) and local antibiotics (1% eye drops). Dress the injured eye with a sterile pad and examine it daily. After 24 hours, if the anterior chamber remains formed, apply atropine 1% and antibiotic eye ointment daily for another week.

If the anterior chamber is flat, apply a bandage for 24 hours. If the anterior chamber does not reform, refer the patient.

Refer patients with perforation of the cornea complicated with iris incarceration or posterior rupture of the globe. Suspect a posterior rupture of the globe if there is low intraocular pressure and poor vision. Instil atropine 1%, protect the injured eye with a sterile pad and shield and refer the patient to an ophthalmologist.

Measurement of intraocular pressure

Measure the pressure by means of a Schiotz tonometer. With the patient prone, instil anaesthetic drops in both eyes. Instruct the patient to look up keeping the eyes steady. With your free hand gently separate the lids without pressing the eyeball and apply the tonometer at right angles to the cornea (Figure 5.20). Note the reading on the scale and obtain the corresponding

5

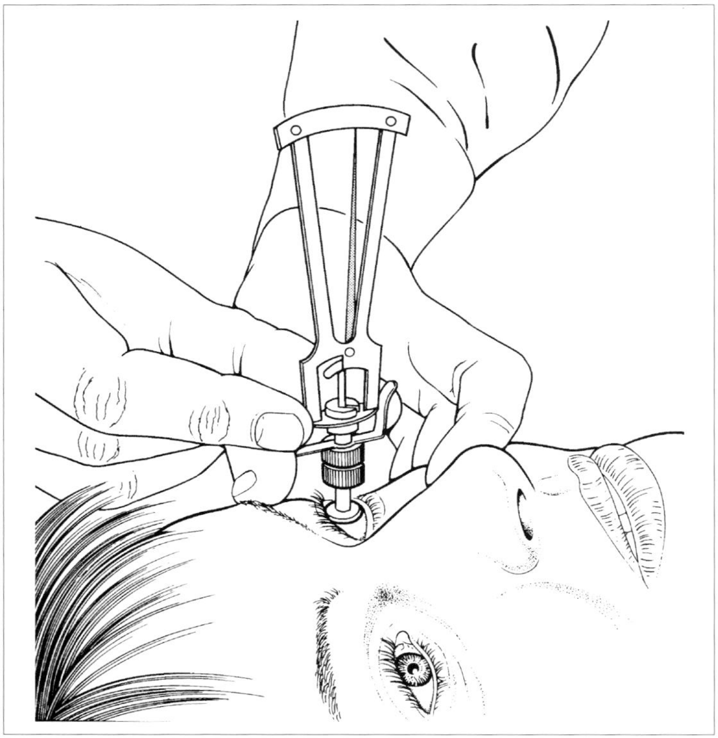

Figure 5.20

value in millimetres of mercury (mmHg) or kilopascals (kPa) from a conversion table. Verify readings at the upper end of the scale by repeating the measurement using the additional weights supplied in the instrument set. Repeat the procedure for the other eye. An intraocular pressure above 25 mmHg (3.33 kPa) is above normal but not necessarily diagnostic. Values above 30 mmHg (4.00 kPa) indicate probable glaucoma, for which the patient will need immediate referral or treatment.

OPEN FRACTURES

Open fractures, also known as compound fractures, are injuries involving both bone and soft tissue. The soft tissue injury allows contamination of the fracture site. All open fractures are contaminated, so primary closure is absolutely contraindicated. Wound closure predisposes to anaerobic infection and chronic osteomyelitis. Treat with wound toilet, debridement and fracture immobilization. Prior to debridement, take a swab for bacteriological examination and administer systemic antibiotics.

When debriding a compound fracture, remove free fragments of bone with no obvious blood supply. Do not strip muscle and periosteum from the fractured bone. Leave vessels, nerves and tendons that are intact. Surgical toilet of these wounds is an emergency. Perform the debridement within 6 hours and do not delay for referral. Osteomyelitis is a grave complication, which can be avoided with proper and expeditious wound toilet.

Stabilize the fracture after wound debridement; perform definitive fracture treatment at a later time.

Achieve stabilization with a well-padded posterior plaster slab, a complete plaster cast split to prevent compartment syndrome, traction or, if available, an external fixator (see Unit 17: *Orthopaedic Techniques*).

TENDON LACERATIONS

Perform immediate repair of tendon lacerations by primary suture for flexor tendons in the forearm; extensor tendons of the forearm, wrist, fingers; extensor tendons on the dorsum of the ankle and foot; and the Achilles tendon. Delay the repair of divided finger flexor tendons within the synovial sheath until the wound is clean and closed and a qualified surgeon is available.

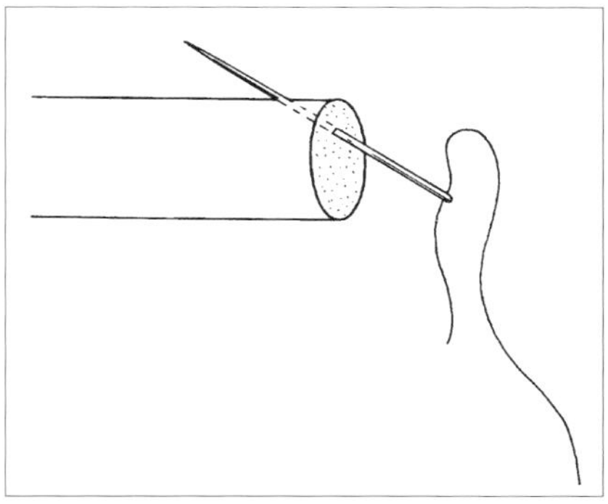

Figure 5.21

To accomplish the repair, use a general or regional anaesthetic. After debriding the wound, pass a loop suture (3/0 non-absorbable or 3/0 polyglycolic acid) on a straight needle into the tendon through the cut surface close to the edge so that it emerges 0.5 cm beyond. Construct a figure-of-8 suture, finally bringing the needle out again through the cut surface (Figures 5.21, 5.22, 5.23). Pull the two ends of the suture to take up the slack, but do not bunch the tendon. Deal similarly with the other end of the tendon and then tie the corresponding suture ends to each other, closely approximating the cut ends of the tendon and burying the knots deep between them (Figure 5.24). Cut the sutures short. Hold the repaired tendons in a relaxed position with a splint for 3 weeks.

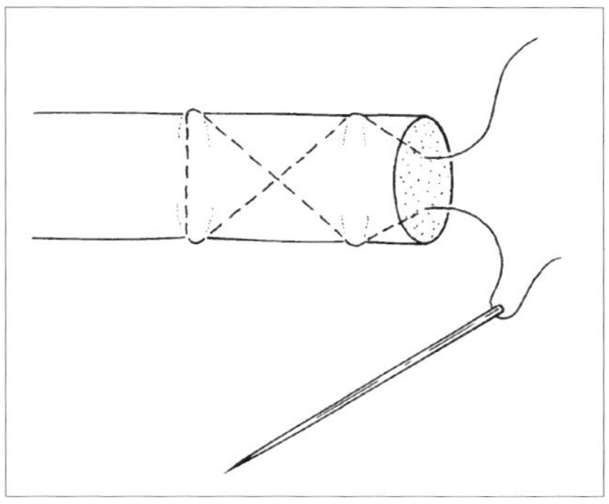

Figure 5.22

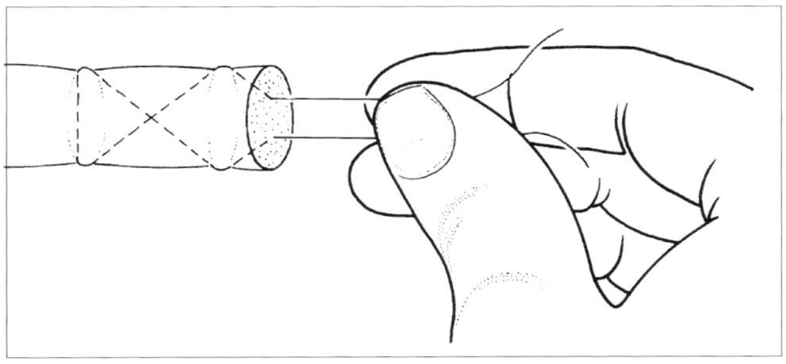

Figure 5.23

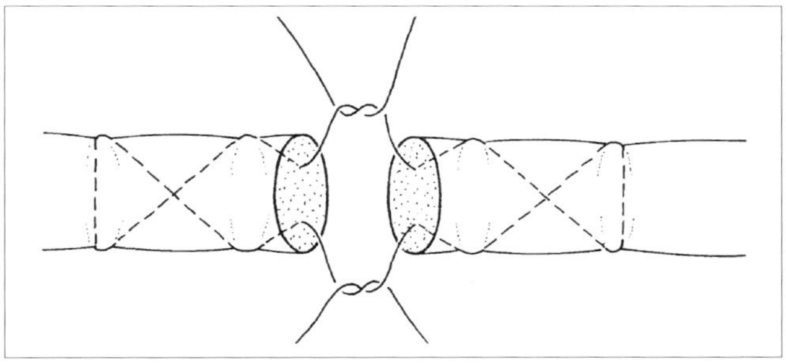

Figure 5.24

ANIMAL BITES

The risks arising from animal bites include:

- Direct tissue damage
- Allergic reactions
- Infection
- Envenomation
- Disease transmission.

First aid includes washing the wound to remove toxins, a sterile dressing, antibiotic and tetanus prophylaxis. Treat allergic reactions with antihistamines or adrenaline.

Dog, cat and human bites

Dog bites occur about the head and neck in children and cause severe tissue damage. Human bites most often involve the hand but can involve the arms, breast or genitalia. The metacarpophlangeal joints or extensor tendons are commonly injured. Treat human bites with aggressive debridement and antibiotics to prevent infection.

Evaluate nerve, tendon and vascular function. Irrigate wounds with saline and remove foreign bodies and devitalized tissue. Assume wound contamination is polymicrobial and give antibiotic coverage for both aerobic and anaerobic organisms. Cat and human bites are particularly prone to infection. Close facial wounds primarily; close extremity wounds and wounds older than 6 hours by delayed primary or secondary closure. Immobilize extremities and elevate the injured part. If underlying structures including bone, joints and tendons are involved, consider specialized care. Determine the need for rabies prophylaxis.

Rabies prophylaxis

Bites from wild and domestic animals are the source of rabies infection with the unvaccinated dog being the major source. If a domestic animal is captured, observe it for 10 days for signs of rabies. If none develops, the animal is considered non-rabid and the patient is safe.

Penetration of the skin by teeth in an unprovoked attack from an animal increases the chance that the animal is rabid. Consider rabies prophylaxis, irrigate and debride the wound.

Post-exposure rabies prophylaxis includes both Human Rabies Immune Globulin (HRIG) and vaccine. There are two types of vaccine:

- Human diploid rabies vaccine
- Absorbed rabies vaccine.

1 ml of either rabies vaccine is given on days 1, 3, 7, 14 and 28 intramuscularly in the deltoid (adults) or the anterior thigh (children). Give HRIG at a dose of 20 IU/kg. Infiltrate half around the wound and give the rest in the gluteal muscle.

HRIG is not indicated in vaccinated individuals or more than 7 days after exposure. Local pain and low grade fever may complicate HRIG or rabies vaccine.

Snakebite

Become familiar with the local poisonous snakes. Venom is a mixture of enzymes and non-enzymatic compounds. Neurotoxins cause respiratory arrest, cardiotoxins cause cardiac arrest and cytotoxins cause soft tissue destruction, infection and renal failure from myoglobinuria. Alterations in coagulation lead to bleeding.

Not all bites from poisonous snakes result in envenomation. The initial bite is not always painful and may or may not have paired fang marks. If no pain or swelling is present within 30 minutes, injection of venom probably did not occur. Non-poisonous bites are less painful and produce rows of punctures which may be associated with local tissue reaction.

Treatment includes:

- First aid
- Wound care
- Systemic support
- Antivenoms.

First aid

The spread of venom occurs via the lymphatic system and can be prevented by applying a pressure bandage (not a tourniquet) to the wound and splinting the extremity. Do not allow the patient to walk.

Wound care

Do not make cuts about the wound; it has no proven value. Give tetanus prophylaxis to the non-immune. If infection is present, give antibiotics and, if there is marked swelling, perform a fasciotomy. If needed, clean the wound and debride necrotic tissue. Neglected cases may require amputation.

Systemic support

Admit to intensive care for observation. Draw a blood sample for crossmatching, assess the coagulation status, evaluate the urine for blood and perform an ECG. Watch for signs of respiratory failure. Treat respiratory failure with intubation and ventilation. If the patient has cranial nerve palsies, administer neostygmine to prevent respiratory failure. Use crystalloid volume expanders to maintain blood pressure and urine output. Use ionotropic support only for life-threatening hypotension.

Antivenom

If systemic spread is suspected give antivenom. If the snake species is known, give a specific monovalent antivenom intravenously over 30 minutes. If there is doubt, give polyvalent antivenom. If the patient has been previously exposed to horse serum give a test dose. When in doubt, give antihistamines and IV steroids prior to the antivenom to prevent allergic reactions. Usually one ampoule (50 ml) of antivenom is sufficient but give repeated doses until the effect of venom is neutralized. In small centres, keep at least two ampoules of the antivenom appropriate for the local snake population.

5.3 BURNS

Thermal burns are a severe form of trauma which cause significant soft tissue injury as well as metabolic changes affecting fluid balance. While most burns are minor and do not require hospitalization, extensive burns are a life-threatening emergency. Extremes of age influence the outcome; the very young and the very old do not tolerate burns well. The circumstances of a burn injury will indicate possible associated injuries.

Begin treatment with airway management and fluid resuscitation. The volume of normal saline or Ringer's lactate required is estimated using the Rule of 9's. Complete the primary and secondary survey and then begin wound treatment (see pages 34–37 in the Annex: *Primary Trauma Care Manual*).

Thermal energy causes coagulation and death of varying levels to the epidermis, dermis and subcutaneous tissues. Viable tissue on the periphery of the burn may be salvaged if tissue perfusion is maintained and infection is controlled.

Classification of depth of burn

The depth of a burn depends upon the temperature of the heat source and the duration of its application. Burns can be classified as superficial, dermal or full-thickness. Flash burns are generally superficial; carbon deposits from smoke may give such burns a charred appearance. House fires, burning clothing, burning cooking oil, hot water scalds and chemicals usually produce mixed full-thickness and dermal burns; whereas molten metal, electric current, and hot-press machines normally cause full-thickness burns.

First degree (superficial) burns

The tissue damage is restricted to the epidermis and upper dermis. Nerve endings in the dermis become hypersensitive and the burn surface is painful. Blister formation is common. If the burn remains free from contamination, healing without scarring takes place in 7–10 days.

Second degree (dermal) burns

The lowest layer of the epidermis, the germinal layer, derives support and nourishment from the dermis. Portions of the germinal layer remain viable within the dermis and are able to re-epithelialize the wound. A deeper burn penetrates into the dermis and fewer epidermal elements survive. The amount of residual scarring correlates with the density of surviving epidermal elements. Healing of deep dermal burns may take longer than 21 days and usually occurs with such severe scarring that skin grafting is recommended. Because the vessels and nerve endings of the dermis are damaged, dermal burns appear paler and are less painful than superficial burns.

Third degree (full-thickness) burns

Full-thickness burns destroy all epidermal and dermal structures. The coagulated protein gives the burn a white appearance, and neither circulation nor sensation are present. After separation of the dead eschar, healing proceeds very slowly from the wound edges. Skin grafting is always required, unless the area is very small. Severe scarring is inevitable.

Mixed depth

Burns are frequently of mixed depth. Estimate the average depth by the appearance and the presence of sensation. Base resuscitation on the total of second and third degree burns and local treatment on the burn thickness at any specific site.

Wound care

First aid

If the patient arrives at the health facility without first aid having been given, drench the burn thoroughly with cool water to prevent further damage and remove all burned clothing. If the burn area is limited, immerse the site in cold water for 30 minutes to reduce pain and oedema and to minimize tissue damage.

If the area of the burn is large, after it has been doused with cool water, apply clean wraps about the burned area (or the whole patient) to prevent systemic heat loss and hypothermia. Hypothermia is a particular risk in young children. The first 6 hours following injury are critical; transport the patient with severe burns to a hospital as soon as possible.

Initial treatment

Initially, burns are sterile. Focus the treatment on speedy healing and prevention of infection. In all cases, administer tetanus prophylaxis (see pages 4–11 to 4–12).

Except in very small burns, debride all bullae. Excise adherent necrotic (dead) tissue initially and debride all necrotic tissue over the first several days. After debridement, gently cleanse the burn with 0.25% (2.5 g/litre) chlorhexidine solution, 0.1% (1 g/litre) cetrimide solution, or another mild water-based antiseptic. Do *not* use alcohol-based solutions. Gentle scrubbing will remove the loose necrotic tissue. Apply a thin layer of antibiotic cream (silver sulfadiazine). Dress the burn with petroleum gauze and dry gauze thick enough to prevent seepage to the outer layers.

Daily treatment

Change the dressing on the burn daily (twice daily if possible) or as often as necessary to prevent seepage through the dressing. On each dressing change, remove any loose tissue. Inspect the wounds for discoloration or haemorrhage which indicate developing infection. Fever is not a useful sign as it may persist until the burn wound is closed. Cellulitis in the surrounding tissue is a better indicator of infection. Give systemic antibiotics in cases of haemolytic streptococcal wound infection or septicaemia. *Pseudomonas aeruginosa* infection often results in septicaemia and death. Treat with systemic aminoglycosides.

Administer topical antibiotic chemotherapy daily. Silver nitrate (0.5% aqueous) is the cheapest, is applied with occlusive dressings but does not penetrate eschar. It depletes electrolytes and stains the local environment. Use silver sulfadiazine (1% miscible ointment) with a single layer dressing. It has limited eschar penetration and may cause neutropenia. Mafenide acetate (11% in a miscible ointment) is used without dressings. It penetrates eschar but causes acidosis. Alternating these agents is an appropriate strategy.

Treat burned hands with special care to preserve function. Cover the hands with silver sulfadiazine and place them in loose polythene gloves or bags secured at the wrist with a crepe bandage. Elevate the hands for the first 48 hours, and then start the patient on hand exercises. At least once a day, remove the gloves, bathe the hands, inspect the burn and then reapply silver sulfadiazine and the gloves. If skin grafting is necessary, consider treatment by a specialist after healthy granulation tissue appears.

Healing phase

The depth of the burn and the surface involved influence the duration of the healing phase. Without infection, superficial burns heal rapidly. Apply split thickness skin grafts to full-thickness burns after wound excision or the appearance of healthy granulation tissue.

Plan to provide long term care to the patient. Burn scars undergo maturation, at first being red, raised and uncomfortable. They frequently become hypertrophic and form keloids. They flatten, soften and fade with time, but the process is unpredictable and can take up to two years.

In children, the scars cannot expand to keep pace with the growth of the child and may lead to contractures. Arrange for early surgical release of contractures before they interfere with growth.

Burn scars on the face lead to cosmetic deformity, ectropion and contractures about the lips. Ectropion can lead to exposure keratitis and blindness and lip deformity restricts eating and mouth care. Consider specialized care for these patients as skin grafting is often not sufficient to correct facial deformity.

Nutrition

The patient's energy and protein requirements will be extremely high due to the catabolism of trauma, heat loss, infection and demands of tissue regeneration. If necessary, feed the patient through a nasogastric tube to ensure an adequate energy intake (up to 6000 kcal a day). Anaemia and malnutrition prevent burn wound healing and result in failure of skin grafts. Eggs and peanut oil are good, locally available supplements.

5.4 FOREIGN BODIES

KEY POINTS

- The removal of a foreign body may be urgent, as in the case of airway compromise or unnecessary, as in the case of some deep metal fragments
- Foreign body removal may be difficult or time-consuming; the patient should therefore be anaesthetized
- X-ray or fluoroscopy is recommended for the removal of radiopaque objects
- Foreign bodies in the cranium, chest or abdomen or in close proximity to vital structures must be removed in an operating room with a team prepared to manage possible complications.

SPECIFIC FOREIGN BODY LOCATIONS

Eye

Conjunctiva

Use sterile saline to wash out a foreign body embedded in the conjunctiva or, after administering a topical anaesthetic, wipe it away with a sterile, cotton tipped applicator. Eversion of the lid may be necessary to expose the foreign body.

Cornea

If the patient complains of the feeling of a foreign body but none is seen, instil two drops of 2% sodium fluorescein. A corneal abrasion, which the patient cannot distinguish from a foreign body, will be confirmed by the retention of green pigment in the abrasion. To remove a superficial corneal foreign body, use a 27-gauge needle. Apply antibiotic eye ointment and an eye patch for 24 hours. Refer patients with corneal foreign bodies that cannot be removed and ones that have corneal inflammation that persists more than 3 days.

Intraocular foreign body

An intraocular foreign body is determined by X-ray or clinical examination. Apply atropine 1%, dress the eye with a sterile pad and shield and refer the patient to an ophthalmologist. Immunize all patients with injuries to the globe for tetanus.

Ear

Children often insert foreign bodies, such as beans, peas, rice, beads, fruit seeds or small stones into their ears. Accumulated ear wax is often confused with foreign bodies. Visualize both the symptomatic and asymptomatic auditory canal to confirm the presence of a foreign body.

Use a syringe to wash the ear; this will remove most foreign bodies, but is contraindicated if the foreign body absorbs water: for example, grain or seeds. If needed, use gentle suction through a soft rubber tube. Rest the suction tip against the object (Figure 5.25).

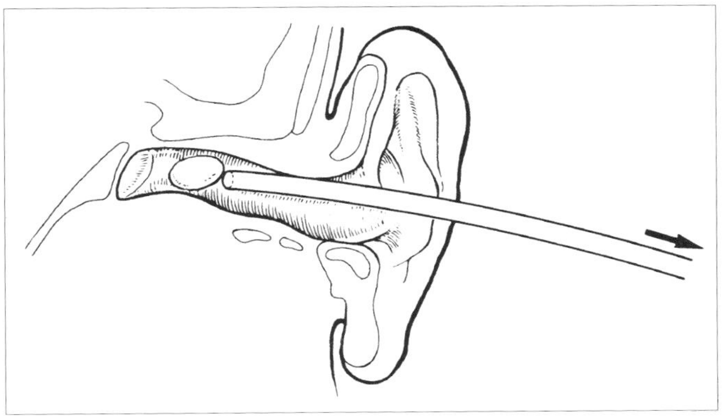

Figure 5.25

As an alternative, pass an aural curette or hook beyond the foreign body and then turn so that the foreign body is withdrawn by the hook (Figures 5.26, 5.27). This requires gentle technique and a quiet patient; children may require a general anaesthetic. To remove a mobile insect from the ear, immobilize it with glycerol irrigation followed by a wash with a syringe.

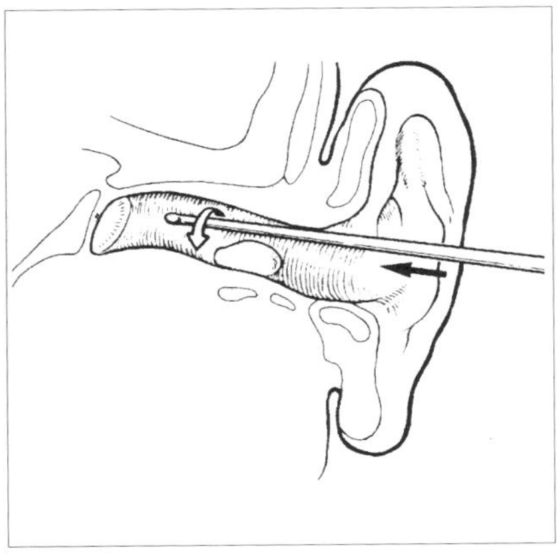

Figure 5.26

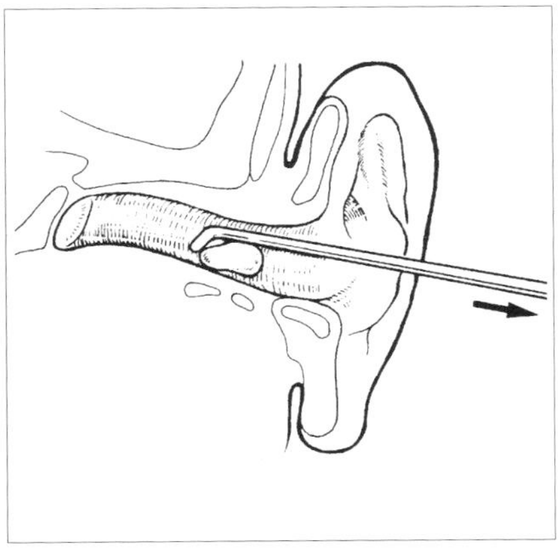

Figure 5.27

To remove accumulated ear wax, syringe the ear with warm water. If the wax remains, instruct the patient to instil glycerol or vegetable oil drops twice daily for 2 days then repeat the syringe wash.

Nose

Visualize nasal foreign bodies to determine their nature and position. Remove a foreign body with rough surfaces with angled forceps or pass a hook beyond it, rotate the hook, and pull the object out. Alternatively, use rubber tube suction.

Airway

Airway foreign bodies are common in children; peanuts are the most frequent object. They usually lodge in the right main stem bronchus and follow an episode of choking while eating. The post aspiration wheeze may be misdiagnosed as asthma and cause a delay in diagnosis. Bronchoscopic removal is indicated.

Obstruction of the upper airway with a bolus of food occurs from improper chewing. It may be associated with poor dentition. Patients present with a sudden onset of respiratory distress while eating. Treatment is the Heimlich manoeuvre (see Unit 13: *Resuscitation and Preparation for Anaesthesia and Surgery*).

Gastrointestinal tract

Oesophageal and stomach foreign bodies in children usually are coins, while bones and boluses of meat are more common in adults. Objects lodge at the cricopharyngeus in the upper oesophagus, the aortic arch in the mid-oesophagus and the gastro-oesophageal junction in the distal oesophagus.

Remove objects in the upper oesophagus with a laryngoscope and Magill forceps. A rigid or flexible oesophagoscope is needed for mid and lower oesophageal objects and the patient should be referred for this treatment.

Superficial lacerations at the oesophageal entrance by fish bones result in a foreign body sensation to the patient. This will resolve in 24 hours, but may need endoscopic examination to rule out the presence of a bone.

Smooth objects that reach the stomach will generally pass through the entire gastrointestinal tract and do not require retrieval. Instruct patients or parents to check the bowel contents to confirm passage of the object. Consider removal of sharp objects by endoscopy. Adults with mental disorders may ingest large objects requiring laparotomy for removal. Treat bezoars (conglomerates of vegetable matter) by dissolving them with proteolytic enzymes (meat tenderizer).

Blunt foreign bodies in the small intestine usually pass and exit the gastrointestinal tract without difficulty. Sharp objects require careful observation with serial X-rays and operative removal if the clinical signs of intestinal perforation present. Catharsis is contraindicated.

Colon and rectum

Sharp foreign bodies may perforate the colon during transit. Remove foreign bodies placed in the rectum using general anaesthesia with muscle relaxation.

Soft tissue

Confirm foreign bodies are present (often pins or needles) in the foot or knee by X-ray. Make one attempt to remove them under local anaesthesia. If that fails, perform the procedure with ketamine or regional anaesthesia with radiological assistance, preferably fluoroscopy.

Remove bullets in subcutaneous tissue or muscle if they are grossly contaminated or if the wound requires exploration for other reasons. Leave deep seated bullets or fragments if vital structures are not in danger. Remove bullets from joint cavities.

Body cavities

Remove foreign bodies that penetrate the head, chest or abdomen in the operating room after the patient's airway has been secured and preparations are made for the consequences of removal, which could include severe haemorrhage.

5.5 CELLULITIS AND ABSCESS

GENERAL PRINCIPLES

Cellulitis and lymphangitis

Cellulitis is a superficial, spreading infection of the skin and subcutaneous tissue and usually follows lacerations and surgical wounds.

The most common causative organism is penicillin sensitive *streptococci*. Cellulitis is characterized by signs of inflammation (local pain, tenderness, swelling and erythema). The border between involved and uninvolved skin is usually indistinct and systemic illness characterized by fever, chills, malaise and toxicity is frequently present.

Lymphangitis is inflammation which tracks along the lymphatics in the subcutaneous tissues. Treat cellulitis and lymphangitis with antibiotics. Failure to respond to antibiotics suggests abscess formation, which requires surgical drainage.

KEY POINTS

- Failure of a superficial infection to respond to medical management may be due to resistance to the antibiotic or to the presence of an abscess cavity
- If an abscess cavity is identified, drain it with a surgical incision
- Adequate surgical drainage requires anaesthesia to ensure that all parts of the abscess cavity are exposed.

Abscess

Treat abscess cavities with incision and drainage to remove accumulated pus. Diagnose by the presence of one or more of the following signs: extreme tenderness, local heat and swelling causing tight, shiny skin. Fluctuation is a reliable sign when present, although its absence does not rule out a deep abscess or an abscess in tissues with extensive fibrous components. These tissues include the breast, the perianal area and finger tips. Be suspicious of deep throbbing pain or of pain which interferes with sleep.

Technique

1 If in doubt about the diagnosis of abscess, confirm the presence of pus with needle aspiration. Prepare the skin with antiseptic, and give adequate anaesthesia. A local anaesthetic field block infiltrating uninfected tissue surrounding the abscess is very effective. Perform the preliminary aspiration using an 18 gauge or larger needle to confirm the presence of pus (Figure 5.28). Make an incision over the most prominent part of the abscess or use the needle to guide your incision. Make an adequate incision to provide complete and free drainage of the cavity. An incision which is too small will lead to recurrence.

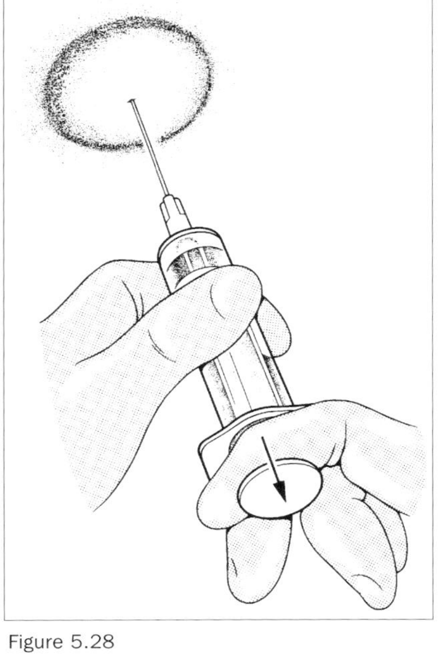

Figure 5.28

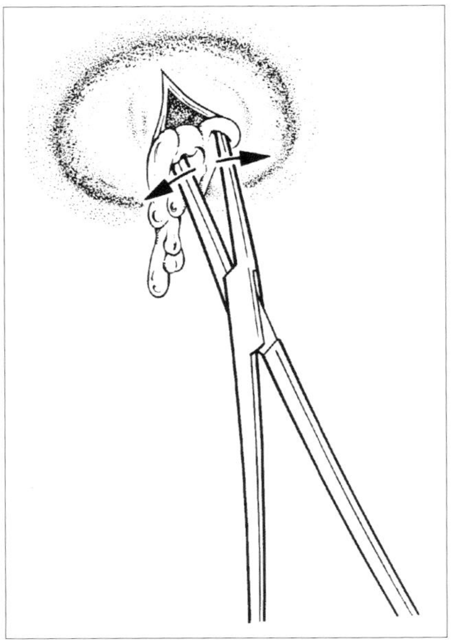

Figure 5.29

2 Introduce the tip of a pair of artery forceps into the abscess cavity and open the jaws (Figure 5.29). Explore the cavity with a finger to break down all septa (Figure 5.30).

3 Extend the incision if necessary for complete drainage (Figure 5.31), but do not open healthy tissue or tissue planes beyond the abscess wall.

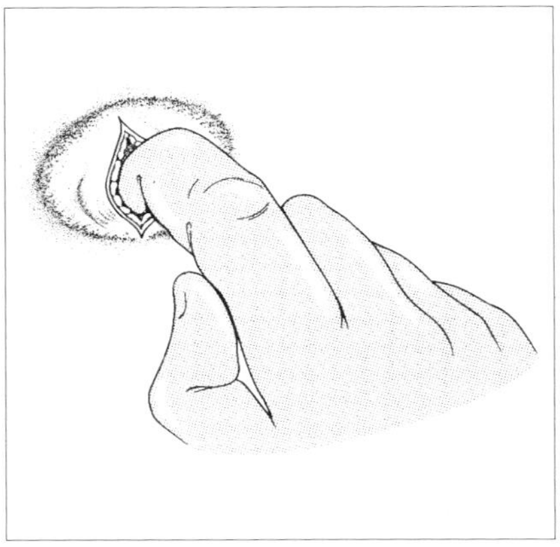

Figure 5.30

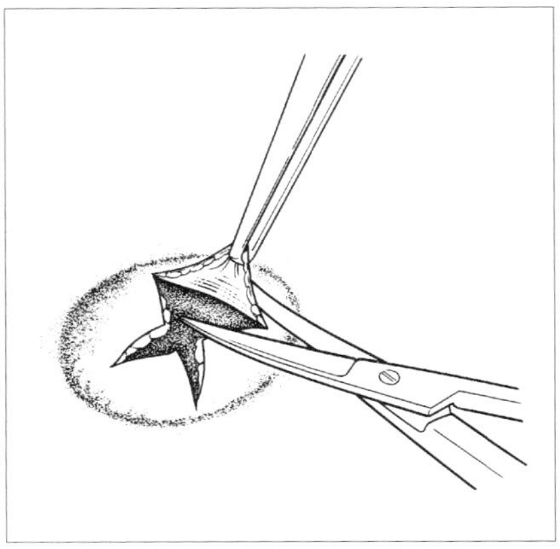

Figure 5.31

4 Culture the abscess wall. Give antibiotics for cutaneous cellulitis, fever or if the abscess involves the hand, ear or throat.

5 Irrigate the abscess cavity with saline and drain or pack open. The objective is to prevent the wound edges from closing, allowing healing to occur from the bottom of the cavity upward. To provide drainage, place a latex drain into the depth of the cavity. Fix the drain to the edge of the wound with a suture and leave in place until the drainage is minimal.

6 Alternatively, pack the cavity open, place several layers of damp saline or petroleum gauze in the cavity leaving one end outside the wound. Control bleeding by tight packing.

SPECIFIC SITES

Cellulitis of the face

Cellulitis following a facial wound carries the risk of cavernous-sinus thrombosis. Monitor the patient closely during antibiotic treatment for signs of increasing facial oedema. Keep the patient in hospital, if necessary. Explain to the patient not to squeeze or manipulate infected foci on the face, even if small. To prevent cavernous-sinus thrombosis, administer heparin by continuous intravenous infusion.

Ocular infection

Panophthalmitis is a complication of a neglected penetrating injury of the eye. When efforts to save the eye have failed and the eye is useless, consider evisceration or enucleation. If possible, refer to an ophthalmologist.

Enucleation of the eye is the surgical removal of the entire globe and requires an ophthalmologist. Evisceration is the surgical removal of the content of the globe and does not require a specialist. This procedure involves excision of the anterior globe and curetting of its contents. If necessary, consider evisceration for uncontrolled panophthalmitis. The eviscerated globe is packed open and treated as an abscess cavity. After healing, refer the patient for a prosthesis.

Ear infection

Middle ear infection presents with chronic drainage of pus from the external meatus. Clean the ear, place a cotton wick and apply a gauze dressing. Continue the administration of antibiotics and give analgesics as needed. Keep the auditory canal dry and change the dressing when necessary.

Acute mastoiditis is usually a complication of acute otitis media. The patient complains of fever and pain in the affected ear, with disturbed hearing. There may be a discharge from the ear. Characteristically there is a tender swelling in the mastoid area, which pushes the pinna forward and out. Definitive treatment is exposure of the mastoid air cells by a qualified surgeon. When this is not possible, initial treatment is to relieve immediate pain with an incision and drainage of the abscess down to the periosteum.

Technique

1. Using a general or local anaesthetic, make a curved incision over the most fluctuant part of the abscess or, if not obvious, at 1.5 cm behind the pinna. Deepen the incision to the periosteum or until pus is found.
2. Take a sample for bacteriological examination and establish free drainage. Apply petroleum gauze or a small latex drain and dress the area with gauze.
3. Continue the administration of antibiotics and analgesics, and change dressings as necessary.
4. Remove the drain after 24–48 hours.

Dental abscess

Treat dental pain initially by cleaning the painful socket or cavity and then packing it with cotton wool soaked in oil of cloves or a paste of oil of cloves and zinc oxide.

Tooth extraction is the best way to drain an apical abscess when there are no facilities for root canal treatment. Remove a tooth if it cannot be preserved, is loose and tender, or causes uncontrollable pain.

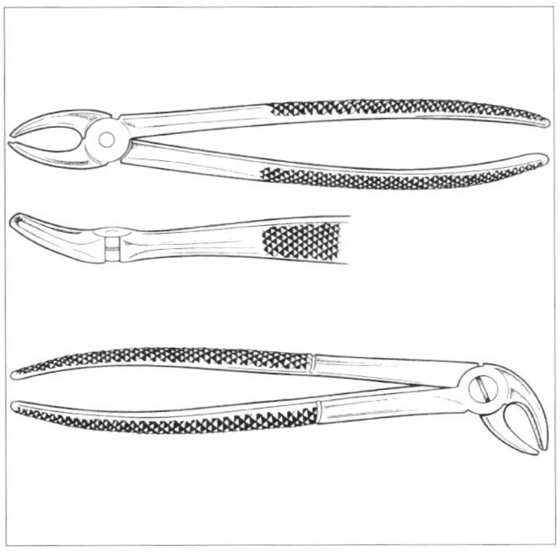

Figure 5.32

Explain the procedure to the patient and obtain permission to remove the tooth. Dental forceps are designed to fit the shape of the teeth including their roots. The inexperienced operator will find it simpler to rely on one pair of universal forceps for the upper jaw and one for the lower (Figure 5.32).

The upper molars have three roots, two buccal and one palatal, whereas the lower molars have two, one medial and one distal. The upper first premolars have two roots side by side, one buccal and one palatal. All the other teeth are single-rooted.

Use local infiltration analgesia for extraction of all but the lower molars, which may require a mandibular nerve block. Occasionally, general anaesthesia is appropriate.

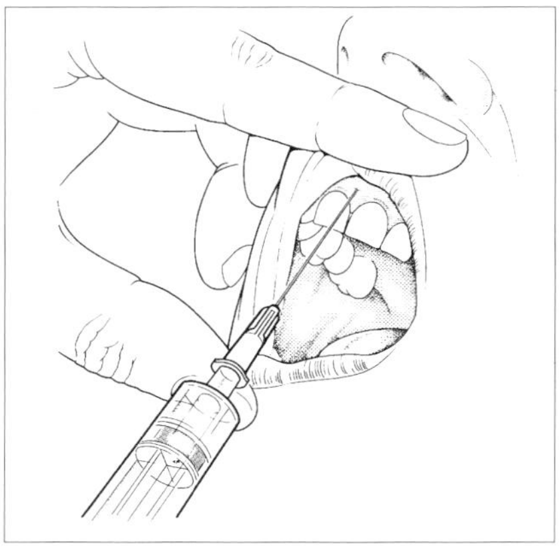

Figure 5.33

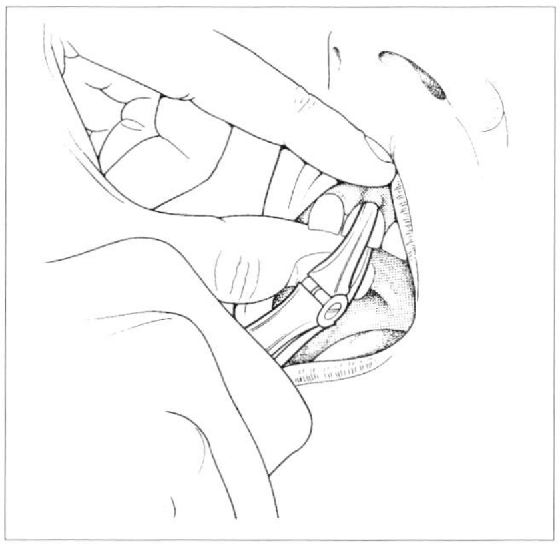

Figure 5.34

Technique

1 Seat the patient in a chair with a high back to support the head. After the patient has rinsed the mouth, swab the gum with 70% ethanol. Insert a 25-gauge, 25 mm needle at the junction of the mucoperiosteum of the gum and the cheek, parallel to the axis of the tooth (Figure 5.33).

Advance the needle 0.5 to 1 cm, level with the apex of the tooth, just above the periosteum. The bevel of the needle should face the tooth. Infiltrate the tissues with 1 ml of 1% lidocaine with adrenaline (epinephrine) and repeat the procedure on the other side of the tooth. Confirm the onset of numbness before handling the tooth.

2 If you are right-handed, stand behind and to the right of the patient when extracting lower right molar or premolar teeth. Face the patient, to the patient's right, when working on all other teeth. Separate the gum from the tooth with a straight elevator. While supporting the alveolus with thumb and finger of your other hand, apply the forceps to either side of the crown, parallel with the long axis of the root. Position the palatal or lingual blade first. Push the blades of the forceps up or down the periodontal membrane on either side of the tooth, depending on which jaw you are working on (Figure 5.34). Successful extraction occurs if you drive the blades of the forceps as far along the periodontal membrane as possible.

Firmly grip the root of the tooth with the forceps and loosen the tooth with gentle rocking movements from buccal to lingual or palatal side. If the tooth does not begin to move, loosen the forceps, push them deeper, and repeat the rocking movements. Avoid excessive lateral force on a tooth, as this can lead to its fracture.

3 Carefully inspect the extracted tooth to confirm its complete removal. A broken root is best removed by loosening the tissue between the root and the bone with a curved elevator. After the tooth has been completely removed, squeeze the sides of the socket together for a minute or two and place a dental roll over the socket. Instruct the patient to bite on it for a short while. After the patient has rinsed the mouth, inspect the cavity for bleeding. Arrest profuse bleeding that will not stop, even when pressure is applied, with mattress sutures of absorbable suture across the cavity.

4 Warn the patient not to rinse the mouth again for the first 24 hours or the blood clot may be washed out, leaving a dry socket. Have the patient rinse the mouth frequently with saline during the next few days. Analgesia may be needed. Warn the patient against exploring the cavity with a finger. If gross dental sepsis occurs, administer penicillin for 48 hours and consider giving tetanus toxoid.

Throat and neck abscesses

Non-emergency operations on the throat, including tonsillectomy, should be performed only by qualified surgeons.

Incision and drainage of peritonsillar abscess

Peritonsillar abscess (quinsy) is a complication of acute tonsillitis. The patient develops progressive pain in the throat which radiates to the ear. The neck is rigid, and there is fever, dysarthria, dysphagia, drooling, trismus, foul breath and lymphadenopathy. Local swelling causes the anterior tonsillar pillar to bulge and displaces the soft palate and uvula. The overlying mucosa is inflamed, sometimes with a small spot discharging pus. The differential diagnosis includes diphtheria or mononucleosis.

Technique

1 Administer antibiotics and analgesics and place the patient in a sitting position with the head supported. Spray the region of the abscess with 2–4% lidocaine. A local anaesthetic is safer than general anaesthesia because of the potential for aspiration with general anaesthetic.

2 Retract the tongue with a large tongue depressor or have an assistant hold it out between a gauze-covered finger and thumb. Perform a preliminary needle aspiration (Figure 5.35) and then incise the most prominent part of the swelling near the anterior pillar (Figure 5.36). Introduce the point of a pair of artery forceps or sinus forceps into the incision, and open the jaws of the forceps to improve drainage (Figure 5.37). Aspirate the cavity with suction and lavage it with saline.

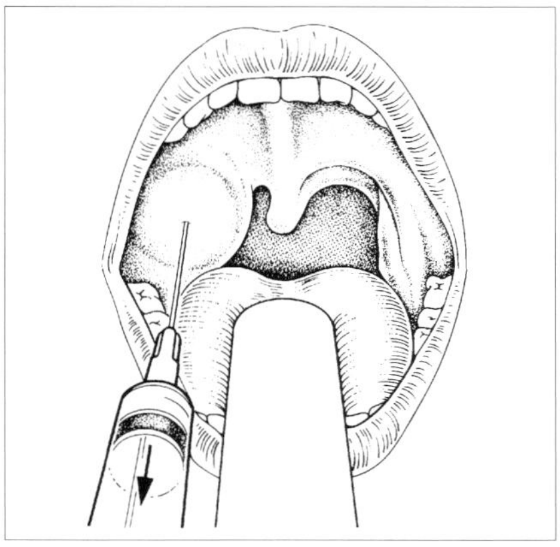

Figure 5.35

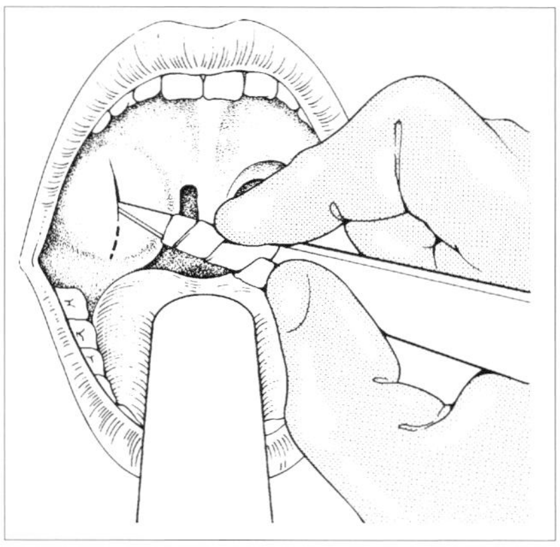

Figure 5.36

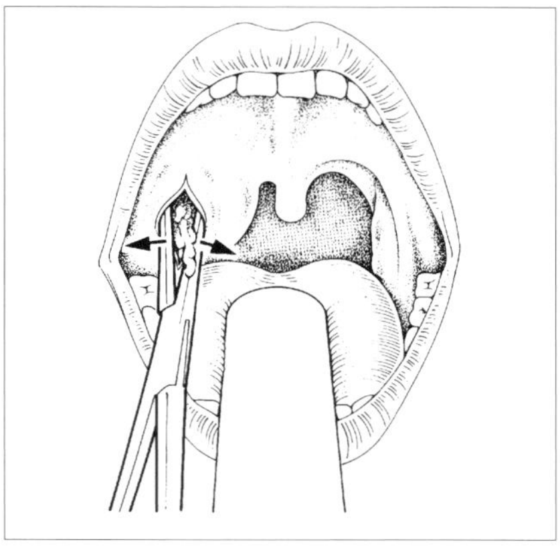

Figure 5.37

Instruct the patient to gargle with warm salt water several times a day for about 5 days. Continue antibiotics for one week and give analgesics as necessary.

Retropharyngeal abscess

Retropharyngeal abscesses occur in children and may compromise the airway. They result from infection of the adenoids or the nasopharynx and must be differentiated from cellulitis. The child cannot eat, has a voice change, is irritable and has croup and fever. The neck is rigid and breathing is noisy. In the early stages of the abscess the pharynx may look normal but, with progression, swelling appears in the back of the pharynx.

A lateral X-ray reveals widening of the retropharyngeal space. The differential diagnosis includes tuberculosis. Obtain a white-cell count and differential, determine the erythrocyte sedimentation rate and test the skin reaction to tuberculin (Mantoux test). Administer antibiotics and analgesics. Treat a patient with tuberculosis with specific antituberculous medication.

Spray the back of the throat with local anaesthetic. While an assistant steadies the patient's head, retract the tongue with a depressor. Incise the summit of

5

the bulge vertically. Introduce the tip of an artery forceps and open the jaws to facilitate drainage. Remove the pus with suction. Instruct the patient to gargle regularly with warm salt water. Administer antibiotics and analgesics.

Acute abscess of the neck

Deep abscesses in the neck arise in lymph nodes. Differentiate abscesses from lymphadenopathy. Examine the patient's mouth and throat, particularly the tonsils and teeth to identify a primary focus. If the abscess is acute and clearly pointing, perform a simple incision and drainage. In children, treat an abscess of the neck by repeated aspiration. For small, superficial abscesses, aspirate the cavity using a syringe with a wide-bore needle.

Perform incision and drainage under general anaesthesia for large abscess cavities. Because of the complexity of the neck, surgical intervention requires a qualified surgeon with adequate support. Place the incision in a skin crease centred over the most prominent or fluctuant part of the abscess. Spread the wound edges with a pair of sinus or artery forceps to facilitate drainage. Take a sample of pus for bacteriological tests, including an examination for tuberculosis. Remove necrotic tissue, but avoid undue probing or dissection. Insert a soft latex drain. Remove the drain after 24–48 hours. Hold gauze dressings in place with tape.

Mastitis and breast abscess

Breast infections, common during lactation, are most often caused by penicillin resistant staphylococcus aureus. The bacteria gain entrance through a cracked nipple causing mastitis (breast cellulitis) which may progress to abscess formation. The features of a breast abscess are pain, tender swelling and fever. The skin becomes shiny and tight but, in the early stages, fluctuation is unusual. Failure of mastitis to respond to antibiotics suggests abscess formation even in the absence of fluctuation. When in doubt about the diagnosis, perform a needle aspiration to confirm the presence of pus.

The differential diagnosis of mastitis includes the rare but aggressive inflammatory carcinoma of the breast. Patients present with an advanced abscess in which the overlying skin has broken down and the pus is discharging. If the woman is not lactating, a neglected carcinoma should not be excluded.

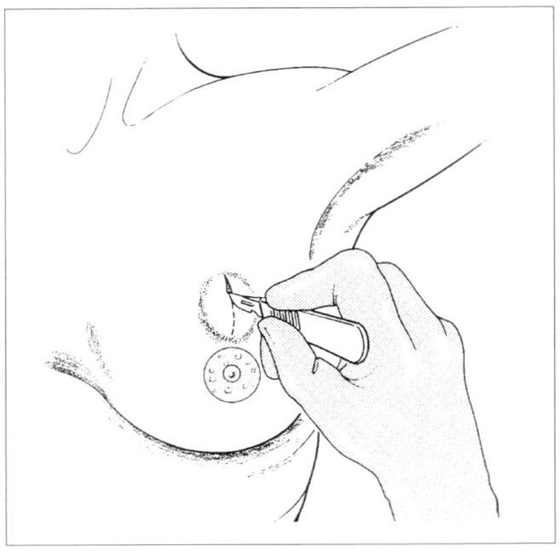

Figure 5.38

Successful drainage of a breast abscess requires adequate anaesthesia; ketamine, a wide field block or a general anaesthetic. Prepare the skin with antiseptic and drape the area. Make a radial incision over the most prominent part of the abscess or the site of the needle aspiration (Figure 5.38).

Introduce the tip of a pair of artery forceps or a pair of scissors to widen the opening and allow the pus to escape (Figure 5.39). Extend the incision if necessary. Obtain cultures for bacteria, fungus and tuberculosis. Break down all loculi with a finger to result in a single cavity (Figure 5.40). Irrigate the cavity with saline and then either pack with damp saline gauze or insert a latex drain through the wound (Figure 5.41).

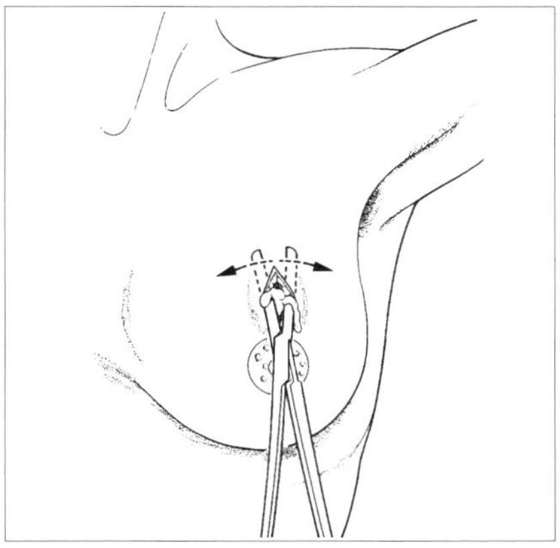
Figure 5.39

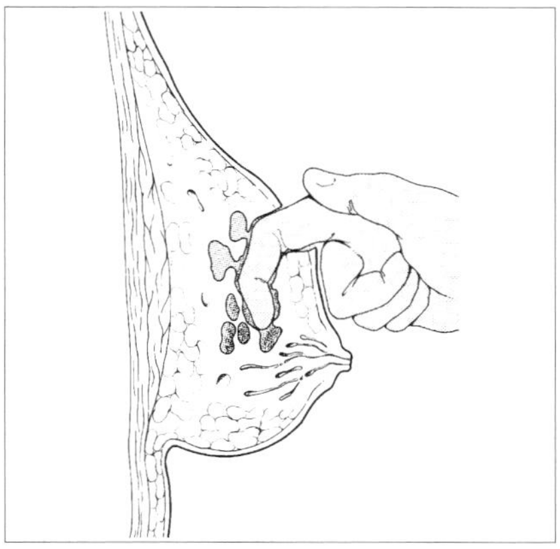
Figure 5.40

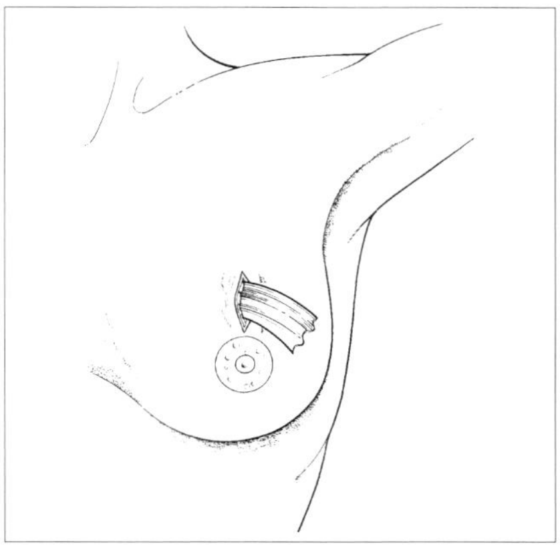
Figure 5.41

Dress the wound with gauze. Give analgesics as required, but antibiotic treatment is unnecessary unless there is cellulitis. Change dressings as necessary, and remove the drain when the discharge is minimal.

Have the patient continue breastfeeding, unless she is HIV positive. The child may feed from both breasts but, if this is too painful for the mother, she may express the milk from the affected breast.

Thoracic empyema

Thoracic empyema is the presence of pus in the pleural cavity. It can complicate lung, mediastinal or chest-wall infections and injuries. Rarely the source is a liver abscess. The infection results from mixed flora including staphylococci, streptococci, coliform bacteria, tuberculosis.

An empyema is either acute or chronic. It can invade adjacent tissues or cause abscesses to form in other organs.

Characteristic features are chest pain, fever and an irritating, dry cough. The affected area is dull to percussion, with an absence of, or markedly reduced, breath sounds. Diagnostic aids include a chest X-ray, white cell count, haemoglobin and urinalysis. A chest X-ray shows evidence of fluid in the pleural cavity, often with features of the underlying disease.

Needle aspiration of the chest is diagnostic. Examine the pus for the infecting organisms. Small acute empyema should be treated by repeated aspiration. Treat a moderate or large collection by placement of a chest tube attached to an underwater seal (see Unit 16: *Acute Trauma Management*). Indications for underwater seal chest drainage at the district hospital are pneumothorax, haemothorax, haemopneumothorax and acute empyema.

Give systemic antibiotics (do not instil them into the pleural cavity) and analgesics. If there is evidence of loculation or failure of lung expansion, refer the patient.

Patients with chronic empyema present with minimal signs and symptoms. Features include finger clubbing, mild chest discomfort and cough. Patients

5

are generally in poor health and may have chronic sepsis, including metastatic abscesses, and malnutrition. The inflamed pleura is thickened and loculated and it is not possible to drain the pleural cavity adequately using underwater seal intercostal drainage. Refer for specialized surgical care.

Pyomyositis

Pyomyositis is an intramuscular abscess occurring in the large muscles of the limbs and trunk, most commonly in adolescent males. It presents with tender, painful muscles and fever. It is usually single but can occur in multiple distantly separated muscle groups. Staphylococcus aureus is the causative organism in over 90% of immune competent patients. Blood cultures are often negative and leukocytosis may be absent. In immune compromised patients, including those who are HIV positive or diabetic, gram negative and fungal pyomyositis may occur.

Aspiration of pus with a large bore needle (14 or 16 gauge) is diagnostic. Treat with incision and drainage. Leave a latex drain in place at least 48 hours.

Infections of the hand

Staphylococci are the organisms commonly responsible for acute infections of the hand. An early infection may resolve with antibiotics alone but incision and drainage are usually needed. Antibiotics should be given until sepsis is controlled.

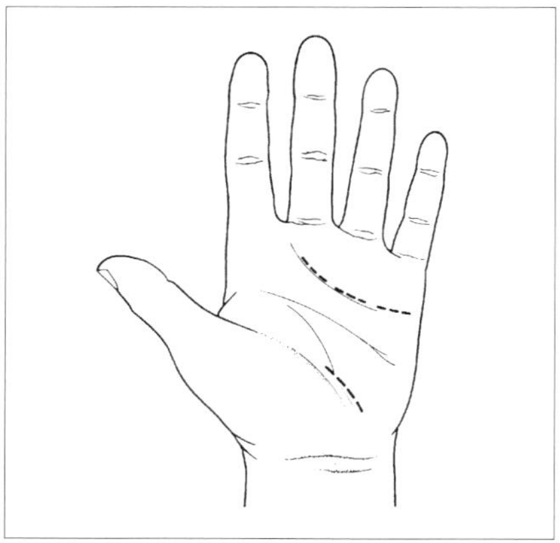

Figure 5.42

Patients present with a history of throbbing pain, warm, tender swelling, a flexion deformity of the finger and pain on movement. Confirm the abscess with needle aspiration. Obtain an X-ray of the hand to determine if there is bone involvement and perform a Gram stain on the pus.

Give general or regional anaesthesia and proceed with incision and drainage. Make an adequate, but not extensive, incision along a skin crease at the site of maximum tenderness and swelling (Figure 5.42).

Aspirate or irrigate away all pus. Open up deeper loculi with artery forceps and insert a latex drain. Obtain a culture. Dress the wound loosely with dry gauze, administer antibiotics and elevate the hand.

Marked swelling on the dorsum of the hand is often due to lymphoedema, which does not require drainage. Infection of the nail bed may necessitate excision of a portion of the nail for effective drainage of pus.

Treat paronychia of the middle finger with an incision over the involved area (Figure 5.43) or excise a portion of the nail (Figure 5.44).

Treat finger tip abscesses with a "hockey stick" incision (Figure 5.45).

Treat acute septic contracture of an involved digit with antibiotics and prompt surgical drainage of the flexor tendon sheath through incisions along the lateral or medial borders of the fingers, preferably the junctional area between the palmar and dorsal skin (Figure 5.46). Infection of the tendon sheaths of the thumb or little finger may spread to the radial or ulnar bursa, respectively (Figure 5.47), necessitating drainage by short, transverse incisions in the distal palmar crease and/or at the base of the palm.

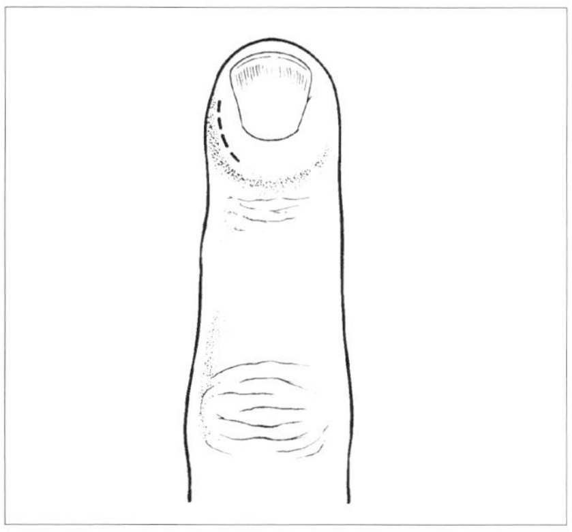

Figure 5.43

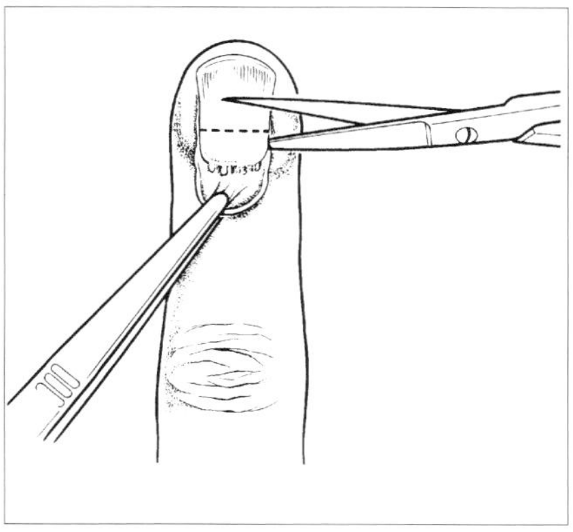

Figure 5.44

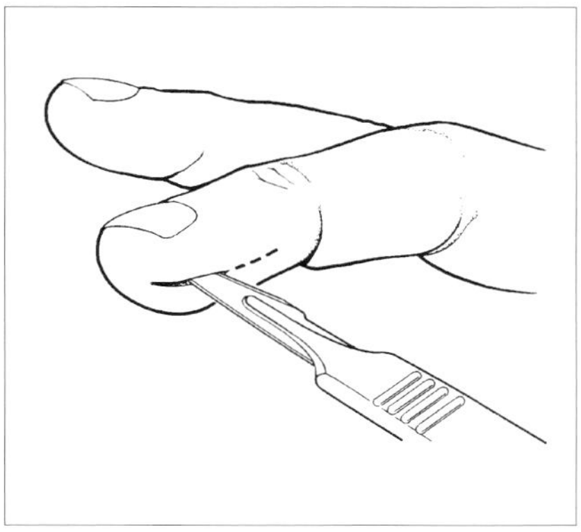

Figure 5.45

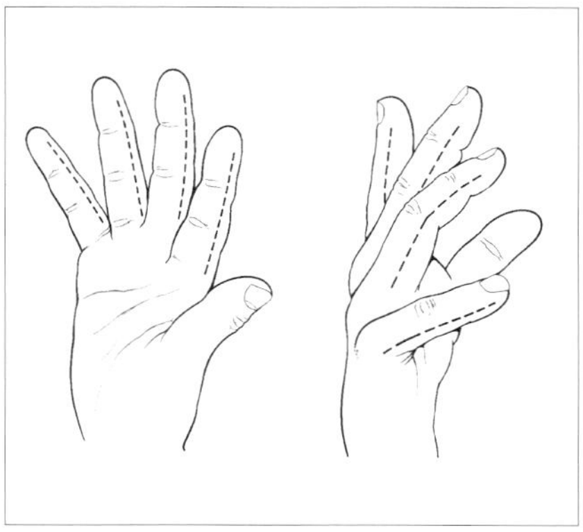

Figure 5.46

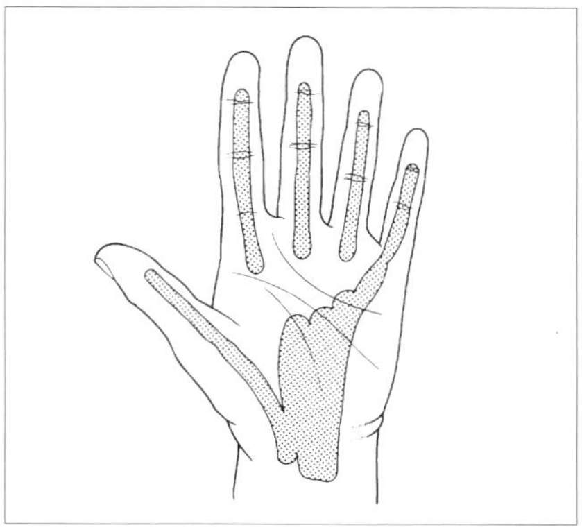

Figure 5.47

Infections of fascial palmar spaces result from extensions of infections of a web-space or a tendon sheath. Drain the affected fascial space through skin incisions directly over the area of maximum swelling and tenderness. Open deeper parts of the abscess with forceps. In general, place incisions for drainage along creases of the palm, along the lateral or medial borders of the fingers, or along the ulnar or radial borders of the forearm (Figure 5.48).

Splint the hand in position of function. Encourage active exercises as soon as possible. Give antibiotics and analgesics and remove the drain in 24–48 hours.

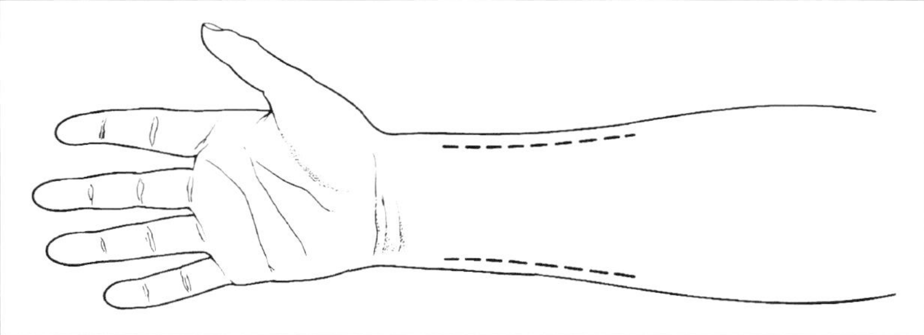

Figure 5.48

PERIANAL, RECTAL AND PILONIDAL SEPSIS

Anus and rectum

The main symptom in perianal septic conditions is throbbing, anal pain with or without fever. Rule out the presence of an abscess in all cases of perianal

5

pain. Perianal, ischiorectal, inter-sphincteric or submucous abscess are identified by location. Patients may be unable to sit. Rectal examination is often diagnostic. For female patients, perform a rectal examination followed by a vaginal examination. The discomfort may be severe and regional or general anaesthesia may be necessary to perform these examinations.

Part the buttocks to inspect the perianal region, the natal cleft and the anal margin. A tightly closed anus suggests spasm, due to a painful anal condition. Palpate any lesions in this area.

Slowly introduce a lubricated, gloved finger into the anus with the palmar surface turned posteriorly. Palpate the posterior anal wall and any anal contents against the curve of the sacrum. Rotate the finger anteriorly to detect any bulge or tenderness suggestive of a pelvic abscess (Figure 5.49). The prostate in the male, and the cervix in the female, will be palpable anteriorly (Figure 5.50). Withdraw the finger and inspect it for stool, mucus or blood. Take specimens for laboratory examination.

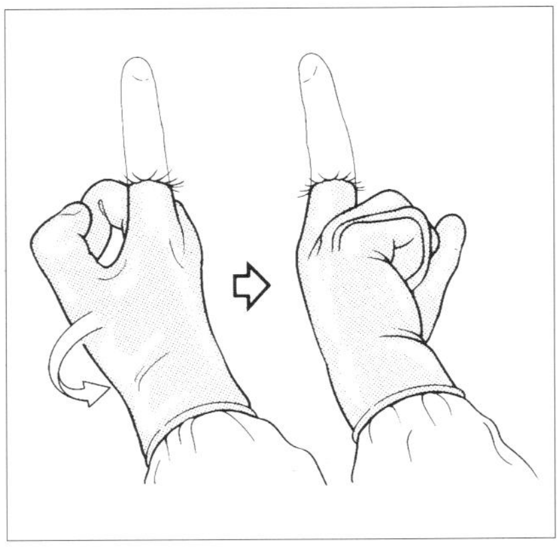
Figure 5.49

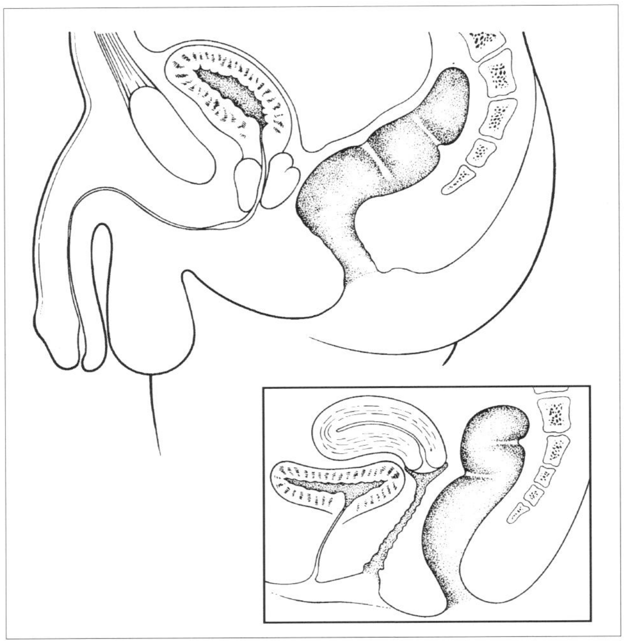
Figure 5.50

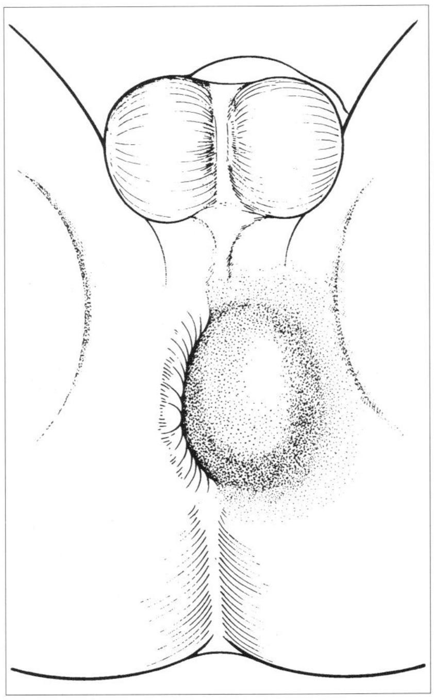
Figure 5.51

Patients with a perianal abscess will have tenderness on rectal examination confined to the anal margin, whereas patients with an ischiorectal abscess will have deep tenderness. If you are in doubt about the diagnosis, perform a diagnostic needle aspiration.

A perianal abscess presents as an extremely tender, inflamed, localized swelling at the anal verge (Figure 5.51). An ischiorectal abscess is indicated by tenderness with a diffuse, indurated swelling in the ischiorectal fossa. Fluctuation in these lesions is rare at an early stage and may not ever occur. Pain is a more reliable feature of perianal or rectal abscess.

Give parenteral antibiotic and administer analgesics. To drain the abscess, place the patient in the lithotomy position. Centre an incision over the most prominent part of the abscess. Take a specimen for culture and gram stain. Break down all loculi with a finger (Figure 5.52). Irrigate the cavity with saline and pack it loosely with petrolatum or saline soaked gauze, leaving it protruding slightly (Figure 5.53). Cover the wound with dry gauze and a bandage.

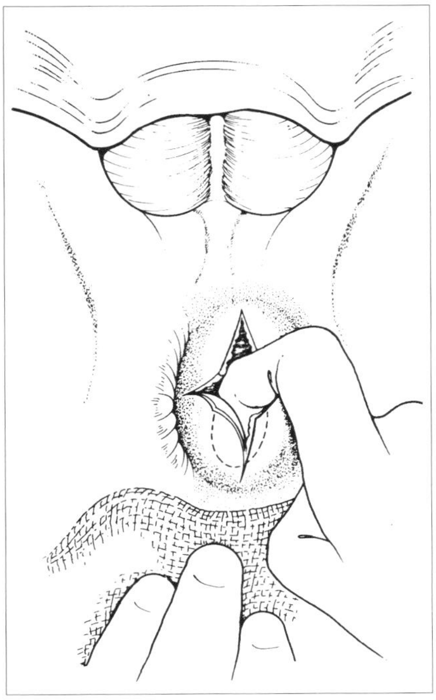

Figure 5.52

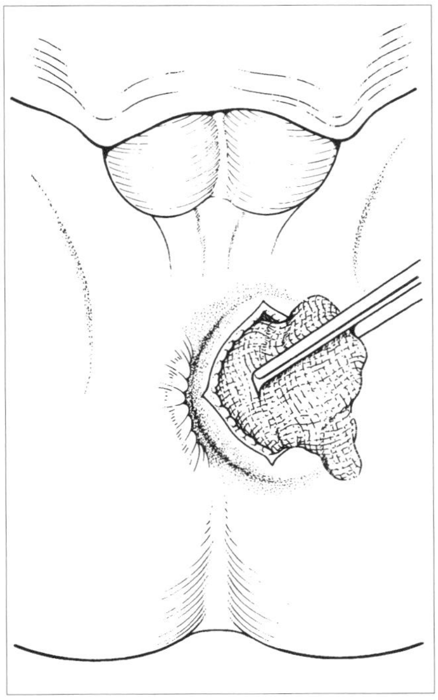

Figure 5.53

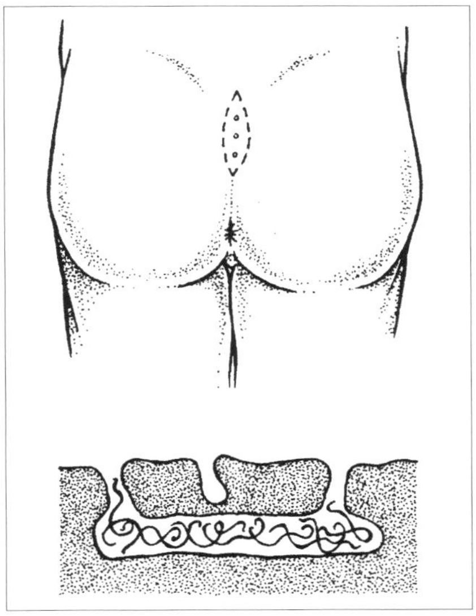

Figure 5.54

Instruct the patient to bathe sitting in warm saline for 15–30 minutes twice a day until the wound is healed, and to change the pack after each bath. Do not allow the wound edges to close. Give a mild laxative, such as liquid paraffin (mineral oil), daily until the bowels move and continue antibiotic treatment for 5 days. Continue analgesics for up to 72 hours.

Recurrence of the abscess is often due to inadequate drainage or to premature healing of the skin wound.

Anal fistula occur as a late complication. Patients presenting with an anal fistula should be referred for surgical correction. The reason this requires referral is that fistulotomy in a high fistula-in-ano will result in incontinence if not managed correctly; expert management is therefore required.

Pilonidal disease and abscess

Pilonidal disease results from ingrown hair causing cutaneous and subcutaneous sinus formation in the post sacral intergluteal cleft overlying the sacrum. The sinus may be single or multiple and presents with single or multiple orifices (Figure 5.54). The disease causes both acute and chronic inflammation. Patients present with pain, swelling and discharge or with an acute abscess. A pilonidal abscess will not respond to antibiotics alone. Treat initially with incision and drainage. For definitive treatment, remove all sinus and hair bearing tissue by excising an ellipse of tissue down to the presacral fascia (Figure 5.55). A field block with 1% lidocaine with epinephrine (adrenaline) gives adequate anaesthesia.

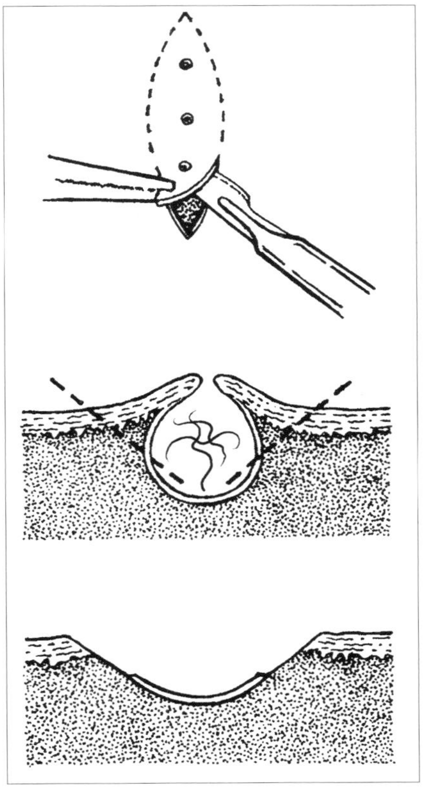

Figure 5.55

KEY POINTS

- Excise benign lesions for treatment and confirmation of the diagnosis
- Establish the diagnosis of malignant disease by biopsy before beginning definitive treatment
- Obtain material for histological examination with:
  - Incisional biopsies when part of the tumour is removed
  - Excisional biopsies when the whole tumour is removed with a margin of surrounding normal tissue
  - Needle biopsies when a core of tissue is removed
- Obtain material for cytolological examination with a fine needle aspiration; false negative results occur if the biopsy does not include the lesion or if the lesion is necrotic
- Necrosis occurs with the use of electrocautery, therefore excise the tumour with a scalpel
- False negative results occur in needle biopsies and aspirates due to sampling error; repeat a biopsy if the results are inconsistent with the clinical context
- Do not refer patients far from home if they have incurable metastatic disease.

5.6 EXCISION AND BIOPSIES

GENERAL PRINCIPLES

Histological and cytological examination

Biopsies require histological or cytological examination. In small centres, a pathologist will not be on site but a pathology unit that will accept specimens and return reports should be available. Specimens must arrive in an acceptable condition, therefore communication with the laboratory is essential on how the specimens are to be prepared and the preservatives, fixatives or solutions that are best for the local situation. Often, the specimens from a remote centre are interesting to the pathologist who will enjoy receiving them. Send specimens to the pathology unit by post or by hospital personnel when they go to the major centre. This process may involve some delay but there are few conditions that will result in deterioration of the patient in 3–5 weeks.

To package both biopsy and cytological preparations, write the name of the patient, the site from which the sample was taken, and the date of collection in pencil on a stiff piece of paper. Place the paper in the specimen bottle. Secure the cap of the bottle with adhesive tape and put the bottle in a metal tube (or box) together with a summary note containing particulars of the patient, clinical state, the tentative diagnosis, the type of tissue sent, and the investigation requested. Place the tube in a wooden or cardboard box, packed well, and dispatch it. If properly prepared, the sample will not deteriorate even if it is a long time in transit.

SPECIFIC PROCEDURES

Skin and subcutaneous lesions

Incise the skin with a scalpel parallel to the direction of the skin lines. Use elliptical incisions making the long axis large enough to close the skin without deformity. To accomplish this, make the long axis twice the length of the short axis and close the incision with two equally spaced sutures. For long incisions, place simple sutures at each end prior to closure. Plan the incision to avoid the need for rotation flaps, v-plasties or grafts (Figure 5.56).

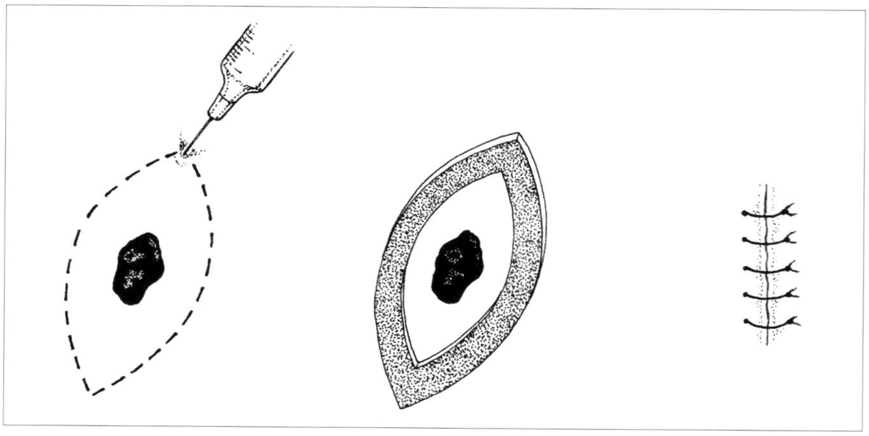

Figure 5.56

Excise subcutaneous lesions after gaining access through the skin incision (Figure 5.57). Do not remove skin unless the subcutaneous mass is adherent. Epidermal inclusion cysts are subcutaneous in location but are epidermal invaginations with a visible punctum on the skin surface where they originate. Failure to remove the punctum with an elliptical incision will result in cyst rupture during excision and possible recurrence due to incomplete excision.

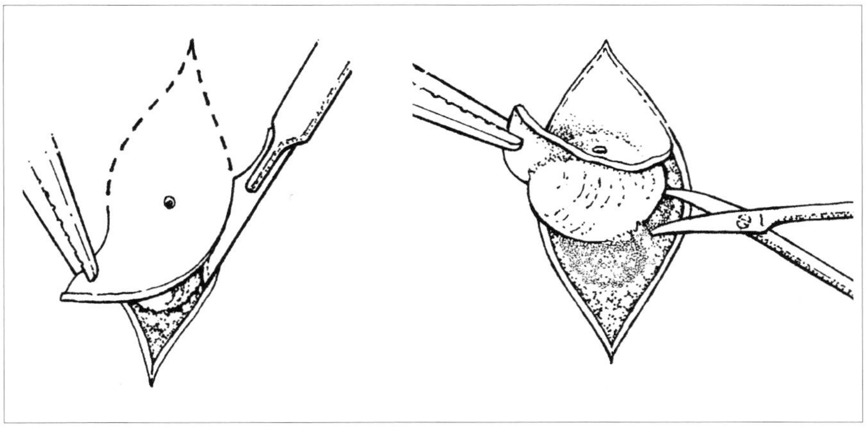

Figure 5.57

Lipomas, benign fatty tumours, are usually subcutaneous and often bother patients because of their inconvenient location or large size. Remove by dissecting the mass from the surrounding subcutaneous tissue. If the mass is large, it is usually difficult to close the subcutaneous tissue without deforming the skin. In this case, use a small latex drain or a pressure dressing to close the dead space instead of subcutaneous sutures.

Send all lesions for pathological examination to check for malignant tissue. Obvious lipomas, epidermal inclusion cysts and ganglions of the wrist are perhaps exceptions.

Basal cell and squamous cell carcinomas are secondary to excess exposure of sensitive skin to the sun. Nordic people and albinos are at particular risk. Because of its benign behaviour, basal cell carcinoma does not require wide excision. Squamous cell carcinoma, however, is life threatening. Treat it with wide local surgical excision.

Naevi are benign tumours of the pigment producing melanocytes; melanomas are malignant tumours from the same cell line. Both are associated with excessive sun exposure but melanomas also occur on the plantar surface of the foot. Melanoma is a life threatening malignancy. Biopsy all suspicious lesions and send to a pathologist for examination. If malignancy is confirmed, arrange for specialized surgical treatment.

Lymph node biopsy

Lymph nodes are located beneath fascia and therefore require deeper dissection than skin or subcutaneous lesion biopsies. A general anaesthetic may be required. Make a cosmetic incision in the skin lines and dissect through the subcutaneous tissue, controlling bleeding as you go. Identify the lymph node

5

with your fingertip and incise the overlying superficial fascia. Dissect the node from surrounding tissue without directly grasping it. Instead, grasp the attached advential tissue with a small artery forceps or place a figure-of-8 suture into the node for traction. Separate all the tissue attached to the node. Control the hilar vessels with forceps and ligate them with absorbable suture after the node has been removed. If you suspect an infectious disease, send a portion of the node for culture (Figure 5.58).

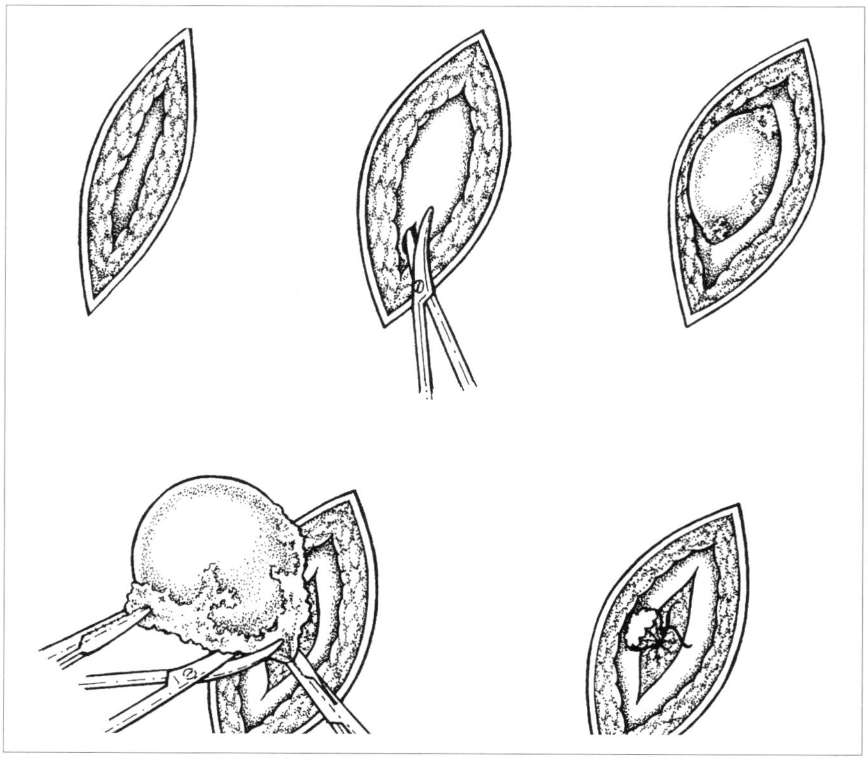

Figure 5.58

Neck and thyroid

Remove skin lesions in the neck as elsewhere in the body. Lymph nodes, congenital cysts, thyroid cysts and tumours are more complex and require a qualified surgeon. Consider using a fine needle aspirate (FNA) for diagnosis of these lesions (see page 5–33). FNA is not useful in the diagnosis of lymphoma as a histological diagnosis is required. FNA of degenerative thyroid cysts is often therapeutic.

Oral cavity

Lesions of the aerodigestive tract present as a white patch (leukoplakia) which is due to chronic irritation, as a red patch (erythroplakia) which may be dysplastic or a squamous cell carcinoma *in situ*. Abuse of alcohol or tobacco or an immunodeficiency syndrome increases the chance of oral malignancy. Perform a complete physical examination of the head and neck, including a mirror examination of the oropharynx. Biopsy questionable lesions. Excise areas of erythroplakia and close the defect with absorbable sutures. If the lesion is large, remove a wedge of tissue including a rim of adjacent normal tissue.

Eye

Chalazion is a chronic inflammatory cyst 2–5 mm in size within one of the tarsal glands of the eyelid. Surgery is indicated if the swelling is long-standing and does not respond to local medical treatment. The condition sometimes recurs in adjacent tarsal glands. After establishing topical anaesthesia with 0.5% tetracaine, inject 1–2 ml of 2% lidocaine around the chalazion through the skin. Apply the chalazion clamp with the solid plate on the skin side and the fenestrated plate around the cyst, tighten the screw, and evert the lid. Incise the cyst at right angles to the lid margin and remove its contents with curettes (Figure 5.59). Remove the clamp and apply pressure on the lid until bleeding stops. Apply antibiotic eye ointment, and dress the eye with a pad and bandage. Apply ointment daily until the conjunctiva heals.

Do not treat small pterygia. If the pterygium extends to the central optical zone of the cornea, consider consultation with an opthalmologist.

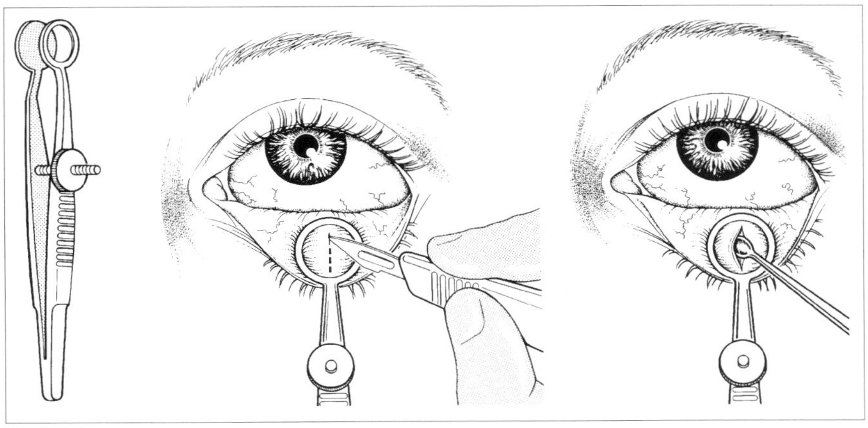

Figure 5.59

Breast biopsy

Breast biopsy is indicated for palpable breast masses and non-palpable lesions visualized on mammography. Excise palpable lesions under local anaesthesia. Non palpable lesions require a specialized surgical technique with the radiological facilities for lesion localization. Treat breast cysts with needle aspiration. If there is a residual tumour noted after cyst aspiration, follow with an excisional biopsy.

Needle aspiration

Use FNA and cytology to make the diagnosis of malignancy in solid tumours of the breast. Insert a 21-gauge needle into the mass and aspirate several times; remove it from the tumour. Take the needle off the syringe and fill the syringe with several millilitres of air. Return the syringe to the needle and use the air to empty the cells within the needle on to a slide. Fix the cells using cytospray or as directed by your local pathologist. (Figure 5.60).

A positive result confirms malignancy while a negative result is non-diagnostic and may be due to sampling error. Repeat the procedure or perform an open biopsy if the result is negative.

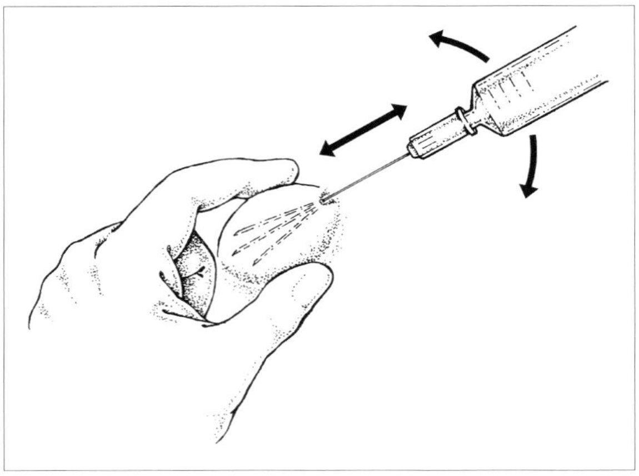

Figure 5.60

Needle biopsy

Needle biopsy is similar to FNA except a core of tissue is removed from the lesion. This is a good method to confirm the clinical impression of a malignancy but, like all needle procedures, is valid only when malignancy is confirmed. (Figure 5.61).

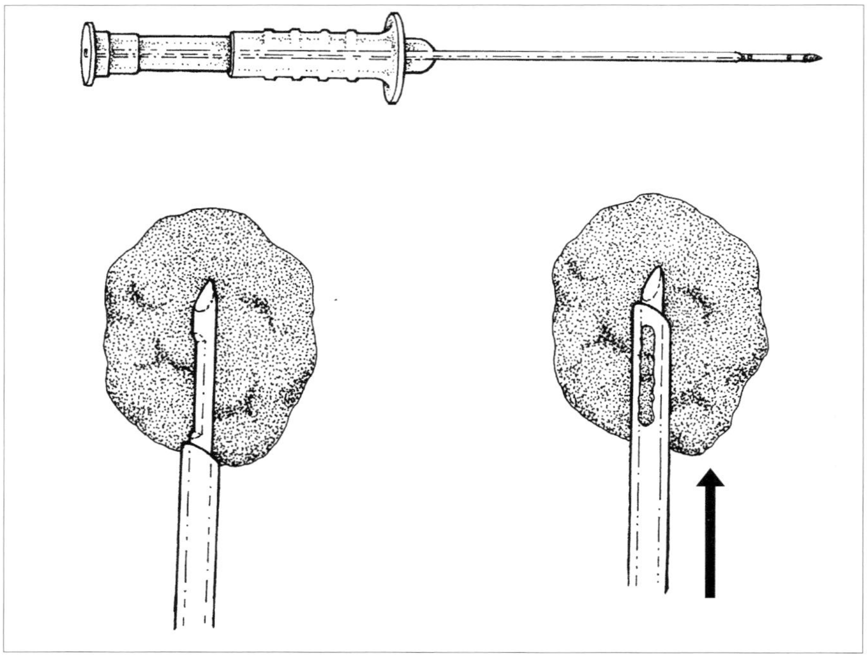

Figure 5.61

Open biopsies

Use excisional or incisional biopsies to obtain breast tissue for histological examination. Place the skin incision in the skin lines. Curvilinear circumareolar incisions give the best cosmetic results but, when making the biopsy approach, consider subsequent surgery, mastectomy or wide excision.

Excisional biopsies

Remove the entire tumour and a rim of normal tissue. This is therapeutic for benign lesions.

Incisional biopsies
Use in large tumours when only a portion of the tumour is being removed. Avoid a biopsy of necrotic tumour as it will be non-diagnostic.

Close deep layers with absorbable sutures and skin with non-absorbable sutures. Subcutaneous sutures may improve the appearance of the final incision. Place a small latex drain at the site and bring it out through the incision. Remove it at 48 hours.

GYNAECOLOGICAL BIOPSIES

Vulval biopsy

Biopsy of vulval lesions is indicated in cases of leukoplakia, carcinoma (*in situ* or invasive) and condylomata. Occasionally, biopsy may identify tuberculosis or schistosomiasis as the cause of a lesion.

Place the patient in the lithotomy position and clean and drape the perineum. Administer a local anaesthetic by infiltration of 1% lidocaine. If the vulval lesion is large, excise a portion of it, ligate any bleeding vessels and approximate the skin. Excise small, localized lesions with a margin of healthy skin. Bleeding is a possible complication.

Cervix cytology

Use cytology for the diagnosis of precancerous lesions. A speculum, wooden spatulae and slides are required. Obtain cytological preparations from the ectocervix and endocervix. After introducing an unlubricated speculum, collect cells under direct vision by scraping with a wooden spatula. Make a smear on the glass slide and apply a fixative.

Cervical biopsy

The indications for cervical biopsy include chronic cervicitis, suspected neoplasm and ulcer on the cervix. Frequent symptoms are vaginal discharge, vaginal bleeding, spontaneous or postcoital bleeding, low backache and abdominal pain and disturbed bladder function. Speculum examination may reveal erosion of the cervix. In cases of invasive carcinoma, the cervix may initially be eroded or chronically infected. Later it becomes enlarged, misshapen, ulcerated and excavated or completely destroyed, or is replaced by a hypertrophic mass. Vaginal examination reveals a hard cervix which is fixed to adjacent tissues and bleeds to the touch. To rule out malignant infiltration, stain the cervix with Lugol's iodine solution. A malignant area will fail to take up the stain.

Perform a punch biopsy as an outpatient procedure. Anaesthesia is not necessary. Place the patient in the lithotomy position, expose the cervix and select the most suspicious area for biopsy. Using punch biopsy forceps, remove a small sample of tissue, making sure that you include the junction of normal and abnormal areas (Figure 5.62). Possible complications include sepsis and haemorrhage. If bleeding is excessive, pack the vagina with gauze for 24 hours.

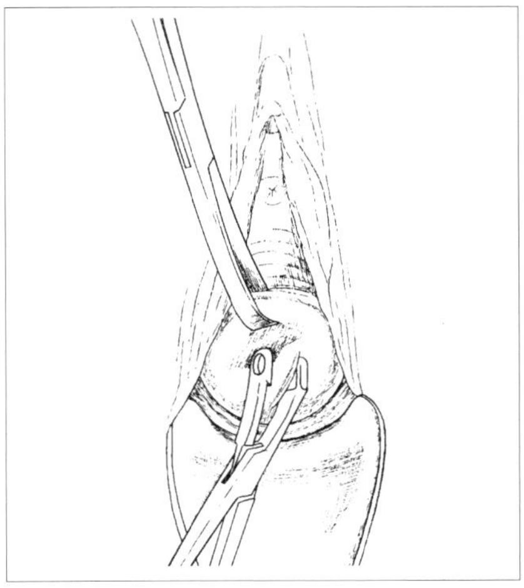

Figure 5.62

Cervical erosion

Cervical erosion is a misnomer for the bright red endocervical epithelium which extends to the ectocervix. It may be associated with contact bleeding. On examination, it is easily recognized as a bright red area continuous with the endocervix. It has a clearly defined outer edge but there is no breach in the surface. On digital examination, it feels soft with a granular surface which produces a grating sensation when stroked with the tip of the finger. It bleeds on touch.

Fix a cervical smear for cytological examination. If symptomatic, treat the lesion with electrocautery. Anaesthesia is unnecessary but a sedative is optional. With electric cautery, make radial stripes in the affected mucosa but leave the cervical canal untouched. There will be an increase in vaginal discharge after cauterization. Have the patient avoid coitus for 3–4 weeks. Possible complications include cervical stenosis (particularly if the endocervix has been inadvertently cauterized) and haemorrhage.

Endometrial biopsy

Perform endometrial biopsy in cases of infertility, to determine the response of the endometrium to ovarian stimulation. Carry out the procedure during the patient's premenstrual phase. Place the patient in the lithotomy position and cleanse the perineum, vagina and cervix. Retract the vaginal walls, grasp the cervix with a toothed tenaculum, and pass a uterine sound. Insert an endometrial biopsy cannula and obtain one or two pieces of the endometrium for histopathological examination (Figure 5.63). Examine for the secretory changes that identify the cycle as ovulatory. Perforation of the uterus and postoperative sepsis are rare complications.

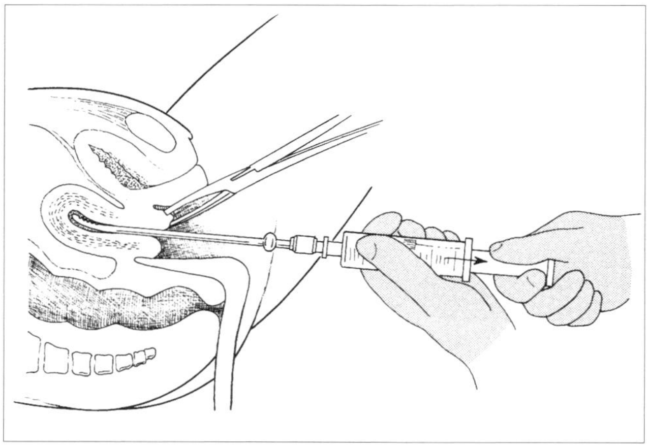

Figure 5.63

Polypectomy

Polypectomy is indicated for the treatment of cervical polyps and of pedunculated endometrial polyps that present through the cervix. Symptoms include vaginal discharge that is mucoid, mucopurulent or serosanguineous, contact bleeding, menorrhagia, intermenstrual bleeding and discharge and uterine colic. Many cervical polyps remain symptomless and are discovered only on routine examination. On speculum examination, a polyp appears through the cervical os as a dull, red and fragile growth. On vaginal examination, it is felt as a soft, fleshy mass that bleeds on touch. Differential diagnosis includes carcinoma and sarcoma botryoides. A polyp can also be confused with extruded products of conception.

Place the patient in the lithotomy position and clean and drape the area. Expose the cervix and grasp its anterior lip with a toothed tenaculum (Figure 5.64).

Grasp the polyp with sponge forceps and remove it by ligating and then cutting the stalk (Figures 5.65, 5.66, 5.67).

Follow the polypectomy by dilatation and curettage with the patient under anaesthesia (see pages 12–18 to 12–19. Look for any other intrauterine source of discharge, such as carcinoma, and treat additional polyps in the cervical canal or the body of the uterus. Send specimens for histological examination.

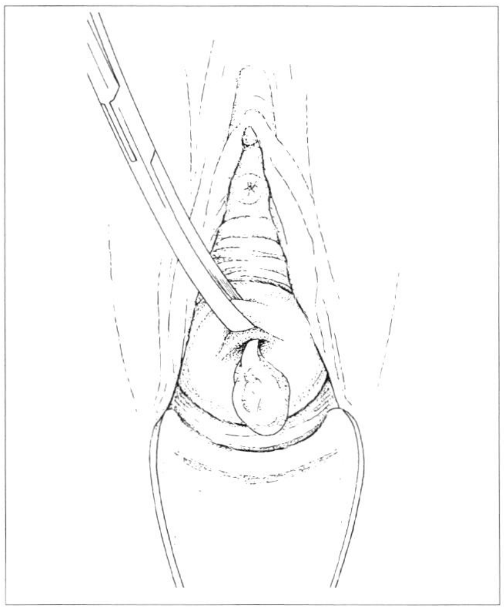

Figure 5.64

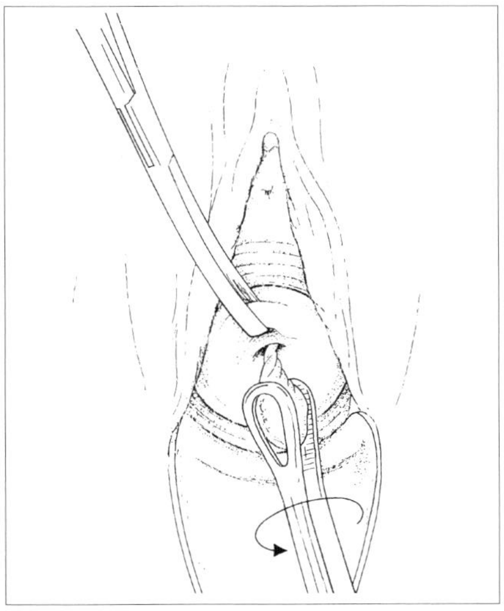

Figure 5.65

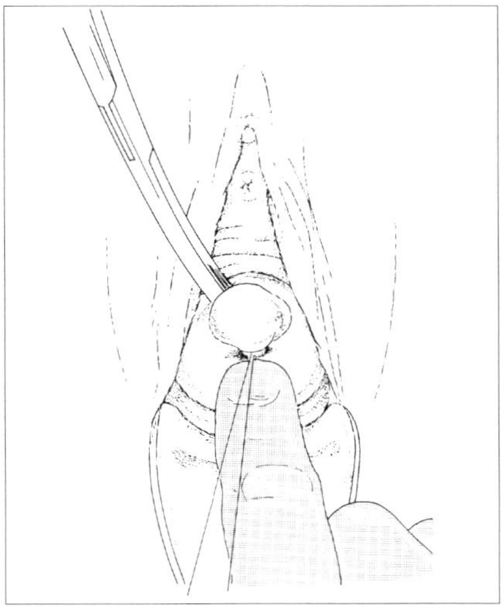

Figure 5.66

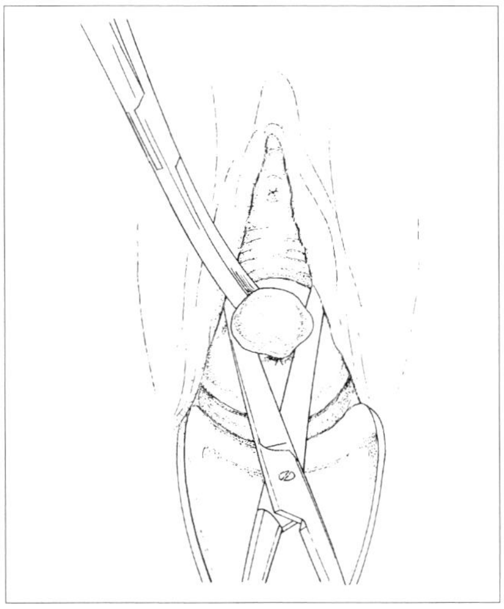

Figure 5.67

ANORECTAL ENDOSCOPY AND SPECIFIC CONDITIONS

Proctoscopy

Proctoscopy enables one to view and biopsy the whole of the anal canal, but only a small part of the rectum is visible at its lower end. Good lighting is essential. It is helpful to obtain the patient's confidence and cooperation. Talk to them throughout the examination. Explain the procedure and its purpose, emphasizing that it should cause only minor discomfort. Do not administer an enema unless the patient is constipated or unless sigmoidoscopy is also required.

Technique

1 Perform a preliminary digital examination. Then, with the patient in the same position, proceed to the proctoscopy to view any lesions that you have just felt. Lubricate and introduce the proctoscope, holding the handle with the fingers and pressing the thumb firmly on the head of the obturator

5

(Figure 5.68). This grip will keep the two parts of the instrument assembled. Point the handle posteriorly.

2 While you introduce the scope to its full length (Figure 5.69), instruct the patient to take deep breaths with the mouth open. Remove the obturator and direct the light into the scope (Figure 5.70).

Remove any faecal material, mucus or blood. Align the scope so that the lumen of the gut just beyond is clearly visible. Slowly withdraw the instrument while maintaining its alignment in the gut so that you can view any mucosal lesions, including haemorrhoidal masses or polyps. Note the appearance of the mucosa and assess its integrity.

3 If reliable facilities for specimen examination exist, take a biopsy sample from any obviously or possibly abnormal area under direct vision, using special biopsy forceps. Remove the tissue sample through the proctoscope. Remember that taking a biopsy sample from the rectal mucosa causes some discomfort and that removal of tissue from the anal lining can produce severe pain. At this examination, do not take tissue from a haemorrhoidal mass or any other lesion that appears to be vascular.

4 Immediately after removal from the patient, fix the tissue sample by total immersion in formaldehyde saline: 10 ml of 37% formaldehyde solution + 90 ml of physiological saline; fixation takes about 48 hours. Alternatively, use a fixative as directed by your local pathologist.

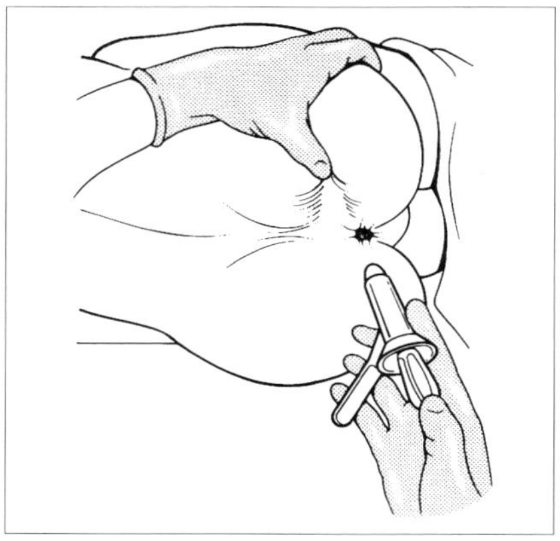

Figure 5.68

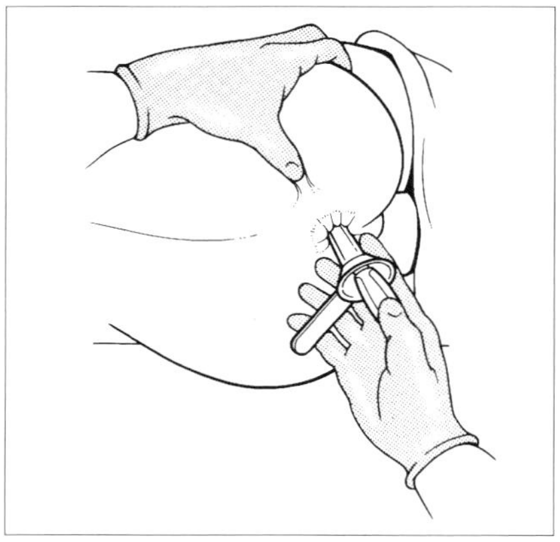

Figure 5.69

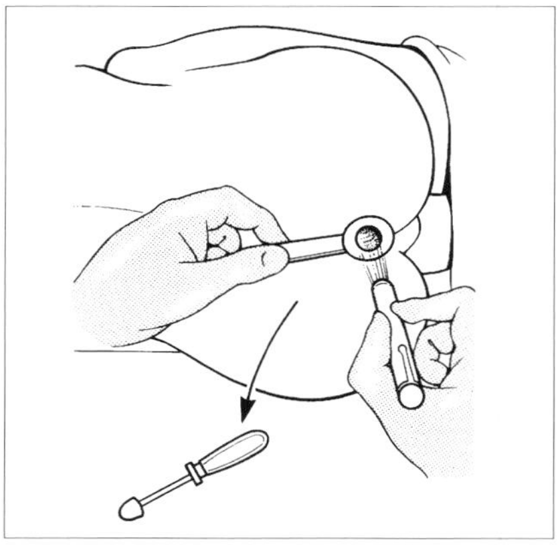

Figure 5.70

Sigmoidoscopy

Sigmoidoscopy is indicated for patients who have symptomatic colorectal disease and have had an inconclusive proctoscopy. It is also indicated following an abnormal proctoscopy to detect additional lesions such as polyposis or rectal schistosomiasis. For amoebic colitis, sigmoidoscopy is useful in assessing the response of proctocolitis to treatment. It can also facilitate the introduction of a rectal tube to decompress and reduce sigmoid volvulus. This examination normally follows a rectal examination and a proctoscopy.

Technique

1 Ask the patient to evacuate the rectum. If they cannot do this spontaneously, give an enema. Check the equipment, particularly the light-head, the eyepiece fitting (window) and the inflation pump (bellows) to ensure that they fit together and that enough light reaches the end of the scope.

2 Lubricate the sigmoidoscope generously before you start and introduce it with the obturator in position. In its initial stages, sigmoidoscopy is similar to proctoscopy (Figure 5.71). Next, point the sigmoidoscope backwards and upwards as you advance it (Figures 5.72, 5.73). Hold the obturator firmly to prevent it being dislodged (Figure 5.74).

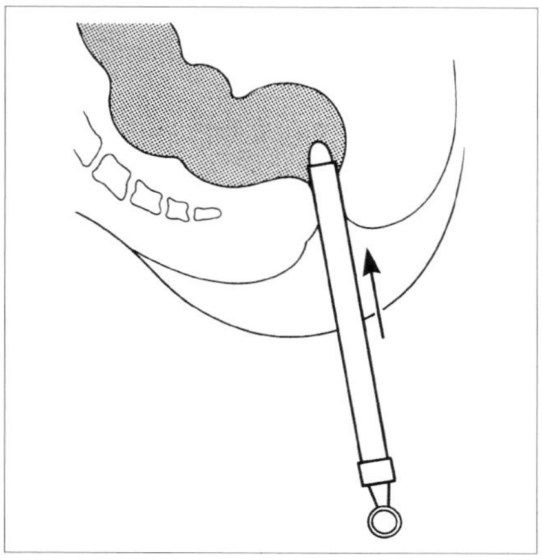

Figure 5.71

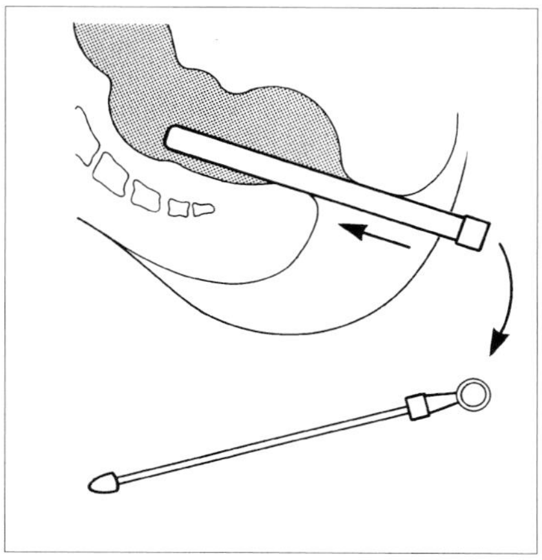

Figure 5.72

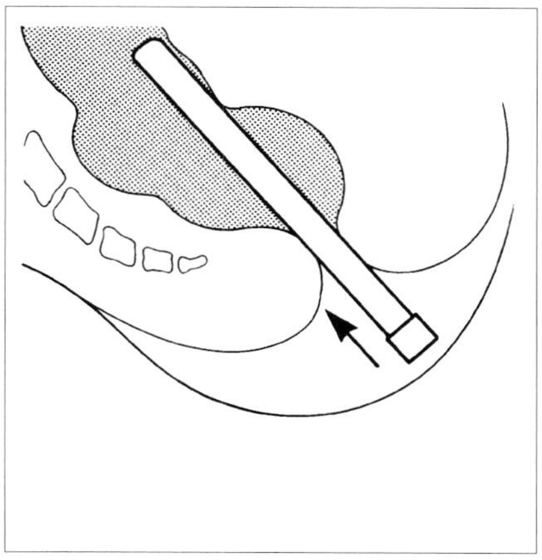

Figure 5.73

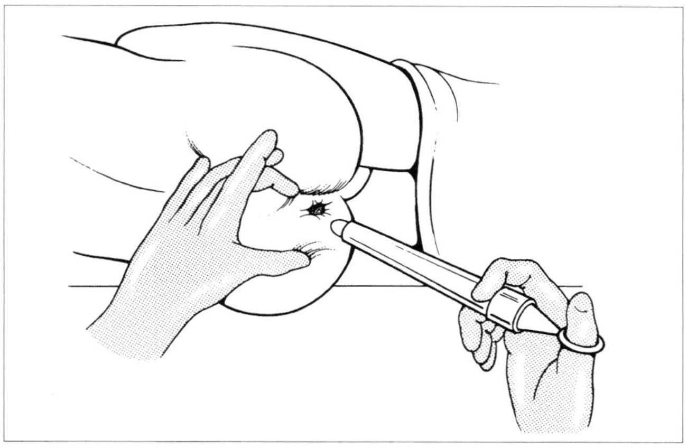

Figure 5.74

3 After introducing the sigmoidoscope about 10 cm, remove the obturator (Figure 5.75). If there is any obstruction before the sigmoidoscope has been inserted 10 cm, remove the obturator at this point. Then attach the

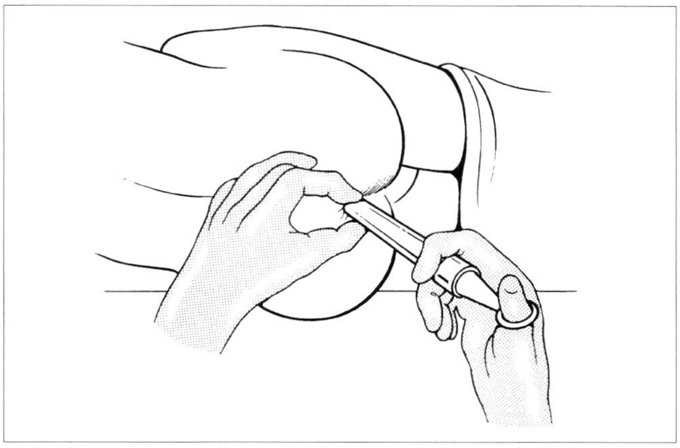

Figure 5.75

eyepiece, which usually carries the light source and pump connections. To view the gut wall and the bowel lumen, introduce a little air and align the scope. Gently advance the instrument, keeping it accurately within the lumen of the bowel. Introduce air at intervals to open up the bowel lumen gradually beyond the scope. Should the view be obscured at any time by rectal contents, remove the eyepiece and evacuate the material using dental rolls held firmly with biopsy forceps.

4 Progressively change the direction of the scope to keep within the lumen. Do not advance the scope unless the lumen of the bowel is in view. The rectosigmoid junction may be difficult to traverse, so do not rush the procedure. If there is much difficulty advancing the scope beyond this level, stop the procedure. Do not use force to introduce the scope or to take a biopsy specimen from the wall of the bowel. Injury or even perforation of the rectal wall can result.

   If the patient experiences discomfort during the examination, check for proper alignment of the sigmoidoscope, release air by removing the eyepiece or by disconnecting the pump tubing, then reassemble the instrument and continue the examination. If necessary, reintroduce the scope and repeat the examination. At the end of each examination, let out the air from the gut before withdrawing the scope.

Perianal haematoma

Perianal haematoma is usually associated with considerable pain. The inflamed area is tense, tender and easily visible upon inspection of the anal verge as a small, tender swelling about the size of a pea.

Management consists mainly of relieving the pain by local or oral administration of analgesics and by helping the patient to avoid constipation. The lesion will resolve slowly over several days or weeks. This can be expedited with hypertonic saline compresses. During this time, the haematoma may spontaneously rupture through the overlying skin, discharging blood clots and providing some pain relief. In the early stages of haematoma formation, surgical evacuation of the clot under local anaesthesia can rapidly relieve pain and discomfort. Drainage is not recommended in the sub-acute or chronic stages of perianal haematoma.

Anal fissure

An anal fissure is a tear in the mucosa of the lower anal canal. It is usually associated with intense pain, especially during and just after defecation. Hard stools precipitate and aggravate the condition.

The anus is tightly closed by spasm, so that the application of a local anaesthetic gel, or occasionally even general anaesthesia, is necessary to allow an adequate examination. The fissure may be acute or chronic, the latter having fibrotic margins.

Non-operative management is recommended, especially for an acute fissure. It should include prescription of a high-fibre diet and administration of a local anaesthetic ointment or suppository. A chronic fissure can be treated by manual dilatation of the anus.

Anal dilatation: technique

1 Before proceeding, empty the rectum by administering an enema. Give the patient a general anaesthetic without a muscle relaxant and use the tone in the anal sphincter to judge the extent to which the anal sphincter should be stretched. Perform a digital, and then proctoscopic, examination to confirm the presence of haemorrhoids (Figure 5.76, 5.77).

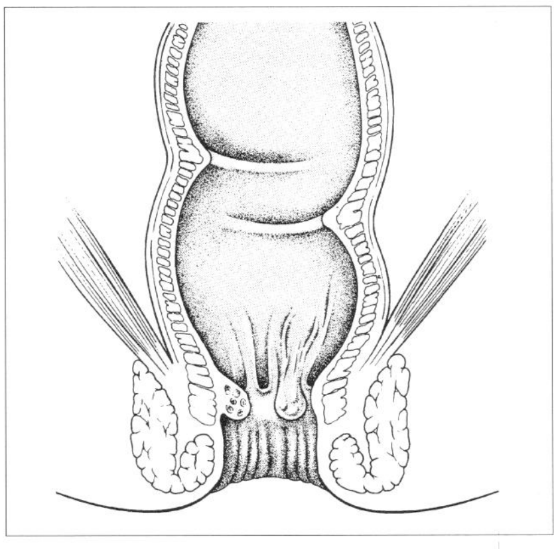

Figure 5.76

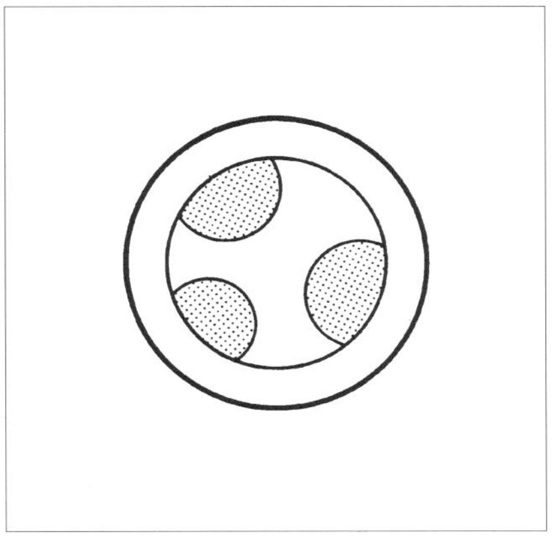

Figure 5.77

The success of the treatment depends largely on adequate dilatation of the anus in the region of the "constricting bands". This is achieved by applying pressure with the fingers but, to avoid over-dilatation and other complications, use no more than four fingers. Do not use any instruments.

2 First, insert the index and middle fingers of the left hand into the anus and press against the wall to assess the degree of constriction caused by the bands in the anal wall (Figure 5.78). Now, dilate the anus by inserting the right index finger and pressing it against the anal wall in the opposite direction to the other two fingers (Figure 5.79). Insert the middle finger of the right hand and repeat the procedure.

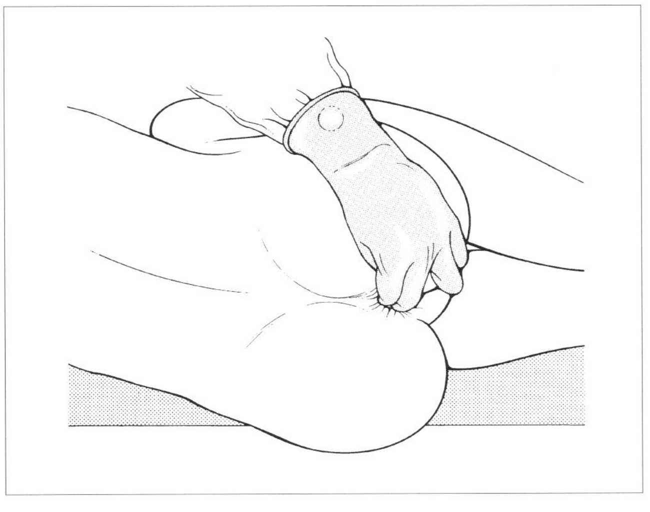

Figure 5.78

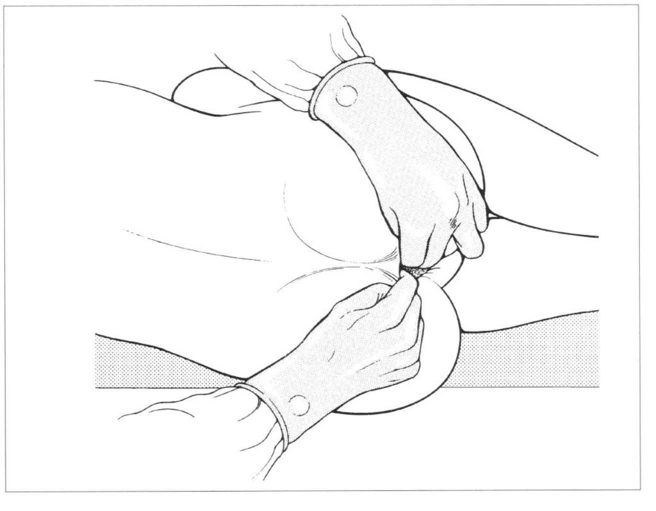

Figure 5.79

3 Finally, insert into the anus a sponge or gauze swab, soaked in a non-irritating antiseptic or saline and wrung out, or a piece of petrolatum gauze. Leave one end of the sponge or gauze protruding.

4 For aftercare, administer analgesics when indicated. Give the patient a mild laxative, such as liquid paraffin (mineral oil), to encourage the regular passing of soft, bulky stools. Instruct the patient to sit in warm water, preferably in which some salt has been dissolved, for about 15–30 minutes at least once a day for 14 days.

Complications can include haematoma formation, incontinence and mucosal prolapse. Provided that no more than four fingers are used for dilatation, no significant complications should arise.

Haemorrhoids

The main symptoms of haemorrhoids are bleeding on passing stools and prolapse of the varicose masses. Pain is not always a significant feature. Haemorrhoids are graded according to whether they prolapse and whether the prolapsed mass reduces spontaneously or must be replaced manually. Rectal examination, proctoscopy and sigmoidoscopy are necessary in diagnosing haemorrhoids and in checking for any associated conditions, in particular carcinoma of the rectum.

Complications of haemorrhoids are anaemia and thrombosis.

Treatment

Many patients benefit from a high-fibre diet which encourages regular, soft, bulky motions and the local application of an analgesic ointment or suppository. This non-operative management is sufficient for the majority of patients.

Patients whose haemorrhoids prolapse (and either return spontaneously or can be replaced) and patients in whom the above regimen has failed to give adequate relief can be treated by manual dilatation of the anus (see anal fissure). This is the only form of surgical treatment recommended for the non surgical specialist. Haemorrhoidectomy undertaken by the inexperienced can be complicated with anal stenosis. If haemorrhoidectomy is required, refer the patient to a qualified surgeon.

Never perform haemorrhoidectomy or anal dilatation on a pregnant or postpartum patient. Hypertonic saline compresses will temporize the discomfort and the haemorrhoids will improve dramatically several weeks after delivery.

Part 3

The Abdomen

Laparotomy and abdominal trauma

6

6.1 LAPAROTOMY

LAPAROTOMY

Use the laparotomy technique to expose abdominal organs. It also allows confirmation or correction of the preoperative diagnosis in a patient presenting with an acute abdomen. Avoid laparotomy in pancreatitis. Be thoroughly familiar with the midline incision, which is simple, causes relatively little bleeding and can be performed rapidly, closed quickly and extended easily.

Make an incision in the upper abdomen to expose:
- The gallbladder
- Stomach
- Duodenum
- Spleen
- Liver.

Use a lower abdominal incision for patients with:
- Intestinal obstruction
- Pelvic problems.

Make an incision from the upper to lower abdomen to:
- Evaluate all abdominal organs in a trauma laparotomy.

Midline incision

1 With the patient in the supine position, prepare the skin and drape the area from the level of the nipples to the pubic region and to the flank on either side. Incise the skin in the midline between the xiphoid process and the umbilicus. Extend the incision below the umbilicus as needed for additional exposure (Figure 6.1).

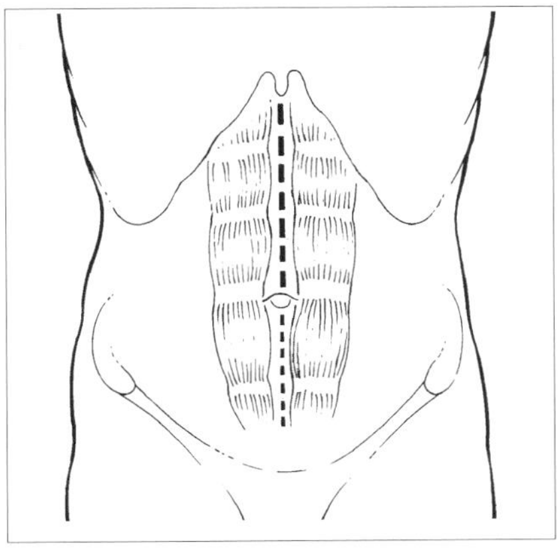

Figure 6.1

KEY POINTS

- Patients with life threatening abdominal conditions, including trauma, should be given life saving treatment at the district hospital, particularly if they are likely to die before arrival at a referral hospital
- Most abdominal emergencies initially present for care at the district hospital and preparations for diagnosis and resuscitation should be in place there
- Appendectomy, drainage of abdominal and pelvic abscesses, small bowel anastomosis, colostomy and elective herniorrhaphy capability should be available at district hospitals
- Laparotomy is used to expose the abdominal organs so as to institute definitive diagnosis and treatment of abdominal trauma and acute abdominal conditions
- At the district hospital, non-specialist practitioners with specific training can capably perform laparotomy and, on occasion, will perform laparotomy on complex cases in order to save lives
- In an emergency, a midline incision is the incision of choice
- A general anaesthetic should be given for an upper midline incision; spinal anaesthesia may be used for low midline incisions in the stable patient
- If there is doubt about the diagnosis, you may use a short paraumbilical incision and extend it up or down in the midline, as indicated.

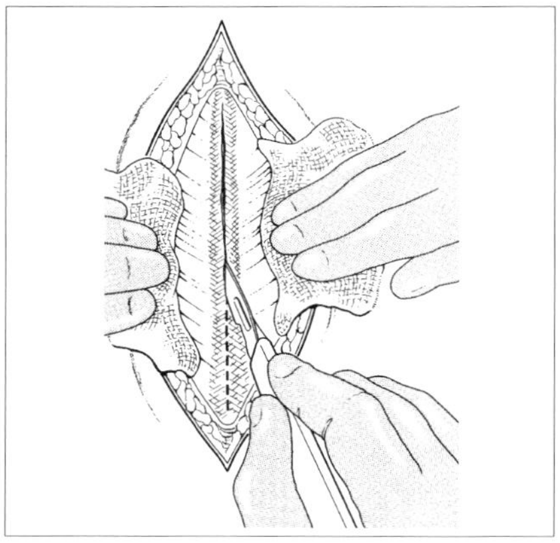

Figure 6.2

2 Incise through the subcutaneous layer and to the loose tissue over the linea alba. Control bleeding with gauze swabs held against the wound edge and ligate persistent bleeding points. Display the linea alba with its longitudinal line of decussating fibres and incise it directly in the midline, exposing the extraperitoneal fat and the peritoneum (Figure 6.2).

3 Exercise care if the incision is through a previous laparotomy scar as the gut may be adherent to the undersurface of the abdominal wall and liable to injury. Clear the extraperitoneal fat laterally with blunt dissection, securing the vessels as necessary.

4 Lift the peritoneum, making it into a "tent" by holding it with forceps on either side of the midline. Squeeze the tent between the fingers and thumb to free any gut on the undersurface, and make a small opening with a knife (Figures 6.3, 6.4).

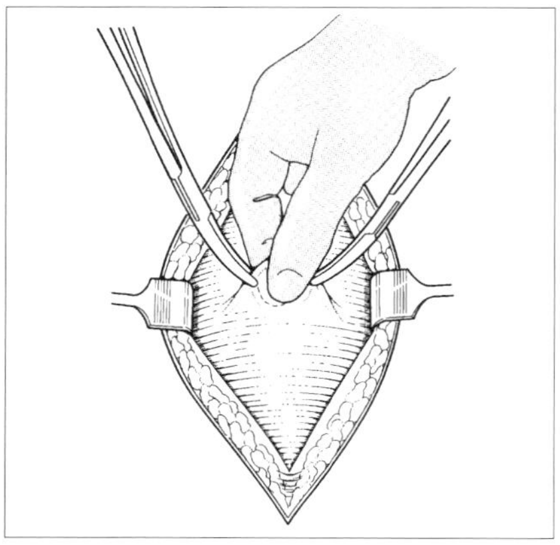

Figure 6.3

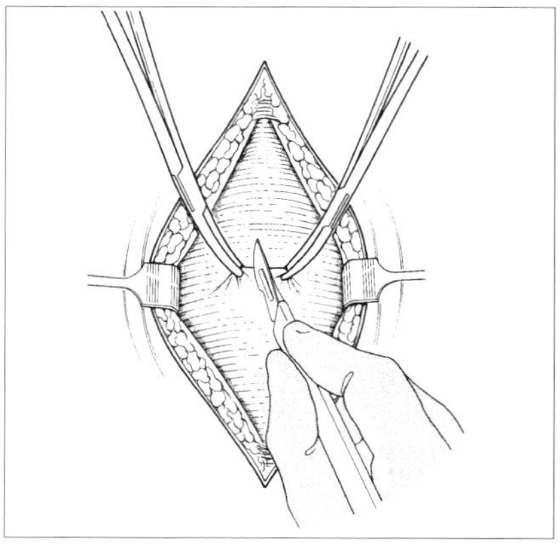

Figure 6.4

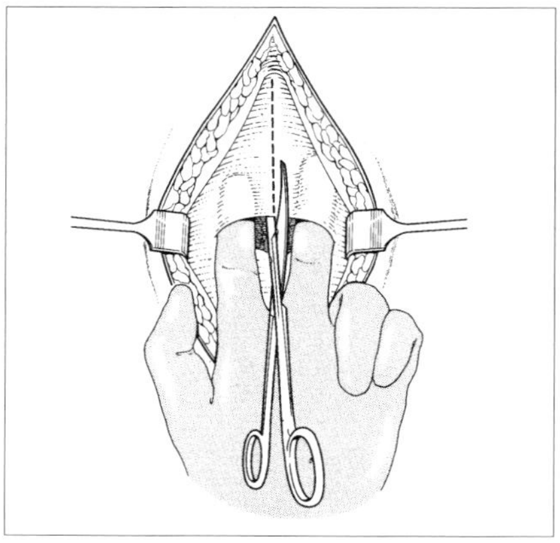

Figure 6.5

5 If the peritoneum opens readily, steady the undersurface with the index and middle fingers and extend the opening with scissors (Figure 6.5). Extend the peritoneal incision the full length of the wound.

6 Examine the abdominal contents to confirm the diagnosis.

Abdominal findings	**Possible cause**
• Greenish fluid and gas	• Perforation of stomach or duodenum
• Free bowel contents and gas in peritoneum	• Bowel perforation
• Free blood in peritoneum: with trauma	• Injury to liver, spleen or mesentery
• Free blood in peritoneum: female, no history of trauma	• Ruptured ectopic pregnancy
• Purulent exudate	• Appendicitis, diverticulitis or perforation of the bowel
• Distended loop of bowel	• Intestinal obstruction or paralytic ileus

7 Systematically examine the abdominal organs for signs of injury or other abnormality:

- Begin examination with the small intestine at the ligament of Trietz, progress along its entire length and then examine the large intestine and rectum

- In the lower abdomen, examine the bladder and uterus
- In the upper abdomen, examine the stomach, duodenum and spleen
- Visualize and palpate the liver and diaphragm and finally examine the retroperitoneum including the pancreas and kidneys
- Plan the appropriate surgical procedure after you have made a complete assessment.

8 Carry out the appropriate procedures as indicated by the pathological findings. These techniques are explained in the following sections.

9 At the end of the operation, close the wound in layers. Use several pairs of large artery forceps to hold the ends and edges of the peritoneal incision. Close the peritoneum with a continuous 0 absorbable suture on a round-bodied needle (Figure 6.6). Maintaining the intestine within the abdominal cavity during the closure is often a problem. If needed, use a muscle relaxant medication or a malleable metal spatula placed under the peritoneum (Figure 6.7).

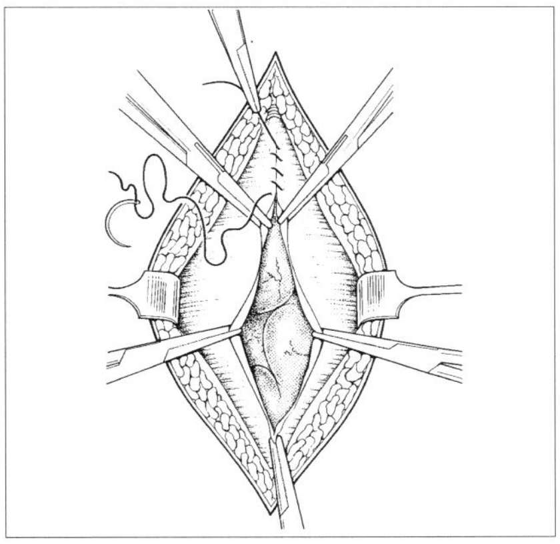

Figure 6.6

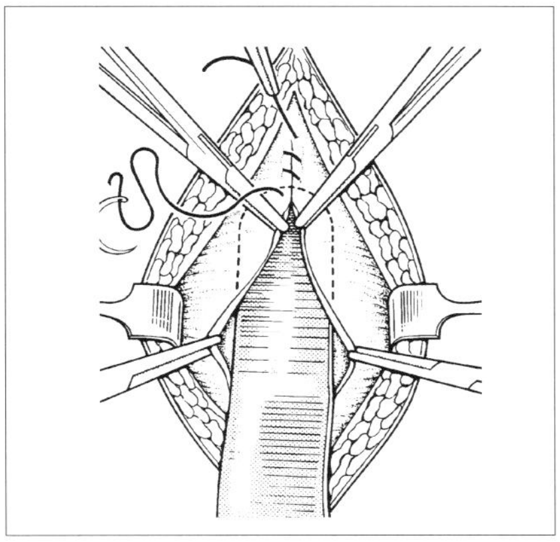

Figure 6.7

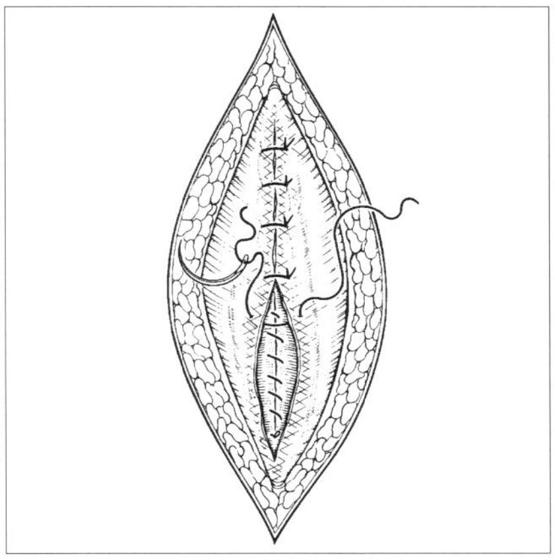

Figure 6.8

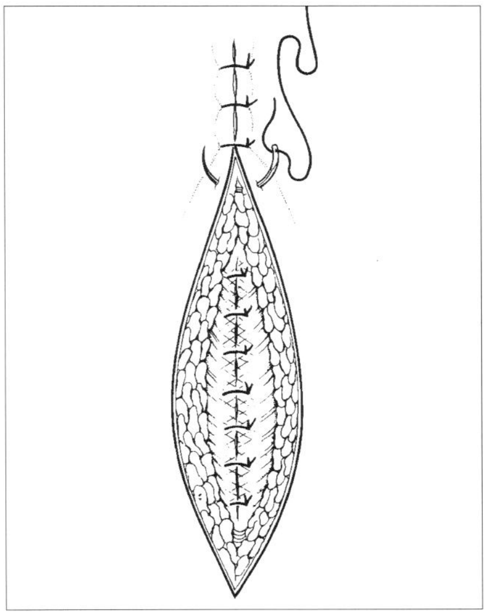

Figure 6.9

10 Close the linea alba with interrupted No. 1 polyglycolic acid or continuous monofilament nylon on a round or trocar needle (Figure 6.8). If the wound is contaminated or infected, use loosely placed No. 1 nylon sutures. Close the skin with interrupted 2/0 stitches, keeping the sutures 1 cm apart and 1 cm from the wound edge (Figure 6.9). Apply a 2 layer gauze dressing.

If closing the abdomen is difficult, check the adequacy of the anaesthesia to reduce abdominal wall tension and empty the stomach with a nasogastric tube. An alternative to multi-layer closure is a simple all-layer retention suture for closure. Retention sutures are indicated in patients debilitated as a result of malnutrition, old age, advanced cancer or HIV/AIDS when healing is likely to be impaired. Monofilament nylon is a suitable material. Insert retention sutures through the entire thickness of the abdominal wall before closing the peritoneum, leaving them untied at first (Figure 6.10). If it is

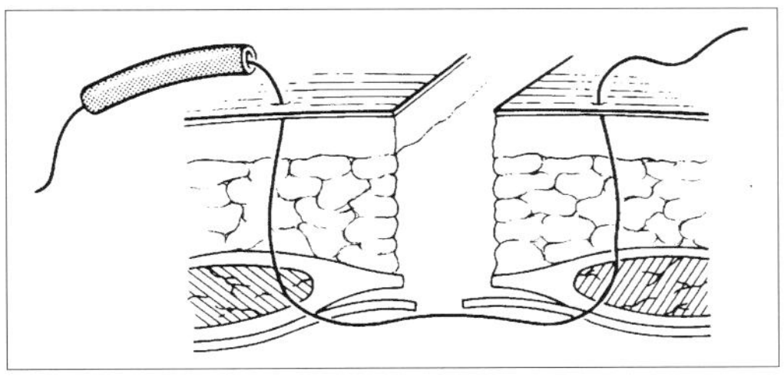

Figure 6.10

6

impossible or very difficult to close the linea alba due to excess intra-abdominal pressure, it is acceptable to close the skin only. Refer the patient to a surgical specialist when stabilized.

KEY POINTS

- Abdominal trauma is classified as blunt or penetrating
- Intra-abdominal bleeding or gastrointestinal perforation may be present without any evidence of abdominal wall injury
- Intra-abdominal bleeding may be confirmed by peritoneal lavage with saline, but a negative result does not exclude injury, particularly in retroperitoneal trauma
- Suspect intra-abdominal bleeding in cases of multiple trauma, especially if hypotension is unexplained
- In the presence of hypovolaemia, the chest, pelvis and femur are alternative sites of major blood loss.

Paediatric cases

- Many blunt abdominal injuries can be managed without operation
- Non-operative management is indicated if the child is haemodynamically stable and can be monitored closely
- Place a nasogastric tube if the abdomen is distended, as children swallow large amount of air.

6.2 ABDOMINAL TRAUMA

Trauma to the abdomen occurs as an isolated injury or associated with high energy polytrauma. The principles of primary trauma care include the abdominal evaluation as a part of the acute resuscitation protocol, see Unit 16: *Acute Trauma Management* and the Annex: *Primary Trauma Care Manual*.

When a patient presents with abdominal injuries, give priority to the primary survey:

1. Establish a clear airway.
2. Assure ventilation.
3. Arrest external bleeding.
4. Set up an intravenous infusion of normal saline or Ringer's lactate.
5. Insert a nasogastric tube and begin suction and monitor output.
6. Send a blood sample for haemoglobin measurement and type and crossmatch.
7. Insert a urinary catheter, examine the urine for blood and monitor the urine output.
8. Perform the secondary survey: a complete physical examination to evaluate the abdomen and to establish the extent of other injury.
9. Examine the abdomen for bowel sounds, tenderness, rigidity and contusions or open wounds.
10. Administer small doses of intravenous analgesics, prophylactic antibiotics and tetanus prophylaxis.

If the diagnosis of intra-abdominal bleeding is uncertain, proceed with diagnostic peritoneal lavage. Laparotomy is indicated when abdominal trauma is associated with obvious rebound, frank blood on peritoneal lavage or hypotension and a positive peritoneal lavage. Serial physical examination, ultrasound and X-rays are helpful in the equivocal case. Repeated examination is an important means of assessing the indeterminate case. Even experienced practitioners should seek the opinion of colleagues to aid in evaluating equivocal abdominal findings and the inexperienced practitioner should not hesitate to do so. X-ray the chest, abdomen, pelvis and any other injured parts of the body if the patient is stable. If you suspect a ruptured viscus, a lateral decubitus abdominal X-ray may show free intraperitoneal air.

Diagnostic peritoneal lavage

After the primary survey, resuscitation and secondary survey have been completed, the findings indicating intra-abdominal bleeding or lacerated viscera may not be adequate to confirm diagnosis. Serial physical examination can be supplemented with diagnostic peritoneal lavage (DPL) to make a decision on whether trauma laparotomy should be performed. The availability of computerized axial tomography in referral centres has reduced the use of DPL, but it is not obsolete and should be available at the district hospital.

Technique

1 Infiltrate a local anaesthetic with epinephrine (adrenaline) into the abdominal wall and peritoneum at an infra-umbilical site (Figure 6.11). The epinephrine reduces abdominal wall bleeding.

2 Make a 2.5 cm midline incision which is carried down through subcutaneous tissue to the linea alba (Figure 6.12). Apply counter traction to the fascia of the linea alba with two stay sutures and make a 3–5 mm incision through the fascia (Figure 6.13). Gently introduce a catheter on a stylet into the peritoneum and advance the catheter over the stylet into the pelvis (Figure 6.14).

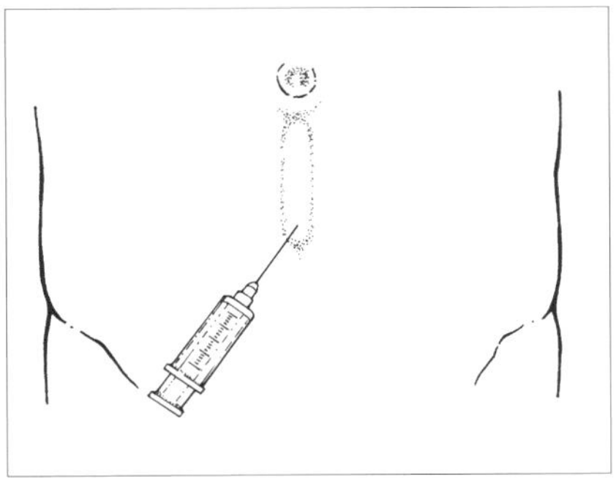

Figure 6.11

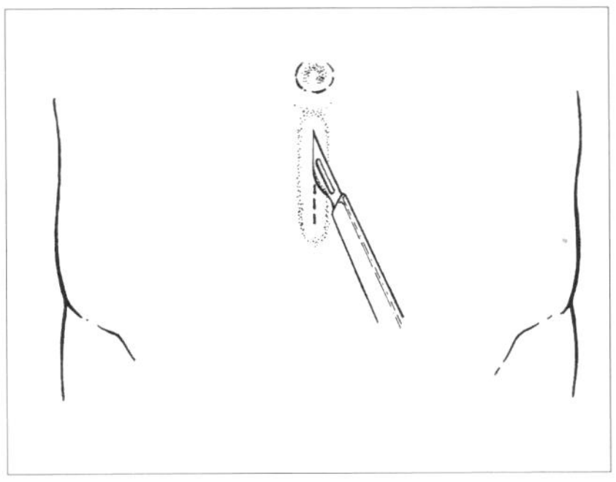

Figure 6.12

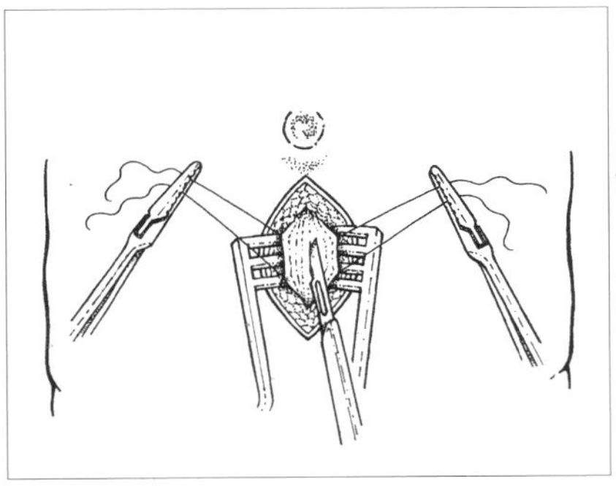

Figure 6.13

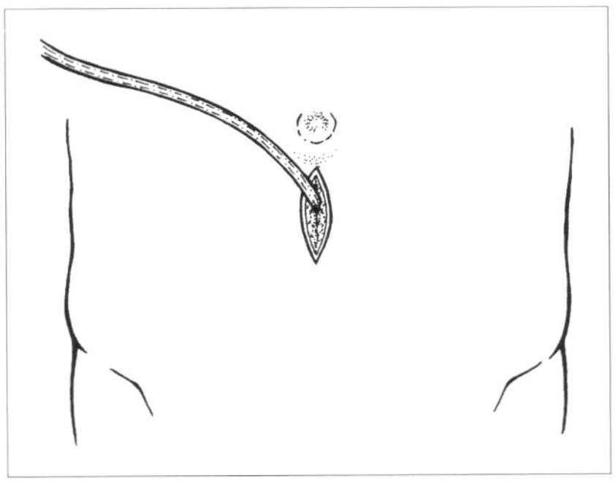

Figure 6.14

Spontaneous return of blood or gross aspiration of blood is an indication for laparotomy.

3 If no blood is returned, infuse 20 ml/kg (1 litre in adults) of intravenous solution (saline or Ringer's lactate) through the catheter (Figure 6.15). Attach the catheter to a closed container and place on the floor. About 100 ml of fluid should flow back into the container (Figure 6.16). If the returning fluid has greater than 100 000 red cells per ml or 500 white cells per ml, consider performing a laparotomy.

KEY POINTS

Diagnostic peritoneal lavage:
- Is indicated when abdominal finding are equivocal in the trauma patient
- Should not be performed if there are indications for immediate laparotomy
- Should be performed only after the insertion of a nasogastric tube and Foley catheter
- Is rapid, sensitive and inexpensive
- Diagnostic peritoneal lavage may rule out significant abdominal trauma in the district hospital where the patient may otherwise be unobserved and unmonitored for extended periods of time
- Gross evaluation of the returned fluid must be performed and decisions made on that evaluation if laboratory evaluation is not available
- Ignore a negative result on diagnostic peritoneal lavage if the patient subsequently develops an acute abdomen: trauma laparotomy is then indicated.

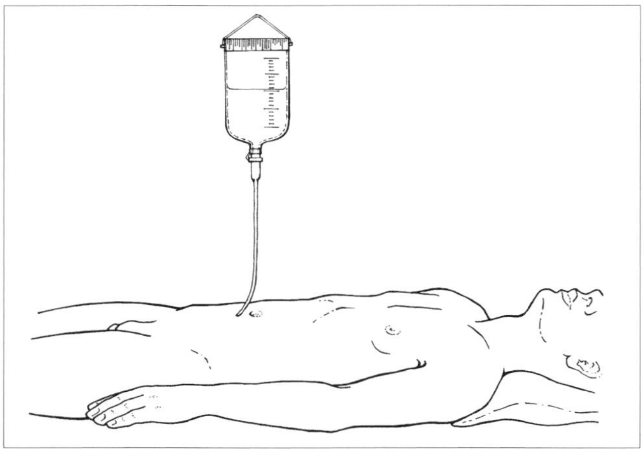

Figure 6.15

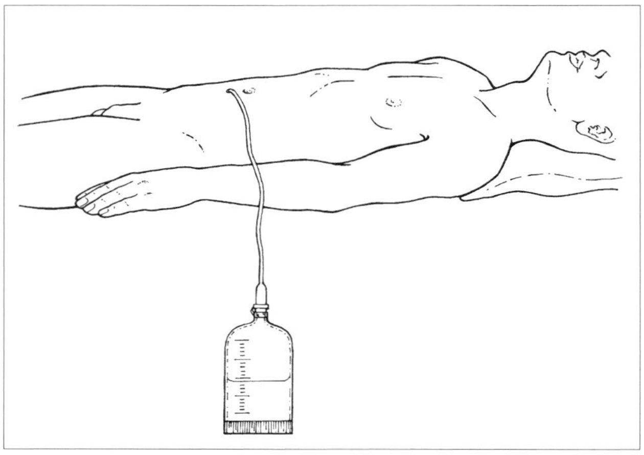

Figure 6.16

The red and white blood cell count can be determined in the laboratory along with an examination for bacteria and amylase. When laboratory evaluation is not available, the approximate laparotomy threshold can be determined by looking at the clarity of the fluid. If you cannot read "newsprint" through the siphoned back solution due to the red colour, there is sufficient blood to indicate the need for a laparotomy. If the fluid is cloudy due to particulate material, it is likely that there is a bowel injury and laparotomy is also indicated.

Penetrating injuries

- Penetrating injuries follow gunshot wounds and wounds induced by sharp objects such as knives or spears
- Laparotomy with intra-abdominal exploration is indicated when the abdomen has been penetrated, regardless of the physical findings
- Signs of hypovolaemia or of peritoneal irritation may be minimal immediately following a penetrating injury involving the abdominal viscera.

Blunt injuries

- Blunt injuries result from a direct force to the abdomen without an associated open wound; they most commonly follow road traffic accidents or assaults
- Following blunt injury, exploratory laparotomy is indicated in the presence of:
  - Abdominal pain and rigidity
  - Free abdominal air, seen on a plain X-ray (lateral decubitus or upright chest)
- Following blunt abdominal trauma, signs that may indicate intra-abdominal bleeding include:
  - Referred shoulder pain
  - Hypotension
- Oliguria associated with suprapubic pain suggests bladder rupture.

Injuries to the diaphragm

- Penetrating trauma to the upper abdomen and lower chest can result in small perforations to the diaphragm which can be closed with simple or mattress 2/0 sutures

- Blunt trauma can result in a large rent in the left diaphragm (the liver protects the diaphragm); the presence of viscera in the chest, identified by auscultation or chest X-ray, is diagnostic.

RUPTURED SPLEEN

In tropical countries, enlargement of the spleen due to malaria or visceral leishmaniasis is common. The affected spleen is liable to injury or rupture as a result of trivial trauma. Delayed rupture can occur up to three weeks after the injury.

Diagnostic features of a ruptured spleen include:

- History of trauma with pain in the left upper abdomen (often referred to the shoulder)
- Nausea and vomiting
- Signs of hypovolaemia
- Abdominal tenderness and rigidity and a diffuse palpable mass
- Chest X-ray showing left lower rib fractures and a shadow in the upper left quadrant displacing the gastric air bubble medially.

Consider conservative management, particularly in children, if the patient is haemodynamically stable and you are able to monitor them closely with bedrest, intravenous fluids, analgesics and nasogastric suction.

If the patient's condition deteriorates, perform a splenectomy.

Perform a laparotomy if you suspect a ruptured spleen and the patient is hypovolaemic. Repair or remove the spleen.

KEY POINTS

- Splenectomy is the treatment for severe injuries to the spleen, but consider preserving the spleen if bleeding is not profuse
- The spleen has blood supplied from the splenic artery and the short gastric arteries
- Vaccination with pneumovax and prophylactic antibiotics are indicated due to the immune deficiency occurring in splenectomized patients.

Technique

1 Place the patient supine on the operating table with a pillow or sandbag under the left lower chest. Open the abdomen through a long midline incision (Figure 6.17). Remove clots from the abdominal cavity to localize the spleen. If bleeding continues, squeeze the splenic vessels between your thumb and fingers (Figure 6.18) or apply intestinal occlusion clamps. Assess the extent of splenic injury and inspect other organs.

2 Make the decision whether to remove or preserve the spleen. If the bleeding has stopped, do not disturb the area. If a small tear is bleeding, try to

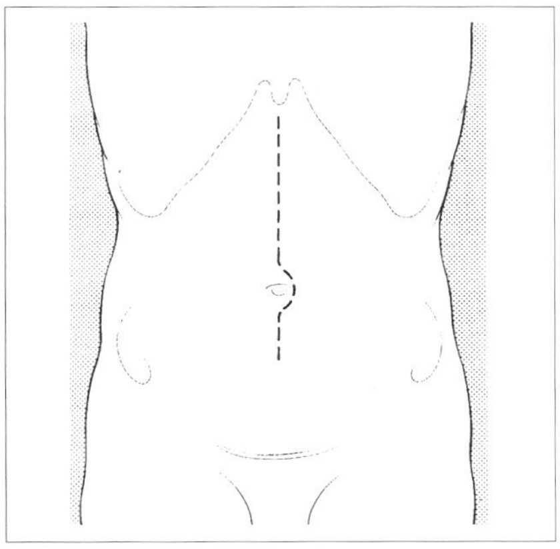

Figure 6.17

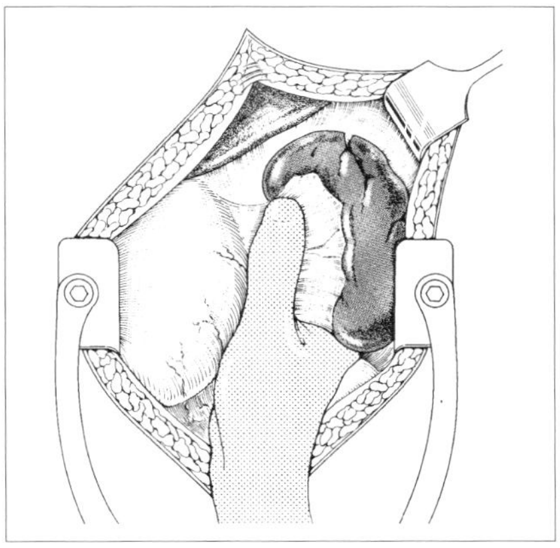

Figure 6.18

control it with 0 absorbable mattress sutures. This is particularly advisable in children.

3 To remove the spleen, lift it into the wound and divide the taut splenorenal ligament with scissors (Figure 6.19). Extend the division to the upper pole of the spleen. Apply a large occlusion clamp to the adjoining gastrosplenic omentum (containing the short gastric vessels) and divide the omentum between large artery forceps (Figures 6.20, 6.21).

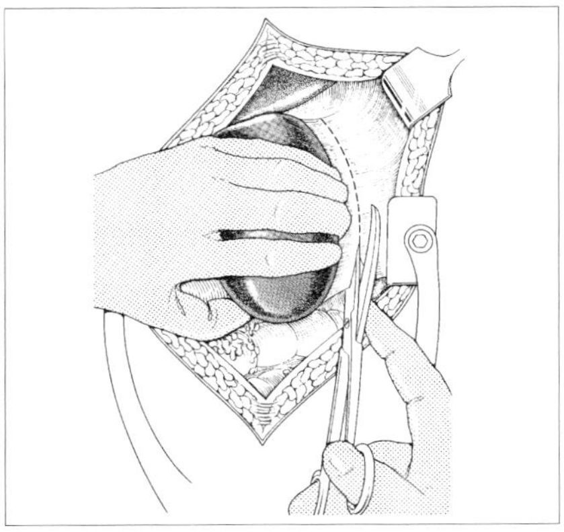

Figure 6.19

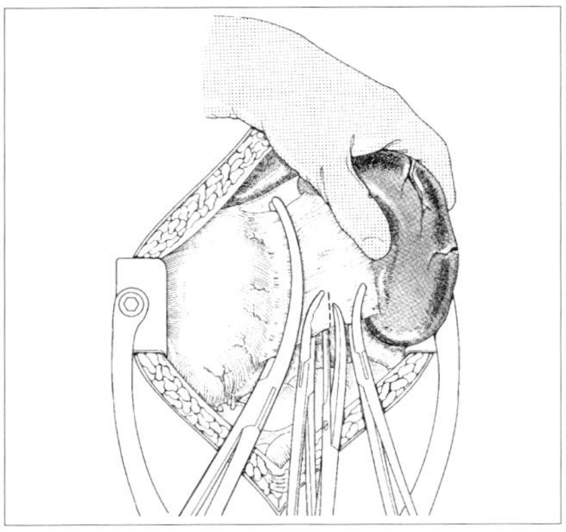

Figure 6.20

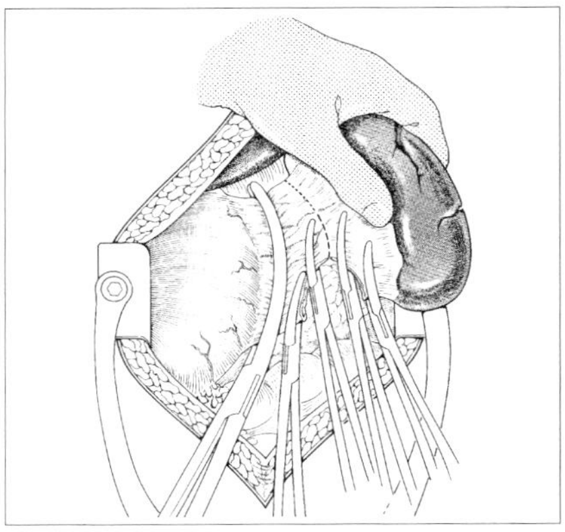

Figure 6.21

4 Ligate the short gastric vessels well away from the gastric wall. Dissect the posterior part of the hilum, identifying the tail of the pancreas and the splenic vessels. Ligate these vessels three times, if possible ligating the artery first, and divide them between the distal pair of ligatures (Figures 6.22, 6.23). Now divide the remaining gastrosplenic omentum between

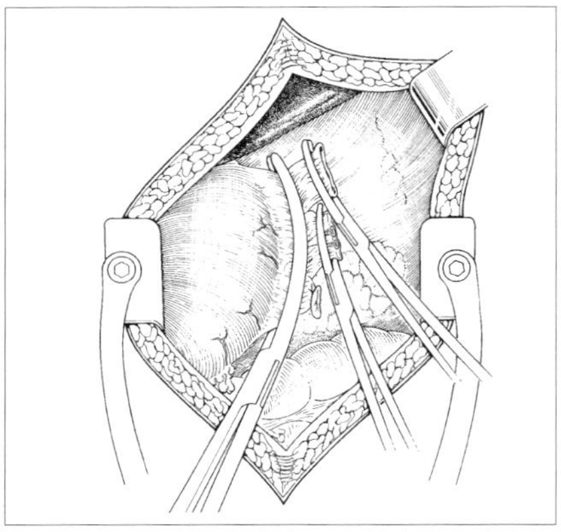

Figure 6.22

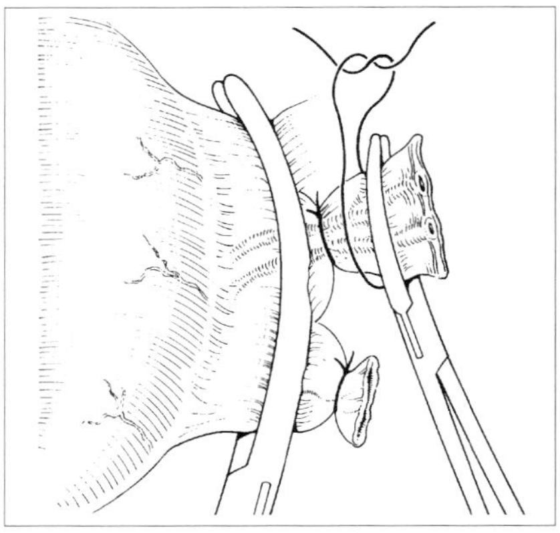

Figure 6.23

several clamps and, finally, divide the anterior layer of the lienorenal ligament.

5 If there is excess bleeding, drain the bed of the spleen with a latex drain brought out through a separate stab wound. Remove the drain at 24 hours, if possible. Close the abdomen in layers.

LACERATION OF THE LIVER

Technique

1 Through a midline incision, examine the liver and gallbladder. Small wounds may have stopped bleeding by the time of operation and should not be disturbed.

2 For moderate wounds or tears that are not bleeding, do not suture or debride the liver. If a moderate wound is bleeding, remove all devitalized tissue and suture the tear with 0 chromic mattress stitches on a large round-bodied needle (Figures 6.24, 6.25). First, place overlapping mattress stitches on both sides of the wound (Figures 6.26, 6.27). Then suture the two sides together (Figure 6.28).

3 If the laceration is large, it should not be sutured. Ligate individual vessels or pack the laceration with a long gauze roll soaked in warm saline. The liver pack should be removed after about 48 hours by a surgical specialist, at repeat laparotomy with the patient under general anaesthesia. Make arrangements for referral of such a patient as soon as condition permits.

KEY POINTS

- Liver injuries follow blunt trauma to the right upper quadrant of the abdomen and may result in significant bleeding
- Many liver injuries stop bleeding spontaneously and you should not suture them as this may result in significant bleeding which is difficult to stop
- Large liver lacerations should not be closed; bleeding vessels should be ligated and the liver defect packed with omentum or, if this is unsuccessful, with gauze
- A large drain is indicated in all patients with liver injuries. It should be removed after about 48 hours unless bile continues to drain.

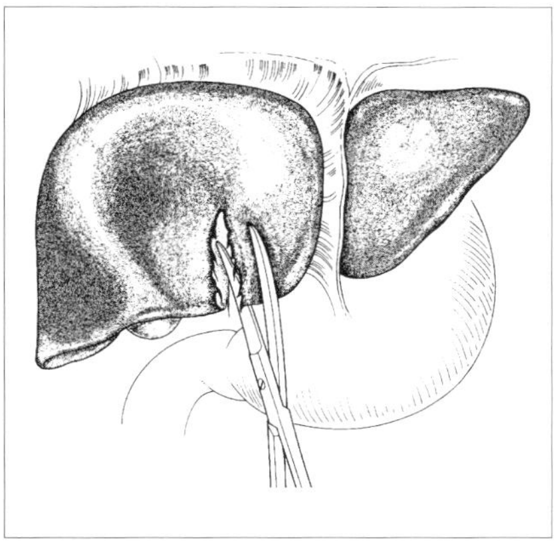

Figure 6.24

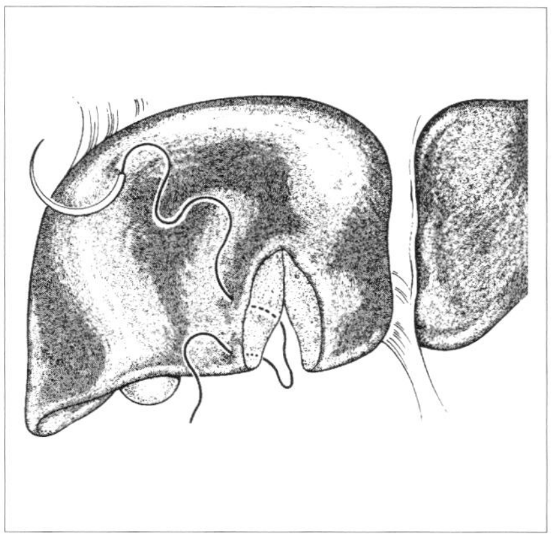

Figure 6.25

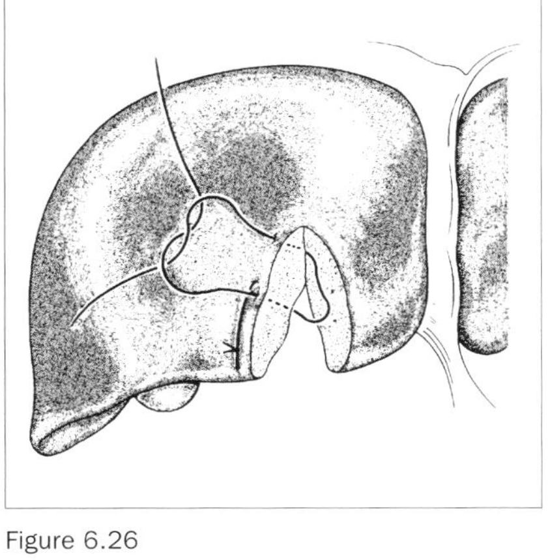

Figure 6.26

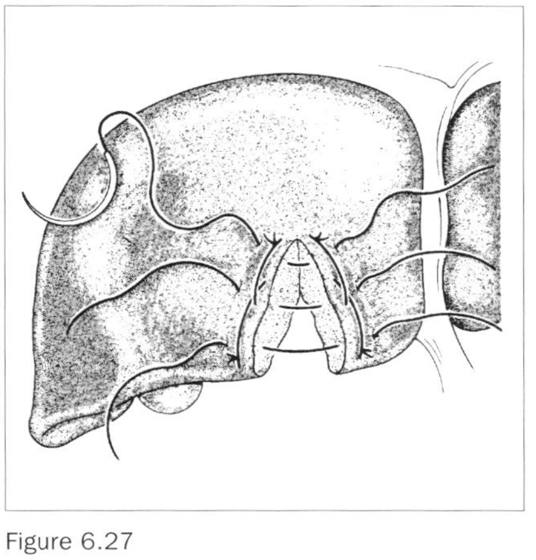

Figure 6.27

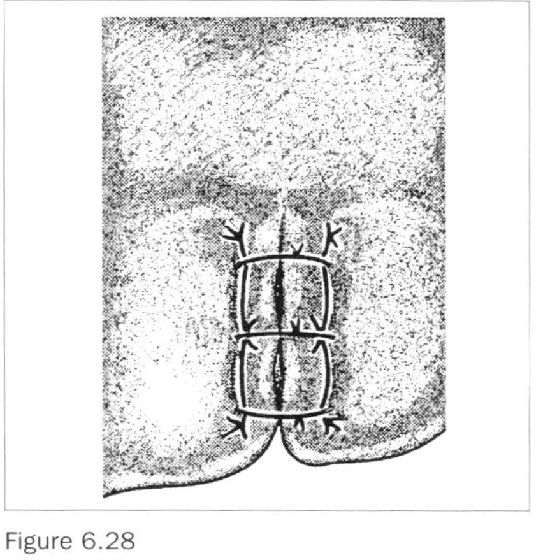

Figure 6.28

KEY POINTS

- The technique for small bowel resection is the same as for trauma and gangrene secondary to hernia or adhesions
- The bacterial count in the small bowel is low so anastomosis is almost always appropriate.

SMALL INTESTINE

In nonviable small intestine:
- Bowel will be black or deep blue without peristalsis
- Mesenteric veins may appear thrombosed
- Arterial pulsation may be absent
- The serosa will have lost its shiny appearance.

Make the decision to resect a part of the small intestine after you have inspected the entire gut. If there is a perforation in the intestine, repair the wound with a purse string invaginating suture or with a transverse two layer invaginating closure.

When several wounds are close together, or if the gut is ischaemic, resect the damaged loop and make an end-to-end anastomosis.

Reasons for resection include:
- Traumatic perforation
- Gangrene
- Tear of the mesentery with an ischaemic loop of bowel.

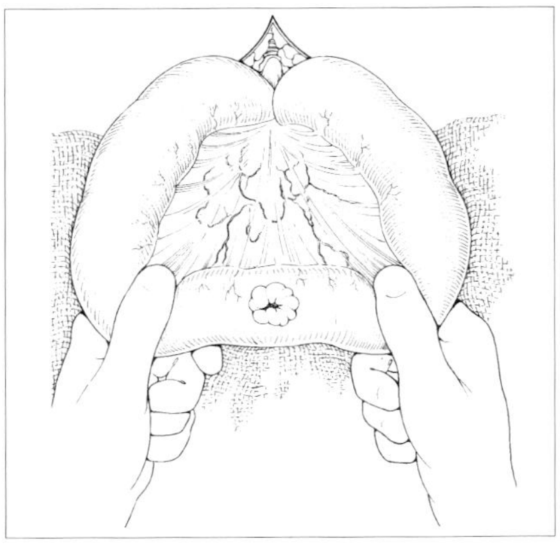

Figure 6.29

Techniques

Closure of a small wound

1 Expose the wounded portion of the intestine (Figure 6.29) and pull the gut transversely with stay sutures (Figure 6.30).

2 Insert the first layer of invaginating sutures to include all layers of the gut wall (Figure 6.31). The second layer, serosa to serosa, completes the repair (Figure 6.32).

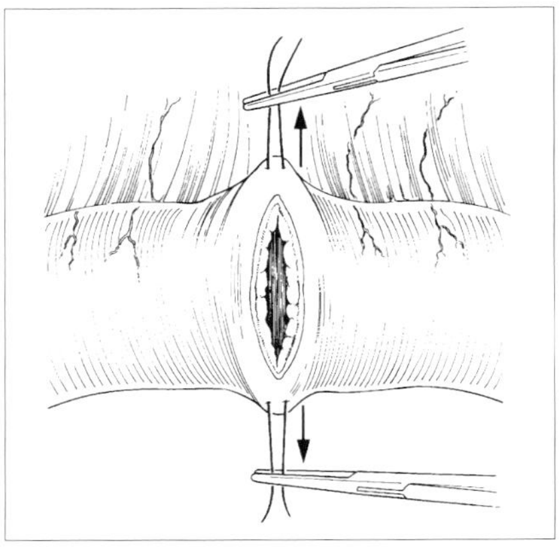

Figure 6.30

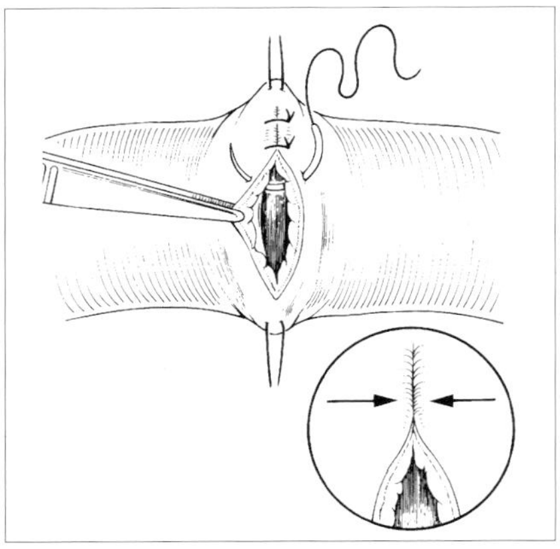

Figure 6.31

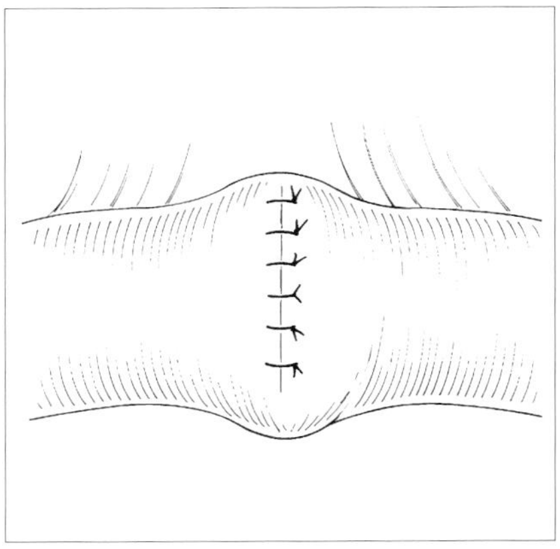

Figure 6.32

Resection

1 Determine the extent of the loop to be resected, including a small margin of healthy gut on either side (Figure 6.33). Hold up the loop so that you can see the mesenteric vessels against the light. Plan to divide the mesentery in a V-fashion or separate it from the intestinal wall, depending upon the length of the mesentery.

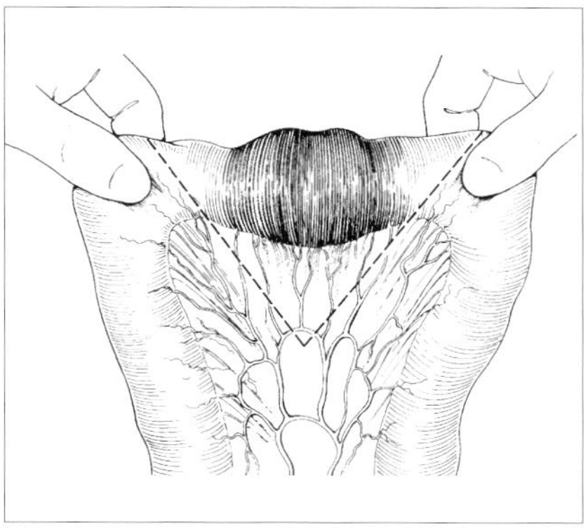

Figure 6.33

2 Isolate the mesenteric vessels by making blunt holes in the mesentery on either side of the vessel. Doubly ligate each vessel and then divide it between the ligatures (Figures 6.34, 6.35). Continue dividing the mesentery until you have isolated the section of gut to be resected.

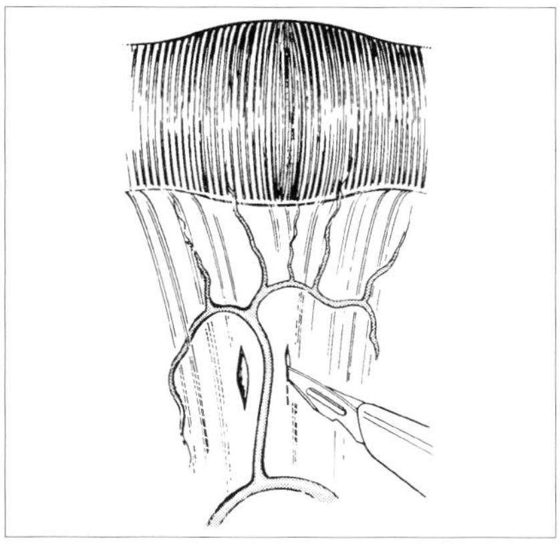

Figure 6.34

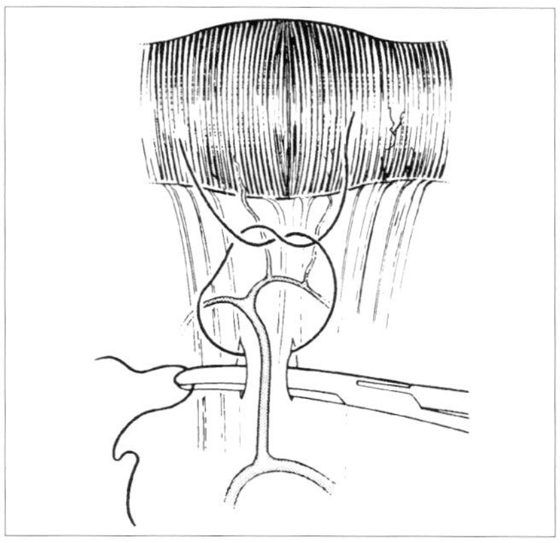

Figure 6.35

3 Apply crushing clamps to both ends of the isolated loop and gently "milk" the normal bowel above and below the loop to move contents away from the planned point of resection. Once these sections of gut have been emptied, apply light occlusion clamps to the bowel 3–4 cm beyond the crushing clamps.

4 Under the loop of bowel, place a swab that has been soaked in saline and wrung out. Holding the knife blade against one of the crushing clamps, divide the gut (Figure 6.36).

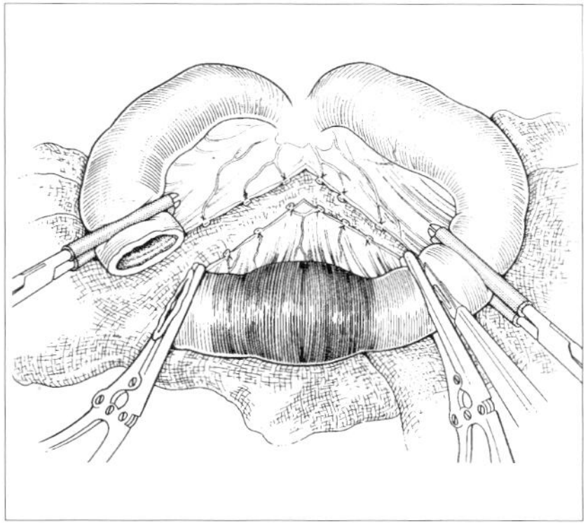

Figure 6.36

5 Clean the exposed part of the lumen and discard the used swab. Temporarily release the occlusion clamp and check to see whether the cut ends of the bowel bleed freely. If so, reapply the clamp. If not, resect the bowel further until it bleeds freely. The healing of the anastomosis depends on a good supply of blood. Confirm that the section of gut between the second pair of clamps also has a good blood supply.

Anastomosis

1 Make the anastomosis carefully using a two-layer technique. Use continuous sutures of 2/0 absorbable suture on a half circle atraumatic needle. First, bring together the occlusion clamps and hold them in position to appose the cut ends of the bowel (Figure 6.37). Check the proper orientation of the

gut and steady the tissues by joining the cut ends with seromuscular stay sutures at each end of the planned anastomosis (Figure 6.38).

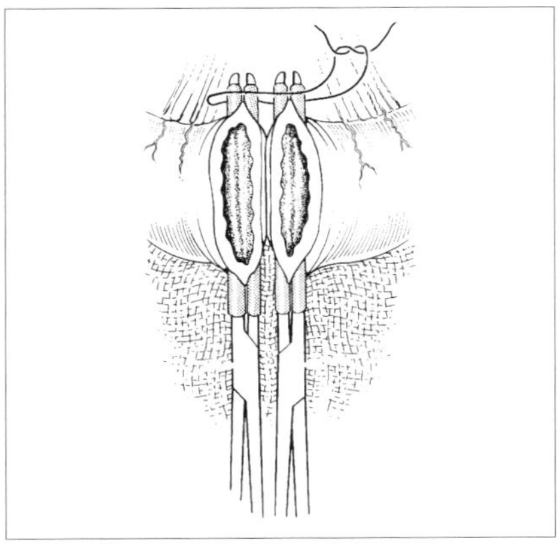

Figure 6.37

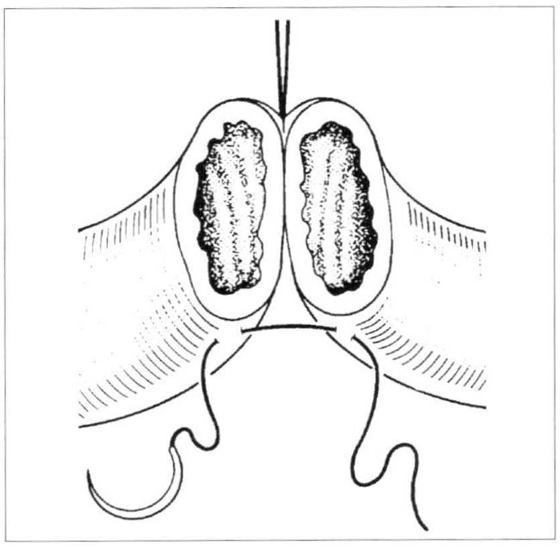

Figure 6.38

2 Begin the anastomosis by inserting the inner layer of absorbable sutures. Start at one corner of the bowel, knotting the suture to anchor it (Figure 6.39). Leave one end long enough to be held with forceps. Use the other end with the needle to make a continuous "over-and-over" stitch through the full thickness of the gut wall (Figure 6.40). When the back is completed, pass the needle out from the mucosa to the serosa on one side and then back from the serosa to the mucosa on the other (Figure 6.41).

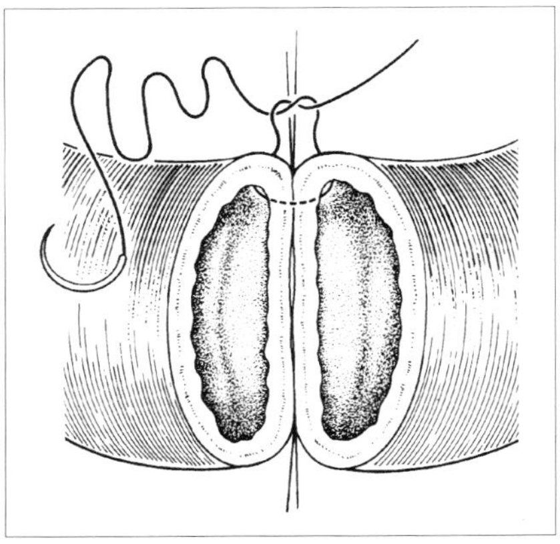

Figure 6.39

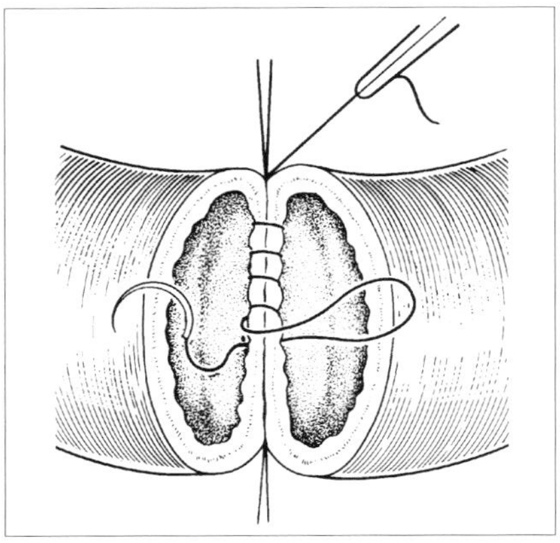

Figure 6.40

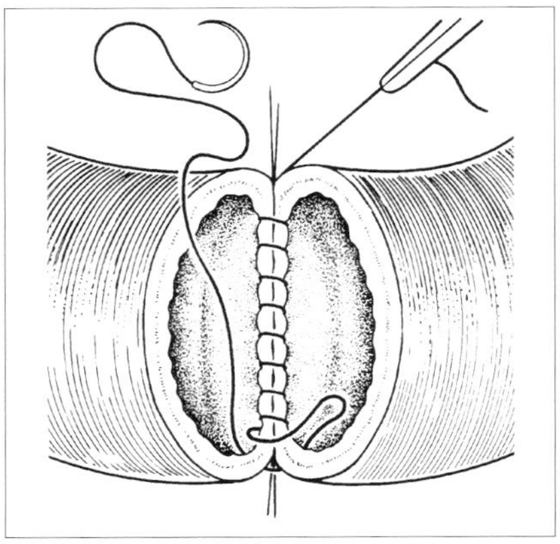

Figure 6.41

Invert the corner by applying traction to the axis of the suture line and suture the anterior wall as an "under-and-under" stitch to invaginate the edge of the bowel (Figures 6.42, 6.43). Continue the stitch back to the origin and knot it to the end that has been left long (Figures 6.44, 6.45). Remove the occlusion clamps.

3 Place a second continuous suture by picking up the serosa and muscle coats on both sides of the bowel, covering the previous suture line (Figure 6.46). Tie this suture to the stay suture at the end and turn the bowel over. Continue the suture to cover the other side of the anastomosis. Cut the ends of the stay sutures. The second layer can also be closed with interrupted absorbable or non-absorbable suture.

4 Close the mesentery with interrupted 2/0 absorbable suture, taking care not to puncture the blood vessels. Check the adequacy of the stoma by

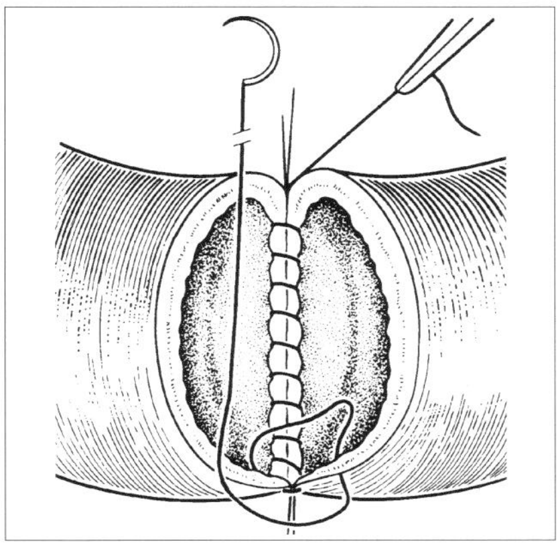

Figure 6.42

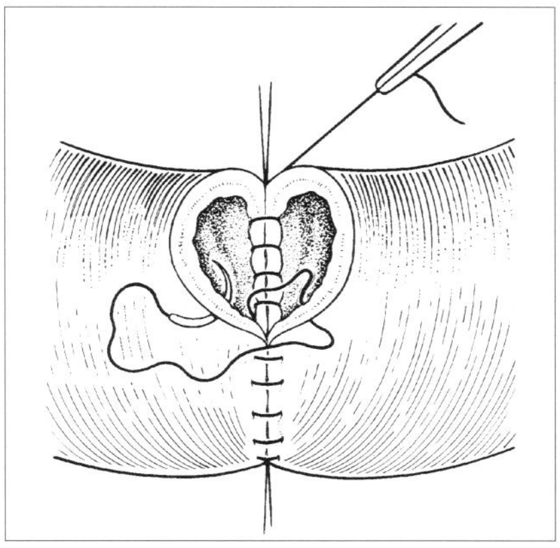

Figure 6.43

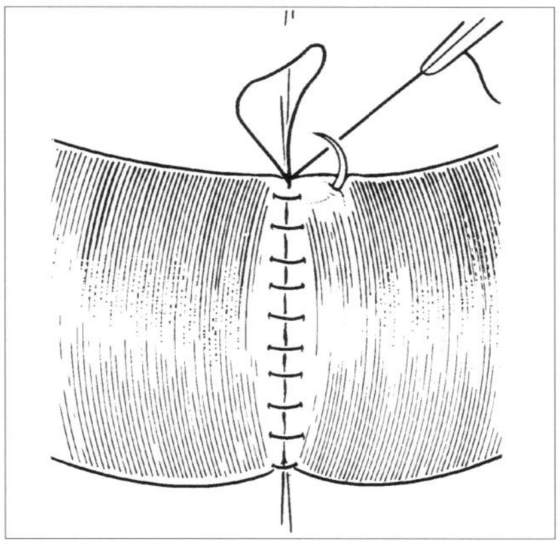

Figure 6.44

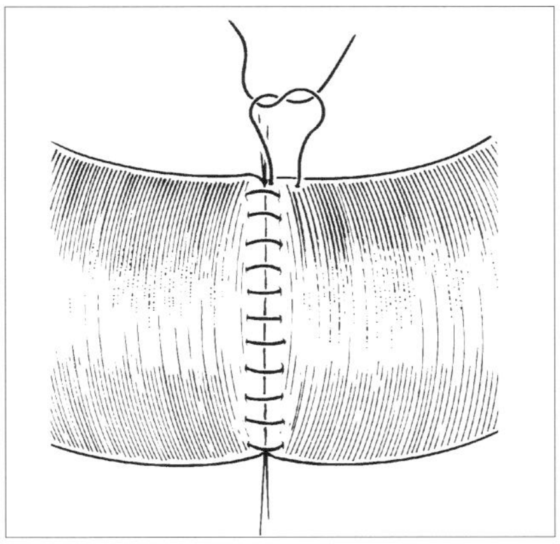

Figure 6.45

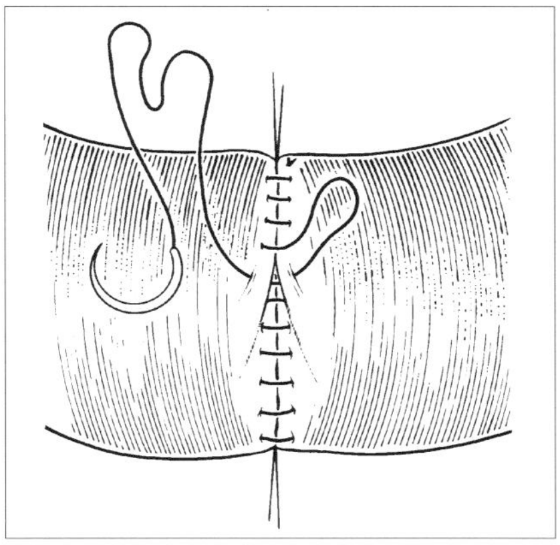

Figure 6.46

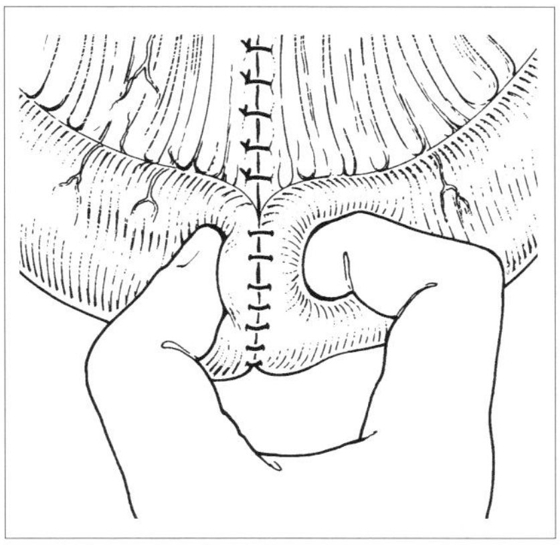

Figure 6.47

palpation: it should admit the tip of the thumb and finger (Figure 6.47). Close the laparotomy incision.

COLON

Treatment of colon injuries is dependent upon the location:

- Treat transverse colon injuries with exteriorization of the site of injury as a colostomy
- Treat left (descending) colon injuries with exteriorization of the injury site through a colostomy; drain the paracolic gutter and the pelvis
- Treat right (ascending) colon injuries with resection of the entire right colon; make an ileostomy and transverse colostomy – do not attempt to repair the injury directly
- An alternative in the treatment of colonic injury or perforation is to defunction the lesion by creating a colostomy or an ileostomy upstream from the lesion, and placing a large latex drain near that lesion
- Patients with colonic trauma require antibiotics.

KEY POINTS

- It is important for the practitioner at the district hospital to be capable of performing a colostomy
- Closing a colostomy may be difficult and should be performed electively by a specialist surgeon
- Colostomy closure should not be performed earlier than 3 months.

Selecting the type of colostomy

- Normally, a loop colostomy is the easiest (Figure 6.48A)
- If you have to resect a piece of colon, perform a double-barrelled colostomy with the two free ends (Figures 6.48B)

6

- Use an end colostomy (Figure 6.48C) when the distal stump is too short to exteriorize after the gangrenous or injured loop has been resected; this is particularly useful in the sigmoid colon and proximal rectum
- Use an end ileostomy after right colon resection when anastomosis is not performed.

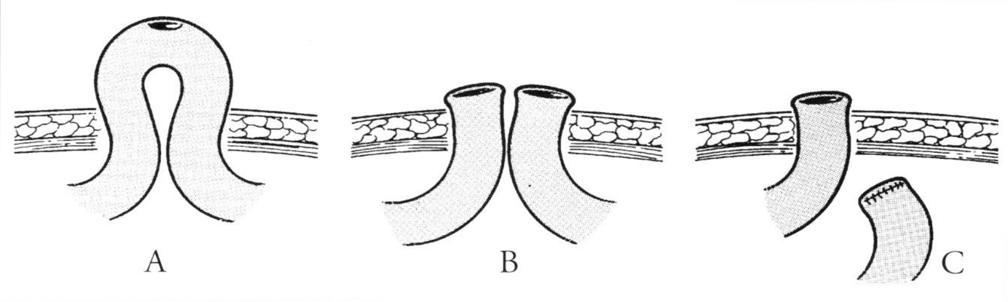

Figure 6.48

Techniques

Determine the site for the colostomy at surgery. Make an incision separate from the main wound in the quadrant of the abdomen nearest to the loop to be exteriorized. Use the greater omentum as a guide to locate the transverse colon.

Loop colostomy

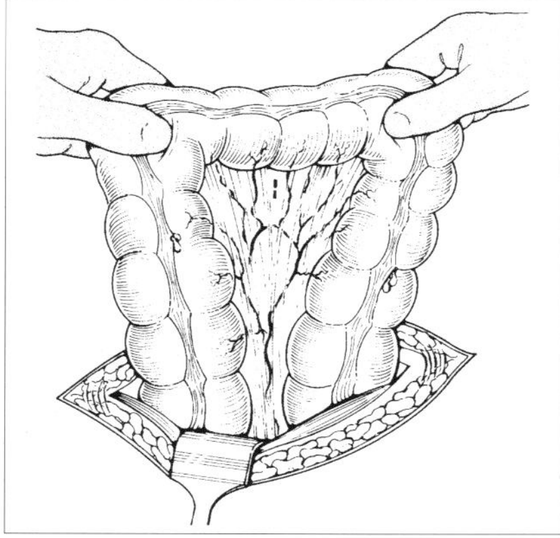

Figure 6.49

1 Bring out the loop of colon without kinking or twisting it (Figure 6.49). Make an opening in the mesocolon just large enough to admit a piece of glass rod. Push the rod halfway through the opening and attach its ends to the ends of a piece of polythene tubing (Figure 6.50, 6.51). As an alternative, insert a catheter through the mesocolon and join the ends with sutures of 2/0 thread. Close the wound around the exteriorized loop of gut.

2 The opening in the colon may be made immediately, provided that extreme care is taken to prevent mechanical contamination of the wound. Alternatively defer making the opening for 8 to 24 hours when there is less risk of wound contamination. Make a cruciate incision in the apex of the loop with a knife or diathermy (Figure 6.52). Pack petroleum gauze and gauze swabs around the colostomy.

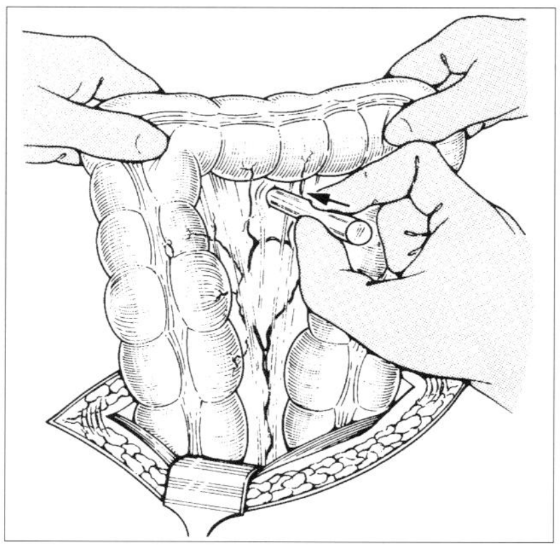

Figure 6.50

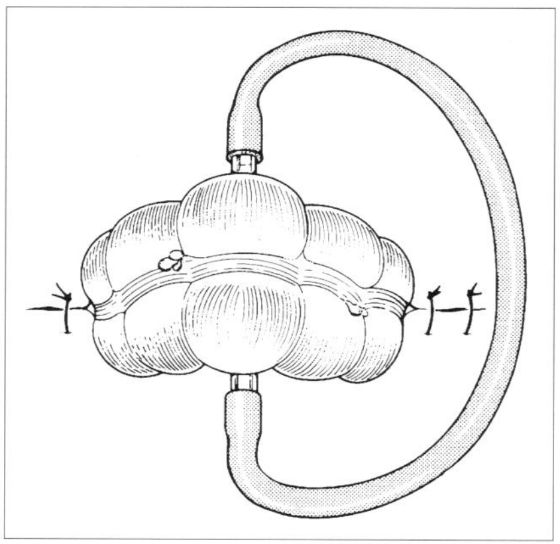

Figure 6.51

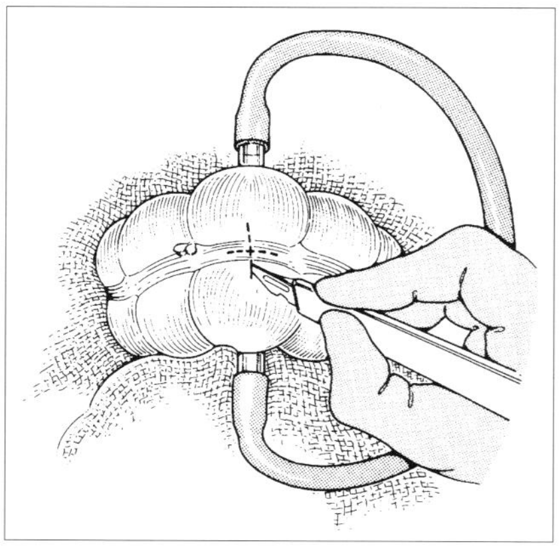

Figure 6.52

Double-barrelled colostomy

1 Resect the gangrenous loop of colon as described for resection of the small intestine (see page 6–10). Mobilize the remaining colon so that the limbs to be used for the colostomy lie without tension.

2 Bring the two clamped ends of bowel out through a stab wound or gridiron incision and keep them clamped until the laparotomy incision has been closed (Figure 6.53). Then remove the clamps and fix the full thickness of the gut edge to the margin of the stab wound. Approximate mucosa to skin edge with interrupted 2/0 absorbable suture (Figures 6.54, 6.55). If a bag is not available, cover the colostomy with generous padding.

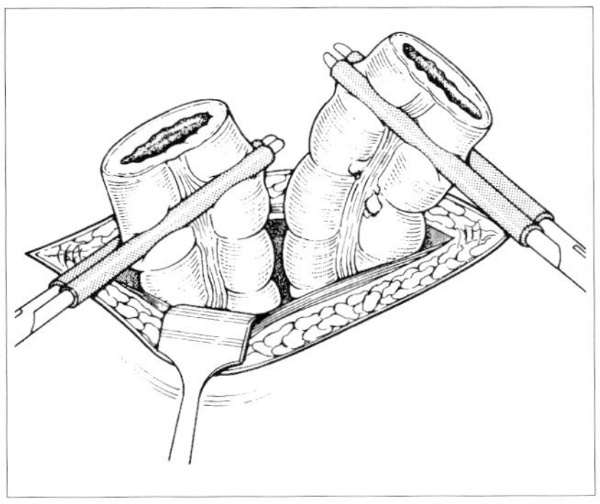

Figure 6.53

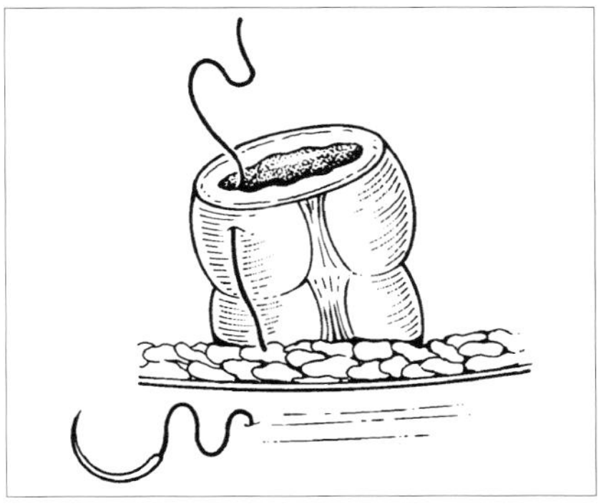

Figure 6.54

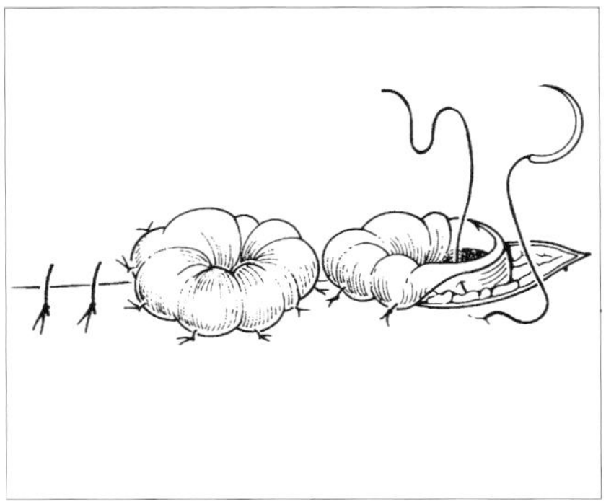

Figure 6.55

End colostomy

1 Bring out the proximal end of the colon through a gridiron incision (Figure 6.56). Close the distal stump of colon without further attempt at mobilization using two layers of stitches: an inner, continuous stitch of 2/0 absorbable suture covered by an outer seromuscular layer of interrupted 2/0 polyglycolic or non-absorbable suture (Figures 6.57 to 6.60). Attach a 5–6 long non-absorbable suture to the distal stump so that it can be found more easily at the time of re-anastomosis.

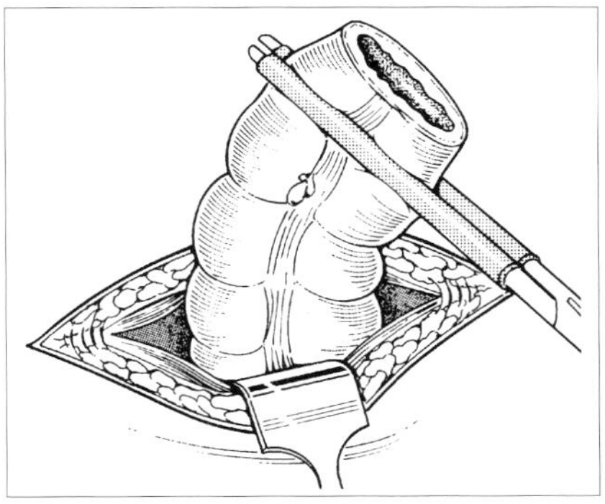

Figure 6.56

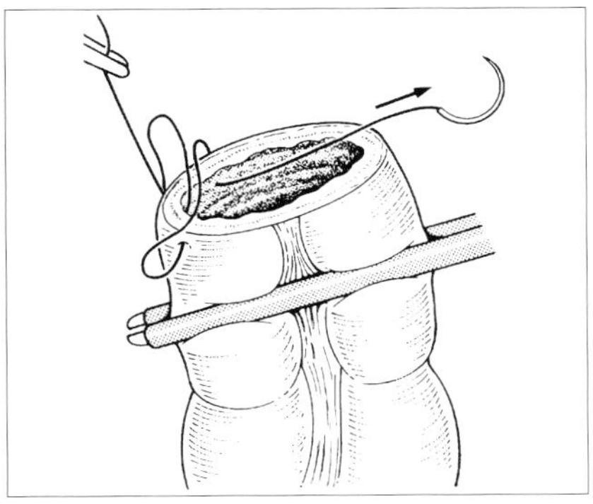

Figure 6.57

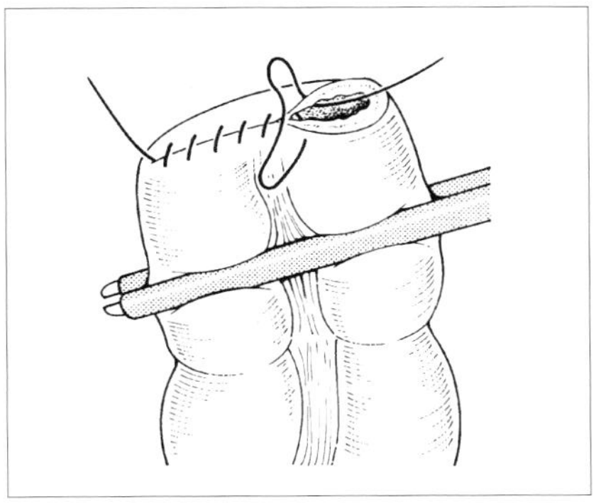

Figure 6.58

2 Drop this end of bowel back into the pelvis. Finally, stitch the proximal end to the margin of the stab wound.

Colostomy bags greatly ease the long-term care of the stoma.

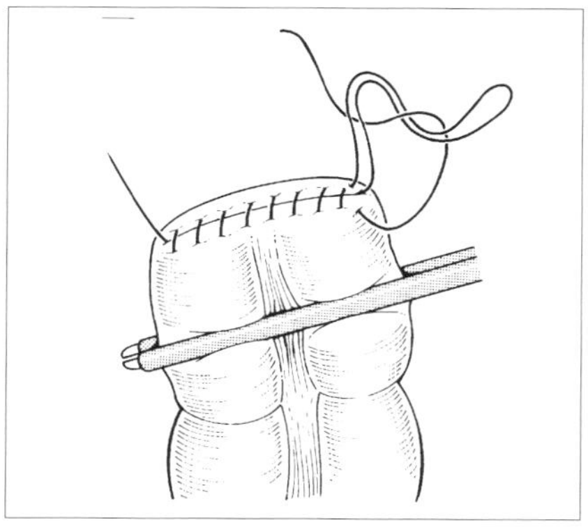

Figure 6.59

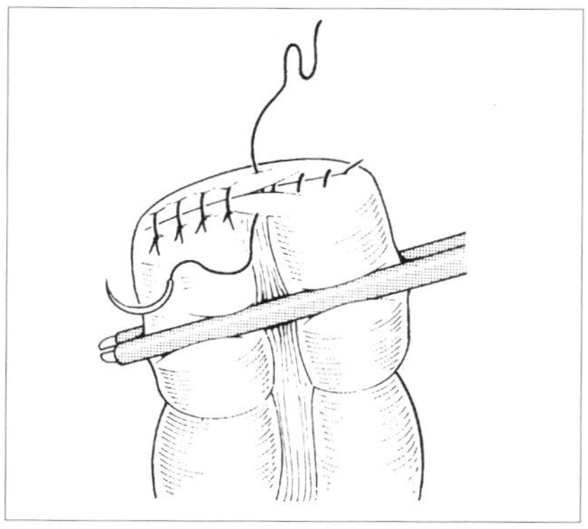

Figure 6.60

RETROPERITONEUM

Haematoma

A retroperitoneal haematoma may indicate trauma to a major vessel. If the patient is stable it should not be opened or disturbed. However, to save life, control and repair of a major vessel should be attempted at the district hospital.

Duodenum

Blunt trauma to the upper abdomen can result in retroperitoneal rupture of the duodenum. Air in the retroperitoneum is diagnostic. The retroperitoneum is opened with blunt dissection and the duodenal perforation closed transversely in two layers. This repair should be protected with a nasogastric tube and, after thorough cleansing of the retroperitoneum, a drain should be placed near but not on the duodenal repair.

Pancreas

Confirm an injury to the pancreas by opening the lesser sac through the gastrocolic (greater) omentum. The only safe procedure at the district hospital is to put a drain at the site of injury. The drain should traverse the lesser sac and come out in the flank. Specialized surgery may be necessary. Make arrangements for referral when the patient is stable.

Kidney

Do not expose the kidney unless there is life-threatening bleeding. An expanding or pulsating haematoma is evidence of such bleeding. Stop the bleeding at the site of the tear with stitches. Consider the need for specialized surgery.

RUPTURE OF THE BLADDER

Extraperitoneal rupture

Extraperitoneal rupture is most commonly associated with fracture of the pelvis, resulting in extravasation of urine (Figure 6.60). The patient may pass only small drops of blood when attempting to pass urine. A significant feature is swollen soft tissues of the groin extending to the scrotum, due to extravasated urine.

KEY POINTS

- Bladder rupture, usually due to trauma, can be extraperitoneal or intraperitoneal
- Extraperitoneal rupture is most commonly associated with fracture of the pelvis
- Intraperitoneal rupture is often the result of a direct blow to the bladder or a sudden deceleration.

Intraperitoneal rupture

Intraperitoneal rupture is often the result of a direct blow to the bladder or a sudden deceleration of the patient when the bladder is distended, for example in a road traffic accident (Figure 6.62). Intraperitoneal rupture presents as "acute abdomen", with pain in the lower abdomen, tenderness and guarding associated with failure to pass urine.

- If possible, urgently refer patients with rupture of the bladder to a surgical specialist
- For extraperitoneal rupture, construct a suprapubic cystostomy; if the rupture is large, also place a latex drain
- For intraperitoneal rupture, close the rupture and drain the bladder with a large urethral catheter or a suprapubic drain; if the rupture is large, also place a latex drain
- Evaluate your patient carefully to ensure that other injuries are not missed. A ruptured bladder is an indication for a full trauma laparotomy to rule out other abdominal injuries.

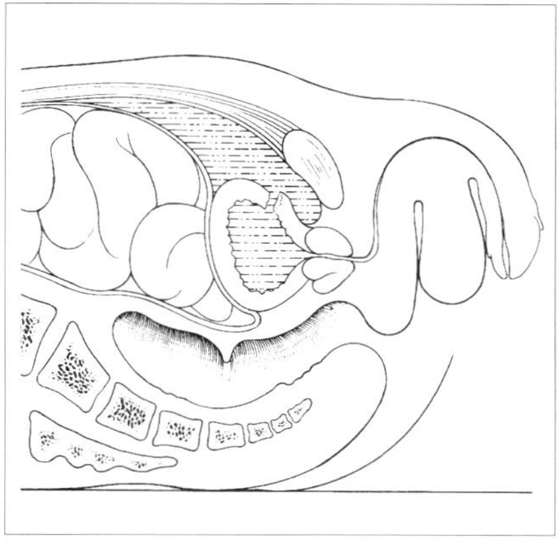

Figure 6.61

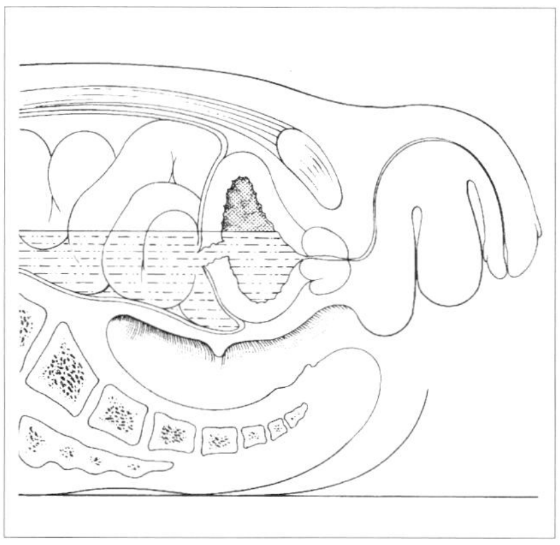

Figure 6.62

MANAGEMENT OF RUPTURED BLADDER

Technique

1 Administer a general anaesthetic. Expose the bladder as in the initial stages of cystostomy with a midline suprapubic incision between the umbilicus and the symphysis pubis. Achieve haemostasis by pressure and ligation. Open the rectus sheath, starting in the upper part of the wound. Continue dissection with scissors to expose the gap between the muscles. In the lower part of the incision, the pyramidalis muscles will obscure this gap. Carry the incision in the linea alba down to the pubis, splitting the pyramidalis muscles. With a finger, break through the prevesical fascia behind the pubis; then sweep the fascia and peritoneum upwards from the bladder surface. Take care not to open the peritoneum if it has not already been torn. Insert a self-retaining retractor to hold this exposure. Cautiously aspirate any blood or urine in the retropubic space, but leave the area unexplored, as uncontrollable bleeding can result.

2 In a patient with intraperitoneal rupture, the bladder will be empty. The site of the tear is usually in the fundus of the bladder. Open the peritoneum, inspect the site of the rupture, and aspirate the fluid in the peritoneal cavity. Introduce a Foley catheter into the bladder through the urethra and then suture the tear with two layers of seromuscular stitches of 0 absorbable suture. Do not include the mucosa in the first layer (Figures 6.63, 6.64, 6.65). After inspecting the other viscera, close the abdomen.

3 Extraperitoneal rupture is usually associated with bladder distension and extravasation, which become obvious when you expose the bladder. Open the bladder, and look for the site of the tear. It may be difficult to find but, if it is clearly visible, close it from within with 2/0 absorbable suture and insert a suprapubic catheter. If no tear is apparent, simply insert a suprapubic catheter. Close the opening in the bladder to construct a suprapubic cystostomy. Insert a latex drain into the retropubic space and close the wound in layers.

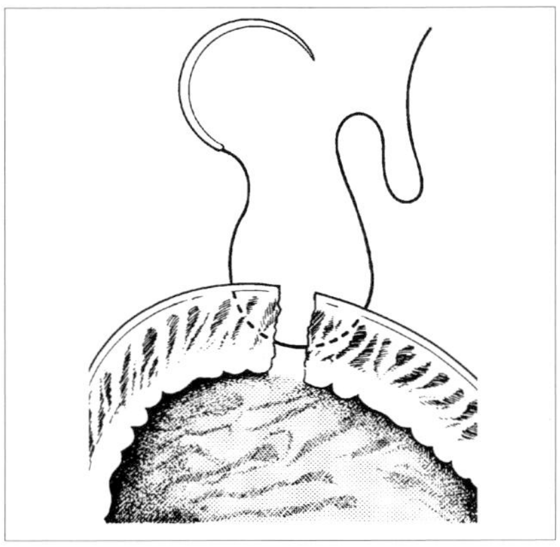

Figure 6.63

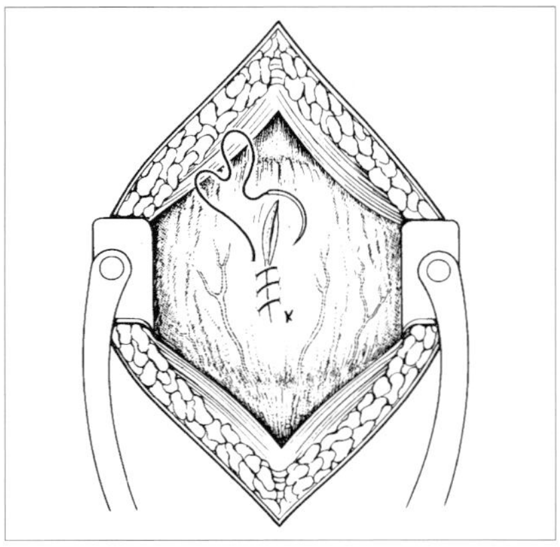

Figure 6.64

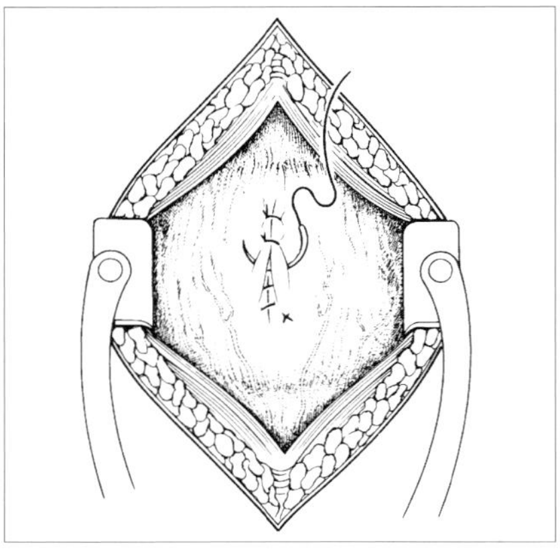

Figure 6.65

Aftercare

1 Administer antibiotics for the first five days and give adequate fluids to maintain the urinary output. The drain can be removed when urine or blood drainage has ceased.

2 For extraperitoneal rupture, clamp the catheter for increasing periods of time, beginning on about the fifth day. The patient with a suprapubic catheter may start passing urine during this period; if so, remove the catheter.

3 In cases of intraperitoneal rupture, remove the urethral catheter after about two days of intermittent clamping, provided that no problems result.

Acute abdominal conditions

7

7.1 ASSESSMENT AND DIAGNOSIS

Referred abdominal pain

Gastrointestinal obstruction, perforation and strangulation are important conditions which usually present with abdominal pain, although pain may also be referred. The location of referred abdominal pain is based on the embryological origin of the affected organ, while the location of peritoneal irritation depends on the anatomical position of the diseased organ. In cases where the diagnosis is not clear, repeated physical examination at frequent intervals will often clarify the need for surgery. It is prudent to seek a second opinion to assist in an equivocal case.

Surgical exploration

The treatment of many acute abdominal conditions includes surgical abdominal exploration. Use laparotomy to expose the abdominal organs and confirm the diagnosis. The patient's history and physical examination should suggest the diagnosis and help determine the site of incision.

Avoid performing a laparotomy for pancreatitis. If surgery is indicated, do not avoid it in vulnerable patients including the young, old or pregnant. The foetus is best protected by providing the mother with optimum care. Use the midline incision which is simple, does not cause much bleeding, can be performed rapidly, closed quickly and extended easily. The midline laparotomy incision is described in Unit 6: *Laparotomy and Abdominal Trauma*. The gridiron incision for appendectomy is described on page 7–11 and the groin incision for hernia in Unit 8: *Abdominal Wall Hernia*. The surgical practitioner at the district hospital who can perform these three incisions can successfully manage most acute abdominal conditions.

Peritoneal irritation

Peritoneal irritation can be localized or generalized. Findings that are important indications for surgery, are:

- Abdominal tenderness, suggesting inflammation of an underlying organ
- Rebound abdominal tenderness elicited by percussion, which confirms peritoneal irritation
- Involuntary contraction of the abdominal wall, a sign of peritoneal irritation, which presents as local guarding or generalized rigidity.

Physical examination

The history and physical examination are crucial to determine the most likely causes of an acute abdomen. The precise location of abdominal pain and

KEY POINTS

- Fore gut pain (stomach, duodenum, gall bladder) is referred to the upper abdomen
- Mid gut pain (small intestine, appendix, right colon is referred to the mid abdomen
- Hind gut pain (mid transverse, descending, sigmoid colon and rectum) occurs in lower abdomen
- Diseased retroperitoneal organs (kidney, pancreas) may present with back pain
- Ureteric pain radiates to the testicle or labia
- Diaphragmatic irritation presents as shoulder tip pain.

7

tenderness helps the practitioner to make a differential diagnosis. Although there are many acute abdominal conditions, only a few causes are common at any facility. Inflammatory bowel disease and colonic cancers are unusual at the district hospital while trauma, hernia and bowel obstruction are common. Become familiar with the patterns in your locality.

When doing a physical examination:

- Determine the vital signs
  - Rapid respiration may indicate pneumonia
  - Tachycardia and hypotension indicate patient decompensation
  - Temperature is elevated in gastrointestinal perforation and normal in gastrointestinal obstruction
- Look for abdominal distension
  - Percuss to differentiate gas from liquid
- Palpate the abdomen
  - Start away from the site of tenderness
  - Check for masses or tumours
  - Determine the site of maximum tenderness
  - Check for abdominal rigidity
- Listen for bowel sounds
  - Absence is a sign of peritonitis or ileus
  - High pitched tinkling indicates obstruction
- Always examine:
  - Groin for incarcerated hernia
  - Rectum for signs of trauma, abscess, obstruction
  - Vagina for pelvic abscess, ectopic pregnancy, distended pouch of Douglas.

7.2 INTESTINAL OBSTRUCTION

KEY POINTS

- In small bowel obstruction, pain is mid-abdominal while in large bowel obstruction the pain is below the umbilicus
- The more proximal the bowel obstruction, the more frequent the vomiting
- The more distal the bowel obstruction, the more distended the abdomen
- For paralytic ileus (non-mechanical obstruction):
  - Provide nasogastric suction and intravenous fluids until gut function returns
  - Maintain fluid and electrolyte balance
  - Treat the underlying cause.

ASSESSMENT

A number of different conditions can cause intestinal obstruction. Intestinal obstruction may be mechanical or non-mechanical (paralytic ileus). Attention to hydration with intravenous fluid resuscitation is vital in all patients with intestinal obstruction. If the obstruction is not resolved, either by non-operative or operative treatment, intestinal gangrene or perforation will occur and lead to peritonitis. Bowel obstruction presents with:

- Abdominal pain, which may be colicky
- Vomiting
- Obstipation (absence of bowel movements and flatus)
- Abdominal distension.

Bowel obstruction is a clinical diagnosis but it is greatly aided by plain erect and supine abdominal X-rays. The normal small bowel does not contain air and is therefore not visualized on X-ray. Distended loops of small bowel with air fluid levels are diagnostic of obstruction. Valvule coniventes cross the entire small bowel lumen and, when seen on X-ray, also indicate that the obstruction is intestinal.

Causes of intestinal obstruction

Mechanical	Non-mechanical
• Adhesion bands (following previous abdominal operation or peritonitis) • Hernia • Volvulus (particularly sigmoid volvulus) • Neoplasms • Intussusception (especially in children) • Bowel ischaemia	• Post-operative paralytic ileus (after abdominal surgery) • Peritonitis • Spinal injury • Drugs, hypokalaemia

NON-OPERATIVE MANAGEMENT OF INTESTINAL OBSTRUCTION

The treatment of simple mechanical small bowel obstruction is initially non-operative. *Failure of non-operative management at 48 hours is an indication for laparotomy.* Non-mechanical obstruction should be treated non-operatively. However, an obstruction caused by an underlying problem like abdominal abscess or generalized peritonitis will require surgery. The resuscitation procedure in non-operative management prepares the patient for surgery if it becomes necessary.

1 Administer intravenous fluids, starting with normal saline or Ringer's lactate and changing on the basis of serum electrolyte results.

2 Insert a nasogastric tube and commence aspirations.

3 Relieve pain with narcotic analgesics.

4 Monitor the response to fluids with vital signs and urinary output. Remember that intestinal obstruction causes dehydration so relatively large volumes of fluid are required to assure adequate urine output.

5 Ascertain from the history, physical examination and plain X-rays the cause of the obstruction.

6 Observe the patient's condition with serial physical examination to determine whether the obstruction is getting better or worse. Do this at least two times per day.

Evidence of improvement includes:

- Reduction in abdominal distension
- Reduction in peristaltic waves (which become less visible)
- Progressive reduction in nasogastric aspirates.

Evidence of deterioration includes:

- Colicky pain that becomes persistent
- Rigid, tender and silent abdomen
- Increasing abdominal distension
- Visible peristaltic waves.

KEY POINTS

In ileus (non-mechanical obstruction):

- Treat the underlying medical cause
- Treat the underlying surgical cause with operation, as indicated.

KEY POINTS

- Gangrene is an indication for small bowel resection
- Strangulated hernia and small bowel obstructions from adhesions can lead to gangrene
- The technique for anastomosis of the small bowel is the same for all indications.

OPERATIVE MANAGEMENT OF SMALL INTESTINAL OBSTRUCTION

The operative management of intestinal obstruction is laparotomy, with specific surgical intervention depending on the findings. Laparotomy should be performed using a midline incision (see pages 6–1 to 6–3).

Division of adhesions to release the obstruction is often the treatment in mechanical small bowel obstruction when non-operative management has failed. If the small intestine is not viable (gangrenous) it should be resected and an anastomosis performed (see pages 6–12 to 6–13).

If the small bowel obstruction is due to inguinal hernia, the hernia should be repaired (see Unit 8: *Abdominal Wall Hernia*). If the small bowel is not viable, it must be resected. If this cannot easily be done through the groin incision, make a lower midline incision and perform the resection through the abdominal approach.

Intestinal gangrene is:

- An indication for laparotomy and intestinal resection
- Suspected when there is continuous abdominal pain
- Associated with tachycardia and fever
- Often associated with reduced blood pressure (shock is a late sign)
- Associated with abdominal tenderness, guarding and absent bowel sounds.

7.3 PERITONITIS

Peritonitis is an acute life-threatening condition caused by bacterial or chemical contamination of the peritoneal cavity. Neglected chemical peritonitis will progress to bacterial peritonitis. The treatment of peritonitis is the treatment of the underlying cause.

Causes

The major causes of peritonitis include:

- Appendicitis
- Perforated peptic ulcer
- Anastomotic leak following surgery
- Strangulated bowel
- Pancreatitis
- Cholecystitis
- Intra-abdominal abscess
- Haematogenous spread of infective agents such as typhoid or tuberculosis
- Typhoid perforation
- Ascending infection: for example, in salpingitis and postpartum infection.

7

Clinical features

Clinical features of peritonitis include:

- Sharp pain, which is worse on movement or coughing
- Fever
- Abdominal distension, tenderness and guarding
- Diminished or absent bowel sounds
- Shoulder pain (referred from diaphragm)
- Tenderness on rectal or vaginal examination (suggests pelvic peritonitis).

These features may be minimal in elderly patients, the very young and those with immune suppression.

Management

1 Make a differential diagnosis of the most likely underlying cause of the peritonitis/abscess.

2 Administer normal saline or Ringer's lactate, depending on the serum electrolyte results.

3 Insert a nasogastric tube and commence aspirations.

4 Give triple antibiotic therapy intravenously, providing aerobic, gram negative and anaerobic coverage. For example, ampicillin 2 g IV every 6 hours plus gentamicin 5 mg/kg body weight IV every 24 hours plus metronidazole 500 mg IV every 8 hours.

5 Record fluid balance and vital signs on the bedside chart every six hours.

Surgical intervention will depend on the diagnosis of the cause of the peritonitis: for example, appendectomy, closure of a perforation or drainage of an abscess.

> Intestinal obstruction may respond to non operative management, but peritonitis indicates gangrene or perforation and therefore requires surgery.

7.4 STOMACH AND DUODENUM

PEPTIC ULCER

Peptic ulceration occurs in the stomach and duodenum and leads to intestinal bleeding, perforation into the abdominal cavity and pyloric obstruction. Initial management of a bleeding ulcer is medical with surgery considered only if medical management fails.

Perforating duodenal ulcers are most often located anteriorly, while stomach ulcers may be at the front or back. Perforation causes a chemical peritonitis followed in about 12 hours by secondary bacterial contamination and sepsis. Treat with surgical closure of the perforation.

KEY POINTS

- Peptic ulcers are caused by helicobacter pylori infection
- The treatment of helicobacter pylori is triple medical therapy:
  - Proton inhibitors
  - Antibiotics
  - Bismuth subsalicylate
- Surgery is indicated for obstruction, bleeding and perforations
- Surgical treatment of bleeding or obstructive complications of peptic ulcer should be performed by a specialist.

7

Medical management of bleeding ulcers

To manage a bleeding ulcer medically:

- Establish a large bore IV line and resuscitate with normal saline or Ringers lactate
- Aspirate blood from the stomach with a nasogastric tube
- Record blood pressure and pulse rate
- Transfuse if the patient is hypotensive or loses more than 1 litre of blood.

Most bleeding stops without surgical intervention. Refer the patient for surgery if the bleeding persists or recurs after it has stopped.

Surgery for bleeding ulcers requires a specialist surgeon.

Perforated peptic ulcer

Diagnosis

The typical history includes:

- Sudden onset of severe abdominal pain
- Intense burning pain in the upper abdomen after the acute episode
- Extreme pain with any movement
- Absent prodromal symptoms.

The major physical findings are:

- Extremely tender, rigid abdomen
- Absent or reduced bowel sounds
- Free gas in the abdominal cavity seen on a left lateral decubitus or erect chest X-ray
- (Later) development of septic shock.

Treatment

A perforated peptic ulcer is an indication for emergency surgery. Delay in operation will adversely affect the prognosis. The delay becomes critical 6 hours after perforation.

The aim of treatment is to close the perforation and to remove the irritant fluid by abdominal lavage and suction.

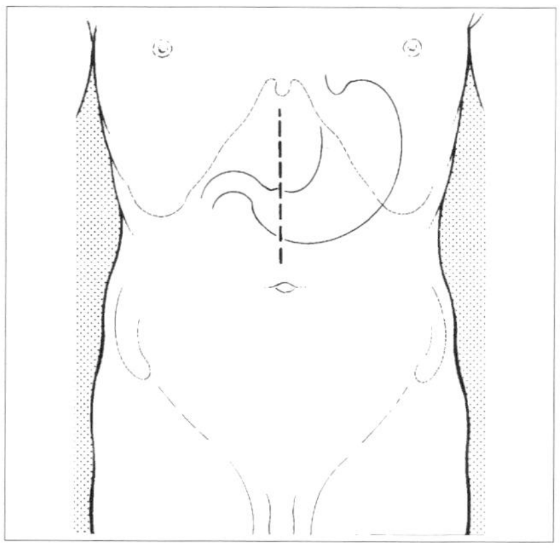

Figure 7.1

Technique

1 Preoperatively administer analgesia, pass a nasogastric tube with suction to remove the stomach contents and place an intravenous line. Give broad-spectrum antibiotics if the history of perforation is longer than 6 hours.

2 In the operating room, have suction available and prepare 5 litres or more of warm saline for peritoneal lavage.

3 Open the abdomen with an upper midline incision (Figure 7.1). Remove all fluid and food debris from the peritoneal cavity using suction and warm, moist abdominal packs. Gently retract the liver up, draw the stomach to the left by gentle traction over a warm pack and identify the perforation. Aspirate fluid, as necessary. Note the appearance of the gut wall adjacent

to the perforation; scarring suggests a chronic ulcer. If a perforation is not obvious, check the posterior wall of the stomach by opening the lesser sac of the peritoneum (Figures 7.2 and 7.3).

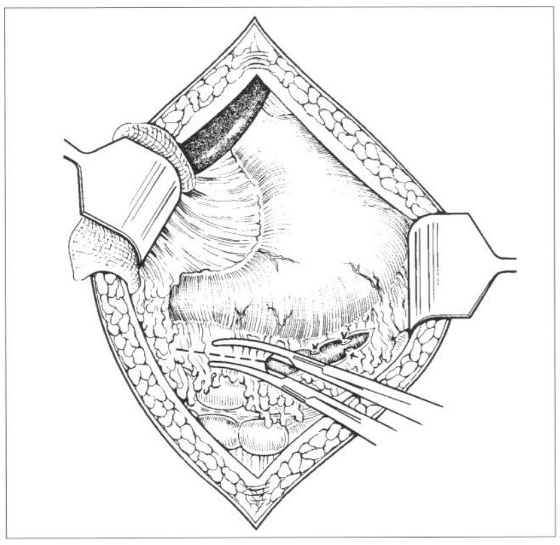

Figure 7.2

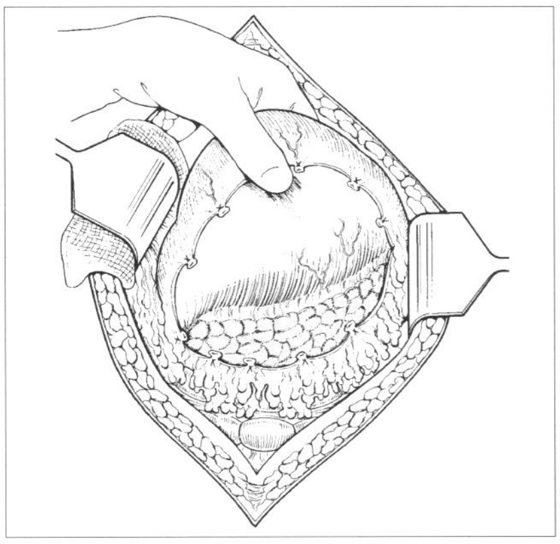

Figure 7.3

4 Insert three 2/0 polyglycolic acid or silk sutures at right angles to the long axis of the duodenum or stomach so that the middle stitch passes across the perforation itself, taking the full thickness of the gut wall about 5 mm from the edge of the perforation. The upper and lower stitches should take a generous seromuscular "bite" of the gut. Tie off the sutures loosely, leaving the ends long (Figures 7.4, 7.5). Draw a piece of adjacent omentum across the perforation and tie the three stitches over it (Figure 7.6).

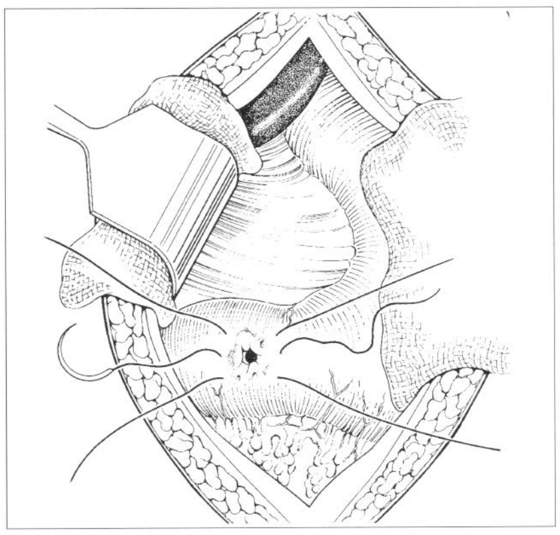

Figure 7.4

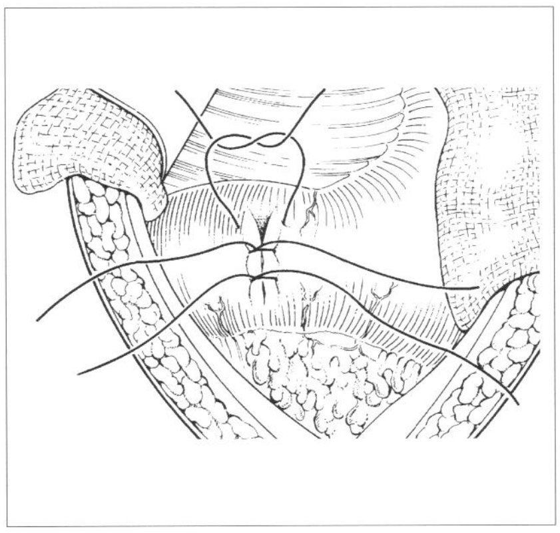

Figure 7.5

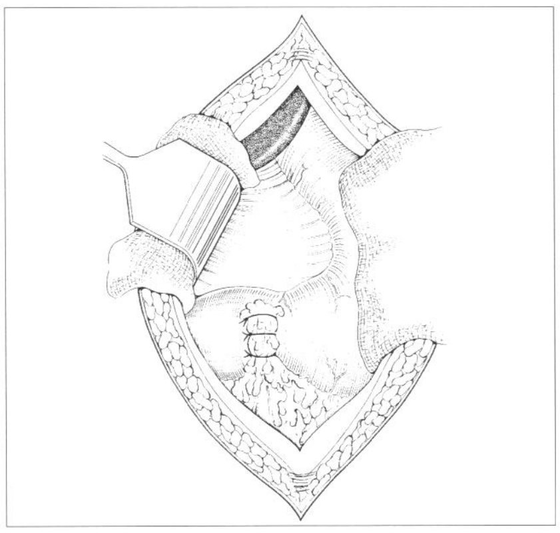

Figure 7.6

Alternatively, the three sutures can be left untied and tied only after the piece of omentum has been placed across the perforation.

5 Repair the greater omentum if you have divided it to locate a posterior perforation (Figure 7.7).

6 Thoroughly cleanse the peritoneal cavity with warm saline irrigation. In particular, pay attention to the subphrenic and pelvic spaces. Repeat saline irrigation and aspiration until the returned aspirate is clear on two consecutive occasions. Close the abdominal wound in layers, except in cases of gross contamination when the skin and subcutaneous tissues are packed open with damp saline gauze in preparation for delayed primary closure two days later.

7 Continue nasogastric aspiration and the intravenous administration of fluids and record fluid balance and vital signs. Give narcotic analgesia.

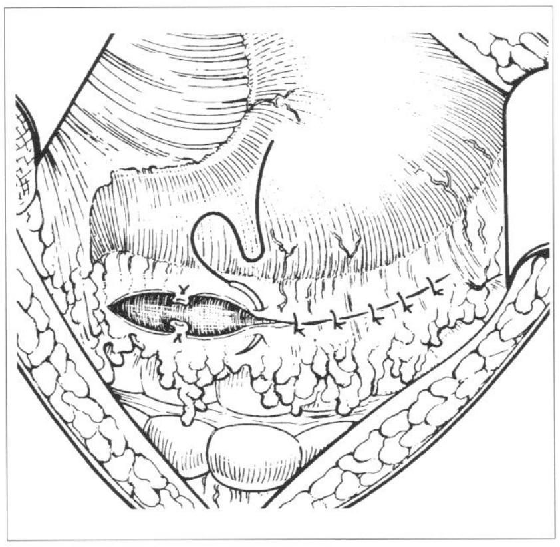

Figure 7.7

Give antibiotics if laparotomy was performed more than 6 hours after duodenal perforation.

Recovery is indicated by:

- Return of bowel sounds
- Passage of flatus
- Reduction in the volume of gastric aspirate
- Adequate urinary output
- Normal pulse, blood pressure and temperature.

After recovery, treat the peptic ulcer and follow the patient to be certain they do not have further symptoms. In most patients, peptic ulceration is secondary to helicobacter infection and medical treatment to eradicate this will prevent recurrence of the ulcer and preclude the need for further surgery.

KEY POINTS

Cholecystitis:

- Is caused by obstruction of the cystic duct by gall stones
- Presents with epigastric cramps then pain which radiates to the right upper quadrant
- May be treated by drainage of the gallbladder (cholecystostomy)
- When complicated with pyogenic infection, requires urgent cholecystostomy and intravenous antibiotics
- Should be referred to a surgical specialist if the patient is jaundiced.

7.5 GALLBLADDER

The indication for cholecystostomy is severe acute cholecystitis with a distended gallbladder that is in danger of rupture.

A relative indication is uncomplicated acute cholecystitis diagnosed by the non-specialist surgical practitioner during laparotomy for an "acute abdomen". The gallbladder will be inflamed, red, oedematous, distended and coated with a film of exudate. It may contain stones. If the gallbladder is tense and appears likely to rupture, proceed with a cholecystostomy. Cholecystectomy should be performed only by a qualified surgeon. For the non-specialist, an alternative to cholecystostomy is to close the abdomen and refer the patient for elective cholecystectomy after the acute attack has subsided.

Technique

Cholecystostomy

1 Begin antibiotics once the diagnosis is made. Pack the gallbladder off with gauze to prevent spillage of infected bile into the peritoneal cavity. Insert 2 purse-string 2/0 absorbable stitches into the fundus (Figure 7.8). Aspirate the infected bile with a needle and syringe to empty the gallbladder (Figure 7.9). Incise the fundus with a pointed knife in the centre of the purse-string sutures (Figure 7.10) and apply suction (Figure 7.11). Extract any stones using suitable forceps (Figure 7.12).

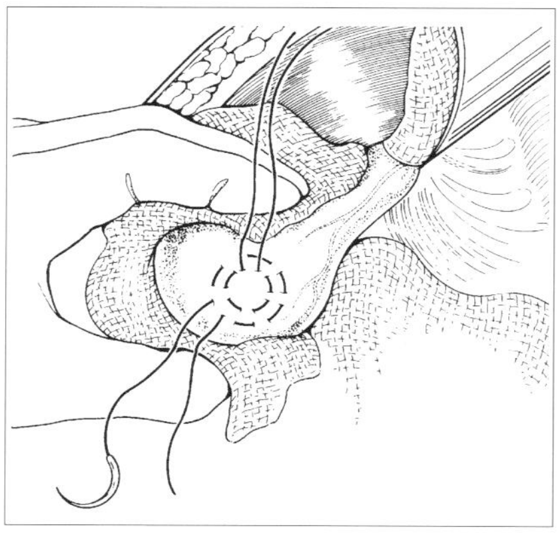

Figure 7.8

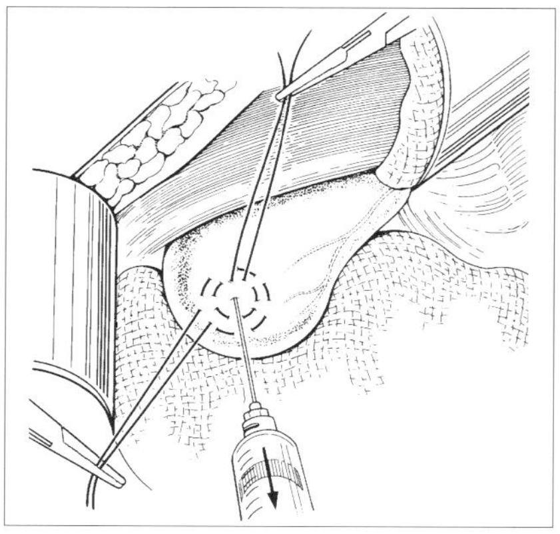

Figure 7.9

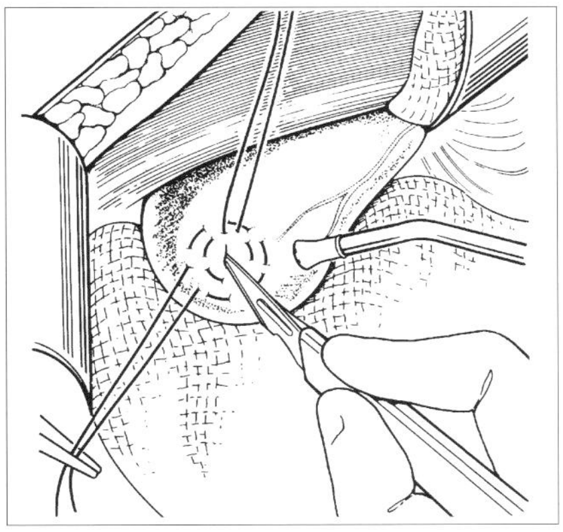

Figure 7.10

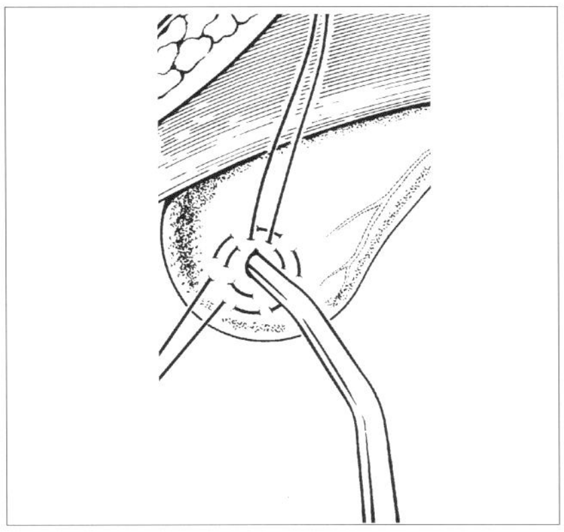

Figure 7.11

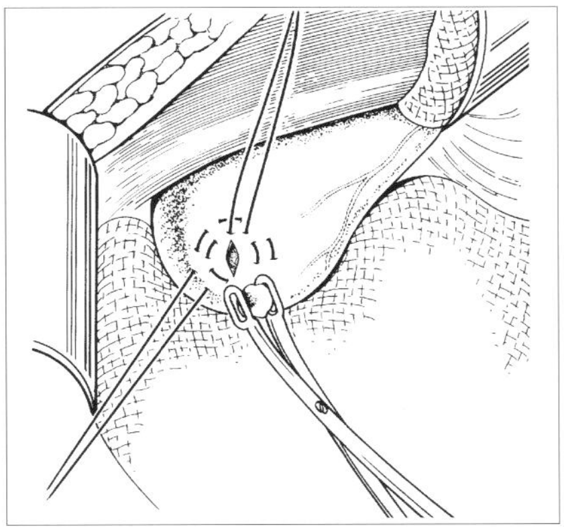

Figure 7.12

2 Introduce the tip of a Foley catheter through a stab wound in the abdominal wall and then into the gallbladder (Figure 7.13). Tie the purse-string sutures, the inner one first, leaving the ends long. Inflate the balloon (Figure 7.14). Bring the ends out through the abdominal wall with the catheter and anchor them to the stab wound. This opposes the gallbladder wall and the cholecystostomy to the abdominal wall. Do not place tension on the gallbladder to bring it into contact with the abdominal wall. The procedure is safe as long as the purse string around the Foley catheter provides a watertight closure. A latex drain may be placed in the hepatorenal pouch and brought out through a separate stab incision. It may be removed after 48 hours.

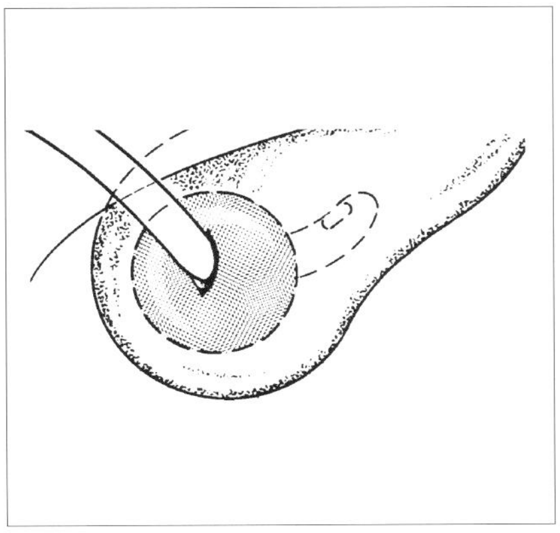

Figure 7.13

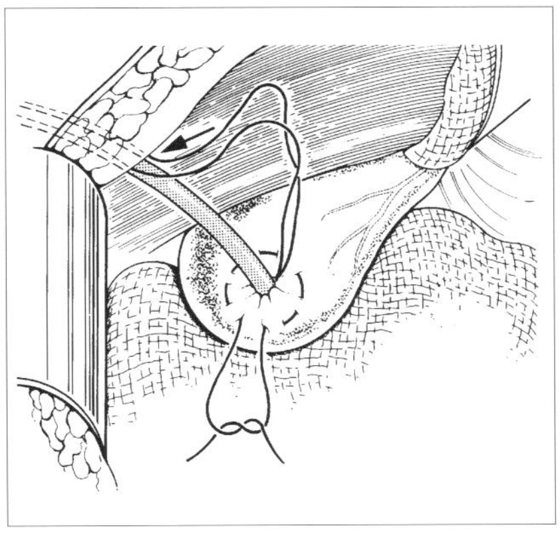

Figure 7.14

3 Close the laparotomy incision. Secure the catheter with the ends of the second purse-string suture and connect it to a sterile closed drainage system.

7

4 Continue antibiotics, nasogastric suction and intravenous fluid administration for 2 to 3 days. After 10 days, intermittently clamp the catheter for increasing periods of time. Remove the catheter when no further leakage occurs. The sinus track will close rapidly. Alternatively, leave the catheter in place and refer the patient for cholecystectomy by a surgical specialist.

KEY POINTS

- Treat acute, gangrenous or perforated appendix with appendectomy
- Treat appendicular mass with medical management
- Treat appendicular abscess with incision and drainage
- Pulse and temperature are normal in early appendicitis
- Tenderness in the right lower quadrant is the most reliable sign
- Retrocaecal and pelvic appendicitis may not have right lower quadrant tenderness
- Rectal examination assists in the diagnosis of a pelvic appendix
- Vaginal examination will help differentiate salpingitis and ectopic pregnancy
- Rectal examination should always be performed
- Abdominal pain in very young, old or pregnant patients may be appendicitis.

7.6 APPENDIX

Acute appendicitis results from bacterial invasion usually distal to an obstruction of the lumen. The obstruction is caused by faecaliths, seeds or worms in the lumen or by invasion of the appendix wall by parasites, such as amoeba or schistosomes. Lymphoid hyperplasia following a viral infection has also been implicated. Untreated, the infection progresses to:

- Local peritonitis with formation of an appendicular mass
- Abscess formation
- Gangrene of the appendix
- Perforation
- General peritonitis.

Clinical features

Symptoms include:

- Central abdominal colic, which settles to a burning pain in the right iliac fossa
- Anorexia, nausea, vomiting and fever.

Physical findings include:

- Tenderness with localized rigidity in the right lower quadrant over McBurney's point
- Rebound tenderness, or tenderness to percussion, in the right lower quadrant
- Pain in the right lower quadrant after pressing deeply in the left lower quadrant
- Right sided tenderness on rectal examination.

The differential diagnosis includes:

- Gastroenteritis
- Ascariasis
- Amoebiasis
- Urinary tract infection
- Renal or ureteric calculi
- Ruptured ectopic pregnancy
- Pelvic inflammatory disease (salpingitis)
- Twisted ovarian cyst
- Ruptured ovarian follicle
- Mesenteric adenitis.

Appendicular mass

This is caused by inflammation and swelling of the appendix, caecum, omentum and distal part of the terminal ileum. Treat conservatively with rest, antibiotics, analgesics and fluids. If the patient's pain and fever either continue or recur, the mass probably includes an abscess which should be incised and drained.

Technique

Emergency appendectomy

1 With the patient in the supine position, place an 8–10 cm incision over McBurney's point or the point of maximum tenderness you have previously marked (Figure 7.15). Note that this incision should be smaller in a child. Deepen the incision to the level of the external oblique aponeurosis and cut through this in line with its fibres (Figure 7.16). Split the underlying muscles along the lines of their fibres using blunt dissection with scissors and large straight artery forceps (Figure 7.17). Use a "gridiron" technique by splitting and retracting the muscle layers until the extraperitoneal fat and the peritoneum are exposed. Lift the peritoneum with two pairs of artery forceps to form a tent and squeeze this with your fingers to displace the underlying viscera. Incise the peritoneum between the two pairs of artery forceps.

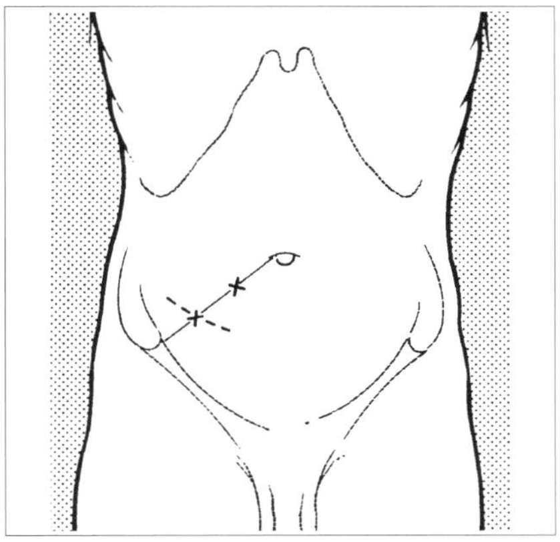

Figure 7.15

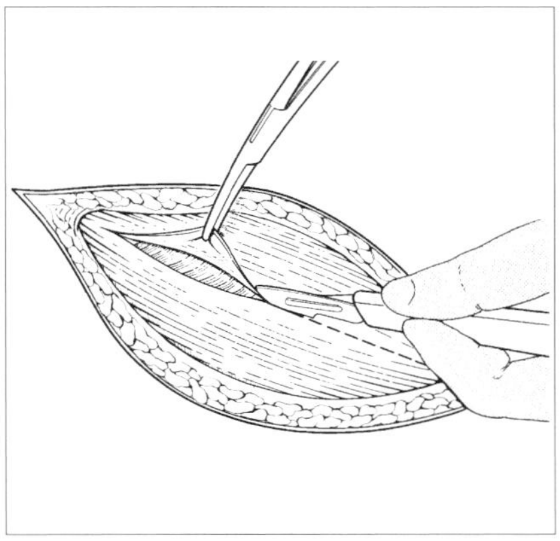

Figure 7.16

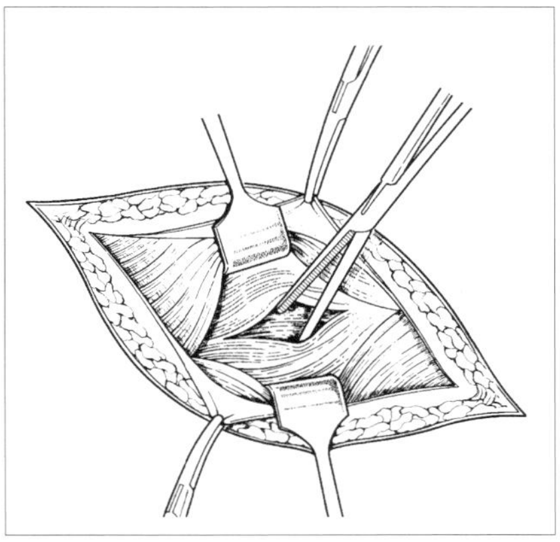

Figure 7.17

2 Aspirate any free peritoneal fluid and take a specimen for bacteriological culture. If the appendix is visible, pick it up with a non-toothed or a Babcock forceps. The appendix may be delivered by gently lifting the caecum with the anterior taeniae coli. An inflamed appendix is fragile so deliver it into the wound with great care. The position of the appendix is variable (Figures 7.18 and 7.19). Locate it by following the taeniae coli to the base of the caecum and lifting both the caecum and the appendix into the wound (Figure 7.20).

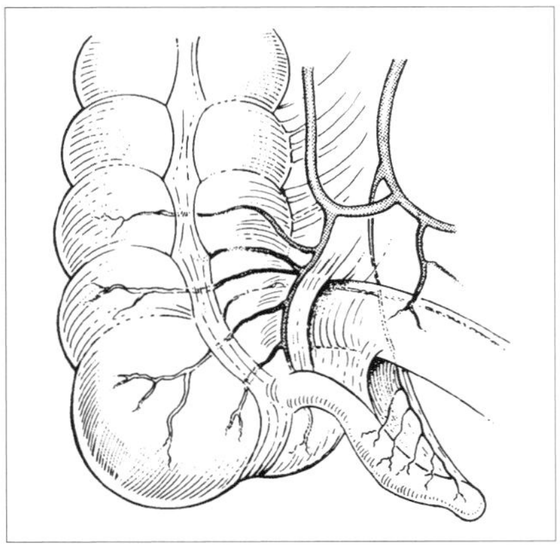

Figure 7.18

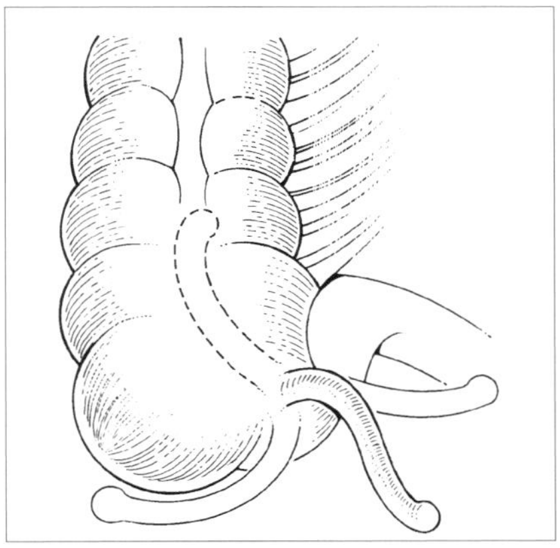

Figure 7.19

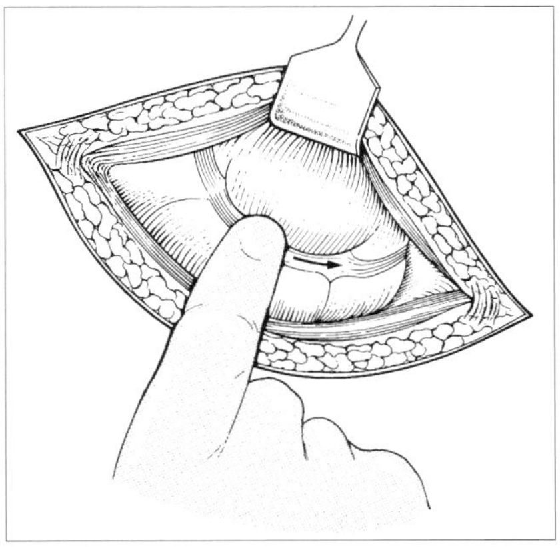

Figure 7.20

7

3 Divide the mesoappendix (containing the appendicular artery) between artery forceps close to the base of the appendix. Ligate it with 0 absorbable suture (Figures 7.21–7.23). Clamp the base of the appendix to crush the wall and reapply the clamp a little further distally (Figure 7.24). Ligate the crushed appendix with 2/0 absorbable suture. Cut the ends of the ligature fairly short and hold them with forceps to help invaginate the appendix stump.

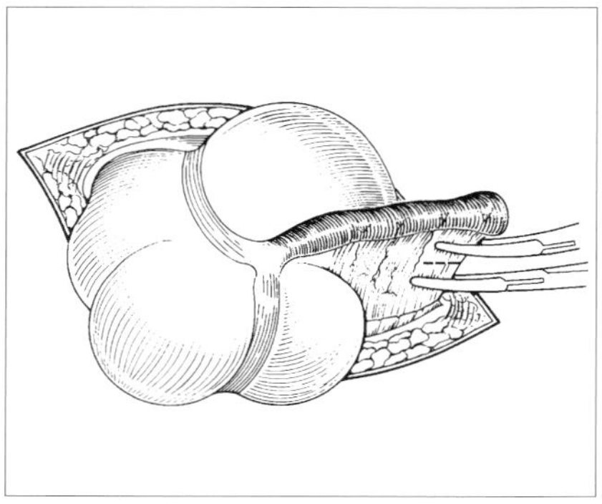

Figure 7.21

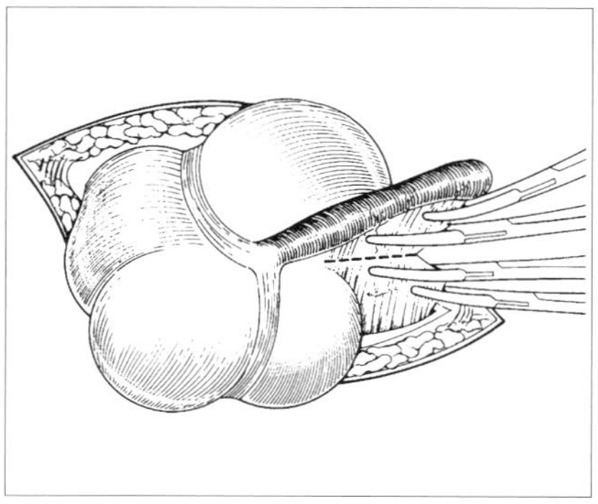

Figure 7.22

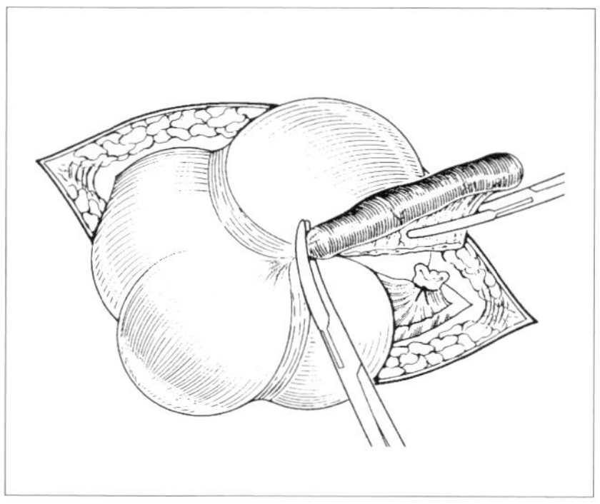

Figure 7.23

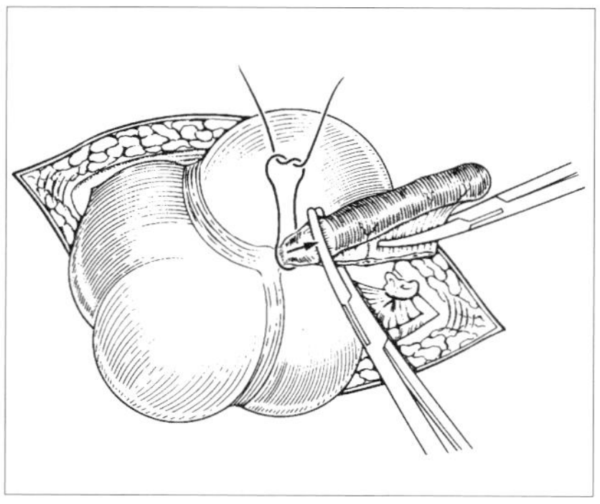

Figure 7.24

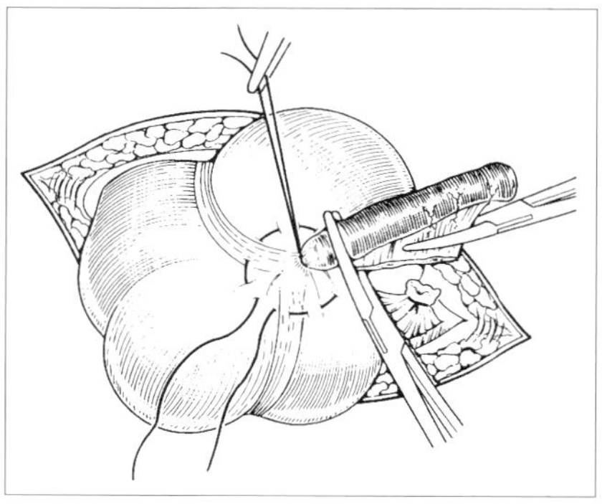

Figure 7.25

Insert a 2/0 absorbable, purse-string suture in the caecum around the base of the appendix (Figure 7.25). Divide the appendix between the ligature and the clamp and invaginate the stump as the purse-string is tightened and tied over it (Figures 7.26 and 7.27). The purse-string is traditional, but optional. Simple ligation is adequate and the preferred technique if insertion of a purse-string is at all difficult.

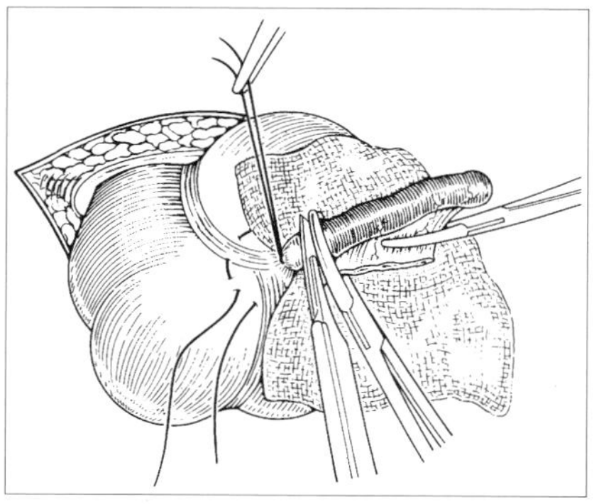

Figure 7.26

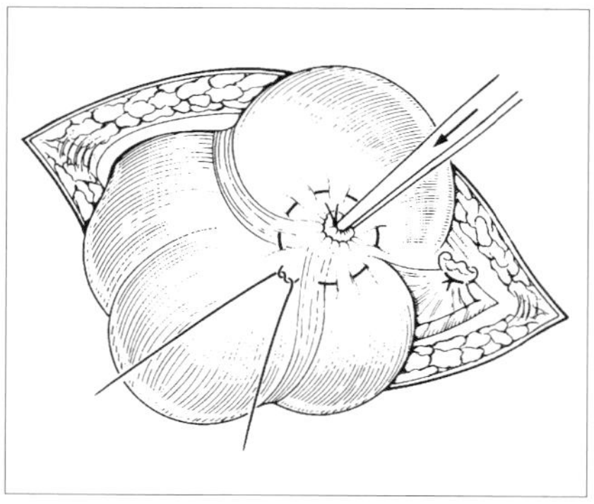

Figure 7.27

4 Close the abdominal wound using:

- Continuous 2/0 absorbable suture for the peritoneum
- Interrupted 0 absorbable sutures for the split muscle fibres

- Interrupted or continuous 0 absorbable for the external oblique aponeurosis
- Interrupted 2/0 monofilament non-absorbable for the skin.

If there is severe inflammation or wound contamination, do not close the skin, but pack the skin and subcutaneous layers with damp saline gauze for delayed primary closure.

Intraoperative problems

Intraoperative problems include:

- Adherent and retrocaecal appendix
- Appendicular abscess.

Adherent and retrocaecal appendix

Mobilize the caecum by dividing its retroperitoneal attachment and then excise the appendix in a retrograde manner. Ligate and divide the base of the appendix, then invaginate the stump, ligate the vessels in the mesoappendix, and finally remove the appendix.

Appendicular abscess

Treat the abscess with incision and drainage. Consider interval appendectomy if symptoms recur.

INTUSSUSCEPTION

Intussusception is a form of intestinal obstruction in which one segment of the intestine telescopes into the next (Figures 7.28).

KEY POINTS

In surgery for intussusception:

- Do not pull on the ileum; rather, squeeze the leading edge through the colon
- Do not perform an incidental appendectomy: if the intussusception recurs, repeat procedures will be compromised
- The last few centimetres of manual reduction are the most difficult – be patient
- Seromuscular splits may occur but are not a problem if the mucosa is intact.

Assessment and preoperative management

Intussusception is most frequent in children less than two years of age.

Diagnosis

- Intermittent crying
- Passing blood and mucus per rectum
- Palpable mass in line with the large bowel (usually right upper quadrant)
- Blood and mucus on rectal examination
- Can be mimicked by dysentery or roundworms.

Medical management

To medically manage intussusception:

- Administer intravenous fluids according to body weight
- Insert a nasogastric tube
- Barium enema can be used to confirm the diagnosis
- Barium enema can be used for non-operative reduction in early intussusception.

Operative technique

1 Give the patient a general anaesthetic with a muscle relaxant. Place the child supine and prepare the skin with antiseptic. Open the abdomen

through a midline incision centred at the umbilicus; make the incision either through or around the umbilicus (Figure 7.29).

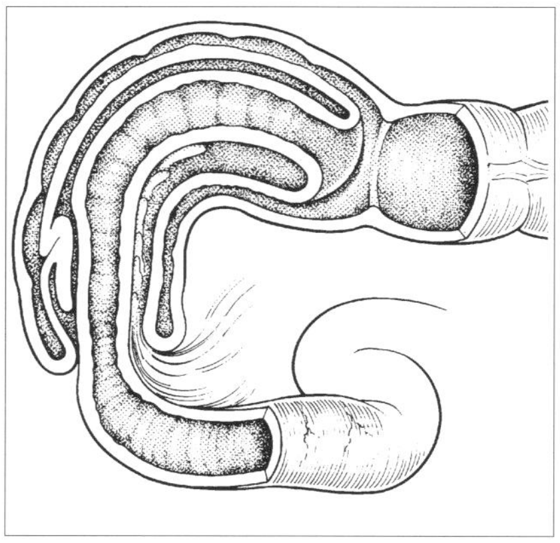

Figure 7.28

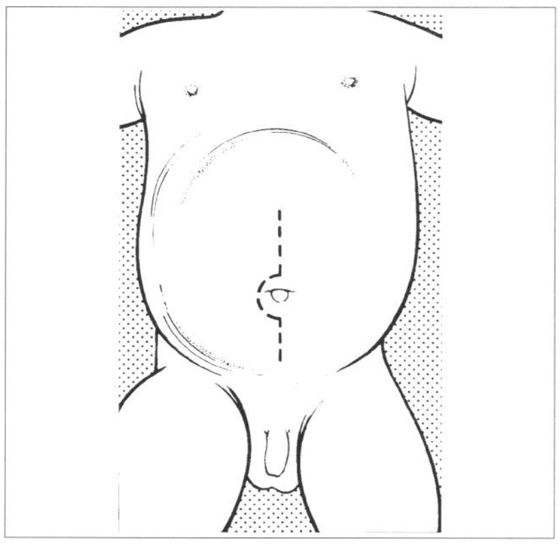

Figure 7.29

2 After opening the peritoneum, locate and examine the intussusception. Make no attempt to reduce the telescoped bowel by pulling on its proximal end, but instead "milk" it in a retrograde manner with the fingers of one hand inside the abdomen pressing against the fingers of the other hand outside the abdomen (Figures 7.30 and 7.31). Once the bowel has been reduced into the ascending colon, deliver the colon through the wound and reduce the remaining intussusception slowly, inspecting the ensheathing layer for serosal and muscular tears (Figure 7.32).

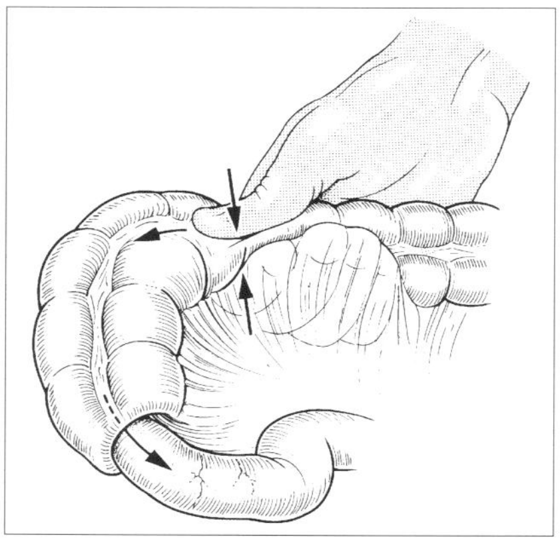

Figure 7.30

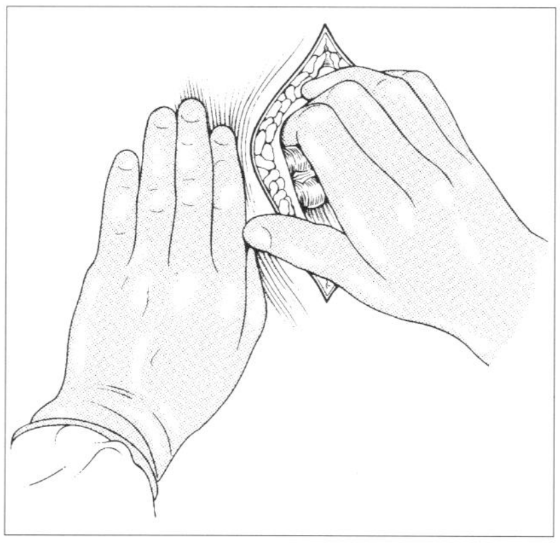

Figure 7.31

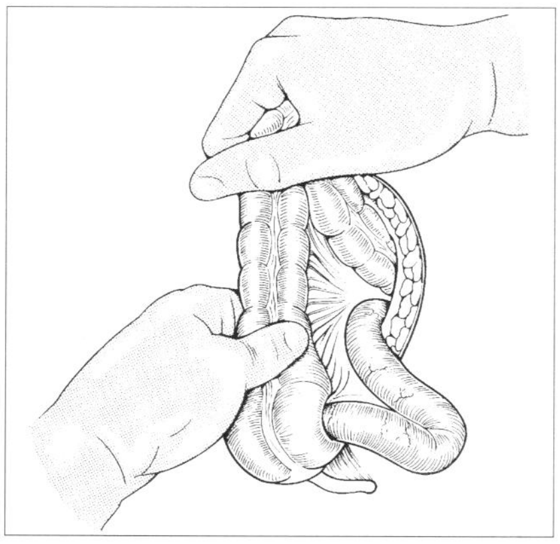

Figure 7.32

3 If the intussusception is not fully reducible, or if the bowel is gangrenous, resect the section of involved bowel. If you are experienced, construct an ileocolic anastomosis. If you are a non specialist practitioner, exteriorize the two ends of the bowel through the abdominal wall, forming an ileostomy and a non-functioning mucous fistula.

4 Close the wound in layers using absorbable suture for the peritoneum and muscle, and non-absorbable suture for the skin. If the bowel ends have been exteriorized, refer the patient for anastomosis by a qualified surgeon. An ileostomy will produce large quantities of fluid. The patient will require fluid based on body weight plus the fluid lost through the ileostomy. Replace the loss with normal saline.

SIGMOID VOLVULUS

Volvulus is the rotation of a loop of bowel on its mesenteric axis, resulting in partial or complete obstruction. The most common portion affected is the sigmoid colon (Figure 7.33). Figure 7.34 shows the X-ray appearance.

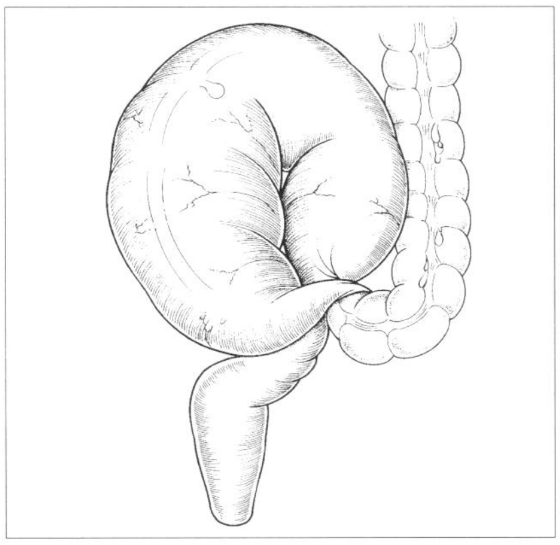

Figure 7.33

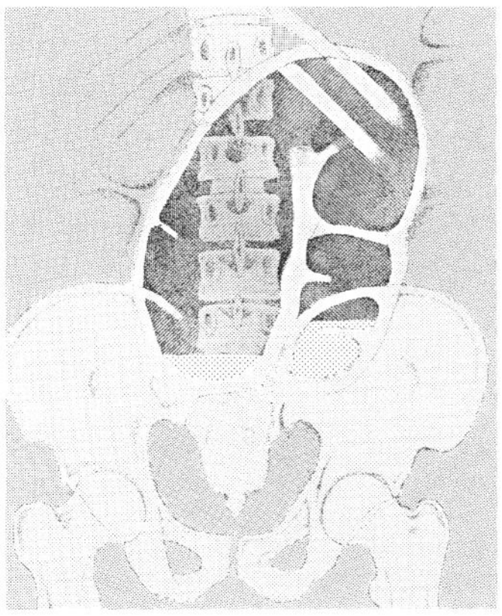

Figure 7.34

Diagnosis

- Sudden onset of severe, colicky abdominal pain
- Absolute constipation
- Rapidly progressive but moderate abdominal distension
- Associated with tachycardia, hypotension and fever
- Empty rectum
- Nausea and vomiting are late symptoms
- Frequently progresses to strangulation and gangrene.

Medical management

Resuscitate dehydrated patients with intravenous fluids and correct anaemia if required. Insert a nasogastric tube if the patient is vomiting. Antibiotics that provide aerobic, gram negative and anaerobic coverage should be administered if the volvulus is suspected to be gangrenous.

Non-operative reduction of subacute volvulus

Subacute volvulus does not require emergency reduction, but should be treated urgently (within 3 hours).

Technique

1 Sedation may be helpful, but do not give an anaesthetic: the patient's reaction to pain, if the sigmoidoscope is incorrectly placed, is a protection against traumatic perforation of the bowel wall. Put on a waterproof apron and place the patient face down in a knee-elbow position (which may itself cause derotation of the bowel) or use the left lateral position.

2 Without using force, pass the well-lubricated sigmoidoscope as high as it can go into the colon with the bowel lumen completely visualized. Lubricate the rectal tube and introduce it through the sigmoidoscope until it meets

KEY POINTS

- Volvulus of the sigmoid colon is:
  - Usually sub-acute
  - Associated with repeated previous episodes
  - The most common cause of large bowel obstruction seen at the district hospital
  - Associated with massive but soft abdominal distension
  - Seen in well hydrated patients
  - Complicated with vomiting and abdominal pain as a late finding
- When neglected, can progress to strangulation and gangrene
- Sub-acute sigmoid volvulus can be reduced by the placement of a rectal tube
- Refer patients after non-operative or operative volvulus reduction for elective surgical management
- Suspect gangrene if you see darkened bowel or blood stained fluid at sigmoidoscopy
- Operate if you suspect gangrene and, if necessary, perform a sigmoid resection with colostomy
- The generalist at the district hospital should be capable of performing a colostomy but should refer patients to a qualified surgeon for colonic anastomosis and colostomy closures.

the obstruction marking the lower part of the twisted loop. Gently rotate the rectal tube, allowing its tip to skip into the distal limb. Keep your face well aside from the tube and the sigmoidoscope at this stage, as successful entry into the volvulus will be evidenced by a sudden profuse outpouring of foul-smelling liquid faeces mixed with gas. If you are not experienced in passing a sigmoidoscope you could still simply pass a well lubricated rectal tube and manoeuvre it as described.

3 After decompression, withdraw the sigmoidoscope, but leave the rectal tube in position strapped to the perineum and buttock. It should be retained in this position for 3 – 4 days, if possible. Should the rectal tube be expelled, gently reintroduce it without using the sigmoidoscope. Indeed, sigmoidoscopy is not essential even for the initial introduction of the tube, though it facilitates the procedure.

4 If this manoeuvre fails to untwist the volvulus, perform laparotomy immediately.

Operative management

1 Anaesthetize the patient and perform a laparotomy with a lower midline incision.

2 At laparotomy, untwist the volvulus.

   If the bowel is viable, have an assistant pass a rectal tube while you guide it along the sigmoid colon. Suture the tube to the buttocks and close the abdomen. Remove the tube after 4 days.

   If the bowel is not viable, resect the dead section, perform an end colostomy and close the rectum in two layers.

After recovery, refer the patient for elective sigmoid colectomy or, in the case of a resection, for closure of the colostomy. Colostomy closure is safely performed 3 months after resection. See pages 6–15 and 6–16 for the description of end colostomy and refer to Figures 6.50 to 6.54.

Abdominal wall hernia

8

An abdominal wall hernia is a protrusion of a viscus or part of a viscus through an abnormal opening in the wall of the abdominal cavity. Inguinal hernia is by far the most common type of hernia in males, accounting for about 70% of all hernias. It is followed in frequency by femoral, umbilical and incisional hernia.

KEY POINTS

- Inguinal hernia bulges above the inguinal ligament, with the hernia neck above and medial to the pubic tubercle
- Femoral hernia bulges below the inguinal ligament in the upper thigh, with the hernia neck below and lateral to the pubic tubercle
- Inguinal hernia is most common in males
- Femoral hernia, which occurs less frequently than inguinal hernia, is more common in women.

8.1 GROIN HERNIAS

Groin hernias include:

- Indirect inguinal hernia: a persistence of a congenital peritoneal tract that follows the indirect path of the spermatic cord
- Direct inguinal hernia: a defect in the floor of the inguinal canal
- Femoral hernia: not an inguinal hernia, but a defect medial to the femoral sheath.

The neck of an inguinal hernia will be above and medial to the pubic tubercle whereas the neck of a femoral hernia will be below and lateral to the pubic tubercle. Surgery is the only definitive treatment for an inguinal or femoral hernia.

Predisposing factors include:

- Congenital failure of obliteration of the processus vaginalis in infants (inguinal hernia)
- Increased intra-abdominal pressure, for example, as a result of chronic cough or straining at micturition
- Previous surgery for ventral hernia.

A hernia is either:

- Reducible: the contents of the sac can be completely pushed back into the abdominal cavity
- Incarcerated: the hernia cannot be completely returned into the abdominal cavity
- Strangulated: the content of the sac has a compromised blood supply with a consequent risk of gangrene.

Assessment

Examine the standing patient. The hernia appears as a visible or palpable mass when the patient stands up or coughs.

A hernia is non-tender and is painless unless it is strangulated. Patients with strangulated hernia require emergency surgery. They will complain of pain in the abdomen and the groin where the hernia is located. Many vomit. The hernia is very tender, tense and incarcerated. Make the diagnosis by physical examination.

Preparation for surgery

A possible complication of hernia repair is recurrence caused by wound infection, haematoma or poor technique.

> Strangulation is the most dangerous complication of a hernia. Recurrence is the commonest complication of hernia operation.

8.2 SURGICAL REPAIR OF INGUINAL HERNIA

The technique described below is for the repair of inguinal hernias in males. In female patients, the procedure is different because the content of the inguinal canal is the round ligament rather than the spermatic cord.

INDIRECT INGUINAL HERNIA

Technique

The aim of the operation is to reduce the hernia, ligate the sac and repair the defect in the posterior inguinal canal.

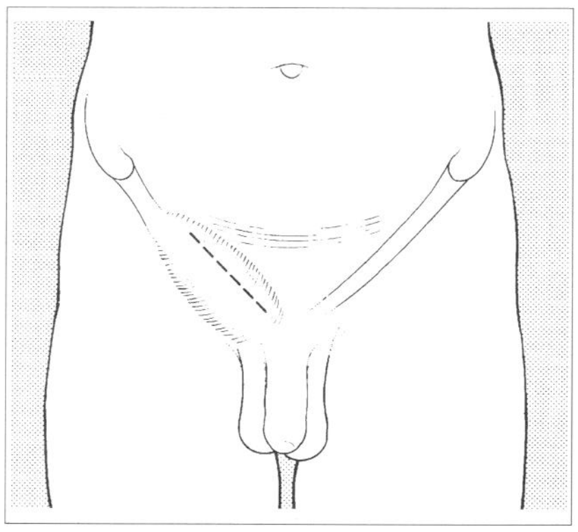

Figure 8.1

1 Make an incision in the inguinal region in a skin crease 1–2 cm above the inguinal ligament, centred midway between the deep ring and the pubic symphysis (Figure 8.1). Divide and ligate the veins in the subcutaneous tissue.
2 Visualize the external oblique aponeurosis with its fibres running in a downward and medial direction. Incise the aponeurosis along its fibres, holding the cut margins with forceps (Figures 8.2 and 8.3). Use these forceps to lift and retract the edges while extending the incision to the full length of the wound. The process of extending the wound also opens the

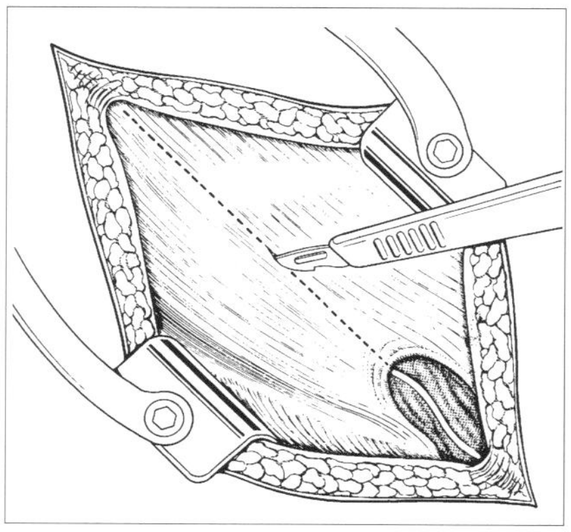

Figure 8.2

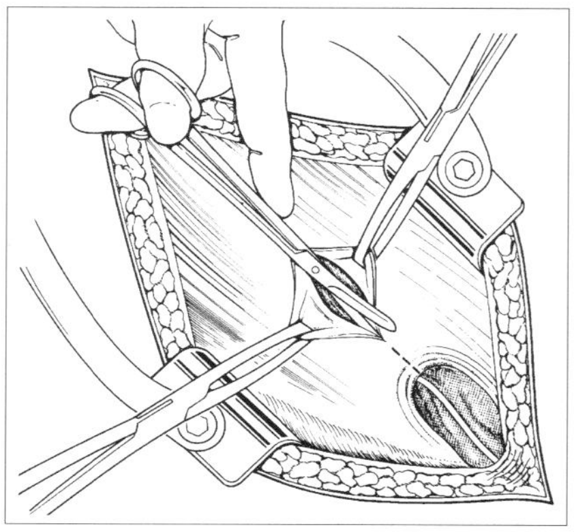

Figure 8.3

external ring. Identify the ilio-inguinal nerve and protect it during surgery by holding it away from the operating field.

3 Using blunt dissection, deliver the spermatic cord together with the hernial sac as one mass and pass a finger around it (Figure 8.4). It is easiest to mobilize the mass by starting medially in the inguinal canal. Secure the mass with a latex drain or gauze (Figure 8.5). Using blunt dissection, separate the sac from the cord (vas deferens and vessels), layer by layer. Do not devascularize the cord. The hernia sac is located in the anteromedial aspect of the cord.

4 Continue to free the hernia sac from the cord (or round ligament in women) up to the internal inguinal ring. Open the sac between two pairs of small forceps and confirm its communication with the abdominal cavity by introducing a finger into the opening (Figure 8.6).

5 Twist the sac to ensure that it is empty (Figure 8.7). Suture ligate the neck with 2/0 suture, hold the ligature and excise the sac (Figures 8.8 and 8.9). If there is adherent gut in the sac, it may be a sliding hernia (see page 8–5). In this situation, do not excise the entire sac.

6 Inspect the stump to be sure that it is adequate to prevent partial slipping of the ligature. When the ligature is finally cut, the stump will recede deeply within the ring and out of view (Figure 8.10).

7 If there is a defect in the posterior inguinal wall, stitch the conjoined muscle and tendon to the inguinal ligament. Do not place sutures too deep medially as the femoral vein will be injured.

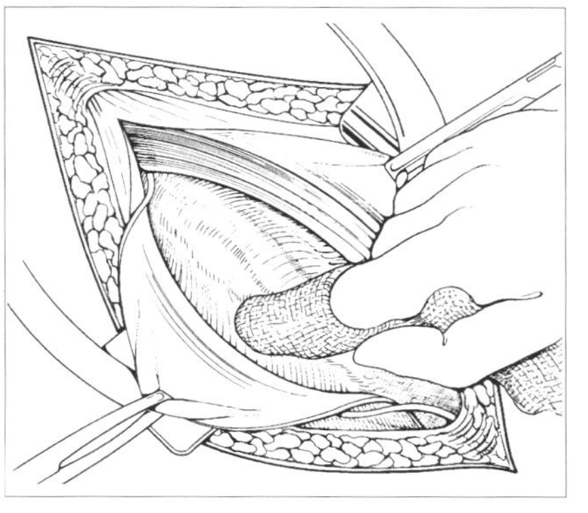

Figure 8.4

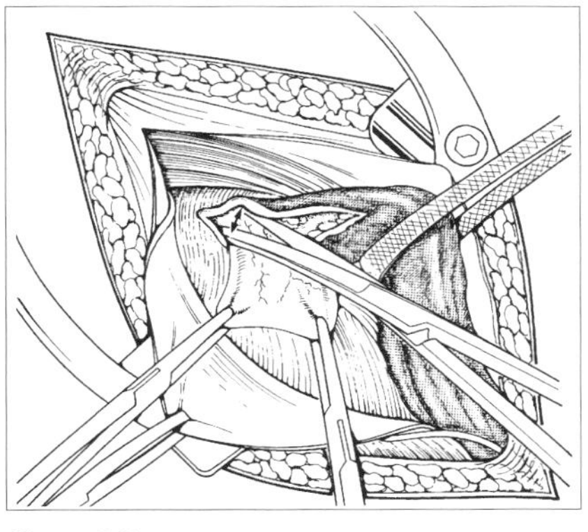

Figure 8.5

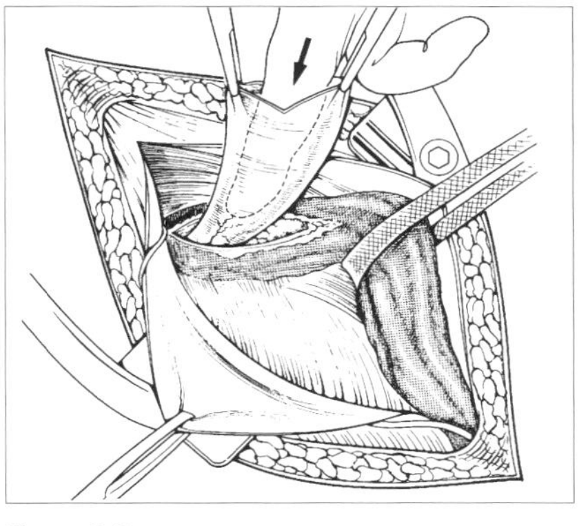

Figure 8.6

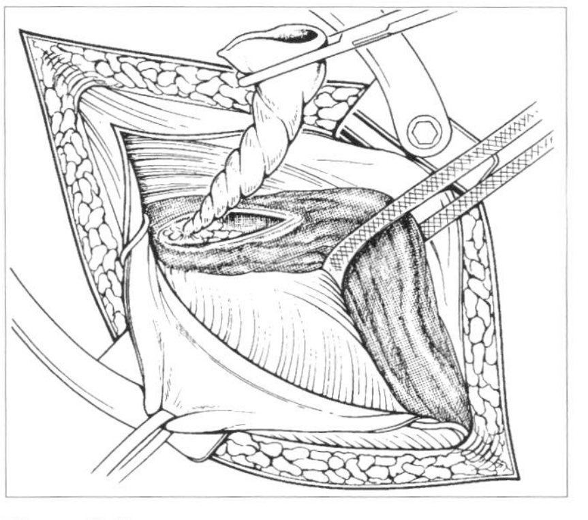

Figure 8.7

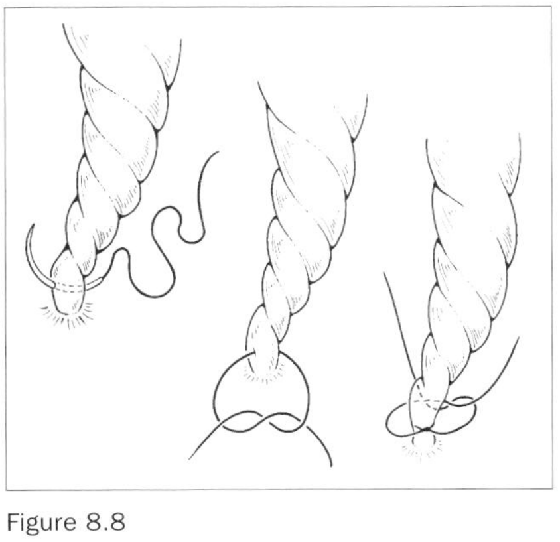

Figure 8.8

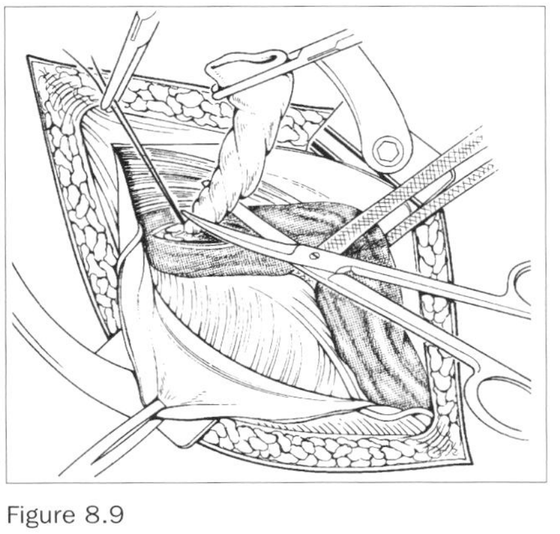

Figure 8.9

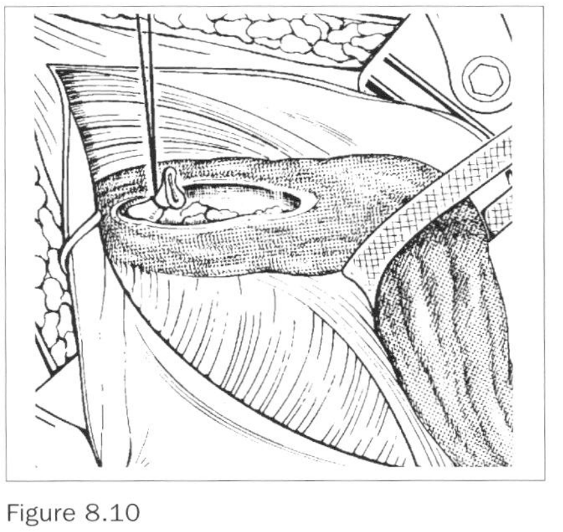

Figure 8.10

- Repair of the posterior wall of the inguinal canal is required in a direct hernia
- If there is a moderate to large defect in the posterior inguinal canal in an indirect hernia, a repair is indicated
- Indirect hernia in children should be treated with a high ligation of the sac and no repair should be performed
- Indirect hernia in young men with a strong inguinal canal should not be repaired. Tightening of the internal ring with one or two sutures is appropriate. The inferior epigastric artery is on the lower edge of the ring and should be avoided.

Begin the repair medially using No. 1 nylon. Insert stitches through the inguinal ligament at different fibre levels, as the fibres tend to split along the line of the ligament.

Insert the first stitch to include the pectineal ligament (Figure 8.11). Insert the next stitch through the conjoined tendon and the inguinal ligament and continue laterally to insert stitches in this manner (Figure 8.12). Leave the stitches untied until all have been inserted. Test the final stitch adjacent to the ring before you start to tie the stitches; it should just allow the tip of the little finger to be passed through the ring along the cord. Then tie the stitches, beginning medially, and cut loose ends (Figure 8.13). As the final stitch is tied, adjust its tension so that the internal ring just admits the tip of your little finger (Figure 8.14). Finally, check the soundness of the repair, inserting additional stitches where necessary.

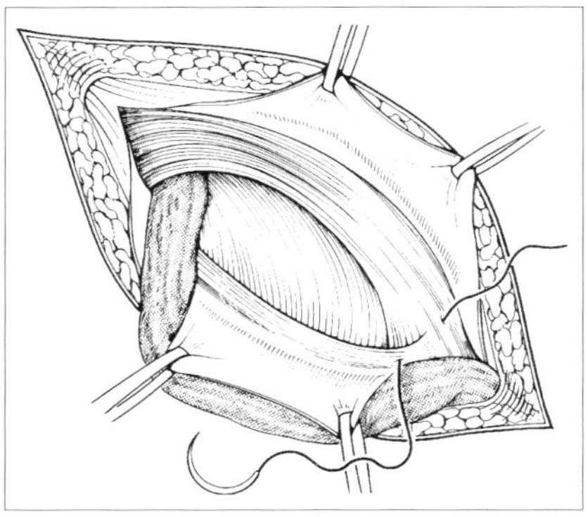

Figure 8.11

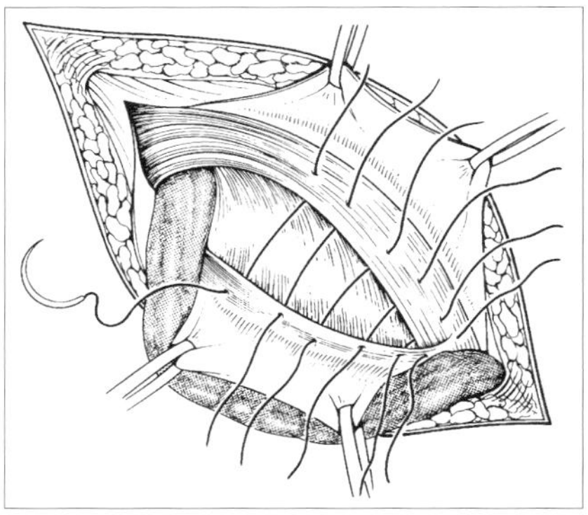

Figure 8.12

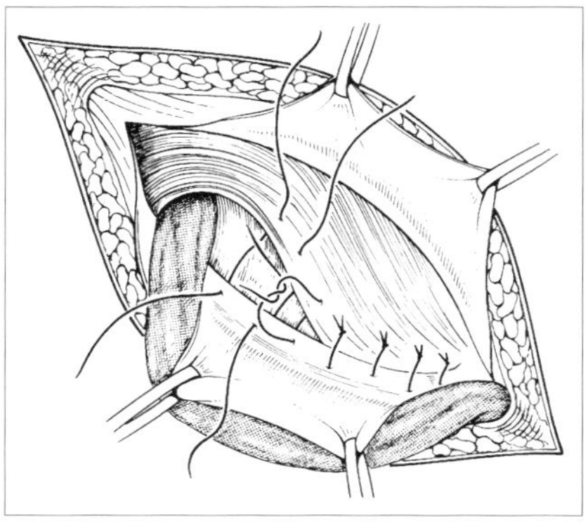

Figure 8.13

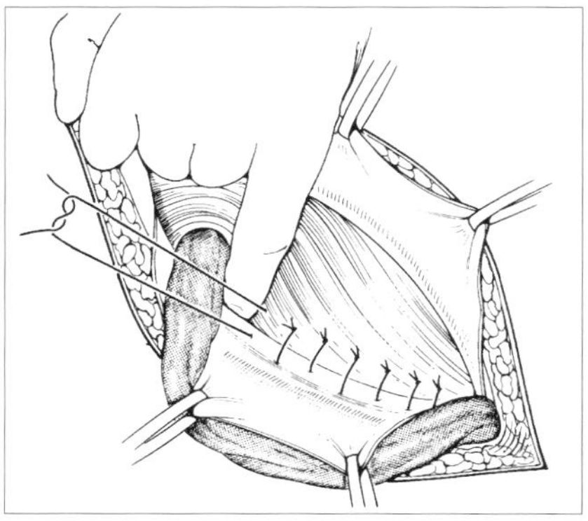

Figure 8.14

8 Close the external oblique aponeurosis with continuous 2/0 absorbable suture (Figure 8.15). Stitch the skin with interrupted 2/0 suture (Figure 8.16). Apply a layer of gauze and hold it in place.

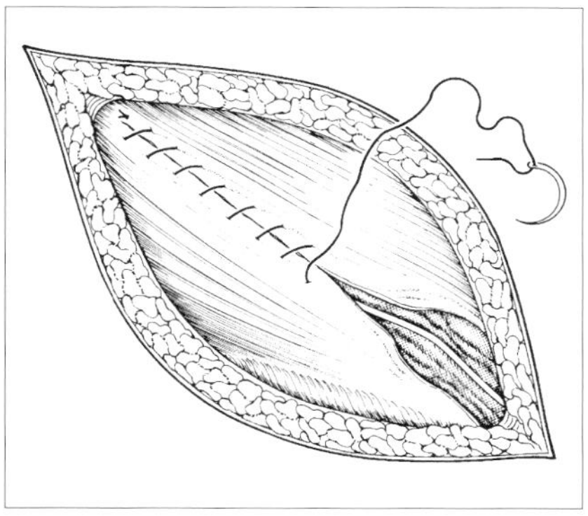

Figure 8.15

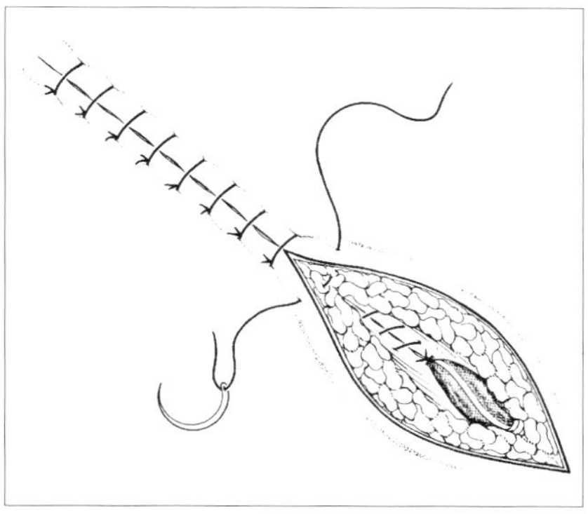

Figure 8.16

Direct inguinal hernia

A direct hernia will appear as a bulge, often covered by fascia transversalis and with a wide neck in the posterior inguinal wall. Once recognized at operation, reduce the hernia but do not open or excise the sac. Cover the reduced sac by completing the repair of the posterior wall of the inguinal canal as described above for indirect hernia (Figures 8.17 and 8.18).

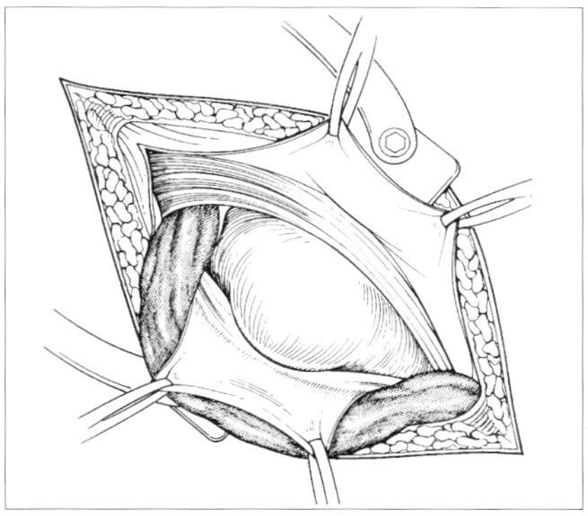

Figure 8.17

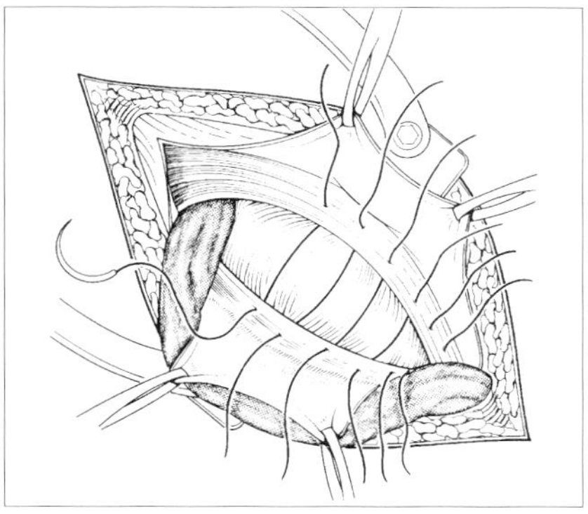

Figure 8.18

Sliding hernia

Diagnosis of a sliding hernia is often intraoperative, becoming apparent once you open the inguinal canal and the hernia sac. A portion of the gut will appear to adhere to the inside wall of the sac: the caecum and appendix if the hernia is in the right groin, and the sigmoid colon if the hernia is on the left. The colon or caecum (depending on where the hernia is located) actually forms part of the posterior wall of the hernia sac. Occasionally the bladder forms part of the sac in a sliding hernia.

Excise most of the sac, leaving a rim of sac below and lateral to the bowel (Figures 8.19 and 8.20). Close the sac with a purse-string suture (Figures 8.21 and 8.22). While tying the suture, push the hernial mass up within the deep inguinal ring. If the hernia fails to reduce completely, make a curved

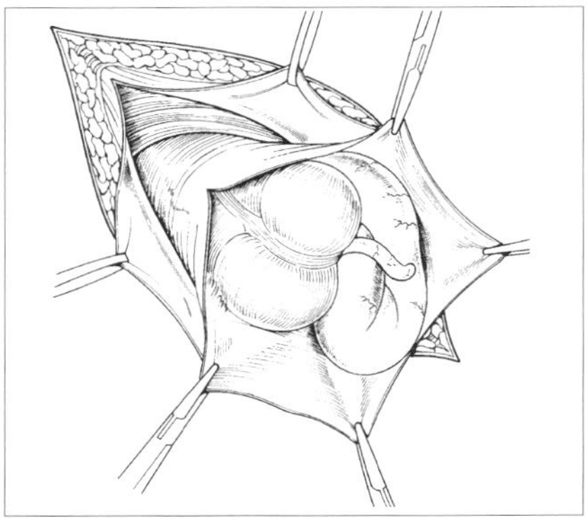

Figure 8.19

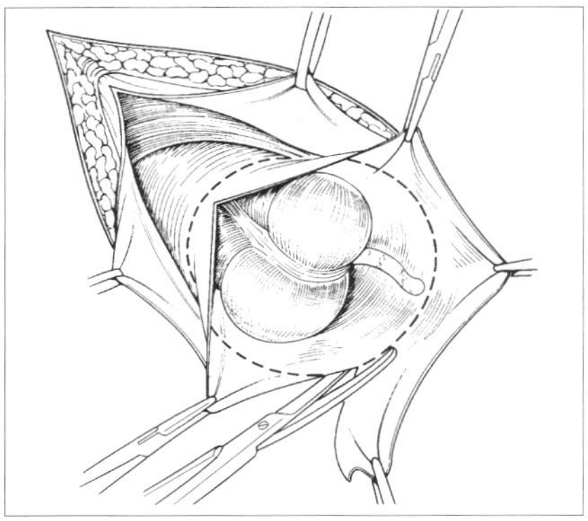

Figure 8.20

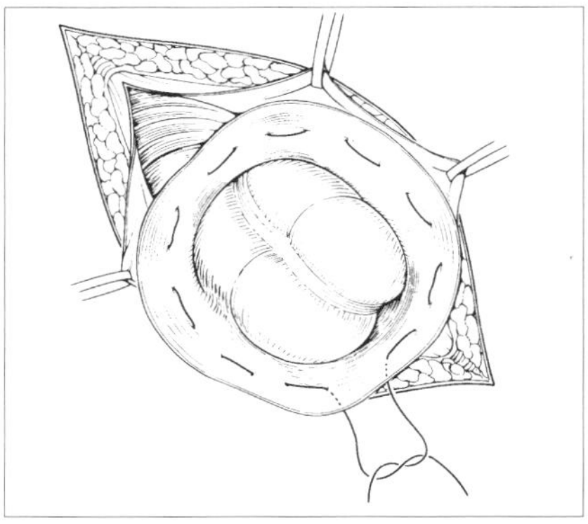

Figure 8.21

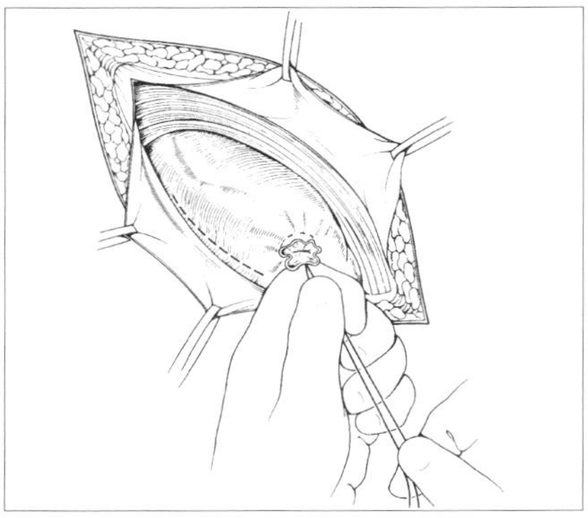

Figure 8.22

incision below and lateral to the caecum to allow the mass to slide back. The skin incision may have to be extended laterally to improve access. Repair the posterior inguinal wall as described for indirect hernia.

Inguinoscrotal hernia

Attempts to excise the scrotal part of the sac can predispose the patient to developing scrotal haematoma. Transect the sac in the inguinal canal and deal with the proximal part as described for indirect inguinal hernia. Leave the distal sac in place, but ensure haemostasis of the distal cut end of the sac.

Recurrent hernia

Operate to repair a recurrent hernia only if it is strangulated; otherwise, refer the patient to a surgeon. Because of previous operations, the inguinal anatomy is often distorted, which makes repair difficult and the risk of further recurrence is increased.

KEY POINTS

- A femoral hernia is below the posterior wall of the inguinal canal
- Open the posterior wall of the inguinal canal with blunt dissection
- Femoral hernia is more common in women.

8.3 SURGICAL REPAIR OF FEMORAL HERNIA

Femoral hernia are groin hernia which have a small opening and are prone to incarceration. If incarcerated, a femoral hernia may be difficult to differentiate from an inguinal hernia. Several operative approaches are used in femoral hernia. However, for the practitioner who is familiar with inguinal hernia repair, the groin approach is easiest. This approach is also helpful if the diagnosis is not certain and in the treatment of combined femoral and inguinal hernia.

Technique

1 In the groin approach for femoral hernia, make the same incision as for an inguinal hernia (Figures 8.1, 8.2, 8.3 on page 8–2). Retract the spermatic cord, taking care to protect the ileo-inguinal nerve (Figure 8.23).

2 The findings and the procedure will now differ from an inguinal hernia. In femoral hernia, the floor of the inguinal canal is intact. Using gentle blunt dissection, open the floor of the inguinal canal, enter the properitoneal space and reduce the femoral hernia (Figure 8.24).

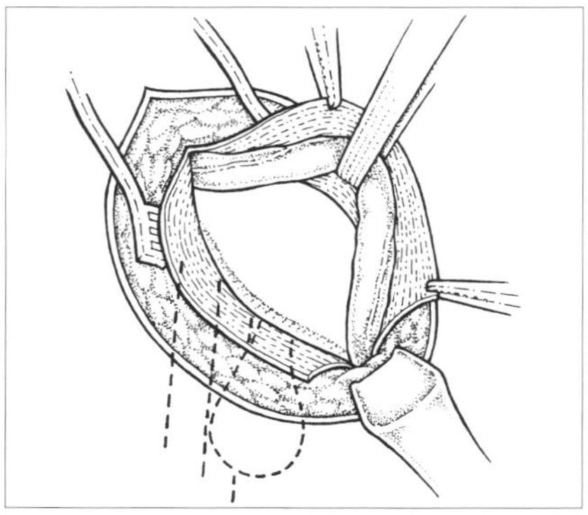

Figure 8.23

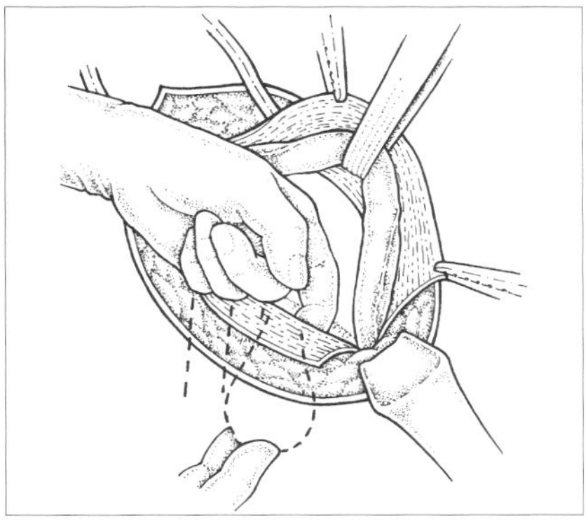

Figure 8.24

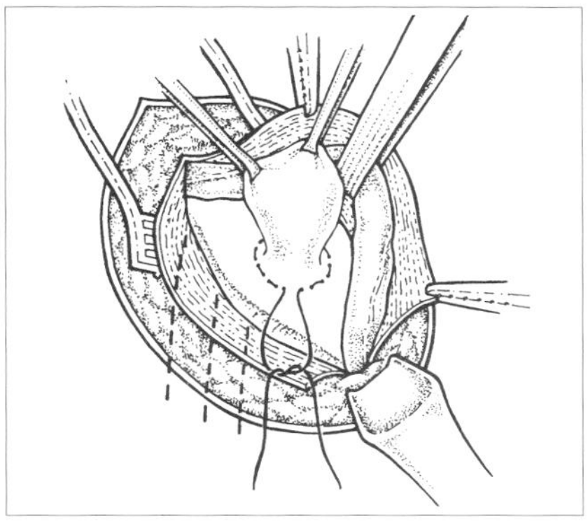

Figure 8.25

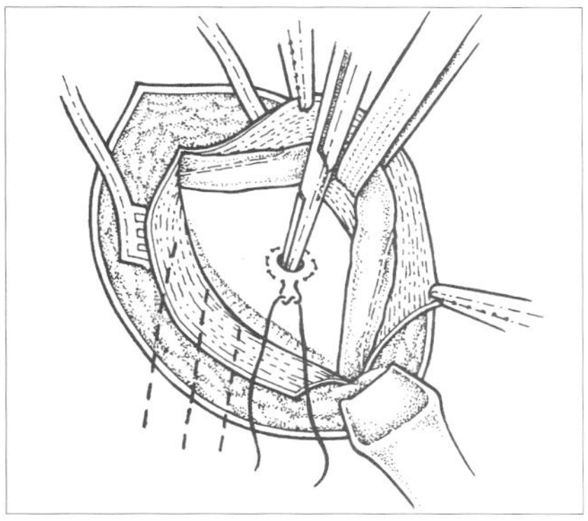

Figure 8.26

3 After reduction, the sac can be managed with a purse-string suture and reduced (Figures 8.25, 8.26). If you are concerned that the sac contents are gangrenous, open the sac and inspect the contents. If the femoral hernia sac cannot be reduced, place an artery forceps at the neck of the sac and divide the overlying inguinal ligament. Take care to cut along the artery forceps to avoid injury to the femoral vessels (Figure 8.27). The sac will then reduce easily.

4 Repair the femoral hernia by attaching the conjoined tendon to the Cooper's ligament, which is the periosteum of the pubic ramus medial to the femoral canal.

5 Close the femoral defect by inserting a transition stitch to include the conjoined tendon, Cooper's ligament and the femoral sheath. Remember that the femoral vein is just under the femoral sheath (Figure 8.28). Figure 8.28 shows how the Cooper's ligament repair and the transition suture are tied.

6 Lateral to the transition suture (untied sutures), reconstruct the inguinal canal by approximating the conjoined tendon to the remnant of the floor and the edge of the inguinal ligament. This type of repair results in excess tension unless a relaxing incision is made. Make an incision in the internal oblique aponeurosis just under the elevated external oblique (Figure 8.29). As in inguinal hernia repair, the internal ring should admit a finger (Figure 8.14). Close the external oblique and skin, as for an inguinal hernia (Figures 8.15, 8.16).

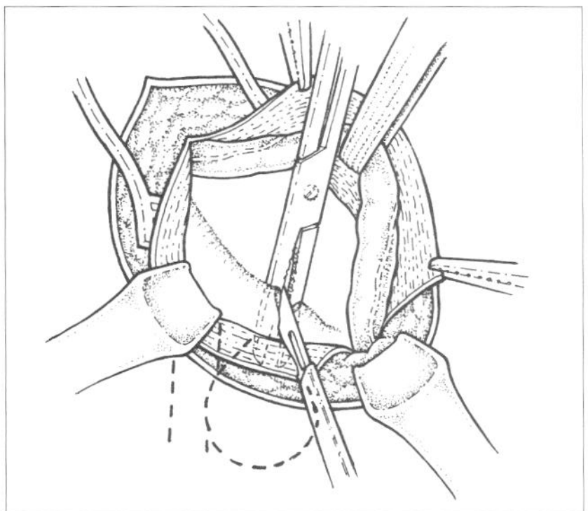

Figure 8.27

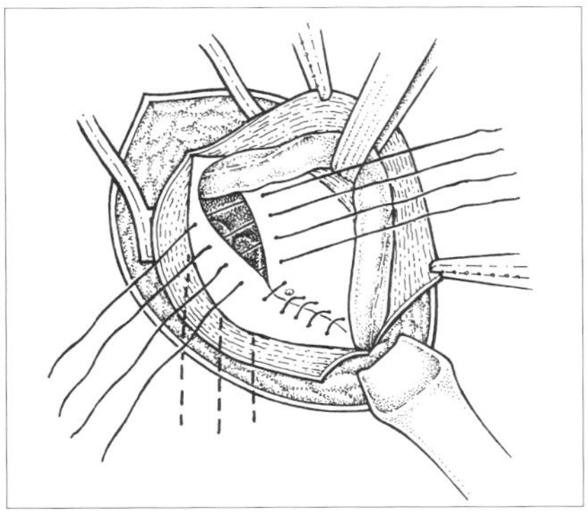

Figure 8.28

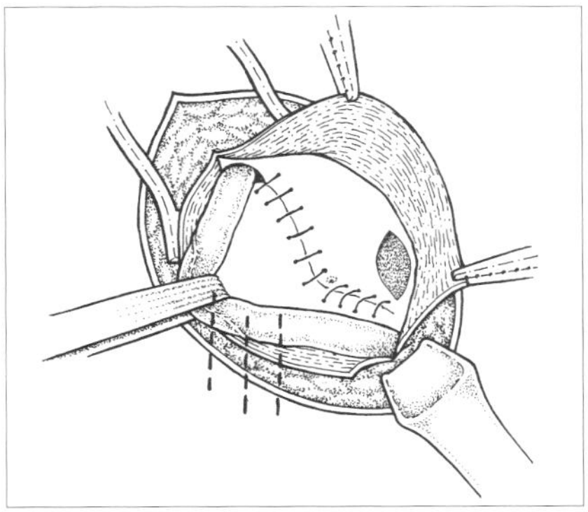

Figure 8.29

In addition to its use in femoral hernia, the Cooper's ligament repair is also an excellent repair for direct inguinal hernia.

KEY POINTS

- In strangulated inguinal hernia, extend the inferior end of the skin incision over the hernia mass
- This incision gives good access to the incarcerated mass
- Always consider strangulated inguinal or femoral hernia as a cause of small bowel obstruction.

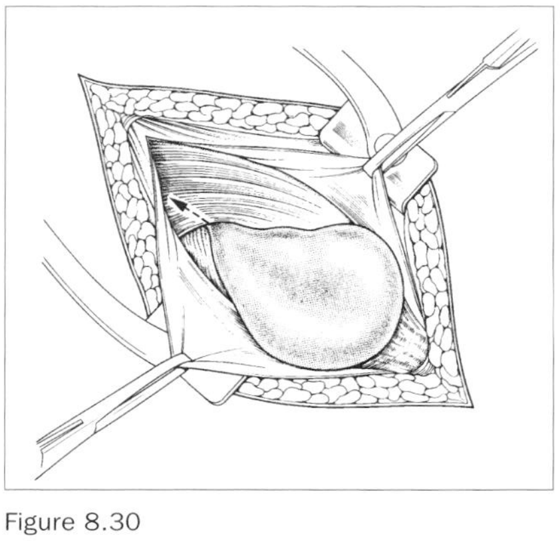

Figure 8.30

8.4 SURGICAL TREATMENT OF STRANGULATED GROIN HERNIA

Provide immediate treatment to patients with a strangulated groin hernia to relieve the obstruction. Begin an intravenous infusion with an electrolyte solution, hydrate the patient, insert a nasogastric tube and aspirate the stomach. If your patient has been vomiting, establish baseline serum electrolyte levels and correct any abnormalities.

Surgical repair

1 Open the skin, subcutaneous tissue and external oblique, as previously described (see Figures 8.1, 8.2 and 8.3). The internal ring may have to be divided to relieve the obstruction in indirect hernia and the inguinal ligament in femoral hernia. In both cases, divide the ring on the superior aspect to avoid underlying blood vessels.

2 Open the sac, being careful to prevent gut from returning to the abdomen, then carefully inspect it for viability. Give particular attention to constriction rings. If bowel falls back into the abdomen prior to assessment of its viability, perform a laparotomy.

3 Apply warm, wet packs to the gut for a few minutes. Gangrenous or nonviable gut will be black or deep blue without peristalsis. The mesenteric veins of the loop will appear thrombosed. There may be no arterial pulsation and the serosa will have lost its shiny appearance.

4 Resect any gangrenous loop of bowel and make an end-to-end anastomosis (see pages 6–11 to 6–13). If the resection of gangrenous bowel can be performed easily and well through the groin incision, continue with that approach. Otherwise, make a lower midline abdominal incision and do the resection using an abdominal approach. Excise the hernial sac and complete the repair as appropriate.

Operation for incarceration can be difficult in children, in patients with recurrent hernias, and in those with large, inguinoscrotal hernias. In these cases, consider non-operative reduction when patients present early with no signs of inflammation in the region of the hernia. To achieve non-operative reduction, place the patient in the Trendelenburg position, support both sides of the neck of the hernia with one hand and apply gentle, firm and continuous pressure to the sac with the opposite hand. Narcotic analgesia may be helpful.

Failure of reduction within 4 hours is an indication for operation. Observe the patient for at least 12 hours after a successful non-operative reduction.

Simple division of the obstructing ring

If non-operative reduction is unsuccessful in children, it may sometimes be prudent simply to divide the obstructing hernial ring (Figure 8.30). The obstructing ring in children is often the external inguinal ring, while in adults it is usually the internal ring. If such temporizing treatment is used, referral to a surgeon is required for definitive treatment.

8.5 SURGICAL REPAIR OF UMBILICAL AND PARA-UMBILICAL HERNIA

Umbilical hernia is common in children. As these congenital hernias usually close spontaneously, they should not be repaired before 5 years of age. Surgical repair of umbilical and para-umbilical hernia is necessary in adults, as strangulation is always a possibility.

Technique

1 Make a transverse incision just below the umbilicus (Figure 8.31).

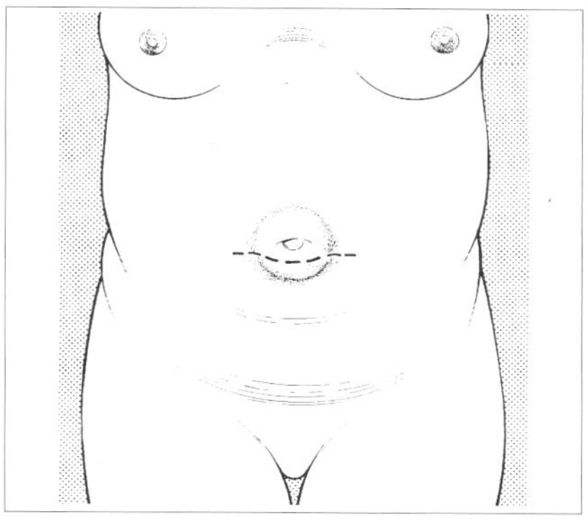

Figure 8.31

2 Clearly define the neck of the sac as it emerges through the linea alba and make an opening in the neck (Figures 8.32 and 8.33). Check for adhesions between the herniated mass and the inside of the sac, using a finger. Complete the division of the neck of the sac while protecting its contents. Carefully examine the contents of the sac (the gut and omentum) and reduce them (Figures 8.34 and 8.35). If the herniated mass consists of omentum alone, divide it in small segments between artery forceps and transfix the remaining tissue. Excise the sac (with any attached omentum) from under the umbilical skin.

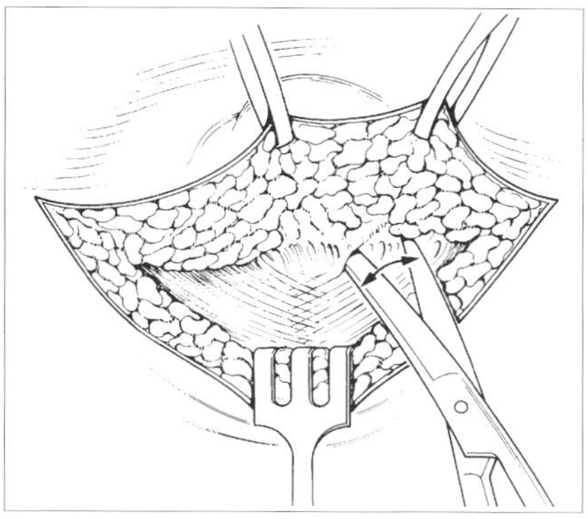

Figure 8.32

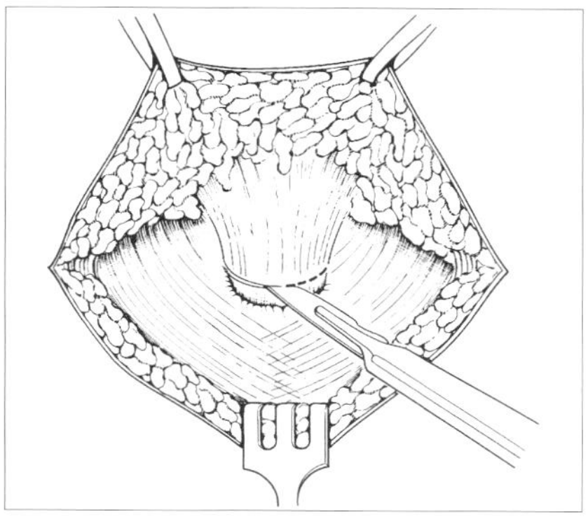

Figure 8.33

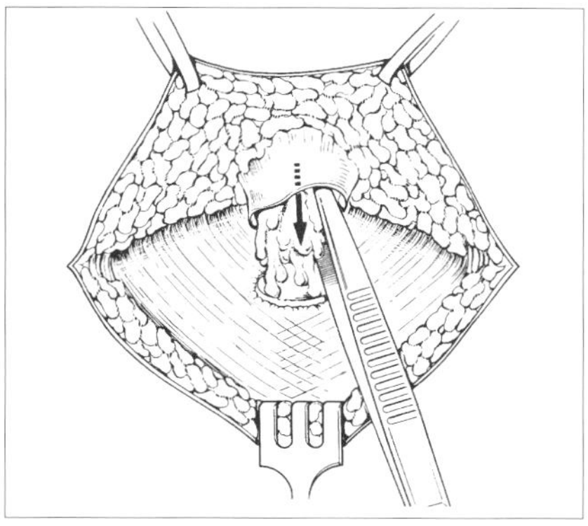

Figure 8.34

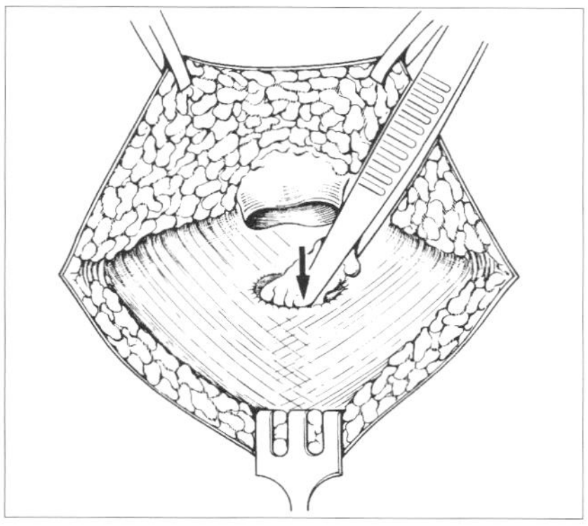

Figure 8.35

3 Using blunt dissection, clearly define the fibrous margins of the defect and enlarge it laterally (Figure 8.36). Make the repair by inserting mattress stitches of 0 non-absorbable suture through all layers of the wound so that the edges overlap; the peritoneum need not be closed separately (Figure 8.37). Apply a further row of stitches to approximate the overlapping edge to the linea alba (Figure 8.38). Complete closure by stitching the skin with 2/0 suture. Then apply a single-layer gauze dressing.

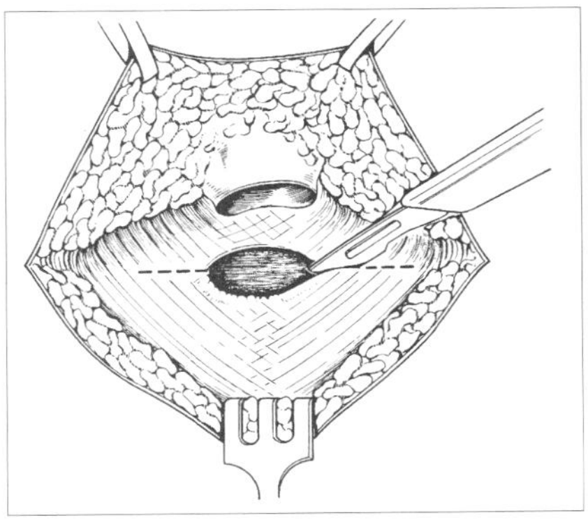

Figure 8.36

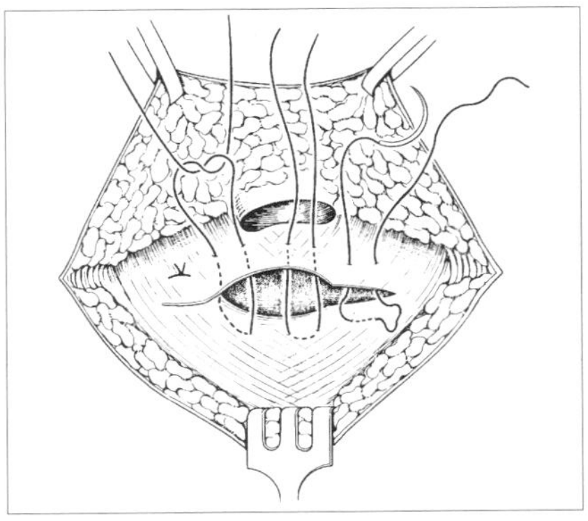

Figure 8.37

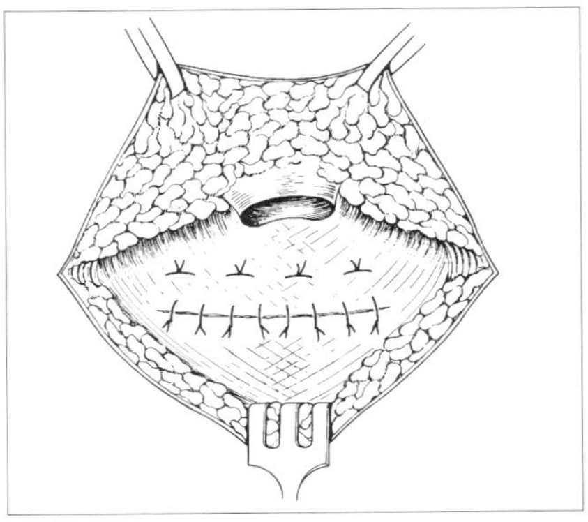

Figure 8.38

Use the same procedure in children, again making a curved incision below the umbilicus. Use simple, interrupted sutures to close small defects.

8.6 SURGICAL REPAIR OF EPIGASTRIC HERNIA

Epigastric hernias are usually protrusions of properitoneal fat, but occasionally contain omentum. They appear through a defect in the linea alba and are normally found in the midline between the xiphisternum and the umbilicus. There is no peritoneal sac.

Technique

1. If the hernia is single, make a transverse incision over the swelling. Make a midline incision over multiple midline epigastric hernias.
2. Dissect the herniated fatty mass down to its neck, make an opening in the neck, and excise both the covering and the extra peritoneal fat. Define the fibrous margins of the defect and close it with interrupted non-absorbable suture as described for para-umbilical hernia.

8.7 INCISIONAL HERNIA

Incisional hernias arise after abdominal surgery and are common after caesarean sections and gynaecological operations. They can be difficult to treat because of adhesions of abdominal viscera to the sac and because the size of the fascial defect may be so large that mesh is required for the repair. All but small incisional hernias should therefore be referred for treatment by a surgeon. Suprapubic incisional hernias are particularly complicated and require a surgical specialist to repair.

In the rare event of strangulation of an incisional hernia, operate to save the patient's life by dividing the fascia and relieving the obstruction. Make your incision through the previous scar. Close the fascia with interrupted monofilament nylon. If this is not possible, close the skin and refer for mesh closure.

Urinary tract and perineum

9

9.1 THE URINARY BLADDER

URINARY RETENTION

Acute retention of urine is an indication for emergency drainage of the bladder. If the bladder cannot be drained through the urethra, it requires suprapubic drainage.

Treatment of chronic retention is not urgent. Arrange to refer patients with chronic urinary retention for further management.

Emergency drainage

Emergency drainage of the bladder in acute retention may be undertaken by:

- Urethral catheterization
- Suprapubic puncture
- Suprapubic cystostomy.

Urethral catheterization or bladder puncture is usually adequate, but cystostomy may become necessary for the removal of a bladder stone or foreign body, or for more prolonged drainage, for example after rupture of the posterior urethra or if there is a urethral stricture with complications.

If a catheter's balloon fails to deflate, inject 3 ml of ether into the tube leading to the balloon. This will rupture the balloon. Cut it off and remove it. Prior to removing the catheter, irrigate the bladder with 30 ml of saline.

KEY POINTS

- Acute retention of urine is an indication for emergency drainage of the bladder
- The common causes of acute retention in the male are urethral stricture and benign prostatic hypertrophy
- Other causes of acute retention are urethral trauma and prostatic cancer
- If the bladder cannot be drained through the urethra, it requires suprapubic drainage
- In chronic retention of urine, because the obstruction develops slowly, the bladder is distended (stretched) very gradually over weeks, so pain is not a feature
- The bladder often overfills and the patient with chronic retention presents with dribbling of urine, referred to as "retention with overflow"
- Treatment of chronic retention is not urgent, but drainage of the bladder will help you to determine the volume of residual urine and prevent renal failure, which is associated with retention. Arrange to refer patients with chronic urinary retention for definitive management.

URETHRAL CATHETERIZATION IN THE MALE PATIENT

Technique

1 Reassure the patient that catheterization is atraumatic and usually uncomfortable rather than painful. Explain the procedure.

2 Wash the area with soap and water, retracting the prepuce to clean the furrow between it and the glans. Put on sterile gloves and, with sterile swabs, apply a bland antiseptic to the skin of the genitalia. Isolate the penis with a perforated sterile towel. Lubricate the catheter with generous amounts of water soluble gel.

3 Check the integrity of the Foley catheter balloon and then lubricate the catheter with sterile liquid paraffin (mineral oil). If you are right-handed, stand to the patient's right, hold the penis vertically and slightly stretched with the left hand, and introduce the Foley catheter gently with the other hand (Figure 9.1).

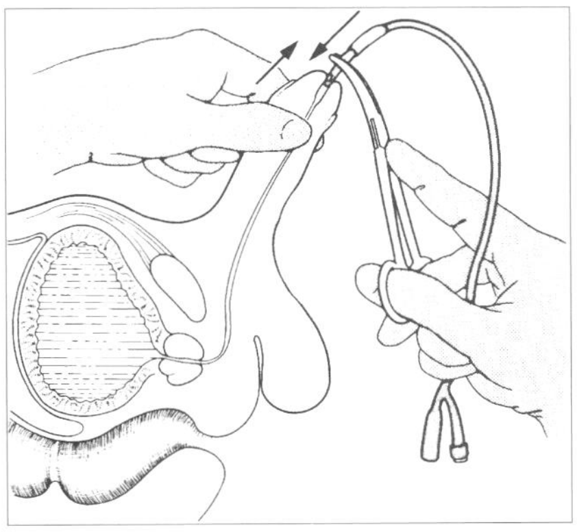

Figure 9.1

At 12–15 cm, the catheter may stick at the junction of the penile and bulbous urethra, in which case angle it down to allow it to enter the posterior urethra. A few centimetres further, there may be resistance caused by the external bladder sphincter, which can be overcome by a gentle pressure applied to the catheter for 20–30 seconds. Urine escaping through the catheter confirms entry into the bladder.

Advance the catheter 5 to 10 cm before inflating the balloon. This prevents the balloon inflating in the prostatic urethra.

4 If the catheter fails to pass the bulbous urethra and the membranous urethra, try a semi-rigid coudé catheter.

5 Pass a coudé catheter in three stages. With one hand, hold the penis stretched and, with the other hand, hold the catheter parallel to the fold of the groin. Introduce the catheter into the urethra and bring the penis to the midline against the patient's abdomen as the "beak" of the catheter approaches the posterior urethra. Finally, position the penis horizontally between the patient's legs as the catheter passes up the posterior urethra over the lip of the bladder neck. At this point, urine should flow from the catheter.

If you fail to pass a catheter, proceed to filiforms and followers (Figure 9.2) or use a Foley catheter with a guide. If these procedures are unsuccessful, abandon them in favour of suprapubic puncture. Forcing the catheter or a metal bougie can create a false passage, causing urethral bleeding and intolerable pain, and increasing the risk of infection.

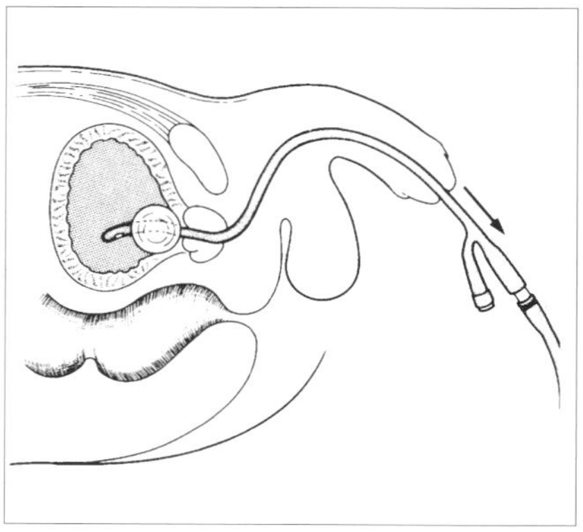

Figure 9.2

Fixation of the catheter

1 If you are using a Foley catheter, inflate the balloon with 10–15 ml of sterile water or clean urine (Figure 9.2). Partially withdraw the catheter until its balloon abuts on the bladder neck.

2 If the catheter has no balloon, knot a ligature around the catheter just beyond the external meatus and carry the ends along the body of the penis, securing them with a spiral of strapping brought forward over the glans and the knot (Figures 9.3, 9.4, 9.5).

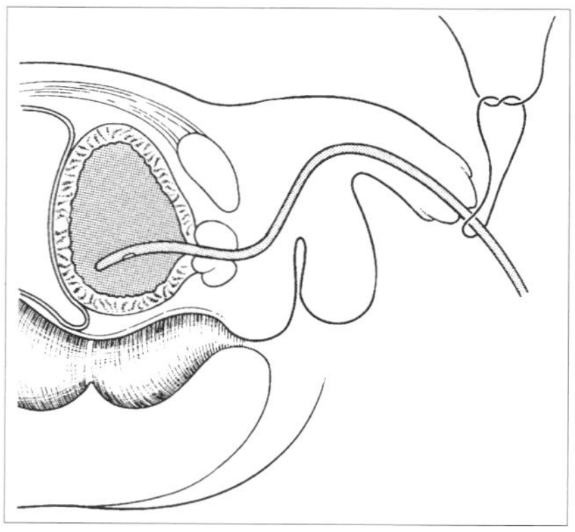

Figure 9.3

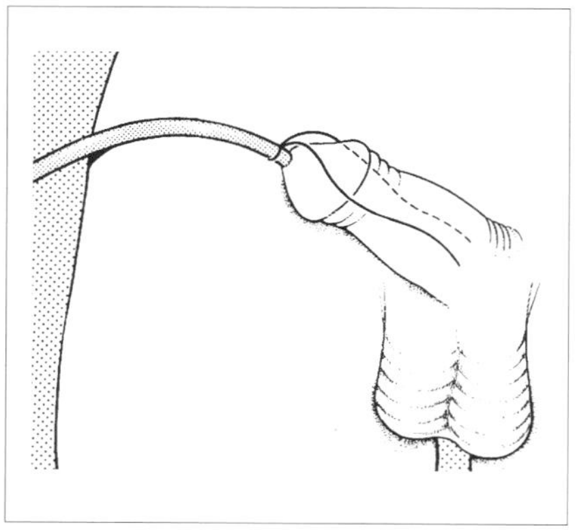

Figure 9.4

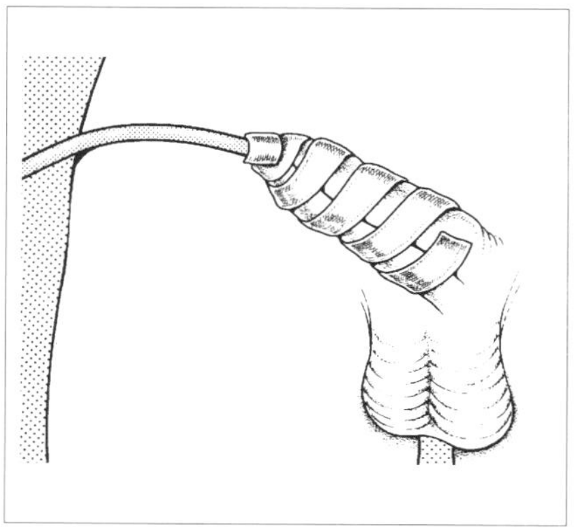

Figure 9.5

Aftercare

- If the catheterization was traumatic, administer an antibiotic with a gram negative spectrum for 3 days
- Always decompress a chronically distended bladder slowly
- Connect the catheter through a closed system to a sterile container (Figure 9.6)
- Strap the penis and catheter laterally to the abdominal wall; this will avoid a bend in the catheter at the penoscrotal angle and help to prevent compression ulceration
- Change the catheter if it becomes blocked or infected, or as otherwise indicated. Ensure a generous fluid intake to prevent calculus formation in recumbent patients, who frequently have urinary infections, especially in tropical countries.

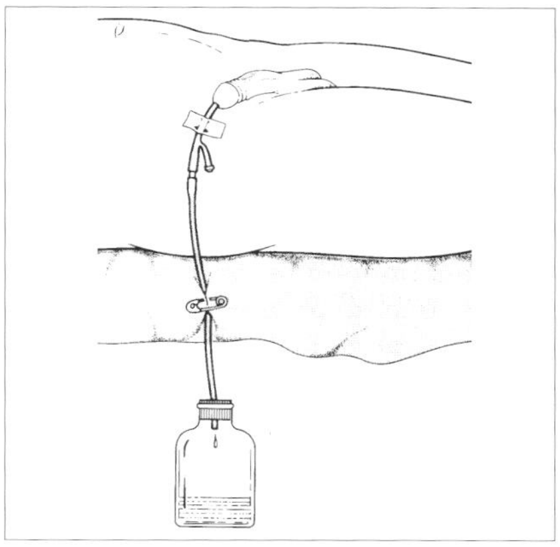

Figure 9.6

SUPRAPUBIC PUNCTURE

Bladder puncture may become necessary if urethral catheterization fails. It is essential that the bladder is palpable if a suprapubic puncture is to be performed.

Technique

1 Assess the extent of bladder distension by inspection and palpation.

2 If you are proceeding to suprapubic puncture immediately after catheterization has failed, remove the perforated sheet that was used to isolate the penis and centre the opening of a new sheet over the midline above the pubis.

3 Make a simple puncture 2 cm above the symphysis pubis in the midline with a wide-bore needle connected to a 50 ml syringe. This will afford the patient immediate relief, but the puncture must be made again after some hours if the patient does not pass urine.

4 It is preferable to perform a suprapubic puncture with a trochar and cannula, and subsequently to insert a catheter. Raise a weal of local anaesthetic in the midline, 2 cm above the symphysis pubis, and then continue with deeper infiltration (Figure 9.7). Once anaesthesia is accomplished, make a simple puncture 2 cm above the symphysis pubis in the midline with a wide bore needle. Introduce the trochar and cannula

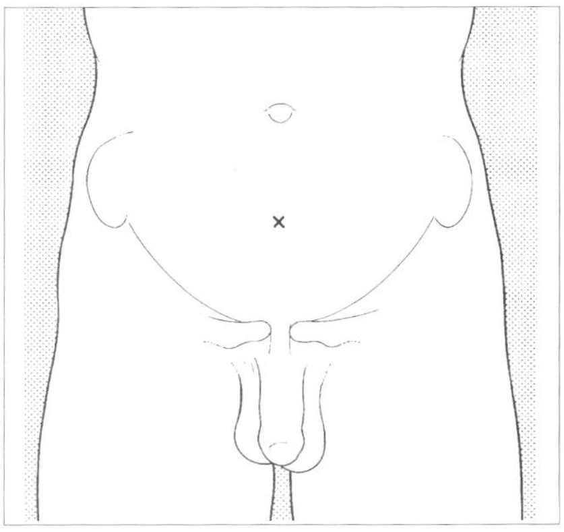

Figure 9.7

and advance them vertically with care (Figure 9.8). After meeting some resistance, they will pass easily into the cavity of the bladder, as confirmed by the flow of urine when the trochar is withdrawn from the cannula.

5 Introduce the catheter well into the bladder (Figure 9.9). Once urine flows freely from the catheter, withdraw the cannula (Figure 9.10).

6 Fix the catheter to the skin with the stitch used to close the wound and connect it to a bag or bottle. Take care that the catheter does not become blocked, especially if the bladder is grossly distended. If necessary, clear the catheter by syringing with saline.

This type of drainage allows later investigation of the lower urinary tract, for example by urethrocystography, to determine the nature of any obstruction.

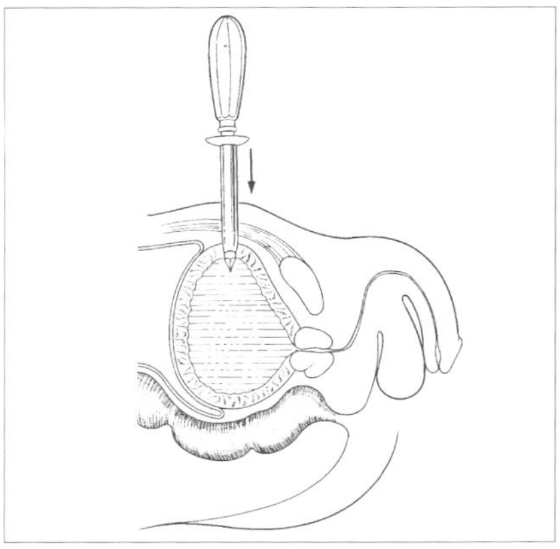

Figure 9.8

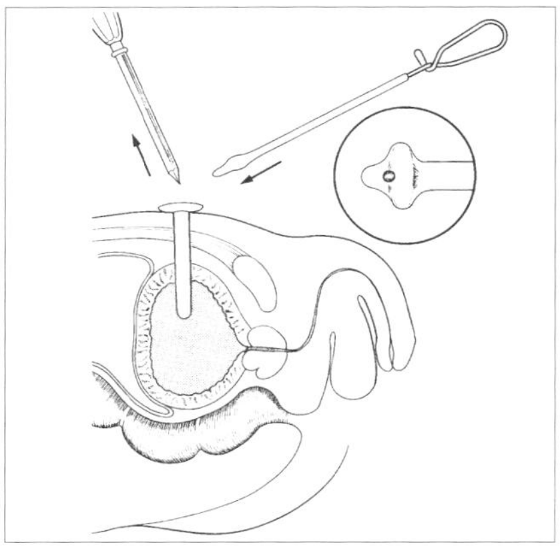

Figure 9.9

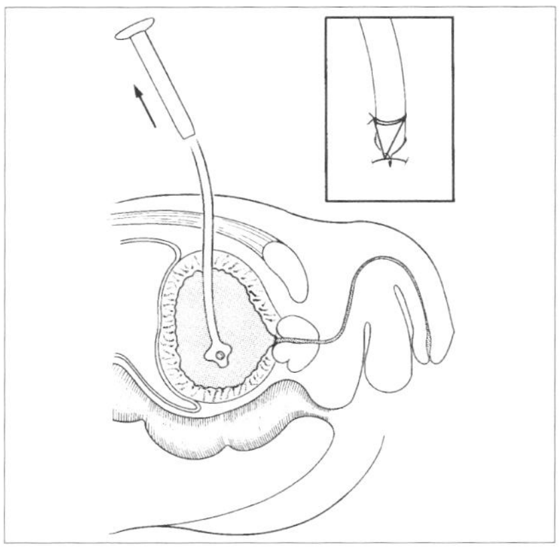

Figure 9.10

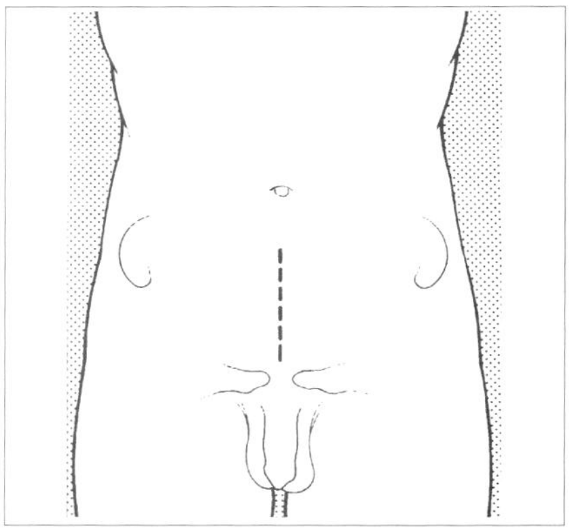

Figure 9.11

SUPRAPUBIC CYSTOSTOMY

The purpose of suprapubic cystostomy is:

- To expose and, if necessary, allow exploration of the bladder
- To permit insertion of a large drainage tube, usually a self-retaining catheter
- To allow suprapubic drainage of a non-palpable bladder.

Technique

1 If the patient is in poor condition, use a local anaesthetic, for example, 0.5% to 1% lidocaine with epinephrine (adrenaline) for layer-by-layer infiltration of the tissues. Otherwise, general anaesthesia is preferable. See page 14 – 4 for dose calculation.

2 Place the patient supine. Centre a midline suprapubic incision 2 cm above the symphysis pubis (Figure 9.11) and divide the subcutaneous tissues. Achieve haemostasis by pressure and ligation

3 Open the rectus sheath, starting in the upper part of the wound. Continue dissection with scissors to expose the gap between the muscles (Figure 9.12). In the lower part of the incision, the pyramidalis muscles will obscure this gap. Finally, expose the extraperitoneal fat.

4 Carry the incision in the linea alba down to the pubis, splitting the pyramidalis muscles. With a finger, break through the prevesical fascia behind the pubis; then sweep the fascia and peritoneum upwards from

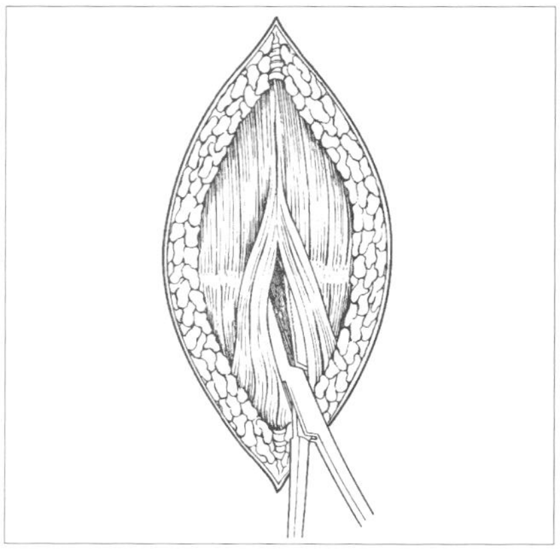

Figure 9.12

the bladder surface (Figure 9.13). Take care not to open the peritoneum. The distended bladder can be recognized by its pale pink colour and the longitudinal veins on its surface. On palpation, it has the resistance of a distended sac. Insert a self-retaining retractor to hold this exposure.

5 Insert stay sutures of No. 1 absorbable suture into the upper part of the bladder on either side of the midline (Figure 9.14). Puncture the bladder between the sutures and empty it by suction (Figure 9.15). Explore the interior of the bladder with a finger to identify any calculus or tumour (Figure 9.16). Note the state of the internal meatus, which may be narrowed by a prostatic adenoma or a fibrous ring.

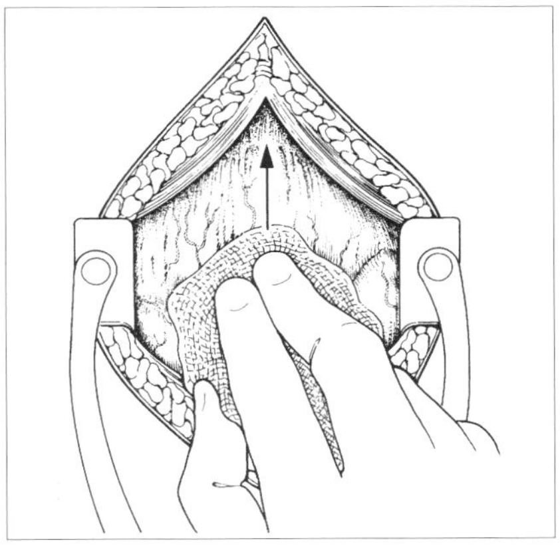

Figure 9.13

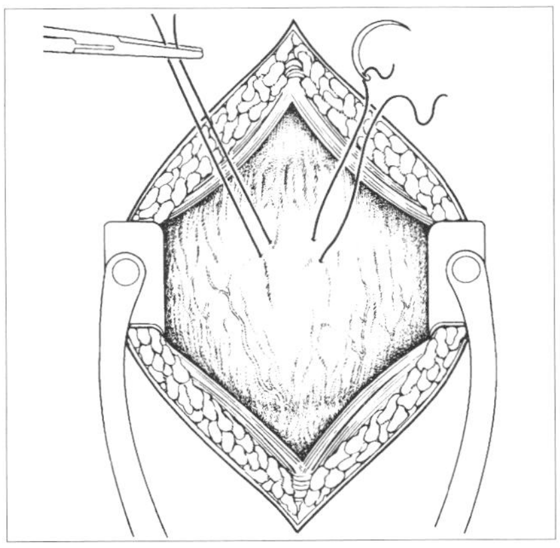

Figure 9.14

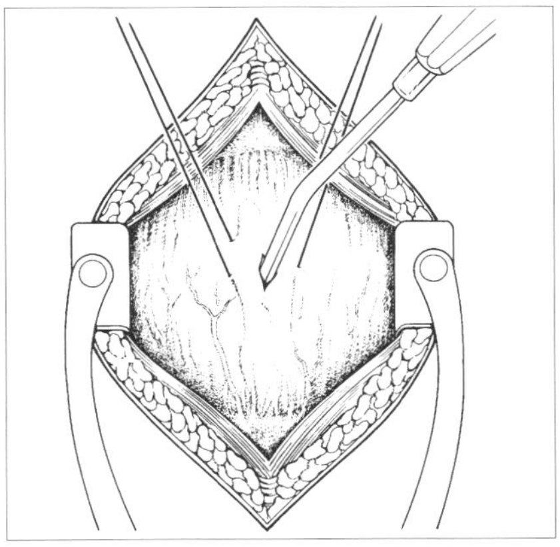

Figure 9.15

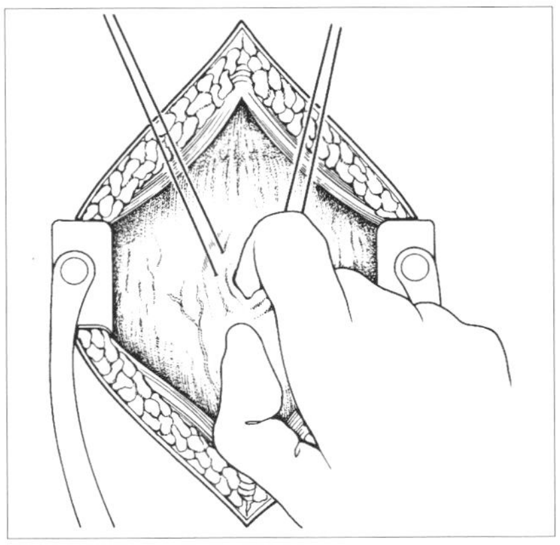

Figure 9.16

6 If the bladder opening must be enlarged to allow you to remove a loose stone, open it 1–2 cm, inserting a haemostatic stitch of 2/0 absorbable suture in the cut edge, if necessary. Close the extended incision partially with one or two stitches of No. 1 absorbable suture, picking up only the bladder muscle. Inspect the interior of the bladder for retained swabs before you introduce the catheter.

7 For insertion of the catheter, hold the edges of the incision with two pairs of tissue forceps, making sure that the mucosa is included so that the catheter does not slip beneath the mucosa (Figure 9.17):

- If you are using a de Pezzer catheter, stretch its head with forceps and introduce the catheter into the bladder between the two pairs of tissue forceps
- If you are using a Foley catheter, introduce it into the bladder and inflate the balloon.

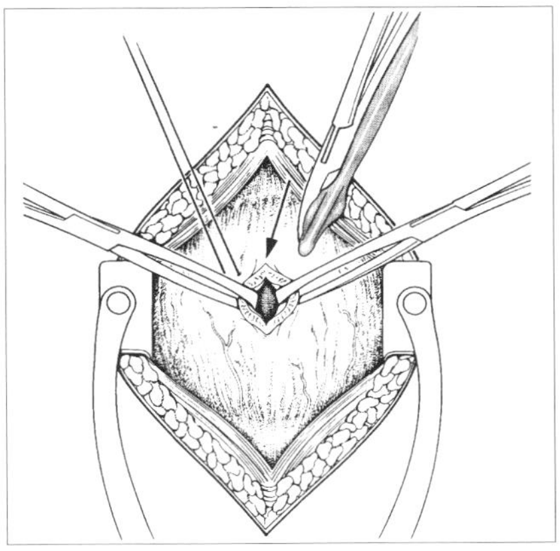

Figure 9.17

8 Insert a purse-string 2/0 absorbable suture in the bladder muscle to ensure a watertight closure around the tube or, if you have made an extended incision in the bladder, secure the catheter with the final stitch needed to close the incision (Figure 9.18).

9 If drainage is to be continued for a long period, fix the bladder to the abdominal wall so that the catheter can be changed. Otherwise, omit this step to allow more rapid healing of the bladder wound. To fix the bladder, pass the traction stitches in the bladder wall out through the rectus sheath (Figure 9.19). Tie them together after closing this layer.

10 Close the linea alba with 0 absorbable suture and the skin with 2/0 non-absorbable suture (Figure 9.20). Connect the tube to a sterile, closed drainage system. Dress the wound every second day until it is healed.

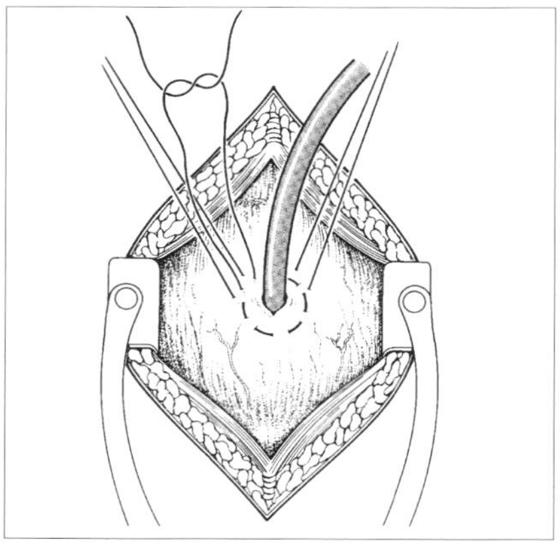

Figure 9.18

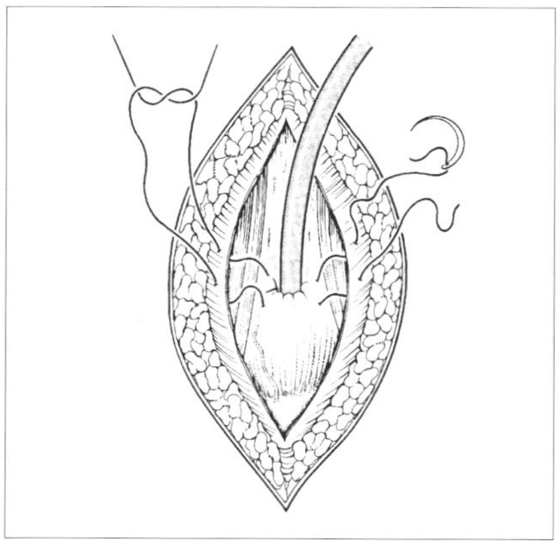

Figure 9.19

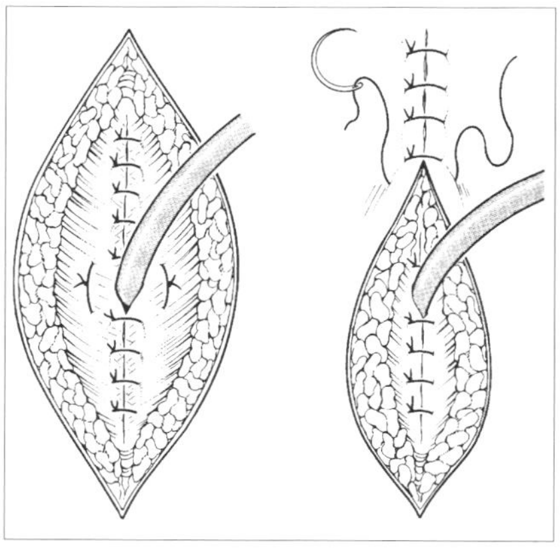

Figure 9.20

KEY POINTS

- Filiforms and followers are the safest means of dilating acute strictures
- Chronic strictures can be managed safely with repeat dilations using metal bougies
- Suprapubic puncture or cystostomy should not be thought of as the last resort and are much preferable to continued instrumentation, which can lead to urethral traumatization.

9.2 THE MALE URETHRA

URETHRAL STRICTURE

Urethral dilatation is indicated for urethral stricture, a problem which is common in certain parts of the world.

Technique

1 Administer appropriate analgesia and sedation before beginning the procedure and start antibiotic treatment, to be continued for three days. Carefully clean the glans and meatus, and prepare the skin with a bland antiseptic. Instil lidocaine gel into the urethra (optional) and retain it for 5 minutes. Drape the patient with a perforated towel to isolate the penis.

2 In the acute stricture, begin by introducing a small filiform; leave it in the urethra and continue to insert filiforms until one passes the stricture. Then progress to dilatation with medium-size followers and gradually work up in size (Figure 9.21).

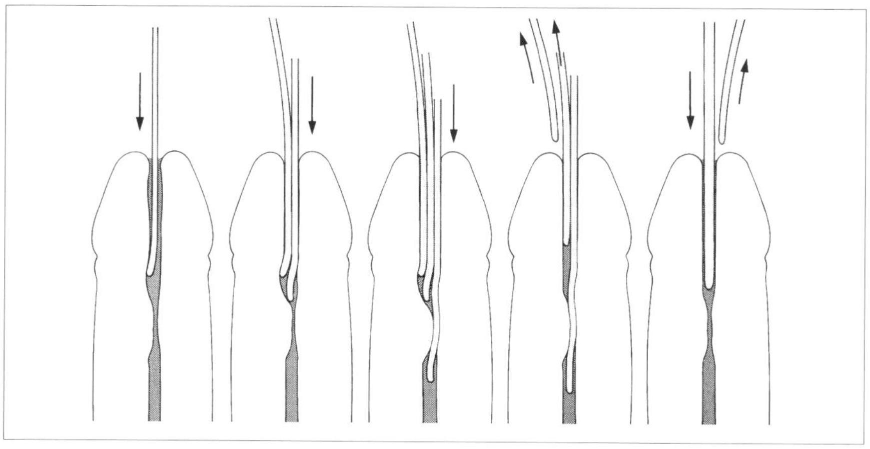

Figure 9.21

For a post-inflammatory stricture that starts in the anterior urethra, always introduce a straight bougie first; this will minimize the risk of urethral damage (Figure 9.22).

9

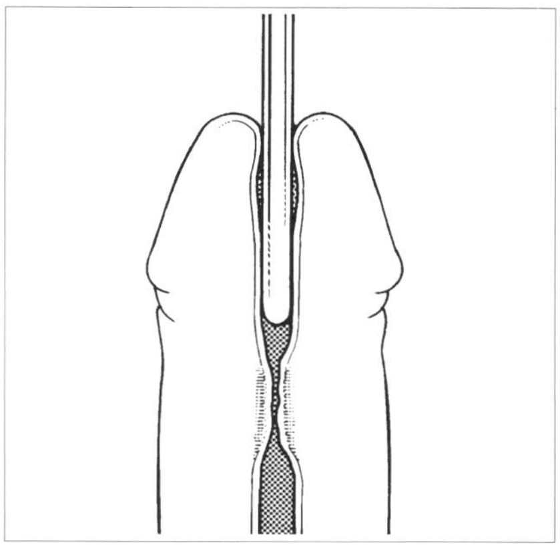

Figure 9.22

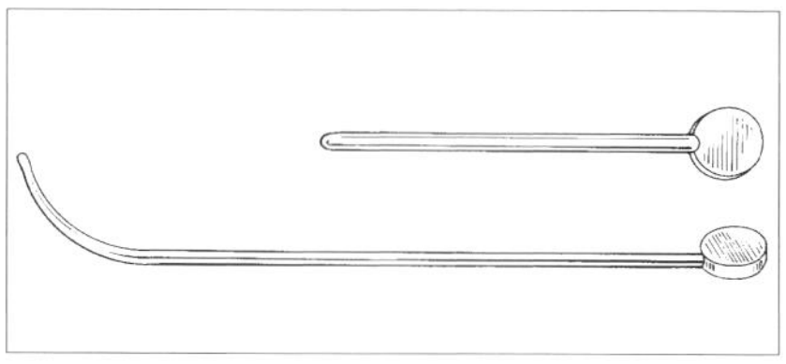

Figure 9.23

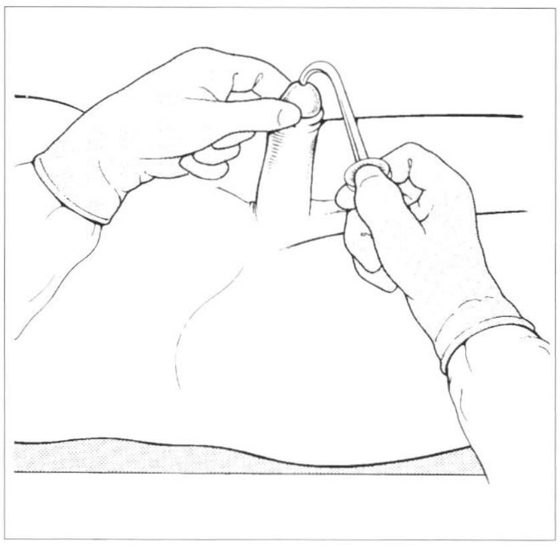

Figure 9.24

After the acute stricture is dilated with filiforms and followers, bouginage can be undertaken at regular intervals, using metal bougies.

Perform dilatation with straight bougies of increasing size, and finally introduce a curved bougie (Figure 9.23). Remember that the small sizes of metal bougies are the most likely to lacerate the urethra. Therefore, in this situation, filiforms and followers should be used.

3 Introduce a curved bougie in three stages:
- Bring the bougie parallel to the crease of the groin and hold the penis taut (Figure 9.24)
- While raising the taut penis to the midline towards the patient's abdomen, slip the bougie into the posterior urethra and let it progress by its own weight (Figure 9.25)
- Finally, bring the penis down to the midline, horizontally between the patient's legs, as the curve of the bougie carries it up the posterior urethra and over the neck of the bladder (Figure 9.26).

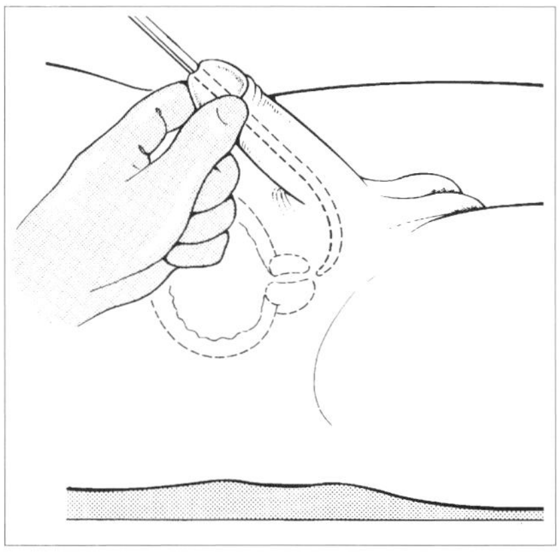

Figure 9.25

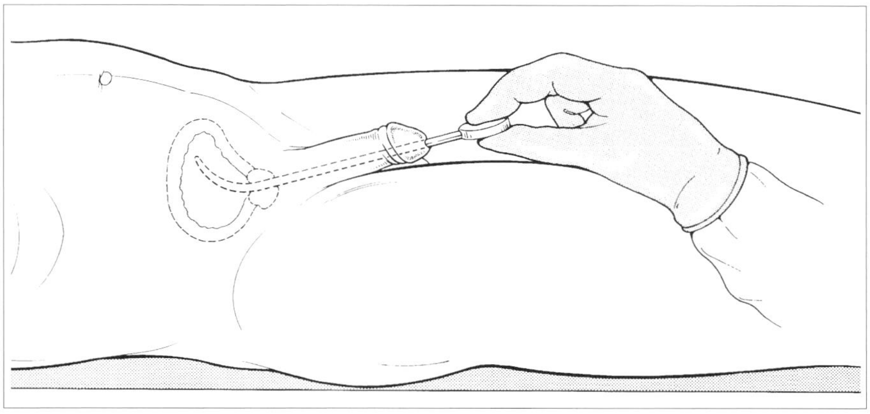

Figure 9.26

4 Initially, dilate the patient's urethra at least twice a week, using two or three sizes of bougie successively at each session. Begin with the smallest sizes (for example, 12) and stop at about 24 Ch. If there is urethral bleeding, skip a session to give the mucosa time to heal. Perform follow-up dilatation:
- Weekly for 4 weeks
- Twice monthly for 6 months
- Every month thereafter.

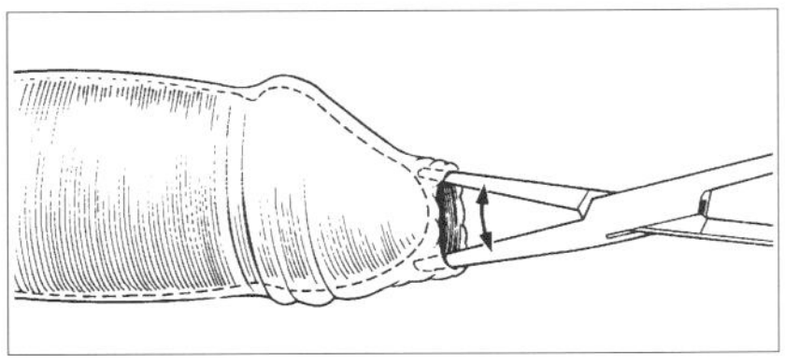
Figure 9.27

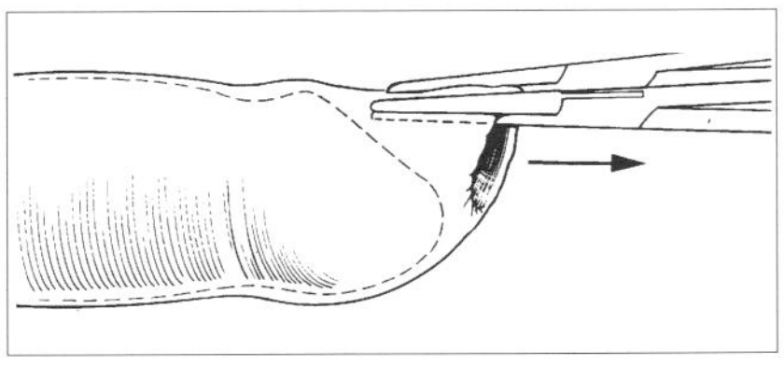
Figure 9.28

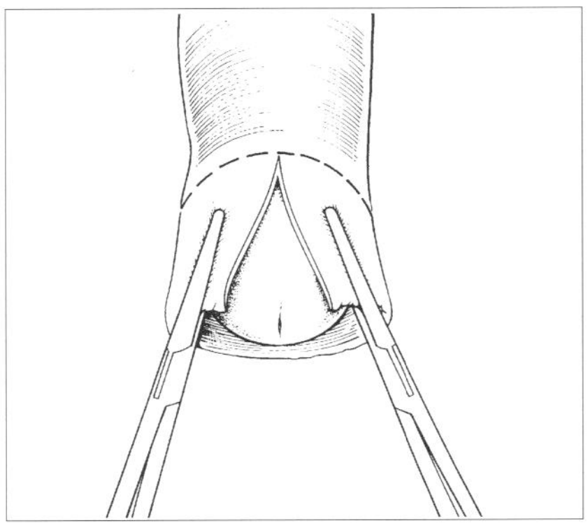
Figure 9.29

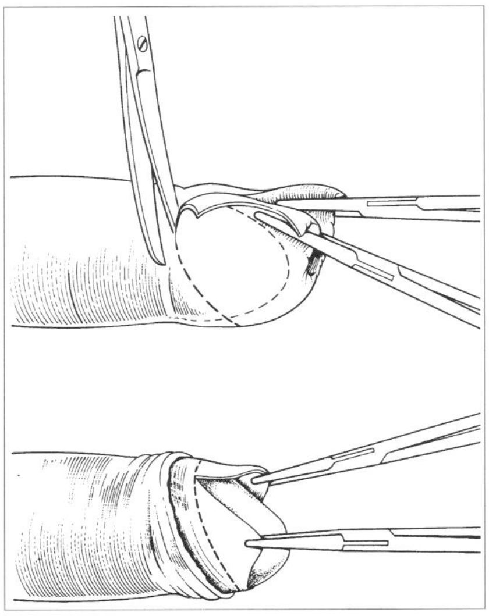
Figure 9.30

Possible complications

- Trauma – bleeding or creation of a false passage
- Bacteraemia
- Septicaemia and septic shock.

Minimize complications by asepsis and the use of antibiotics.

THE PREPUCE

Diseases of the penile foreskin include:

- Phimosis
- Paraphimosis
- Recurrent balanitis
- Injury to the foreskin.

Male circumcision

The resection of the prepuce is the definitive surgical treatment. The purpose of the operation is to resect the prepuce obliquely at the level of the corona of the glans, allowing the glans to be fully exposed while preserving enough of the frenulum to permit erection.

Technique

1 Conduction anaesthesia can be used for circumcision. Dorsal nerve block is reinforced by infiltration of the underside of the penis between the corpus spongiosum and the corpora cavernosa.

2 Prepare all the external genitalia with an antiseptic. If the prepuce can be retracted, carefully clean the glans and the preputial furrow with soap and water. If the prepuce cannot be retracted, gently stretch the preputial opening by inserting the blades of a pair of artery forceps and slowly opening them until the area can be properly cleaned (Figure 9.27). Break down any fine adhesions between the glans and replace the prepuce. Isolate the penis with a perforated towel.

3 Take hold of the prepuce dorsally in the midline with pairs of forceps and cut down between the forceps with scissors until the blades nearly reach the corona (Figures 9.28, 9.29). Check that the lower blade really is lying between the glans and prepuce and has not been inadvertently passed up the external meatus. Then excise the prepuce by extending the dorsal slit obliquely around on either side to the frenulum, and trim the inner preputial layer, leaving at least 3 mm of mucosa (Figure 9.30).

4 Catch the cut edges of the frenulum and the bleeding artery of the frenulum with absorbable suture, leaving the suture long as a traction stitch to steady the penis (Figure 9.31). Insert a similar traction stitch to unite the edges of the prepuce dorsally (Figure 9.32). Catch and tie any bleeding vessels on either side of the raw area. Unite the edges of the prepuce with interrupted stitches and cut the stitches short (Figures 9.33, 9.34).

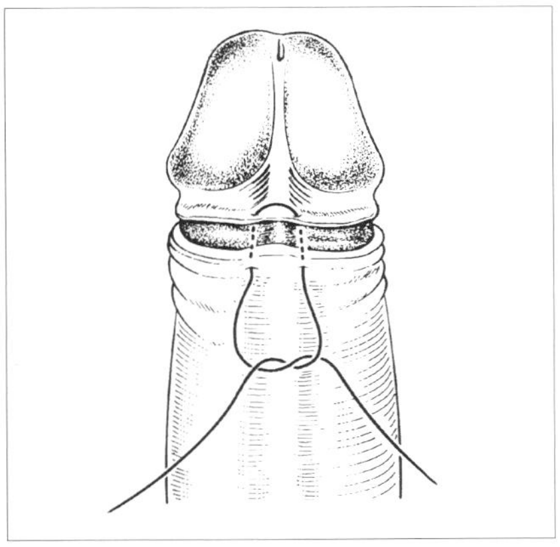

Figure 9.31

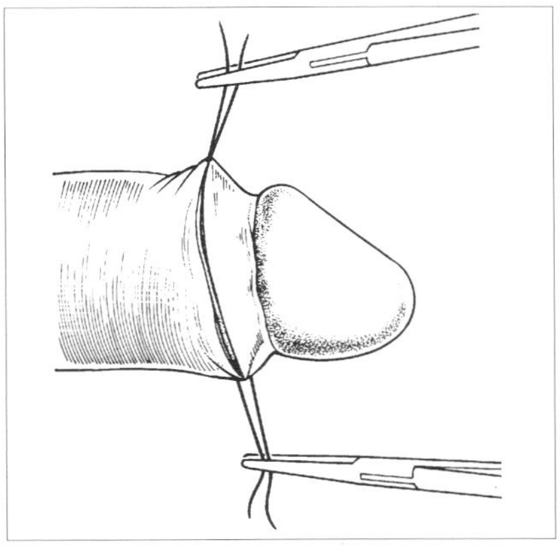

Figure 9.32

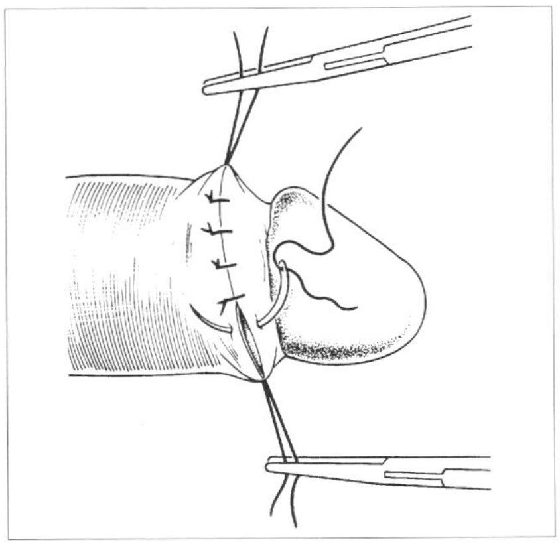

Figure 9.33

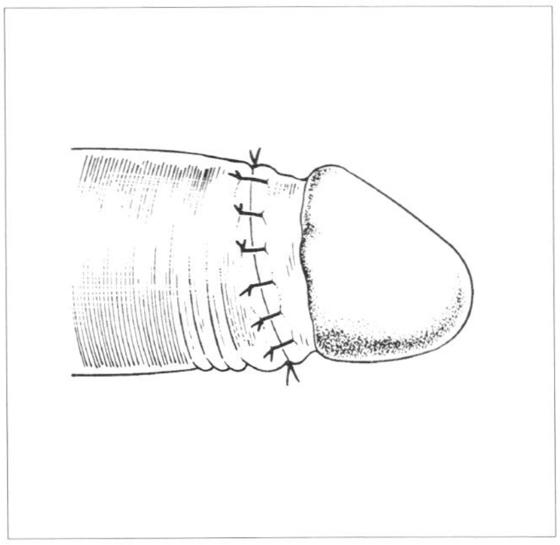

Figure 9.34

Aftercare

Dressing the penis with loose layers of petroleum gauze covered with dry gauze is optional. The alternative is open management without dressing. The stitches should dissolve in 10–15 days.

Complications

The most serious complication of operation is haematoma due to failure to secure the artery to the frenulum sufficiently or to dehiscence of the stitches as a result of an early morning erection.

PARAPHIMOSIS

Paraphimosis occurs most commonly in children. Diagnose it by recognizing a retracted, swollen and painful foreskin. The glans penis is visible, and is surrounded by an oedematous ring with a proximal constricting ring (Figure 9.35).

Differential diagnosis includes:

- Inflammation of the foreskin (balanitis) due, for example, to infection
- Swelling caused by an insect bite.

In such cases, the glans is not visible.

KEY POINTS

- Paraphimosis should be treated urgently with manual reduction of the foreskin or dorsal slit
- Phimosis is prevented by reduction of the foreskin and cleansing of the glans penis on a regular basis
- Phimosis may be treated definitively by circumcision or with a dorsal slit, if necessary.

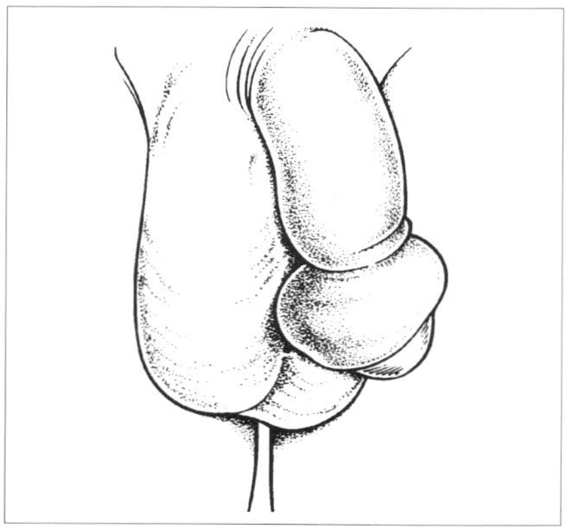

Figure 9.35

Treat paraphimosis by reduction of the foreskin or, if this fails, by dorsal slit or circumcision.

Reduction of the foreskin

1 Sedate the child and prepare the skin of the genitalia with a bland antiseptic. Isolate the penis with a perforated towel and inject local anaesthetic in a ring around its base (Figure 9.36).

2 Once local anaesthesia is achieved, take hold of the oedematous part of the penis in the fist of one hand and squeeze firmly; a gauze swab may be necessary for a firm grip (Figure 9.37). Exert continuous pressure, changing hands if necessary, until the oedema fluid passes proximally under the constricting band to the shaft of the penis (Figure 9.38). The foreskin can usually then be pulled over the glans (Figure 9.39).

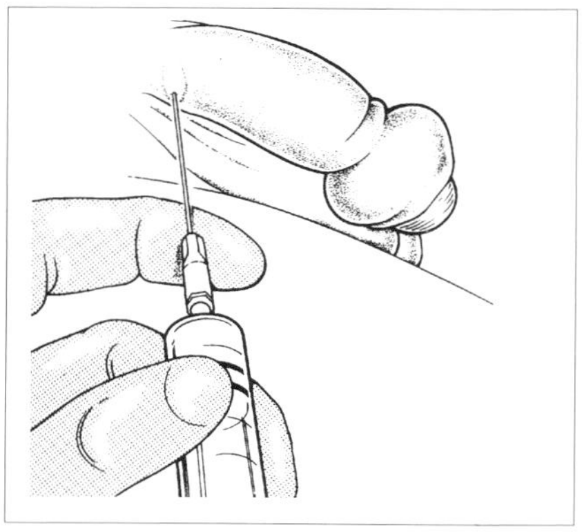

Figure 9.36

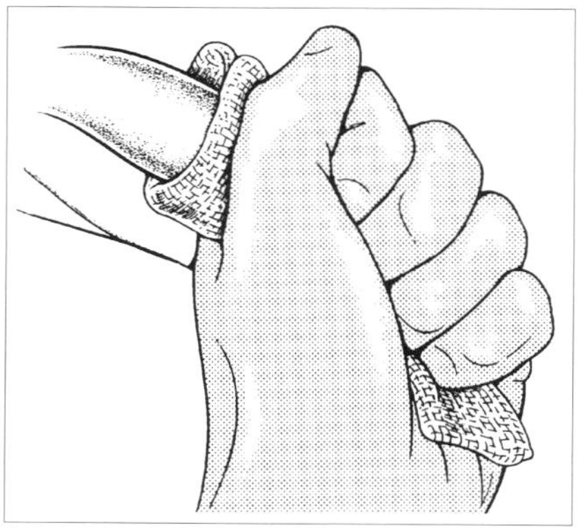

Figure 9.37

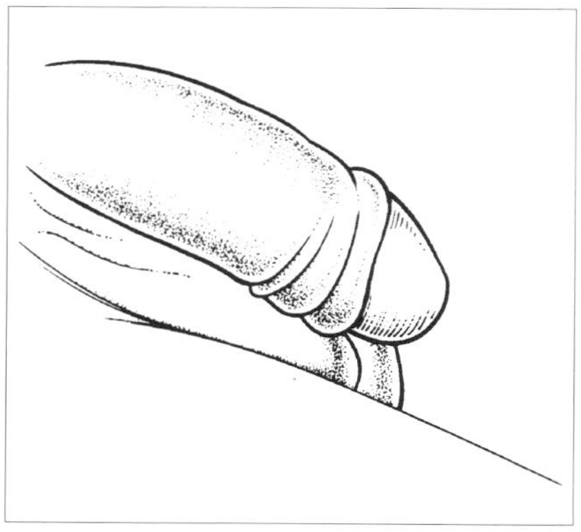

Figure 9.38

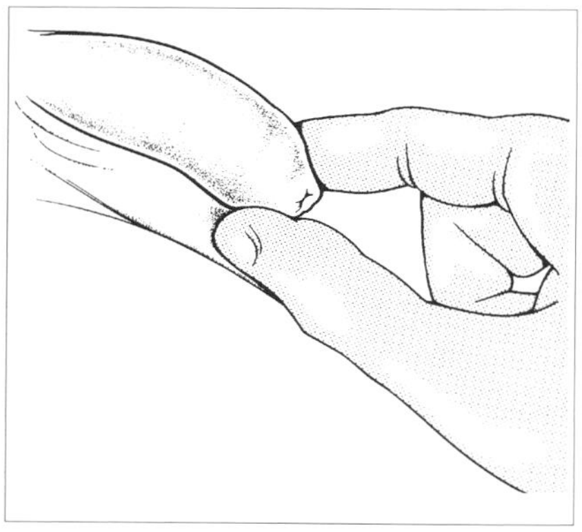

Figure 9.39

Aftercare

Have the patient wear a scrotal support for 48 hours after the operation.

- Phimosis and paraphimosis are definitively treated with circumcision, but can be treated with a dorsal slit of the foreskin
- Dorsal slit can be performed with direct infiltration of the foreskin with xylocaine 1% without epinephrine (adrenaline)
- Clamp the foreskin with two artery forceps and make an incision between them (Figure 9.40).

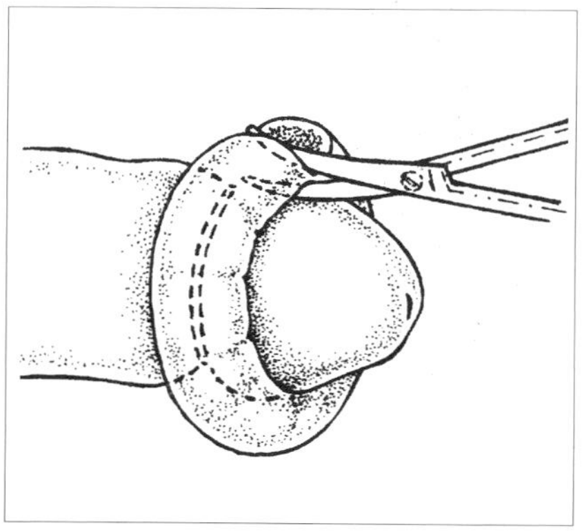

Figure 9.40

TORSION OF THE TESTIS

Torsion of the testis is seen most commonly in children and adolescents. The predisposing factors are congenital scrotal abnormalities which include:

- Long mesorchium, a horizontal lie of the testis within the scrotum
- Ectopic testis.

The presentation is one of sudden onset of lower abdominal pain, pain in the affected testis and vomiting. The affected testis and cord are markedly tender. The testis is often swollen and drawn upwards. Important differential diagnoses include:

- Epididymorchitis: the patient often has urinary symptoms, including urethral discharge
- Testicular tumour: the onset is not sudden.

Treatment

The treatment is urgent surgery to:

- Untwist the torsion
- Fix the testis
- Explore the other side and similarly fix the testis to prevent the normal testis from undergoing torsion subsequently.

Operate on torsion of the testis without delay. Make every effort to save the testis. Do not rush into performing orchidectomy even if, at exposure, you think that the testis is already gangrenous. Always ask for a second opinion in such circumstances.

Wrap the affected testis with warm wet swabs, wait for a minimum of 5 minutes and check for any improvement in colour. Do not hurry this stage; give yourself plenty of time, provided you have already untwisted the torsion. However, if the testis is dead, it should be removed, as autoimmune responses can result in loss of function of the other testis.

KEY POINTS

- In torsion, the testicle can become gangrenous in 4 hours; treatment is thus an emergency
- The non-affected side should be fixed at the same time as the subsequent incidence of torsion on the opposite side is high
- When the testis is dead, orchidectomy should be performed to protect the other testis from loss due to autoimmune disease
- One testicle is enough for normal fertility.

SCROTAL HYDROCOELE

Scrotal hydrocoele is an abnormal accumulation of fluid in the tunica vaginalis sac (Figure 9.41). The swelling that results is often enormous and usually uncomfortable. In adults, the hydrocoele fluid is located entirely within the

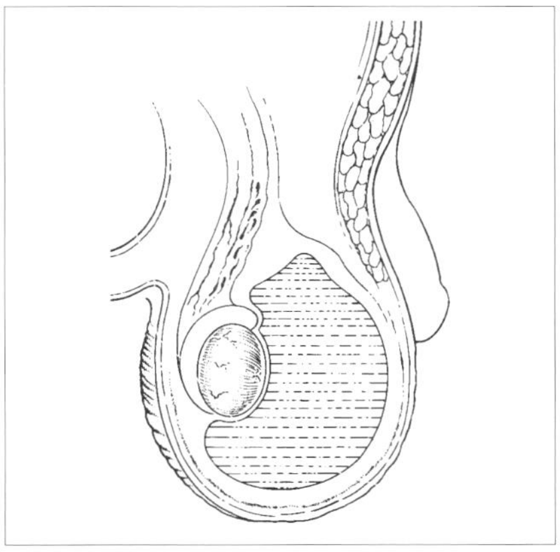

Figure 9.41

KEY POINTS

A hydrocoele is differentiated from hernia in that it:

- Does not extend above the inguinal ligament
- Transilluminates
- Does not reduce
- Does not transmit a cough impulse
- In children, the hydrocoele often communicates with the peritoneal cavity; it is a variation of hernia and is managed as a hernia
- Non-communicating hydrocoeles in children under the age of 1 year often resolve without intervention
- The surgical management of adult hydrocoele is not appropriate for children.

9

scrotum; the surgical treatment is straightforward and can be performed by a non specialist.

Diagnosis

Palpation will confirm that the swelling is scrotal; it will be soft or tense, fluctuant and may mask the testis and epididymis.

Lymphoedema of the scrotum is characterized by thickened skin.

Treatment

Aspiration is not recommended, as the relief is only temporary and repeated aspirations risk infection. Injection of sclerosants is not recommended, as it is painful and, although inflammation is reduced, it does not effect a cure. Surgery is the most effective treatment.

Of the various alternative operations, eversion of the tunica vaginalis is the simplest, although recurrences are still possible.

Wash the scrotal skin and treat any lesions, for example wounds made by traditional healers, with saline dressings. The presence of skin lesions is not a contraindication to surgical treatment, so long as there are healthy granulations with little or no infection.

Technique

1 Perform the procedure with local infiltrate, spinal or general anaesthesia. Prepare the skin widely with antiseptic. Place a sterile towel under the scrotum (Figure 9.42); elevating the scrotum with tissue forceps will facilitate this. Stand on the side of the lesion.

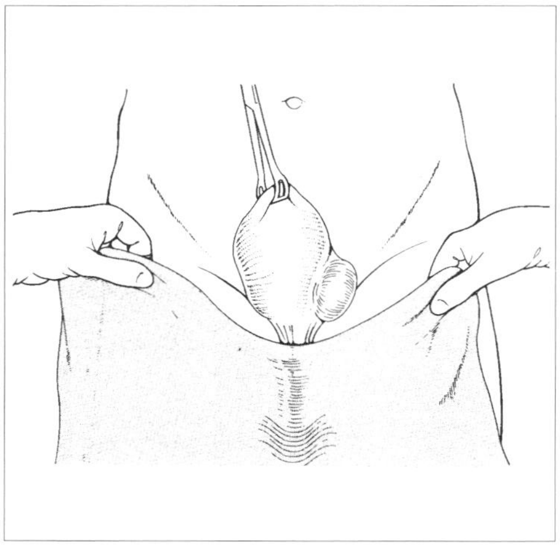

Figure 9.42

2 Press on the hydrocele to render it tense, make an oblique incision over the hydrocele in a skin crease (Figure 9.43) or in the midline, which is less haemorrhagic. Continue incising through the layers of the scrotal wall down to the tunica vaginalis. This is normally recognized by a lattice of fine blood vessels in a thin, translucent membrane unless the membrane

has been thickened by previous infection or trauma. Ligate all vessels encountered with 2/0 absorbable suture (Figure 9.44).

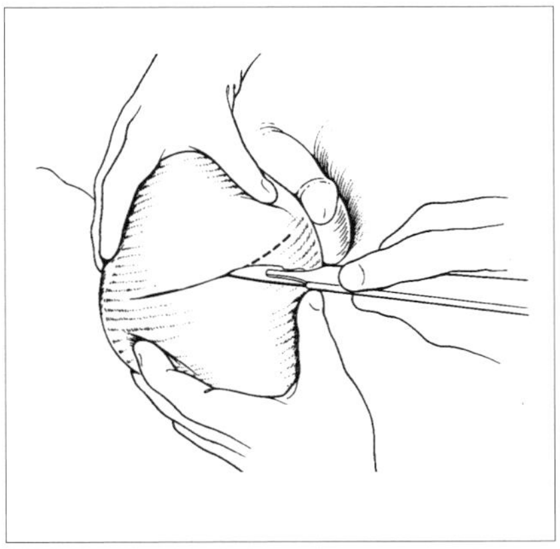

Figure 9.43

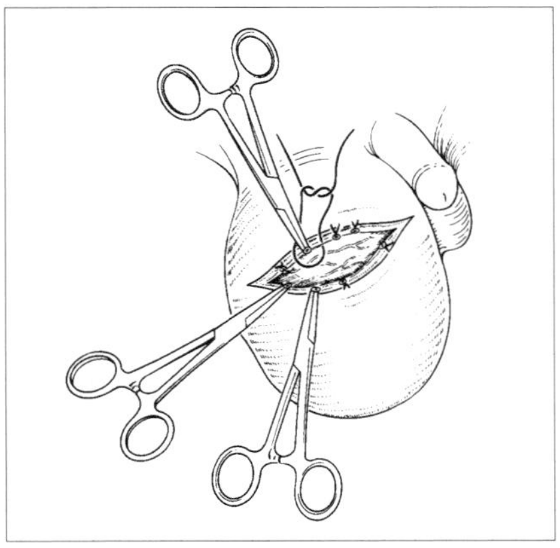

Figure 9.44

3 By means of blunt dissection with scissors, find a plane of cleavage between the sac and the fibrous coverings. With gauze and scissors, continue separation to the termination of the spermatic cord where it is attached to the hydrocele (Figures 9.45, 9.46). If the sac is inadvertently opened, catch the edges of the opening with forceps and introduce a finger into the sac to stretch it and the overlying tissues as an aid in dissection. Puncture the sac and collect the fluid in a dish (Figure 9.47). Catch the edge of the hole with forceps and, after making sure that the epididymis is not adherent to its posterior surface, slit the sac vertically with scissors (Figure 9.48).

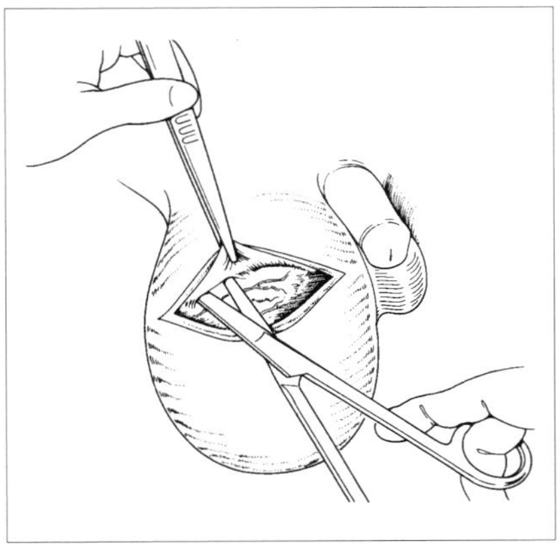

Figure 9.45

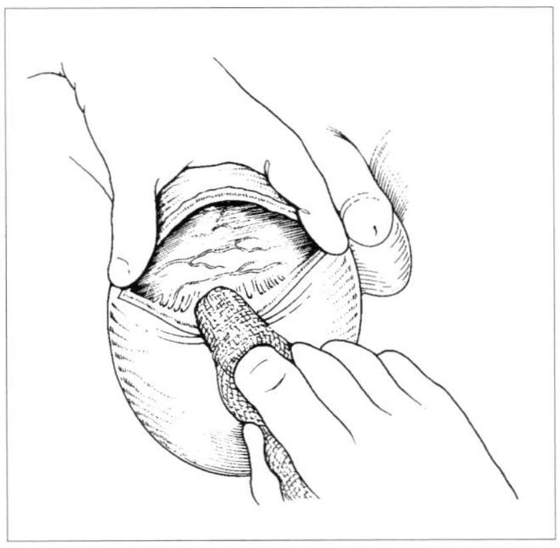

Figure 9.46

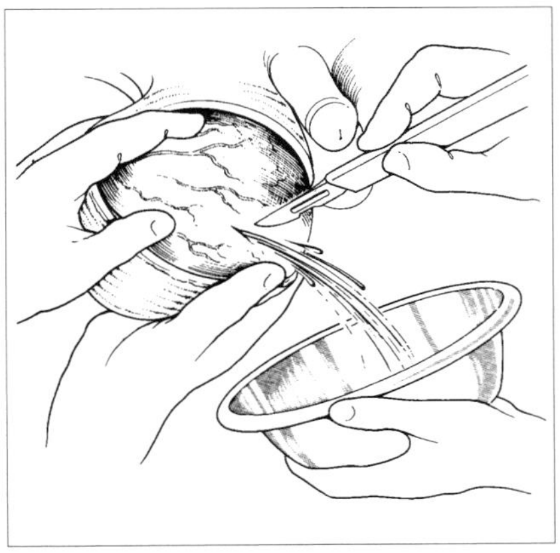

Figure 9.47

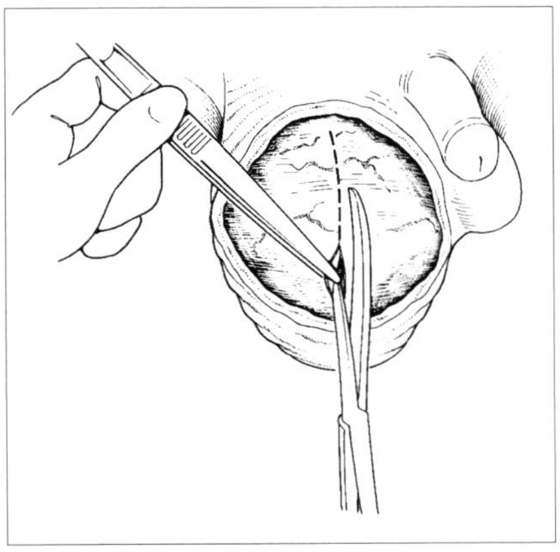

Figure 9.48

4 Evert the testis and the epididymis through the hole and inspect them for tuberculosis, schistosomiasis and cancer. If cancer is present, do not return the testicle to the scrotum. Clamp and divide the cord structures and remove the testis. Biopsy the testicle, then refer the patient if tuberculosis or schistosomiasis is suspected.

Reunite the edges of the everted sac behind the cord and epididymis with a few interrupted stitches of 2/0 absorbable suture (Figure 9.49). Maintain careful haemostasis throughout; it is important to stop even the slightest bleeding to minimize the risk of haematoma formation. Insert a latex drain, bringing it out inferiorly through a counter incision, and fix it to the skin with a stitch (Figure 9.50, 9.51).

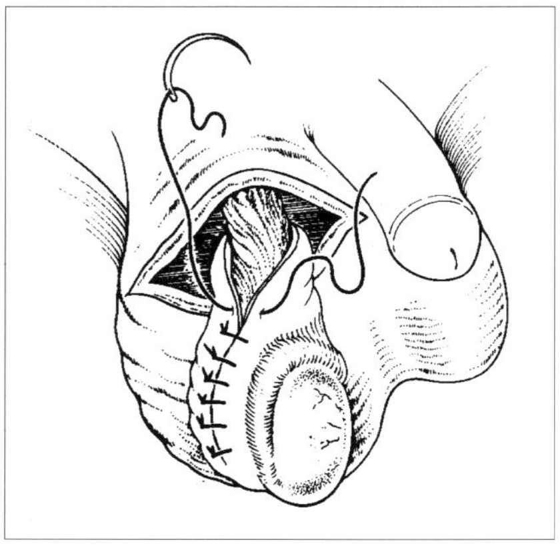

Figure 9.49

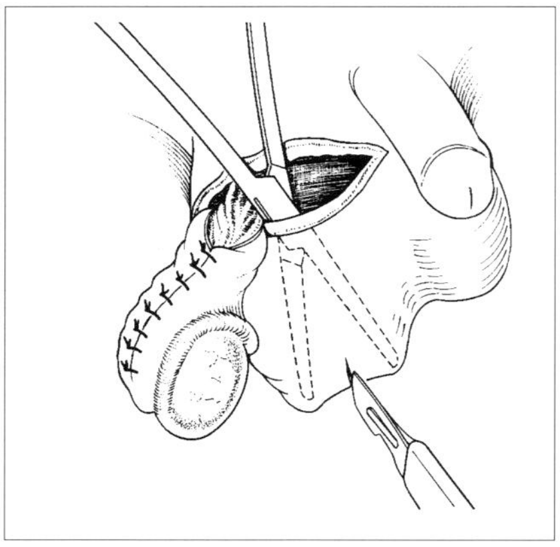

Figure 9.50

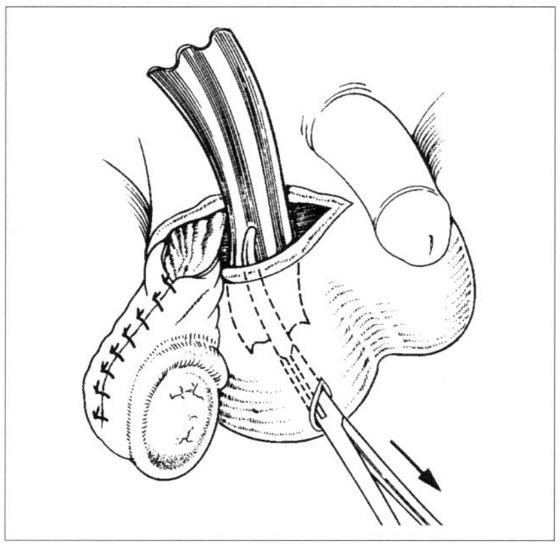

Figure 9.51

5 Replace the testis and the cord. Close the dartos muscle with interrupted 2/0 absorbable suture and the skin with interrupted 2/0 non-absorbable suture (Figure 9.52, 9.53). Apply a compression dressing of gauze and then a T-bandage.

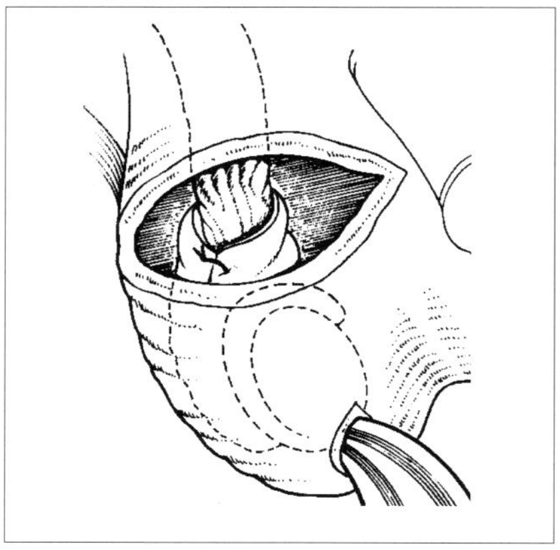

Figure 9.52

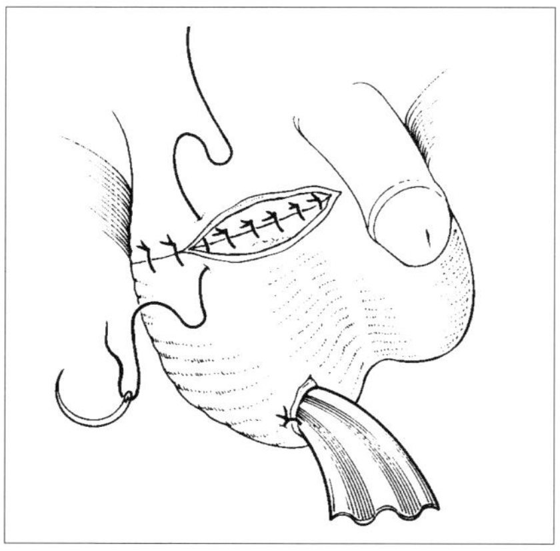

Figure 9.53

Aftercare

Support the scrotum in an elevated position. Remove the drain after 24–48 hours.

Complications

Possible complications include haematoma formation, infection and recurrence. If haematoma develops despite every care having been taken to stop bleeding during surgery, remove a few stitches from the wound, open the edges with a pair of large artery forceps and express the clots from the wound. This procedure may need to be repeated over several days. Antibiotics do not always prevent infection; if it does occur, give appropriate antibiotic therapy and drain the wound. Even with treatment, however, an infection may take up to 2 months to clear.

VASECTOMY

Vasectomy is a method of sterilization in the male. Explain to the patient that the operation is irreversible and permanent. Emphasize that the operation is almost always successful, but that sterility cannot be guaranteed since there is a small chance of failure. Spontaneous recanalization can occur, even after meticulous surgery. Stress that sterility will not be immediate; it can take up to 8 weeks for the patient to become completely sterile. Always observe local legal formalities. Following vasectomy, carry out a semen analysis at 6–8 weeks to confirm sterility.

Technique

1 Vasectomy is usually carried out with the patient under local anaesthesia.

2 Place the patient in a supine position. Cleanse and shave the pubis and external genitalia. If you are using local anaesthesia, inject a weal of 1% lidocaine and make an incision of 2–3 cm in the scrotal raphe (Figure 9.54). Infiltrate the deeper tissues, picking up each layer in turn to inject anaesthetic. At each stage, allow a few minutes for the local anaesthetic to take effect.

3 Hold up the vas from one side with a pair of tissue forceps and infiltrate its connective tissue sheath with lidocaine (Figure 9.55). Open the sheath, isolate the vas with artery forceps (Figure 9.56) and excise about 1 cm (Figure 9.57). The cut ends will be characteristically conical, with the outer fibromuscular tissues retracting from the lumen.

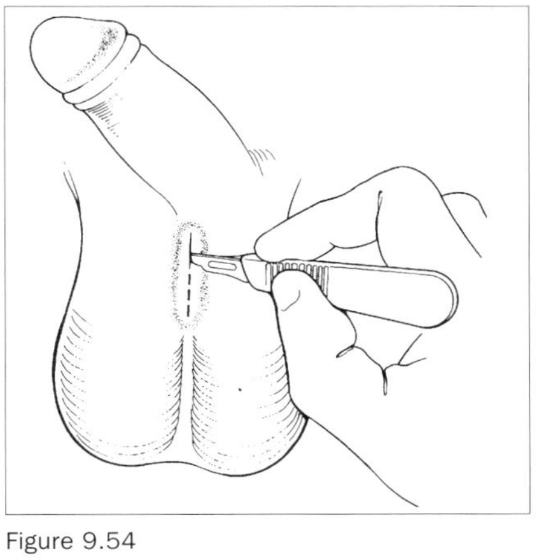

Figure 9.54

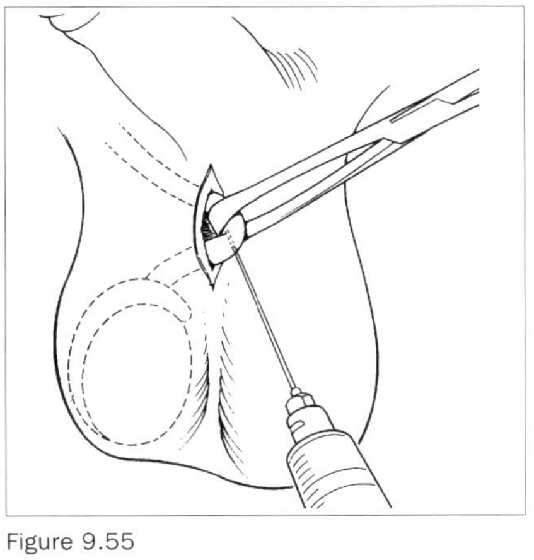

Figure 9.55

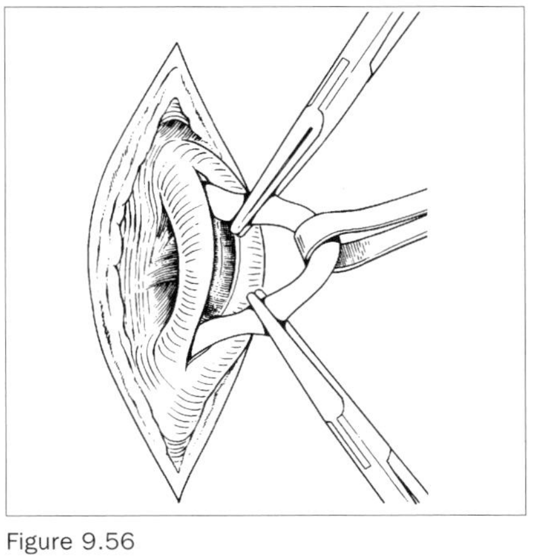

Figure 9.56

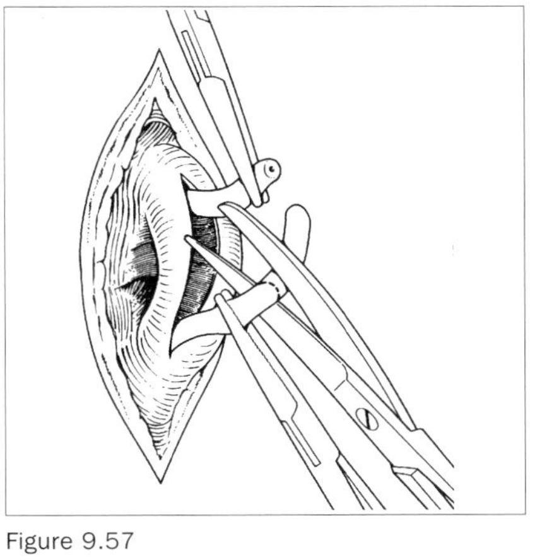

Figure 9.57

9

4 Ligate the testicular end and replace it within the connective tissue sheath (Figure 9.58). Turn the proximal end back on itself and ligate it so that it lies outside the sheath. Repeat the procedure on the other vas. Close the scrotal wound with a few 2/0 absorbable stitches, making sure to include the dartos layer (Figure 9.59).

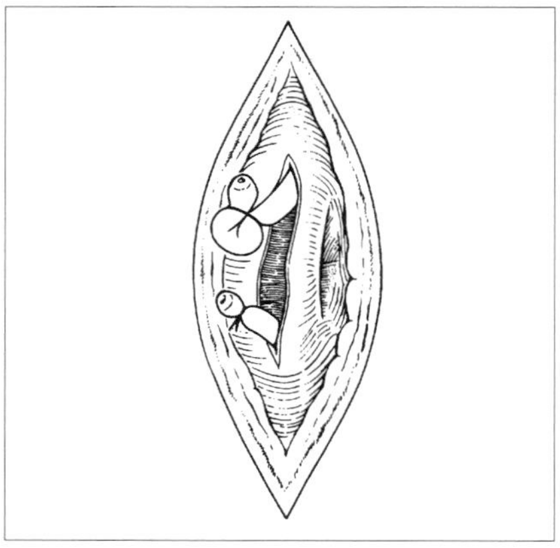

Figure 9.58

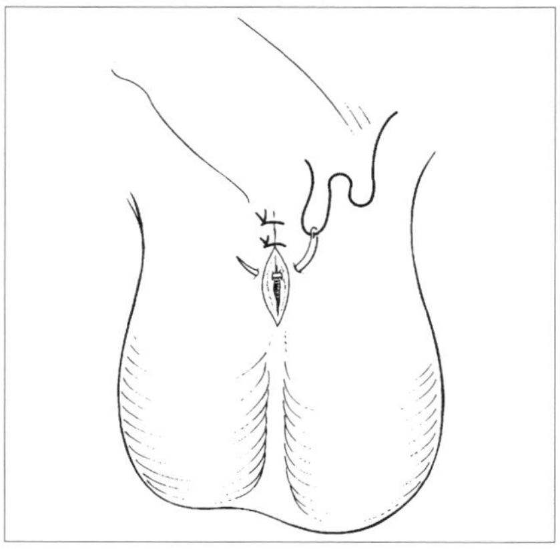

Figure 9.59

This technique is widely used and allows a rapid turnover of patients in outpatient clinics. The less experienced practitioner may find it easier to identify the vas by pinching it between the thumb and finger at the lateral side of the neck of the scrotum, incising the skin directly above it, catching the vas with a pair of tissue forceps before it slips away.

As an alternative, fix each vas under the skin by inserting a hypodermic needle after effecting local anaesthesia with 1% lidocaine. Make a vertical incision 1 cm long over the vas on one side, and hook it out with forceps. Proceed to divide and ligate the vas, as described above. Then make an incision over the other vas and repeat the procedure.

9.3 THE PERINEUM

FEMALE GENITAL INJURY

Injuries result from unintentional trauma, sexual assault and, in some regions, female genital mutilation.

Technique

1 Conduct a local examination of the genital area. Check for associated injuries. Obtain information about the nature of the object causing injury; sharp objects may have penetrated adjacent organs.

2 Catheterize the bladder if the patient has urinary retention. Repair all lacerations unless they are very superficial. Anaesthesia may be required to perform a thorough examination and repair of severe injuries.

3 Check for tears of the hymen then introduce a speculum and examine all the vaginal walls, fornices and the cervix.

4 Thoroughly clean the skin with soap and water, irrigate lacerations with saline and ligate bleeding vessels. Excise only devitalized tissues.

5 Repair deep lacerations with absorbable suture without tension and the skin with non-absorbable suture.

6 Perform a laparotomy if the peritoneum is penetrated. For vulval haematomas, infiltrate the area with local anaesthesia and evacuate the clots.

Complications

Complications include:

- Infection
- Haematoma in the parametrium
- Rectovaginal fistula
- Dyspareunia.

These can be prevented by proper haemostatis and laceration repair.

Rape

If there is allegation of rape, make detailed records of your findings and comply fully with local legal requirements. Give a dose of penicillin to protect the patient against bacterial infection. Protect the patient against pregnancy; use an IUD or emergency contraception with two birth control pills immediately and two more in 12 hours. Give an anti-emetic with the birth control pills. Arrange psychological counselling.

FEMALE GENITAL MUTILATION

Female genital mutilation (FGM) continues to be performed in some parts of the world. The majority of cases are performed with non-sterile razors by untrained personnel. Tradition rather than religion is the reason for these acts. There is no health indication for FGM.

The procedure varies from amputation of the clitoris (type I), excision of the clitoris and labia minor (type II), and complete excision of the clitoris, labia minora and portions of the labia majora (type III). Type III is very destructive and healing creates an epidermal cover over the urethra and the vagina.

Treatment

1 Treat as other genital injuries with wound debridement, saline irrigation and removal of all foreign material.

2 Remove minimal tissue and drain abscesses. Administer antibiotics for infected wounds, cellulitis or abscesses.

3 Catheterize the bladder to provide adequate drainage and administer tetanus prophylaxis to non-immune patients.

4 Excise the epidermal tissue to permit urine flow and sexual intercourse.

5 For childbirth, consider Caesarean section in severe cases. Healed mutilation wounds with vaginal or perineal stenosis may need specialized gynaecology care.

KEY POINTS

Female genital mutilation:

- Acute complications include:
  - Haemorrhage
  - Shock
  - Urinary retention
  - Damage to the urethra and anus
  - Cellulitis
  - Abscesses
- Chronic complications include:
  - Sexual dysfunction
  - Psychological disturbance
  - Urinary obstruction
  - Keloids
  - Large epidermal inclusion cysts
  - Difficult micturation
  - Vaginal stenosis, which can cause obstructed labour, often complicated by vesical or rectal vaginal fistulae.

PERINEAL ABSCESSES

Bartholin's abscess

The patient complains of a painful, throbbing and tender swelling in the vulva on the posterior and middle parts of the labia majora. Differential diagnosis of labial masses includes:

- Cysts of the vaginal process
- Labial hernia.

These conditions are lateral to Bartholin's gland. Take a smear of vaginal discharge to examine for gonococci and other bacteria. Treat Bartholin's cysts with marsupialization but, if an abscess is present, incision and drainage is sufficient. Interference with sleep is an indication for urgent intervention.

An abscess is diagnosed by evidence of:

- Localized pus
- Throbbing pain
- Marked tenderness
- Fluctuation.

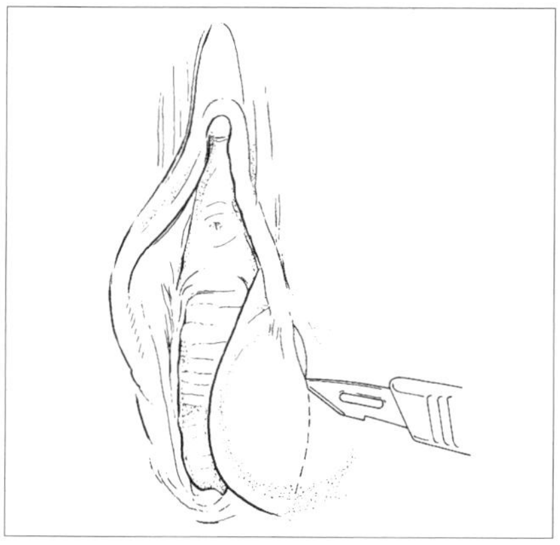

Figure 9.60

Technique

Incision and drainage is easy to perform, almost bloodless and provides the best chance of a cure.

1 Place the patient in the lithotomy position and clean and drape the perineum.

2 Make a longitudinal incision in the most prominent part of the abscess at the junction of the vulva and vagina (Figure 9.60).

3 Deepen the incision and open the abscess widely. Drain the pus and take a specimen for bacteriological examination. Pack the cavity with petroleum or saline soaked gauze and apply an external gauze dressing.

HAEMATOCOLPOS

Haematocolpos occurs in cases of imperforate hymen, but may also present in cases of vulval stenosis resulting from exposure to irritant substances or from infection, trauma or dystrophy. The latter are best referred for specialized treatment.

The patient complains of amenorrhoea with cyclical abdominal pain or acute retention of urine. Examination reveals a mass in the lower abdomen that is dull to percussion. This is the distended vagina with the uterus on top. Differential diagnosis includes:

- Pregnancy
- Tuberculous peritonitis
- Pelvic kidney
- Ovarian cyst.

Technique

Treat haematocolpos due to imperforate hymen surgically with incision and drainage under a general or regional anaesthetic.

1 With the patient in the lithotomy position, clean and drape the perineum.

2 Make an incision over the bulging membrane. Evert the edges of the wound and stitch them to the adjacent vaginal tissue with interrupted sutures of 2/0 absorbable suture (Figures 9.61, 9.62).

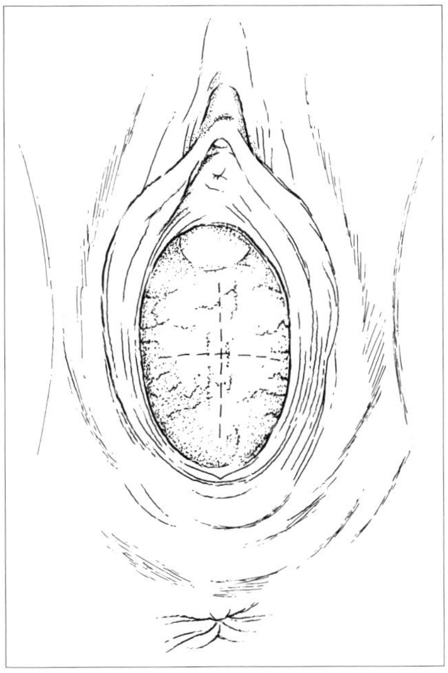

Figure 9.61

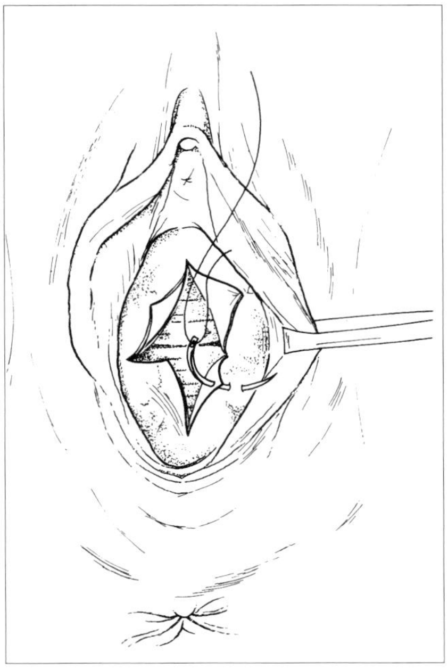

Figure 9.62

3 Allow the blood to drain and apply a sterile pad. Administer antibiotics for 48 hours.

4 Avoid vaginal examination for 1–2 months after the operation.

Complications

Complications include:

- Salpingitis
- Peritonitis.

MALE PERINEAL INFECTIONS

Fournier's gangrene

Fournier's gangrene is a necrotizing fasciitis of perineal areas most commonly affecting the scrotum of adults. The source of infection is the genitourinary or gastrointestinal tract with E. coli as the predominant aerobe and *Bacteroides* as the predominant anaerobe.

Urethral obstruction is a frequently associated urinary sepsis. Patients present with scrotal swelling and with pain out of proportion to the physical findings. A feculant odour may be present. The scrotal skin may be normal but is usually discoloured and oedematous. If black areas develop, trans-scrotal necrosis may ensue. Gas gangrene is unusual. Systemic findings are fever, dehydration and tachycardia.

Treatment

Treat with systemic broad spectrum antibiotics, fluid resuscitation, tetanus prophylaxis and complete surgical debridement, which may need to be extensive. Perform multiple daily debridements, as required, to remove all necrotic tissue.

Uncontrolled sepsis may lead to death, but the prognosis is generally good. The scrotum has a great ability to heal by secondary intention. Use skin grafts to cover healthy granulation tissue.

Periurethral abscesses

Infections of the male periurethral glands secondary to gonococcal urethritis or urethral stricture may lead to abscess formation.

Treatment

Treat with antibiotics and drainage. Needle aspiration may be sufficient in small gonococcal abscesses. Use suprapubic urinary diversion for large abscesses and for urinary fistula.

Part 4

Emergency Obstetric Care

Hypertension in pregnancy

10

10.1 HYPERTENSION

> **KEY POINTS**
>
> - Untreated hypertension in pregnancy can cause maternal and perinatal deaths
> - Delivery is the only cure for pre-eclampsia and eclampsia.

Hypertensive disorders in pregnancy are major contributors to maternal and perinatal morbidity and mortality, affecting 10% of all pregnant women. Hypertension most often appears for the first time in women who have had normal blood pressure before pregnancy and may be associated with proteinuria and convulsions. The causes of hypertension in pregnancy are still largely unknown.

Hypertensive disorders in pregnancy include:

- Pregnancy induced hypertension
- Chronic hypertension
- Pre-eclampsia
- Eclampsia.

Hypertension is diagnosed when the systolic blood pressure is 140 mmHg and/or the diastolic blood pr essure is 90 mmHg on two consecutive readings taken 4 hours or more apart. A time interval of less than 4 hours is acceptable if urgent delivery must take place, or if the diastolic blood pressure is equal to or greater than 110 mmHg.

Diastolic blood pressure is a good indicator of prognosis for the management of hypertensive diseases in pregnancy. Diastolic blood pressure is taken at the point the arterial sound disappears. A falsely high reading is obtained when the inflatable part of the cuff does not encircle at least three-quarters of the circumference of the arm. Use a wider cuff when the width of the upper arm is more than 30 cm.

Hypertension is classified as pregnancy induced hypertension if it occurs for the first time:

- After 20 weeks of gestation
- During labour and/or within 48 hours after delivery

If it occurs before 20 weeks of gestation, it is classified as chronic hypertension. If the blood pressure prior to 20 weeks of gestation is unknown, differentiation may be impossible; in this case, manage as pregnancy induced hypertension.

The presence of *proteinuria* changes the diagnosis from pregnancy induced hypertension to *pre-eclampsia.*

Other conditions that cause proteinuria or false positive results include:

- Urinary infection
- Severe anaemia

- Heart failure
- Difficult labour
- Blood in the urine due to catheter trauma
- Schistosomiasis
- Contamination from vaginal blood
- Vaginal secretions or amniotic fluid contaminating urine specimens.

Only clean catch mid-stream specimens should be used for testing. Catheterization for the sole purpose of testing is not justified due to the risk of urinary tract infection.

CLINICAL FEATURES

Pregnancy induced hypertension is more common among women who are pregnant for the first time. Women with multiple pregnancies, diabetes and underlying vascular problems are at higher risk of developing pregnancy induced hypertension. The spectrum of the disease includes:

- Hypertension without proteinuria
- Mild pre-eclampsia
- Severe pre-eclampsia
- Eclampsia.

Women with pregnancy-induced hypertensive disorders may progress from mild disease to a more serious condition. Mild pre-eclampsia is often symptomless. Rising blood pressure may be the only clinical sign. A woman with hypertension may feel perfectly well until seizure suddenly occurs.

Proteinuria is a later manifestation of the disease process. When pregnancy induced hypertension is associated with proteinuria, the condition is called pre-eclampsia. Increasing proteinuria is a sign of worsening pre-eclampsia. Mild pre-eclampsia could progress to severe pre-eclampsia; the rate of progression could be rapid. The risk of complications, including eclampsia, increases greatly in severe pre-eclampsia.

Eclampsia

Eclampsia is characterized by convulsions, together with signs of pre-eclampsia. Convulsions can occur regardless of severity of hypertension, are difficult to predict and typically occur in the absence of hyperreflexia, headache or visual changes. Convulsions are tonic-clonic and resemble grand-mal seizures of epilepsy. Seizures may recur in rapid sequence, as in status epilepticus, and end in death. Convulsion may be followed by coma that lasts minutes or hours, depending on the frequency of seizures. 25% of eclamptic fits occur after delivery of the baby.

Eclampsia must be differentiated from other conditions that may be associated with convulsions and coma, including epilepsy, cerebral malaria, head injury, cerebrovascular accident, intoxication (alcohol, drugs, poisons), drug withdrawal, metabolic disorders, meningitis, encephalitis, hypertensive encephalopathy, water intoxication and hysteria.

In general, convulsions in a woman who is pregnant or has been recently delivered (within 48 hours after delivery) should be managed as eclampsia, unless proved otherwise.

10.2 ASSESSMENT AND MANAGEMENT

KEY POINTS

- Protect the mother by lowering blood pressure and preventing or controlling convulsions
- Magnesium sulfate is the preferred drug for preventing and treating convulsions.

SPECIFIC MANAGEMENT

Pregnancy induced hypertension

Pregnancy induced hypertension can be managed on an outpatient basis:

- Monitor blood pressure, urine (for proteinuria) and fetal condition weekly
- If blood pressure rises or proteinuria occurs, manage as mild pre-eclampsia
- If there are signs of fetal compromise, admit the woman to the hospital for assessment and possible expedited delivery
- Counsel the woman and her family about danger signals indicating pre-eclampsia or eclampsia
- If all observations remain stable, allow to proceed with normal labour and childbirth.

Mild pre-eclampsia

Gestation less than 36 weeks

If signs remains unchanged or normalize, follow up twice a week as an outpatient:

- Monitor blood pressure, urine (for proteinuria), reflexes and fetal condition
- Counsel the woman and her family about danger signals indicating pre-eclampsia or eclampsia
- Encourage the woman to eat a normal diet; discourage salt restriction
- Do not give anticonvulsants, antihypertensives, sedatives or tranquillizers.

If follow-up as an outpatient is not possible, admit the woman to the hospital or set up a hostel beside your hospital where high risk mothers may stay and attend the hospital for regular checks

- Provide a normal diet without salt restriction
- Monitor blood pressure (twice daily) and urine for proteinuria (daily)
- Do not give anticonvulsants, antihypertensives, sedatives or tranquillizers unless blood pressure increases
- Do not give diuretics; these are harmful and only indicated for use in pre-eclampsia with pulmonary oedema or congestive heart failure

If diastolic pressure decreases to normal levels or the woman's condition remains stable, send her home:

- Advise her to rest and watch out for significant swelling or symptoms of severe pre-eclampsia
- See her twice weekly to monitor blood pressure, proteinuria and fetal condition and to assess for symptoms and signs of severe pre-eclampsia
- If diastolic pressure rises again, readmit her.

If the signs remain unchanged and if outpatient monitoring is not possible, keep the woman in the hospital

- Continue the same management and monitor fetal growth by symphysis-fundal height
- If there are signs of growth restriction, consider early delivery; if not, continue hospitalization until term
- If urinary protein level increases, manage as severe pre-eclampsia.

Gestation more than 36 weeks

- If there are signs of fetal compromise, assess the cervix and expedite delivery
- If the cervix is favourable (soft, thin, partly dilated), rupture the membranes with an amniotic hook or a Kocher clamp and induce labour using oxytocin or prostaglandins
- If the cervix is unfavourable (firm, thick, closed), ripen the cervix using prostaglandins or Foley catheter or deliver by caesarean section.

Severe pre-eclampsia and eclampsia

Severe pre-eclampsia is present if one or more of the conditions in column three of the table below are present.

	Mild pre-eclampsia	Severe pre-eclampsia
Diastolic blood pressure	<110	110
Proteinuria	Up to 2+	3+ or more
Headache	No	One or more of these conditions may be present
Visual disturbances	No	
Hyperreflexia	No	
Urine output <400 ml in 24 hours	No	
Epigastric or right upper quadrant pain	No	
Pulmonary oedema	No	

Severe pre-eclampsia and eclampsia are managed similarly, with the exception that delivery must occur within 12 hours of the onset of convulsions in eclampsia.

> *All* cases of severe pre-eclampsia should be managed actively. Symptoms and signs of "impending eclampsia" (blurred vision, hyperreflexia) are unreliable and expectant management is not recommended.

Management

Immediate management of a pregnant woman or a recently delivered woman who complains of severe headache or blurred vision, or if a pregnant woman or a recently delivered woman is found unconscious or having convulsions:

SHOUT FOR HELP

1 Make a quick assessment of the general condition of the woman, including vital signs (pulse, blood pressure, respiration) while simultaneously finding out the history of her present and past illnesses from her or her relatives:
- Check airway and breathing
- Position her on her side
- Check for neck rigidity and temperature.

2 If she is not breathing or her breathing is shallow:
- Open airway and intubate, if required
- Assist ventilation using an Ambu bag and mask
- Give oxygen at 4–6 L per minute.

3 If she is breathing, give oxygen at 4–6 L per minute by mask or nasal cannulae.

4 If she is convulsing:
- Protect her from injury, but do not actively restrain her
- Position her on her side to reduce the risk of aspiration of secretions, vomit and blood
- After the convulsion, aspirate the mouth and throat as necessary. Look in the mouth for a bitten tongue: it may swell.

5 Give magnesium sulfate (see page 10–6). If a convulsion continues in spite of magnesium sulfate, consider diazepam 10 mg IV.

6 If diastolic blood pressure remains above 110 mmHg, give antihypertensive drugs (see page 10–6). Reduce the diastolic pressure to less than 100 mmHg, but not below 90 mmHg.

7 Fluids:
- Start an IV infusion
- Maintain a strict fluid balance chart and monitor the volume of fluids administered and urine output to ensure that there is no fluid overload
- Catheterize the bladder to monitor urine output and proteinuria
- If urine output is less than 30 ml per hour:
  - Withhold magnesium sulfate until urine output improves
  - Infuse a maintenance dose of IV fluids (normal saline or Ringer's lactate) at 1 L in 8 hours
  - Monitor for the development of pulmonary oedema.

Never leave the woman alone. A convulsion followed by aspiration of vomit may cause death of the woman and fetus.

---

8 Observe vital signs, reflexes and fetal heart rate hourly.

9 Auscultate the lung bases hourly for rales indicating pulmonary oedema. If rales are heard, withhold fluids and give frusemide 40 mg IV once.

10 Assess clotting status.

10

Anticonvulsant drugs

Adequate administration of anticonvulsive drugs is a key factor in anticonvulsive therapy. Convulsions in hospitalized women are most frequently caused by under-treatment. Magnesium sulfate is the drug of first choice for preventing and treating convulsions in severe pre-eclampsia and eclampsia.

Magnesium sulfate schedules for severe pre-eclampsia and eclampsia

Loading dose

- Magnesium sulfate 20% solution 4 g IV over 5 minutes
- Follow promptly with 10 g of 50% magnesium sulfate solution, 5 g in each buttock, as deep IM injection with 1.0 ml of 2% lidocaine in the same syringe
- Ensure that aseptic technique is practised when giving magnesium sulfate deep IM injection; warn the woman that a feeling of warmth will be felt when magnesium sulfate is given
- If convulsions recur after 15 minutes, give 2 g magnesium sulfate (50% solution) IV over 5 minutes

Maintenance dose

- 5 g magnesium sulfate (50% solution) + 1 ml lidocaine 2% IM every 4 hours into alternate buttocks
- Continue treatment with magnesium sulfate for 24 hours after delivery or the last convulsion, whichever occurs last.
- Before repeat administration, ensure that
  - Respiratory rate is at least 16 per minute
  - Patellar reflexes are present
  - Urinary output is at least 30 ml per hour over the last 4 hours
- Withhold or delay drug if:
  - Respiratory rate falls below 16 per minute
  - Patellar reflexes are absent
  - Urinary output falls below 30 ml per hour over preceding 4 hours
- In case of respiratory arrest:
  - Assist ventilation (mask and bag; anaesthesia apparatus; intubation)
  - Give calcium gluconate 1 gm (10 ml of 10% solution) IV slowly until the drug antagonizes the effects of magnesium sulfate and respiration begins

Diazepam schedules for severe pre-eclampsia and eclampsia

Intravenous administration

Loading dose

- Diazepam 10 mg IV slowly over 2 minutes
- If convulsions recur, repeat loading dose

Maintenance dose

- Diazepam 40 mg in 500 ml IV fluids (normal saline or Ringer's lactate) titrated to keep the patient sedated but rousable
- Do not give more than 100 mg in 24 hours

Use diazepam if magnesium sulfate is not available, although there is greater risk for neonatal respiratory depression because diazepam passes the placenta freely.

A single dose of diazepam to abort a convulsion seldom causes neonatal respiratory depression. Long-term continuous IV administration increases the risk of respiratory depression in babies who may already be suffering from the effects of utero-placental ischaemia and preterm birth. The effect of diazepam may last several days.

Use diazepam only if magnesium sulfate is not available.

Antihypertensive drugs

If the diastolic pressure is 110 mmHg or more, give antihypertensive drugs. The goal is to keep the diastolic pressure between 90 mmHg and 100 mmHg to prevent cerebral haemorrhage. Avoid hypotension.

Hydralazine is the drug of choice:

1 Give hydralazine 5 mg IV slowly every 5 minutes until blood pressure is lowered. Repeat hourly as needed or give hydralazine 12.5 mg IM every 2 hours as needed.

2 If hydralazine is not available:
   - Give labetolol 10 mg IV:
     - If response is inadequate (diastolic blood pressure remains above 110 mmHg) after 10 minutes, give labetolol 20 mg IV
     - Increase dose to 40 mg and then 80 mg if satisfactory response is not obtained within 10 minutes of each dose

   Or
   - Nifedipine 5 mg chewed and swallowed or injected into the oropharynx; may be repeated at 10-minute intervals

   Or
   - Nicardipine 1–2 mg at one minute intervals until control is obtained. Then 1–2 mg every hour.

Rectal administration of drugs

1 Give diazepam rectally when IV access is not possible. The loading dose of 20 mg is taken in a 10 ml syringe.

2 Remove the needle, lubricate the barrel and insert the syringe into the rectum to half its length. Discharge the contents and leave the syringe in place, holding the buttocks together for 10 minutes to prevent expulsion of the drug. Alternatively, instill the drug in the rectum through a urinary catheter.

3 If convulsions are not controlled within 10 minutes, inject an additional 10 mg per hour or more, depending on the size of the woman and her clinical response.

10.3 DELIVERY

Delivery should take place as soon as the woman's condition has been stabilized. Delaying delivery to increase fetal maturity will risk the lives of both the woman and the fetus. Delivery should occur regardless of the gestational age.

10

- Assess the cervix
- If the cervix is favourable (soft, thinned, partially dilated), rupture the membranes with an amniotic hook or Kocher clamp and induce labour using oxytocin or prostaglandins
- If vaginal delivery is not anticipated within 12 hours (for eclampsia) or 24 hours (for severe pre-eclampsia), deliver by caesarean section
- If there are fetal heart rate abnormalities (less than 100 or more than 180 beats per minute), deliver by caesarean section
- If the cervix is unfavourable (firm, thick, closed) and the fetus is alive, deliver by caesarean section.

Spinal anaesthesia is suitable for most pre-eclamptic patients if there is no clinical evidence of abnormal bleeding (see pages 14–29 to 14–30). A general anaesthetic raises the risks of a hypertensive disaster (stroke or left ventricular failure) at intubation or airway problems from laryngeal oedema (see page 14–30).

Get skilled anaesthetic help early; this will also aid the management of hypertensive crises and fits.

If safe anaesthesia is not available for caesarean section or if the fetus is dead or too premature for survival, aim for vaginal delivery.

If the cervix is unfavourable (firm, thick, closed) and the fetus is alive, ripen the cervix using prostaglandins or Foley catheter.

KEY POINT

- Life threatening complications can still occur after delivery; monitor carefully until the patient is clearly recovering.

10.4 POSTPARTUM CARE

- Continue anticonvulsive therapy for 24 hours after delivery or last convulsion, whichever occurs last
- Continue antihypertensive therapy as long as the diastolic pressure is 110 mmHg or more
- Continue to monitor urine output
- Watch carefully for the development of pulmonary oedema, which often occurs after delivery.

Referral for tertiary level care

Consider referral of women who have:

- Oliguria (less than 400 ml urine output in 24 hours) that persists for 48 hours after delivery
- Coagulation failure (e.g. coagulopathy or haemolysis, elevated liver enzymes and low platelets [HELLP] syndrome)
- Persistent coma lasting more than 24 hours after convulsion.

10.5 CHRONIC HYPERTENSION

Encourage additional periods of rest.

High levels of blood pressure maintain renal and placental perfusion in chronic hypertension; reducing blood pressure will result in diminished perfusion. Blood pressure should not be lowered below its pre-pregnancy level. There is no evidence that aggressive treatment to lower the blood pressure to normal levels improves either fetal or maternal outcome:

- If the woman was on antihypertensive medication before pregnancy and the disease is well controlled, continue the same medication if acceptable in pregnancy
- If diastolic blood pressure is 110 mmHg or more, or systolic blood pressure is 160 mmHg or more, treat with antihypertensive drugs: e.g. methyldopa
- If proteinuria or other signs and symptoms are present, consider superimposed pre-eclampsia and manage as pre-eclampsia
- Monitor fetal growth and condition
- If there are no complications, deliver at term
- If there are fetal heart rate abnormalities (less than 100 or more than 180 beats per minute), suspect fetal distress
- If fetal growth restriction is severe and pregnancy dating is accurate, assess the cervix and consider delivery
- If the cervix is favourable (soft, thin, partially dilated) rupture the membranes with an amniotic hook or a Kocher clamp and induce labour using oxytocin or prostaglandins
- If the cervix is unfavourable (firm, thick, closed), ripen the cervix using prostaglandins or Foley catheter
- Observe for complications including abruptio placentae and superimposed pre-eclampsia.

10.5 COMPLICATIONS

Complications of hypertensive disorders in pregnancy may cause adverse perinatal and maternal outcomes. Complications are often difficult to treat so make every effort to prevent them by early diagnosis and proper management. Be aware that management can also lead to complications.

Management

- If fetal growth restriction is severe, expedite delivery
- If there is increasing drowsiness or coma, suspect cerebral haemorrhage
- Reduce blood pressure slowly to reduce the risk of cerebral ischaemia
- Provide supportive therapy
- If you suspect heart, kidney or liver failure, provide supportive therapy and observe

- Suspect coagulopathy if:
  - A clotting test shows failure of a clot to form after 7 minutes or a soft clot that breaks down easily
  - Continued bleeding from venepuncture sites
- A woman who has IV lines and catheters is prone to infection; use proper infection prevention techniques and closely monitor for signs of infection
- If the woman is receiving IV fluids, she is at risk of circulatory overload. Maintain a strict fluid balance chart and monitor the amount of fluids administered and urine output.

Management of slow progress of labour

11

11.1 GENERAL PRINCIPLES

Labour is a physiological event that usually ends with the birth of a baby and expulsion of the placenta. While normal labour usually ends within 12 hours, labour may be prolonged in some cases. Prolonged labour can lead to serious maternal problems including:

- Infection
- Uterine rupture
- Genital fistulas
- Maternal death.

Problems for the baby include:

- Infection
- Asphyxial and traumatic injury to the baby
- Stillbirth
- Neonatal death.

These problems can be largely prevented by good management of labour.

LABOUR

Labour is the process in which uterine contractions lead to progressive dilatation of the cervix and delivery of the baby and placenta.

Suspect or anticipate labour if a pregnant woman has:

- Intermittent abdominal pain after 22 weeks gestation
- Blood stained mucus discharge or "show"
- Watery vaginal discharge or a sudden gush of water with or without pain.

These symptoms are not, by themselves, diagnostic of labour. Confirm the onset of labour only if intermittent uterine contractions are associated with progressive changes in the cervix:

- Cervical effacement: the progressive shortening and thinning of the cervix in labour; the length of the cervix at the end of normal pregnancy is variable (a few millimetres to 3 cm); with the onset of labour, the length of the cervix decreases steadily to a few millimetres when it is fully effaced
- Cervical dilatation: the increase in diameter of the cervical opening, measured in centimetres (Figure 11.1).

KEY POINTS

- Prolonged labour may cause maternal and perinatal death and disability
- Ineffective uterine contractions are the most common reason for slow progress of labour in a primagravida
- Good management of labour may prevent problems associated with prolonged labour
- Recognize slow progress in labour with a partograph
- If labour is not obstructed, use oxytocin to augment ineffective uterine contractions.

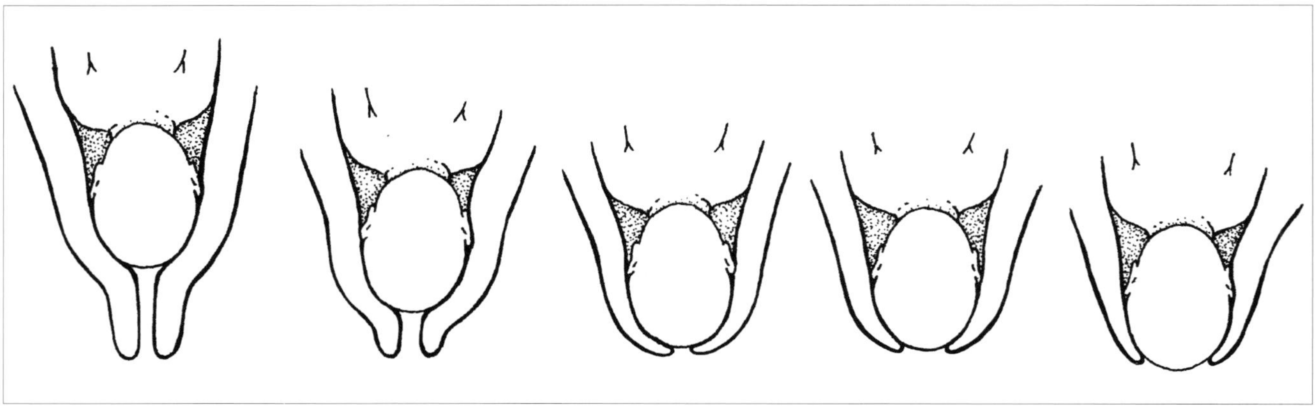

Figure 11.1

First stage

In early labour (the latent phase), effacement and slow dilatation occur. Effacement is usually complete by the time the cervix is 3–4 cm dilated. After this phase, the cervix dilates rapidly (the active phase) until it is 10 cm (fully dilated). The latent phase and the active phase together constitute the first stage of labour.

Second stage

The second stage of labour begins after full cervical dilatation is reached. Fetal descent through the birth canal occurs towards the latter part of the active phase and after the cervix is fully dilated. Once the fetus touches the pelvic floor, the woman usually has the urge to push (the expulsive phase).

Fetal descent

Fetal descent may be assessed by abdominal palpation and vaginal examination

Abdominal palpation

Fetal descent into the pelvis may be assessed in terms of fifths of head palpable above the symphysis pubis (Figures 11.2–11.3):

- 5/5 refers to a head that is entirely above the inlet of the pelvis
- 0/5 refers to a head that is deep within the pelvis.

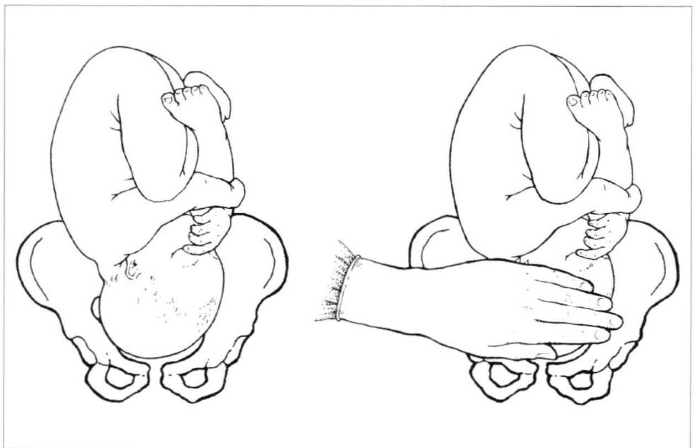

Figure 11.2

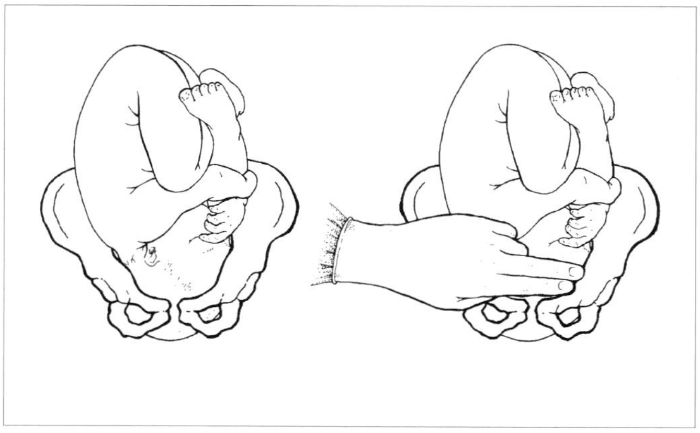

Figure 11.3

Vaginal examination

Fetal descent can also be quantified by relating the level of the fetal presenting part to a bony reference point in the maternal pelvis. Conventionally the ischial spines provide such a reference point (Figure 11.4: 0 = level of ischial spine).

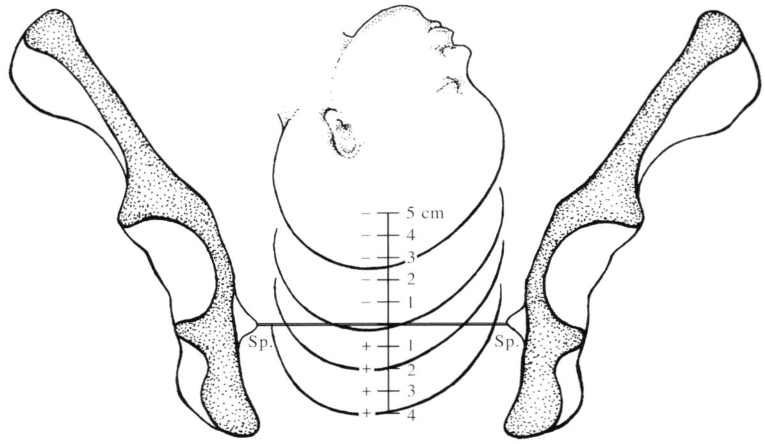

Figure 11.4

Third stage

The third stage of labour begins with the delivery of the baby and ends with the expulsion of the placenta.

11.2 SLOW PROGRESS OF LABOUR

Slow progress of labour has three fundamental causes:

- Poor uterine contractions
- Malpresentations and malpositions
- Disproportion between the fetal size and pelvic size.

These are often interrelated. Poor contractions are the most common cause of slow progress of labour.

> Exclude malpresentations and poor contractions before making a diagnosis of disproportion.

Uterine contractions

"Good contractions" are characterized by:

- A frequency of 2 to 4 in 10 minutes
- A duration of 30 to 60 seconds
- Progressive effacement and dilatation in the latent phase
- Progressive dilatation of at least 1 cm/hour in the active phase
- Progressive descent of the fetal presentation.

11

Poor contractions lack the above characteristics. They may occur at any stage of labour. If you have excluded malpresentation and labour fails to progress in spite of good contractions, assume the cause to be disproportion. Poor contractions in the latent phase may represent false labour; do not confuse them with abnormal labour.

Malpresentations and malpositions

The most frequent and most favourable presentation is a well flexed head in the occipito-anterior position. In a malpresentation, there is usually a poor fit between the presenting part and the maternal pelvis. The presenting part is poorly applied to the cervix. Contractions are usually ineffective in achieving progress of labour.

Disproportion

If labour persists with disproportion, it may become arrested or obstructed. Disproportion occurs because:

- The baby is too large
- The pelvis is too small.

You may be able to identify disproportion early in some cases: for example, with a hydrocephalic head or a large baby in a woman with an abnormal pelvis because, for instance, of a history of malformation or trauma to the pelvis. In most cases, however, disproportion is a diagnosis of exclusion: that is, after you have excluded poor uterine contractions and malpresentations.

> The best test for an adequate pelvis is a trial of labour. Clinical pelvimetry is of limited value.

Chart progress on the partograph (Figure 11.5, pages 11–6 and 11–7) to obtain early warning of disproportion. When arrested labour is not recognized and becomes prolonged, cephalopelvic disproportion leads to obstruction. Evidence of obstructed labour includes arrested dilatation or descent with:

- Large caput and excessive moulding
- Presenting part poorly applied to cervix or cervix is oedematous
- Ballooning of the lower uterine segment and formation of a retraction band
- Maternal and fetal distress
- Prolonged labour without delivery.

ASSESSMENT AND DIAGNOSIS

When a woman presents with intermittent abdominal pains, ask the following questions:

- Is this woman in labour?
- If she is in labour, what is the phase of labour?
- What is the presentation of the fetus?
- Are the membranes ruptured? If so, how long ago?

Assess the woman's general condition:

- Is she in pain? Is she distressed?
- Check pulse, blood pressure and hydration (tongue, urine output), temperature
- Does she have any medical problems?

Palpate for uterine contractions. If the woman has at least 2 uterine contractions lasting more than 20 seconds over 10 minutes, do a vaginal examination to assess cervical effacement and dilatation.

If the cervix is not dilated on first examination, it may not be possible to make a diagnosis of labour. If contractions persist, re-examine the woman after 4 hours for cervical changes. At this stage, if there is effacement and dilatation, the woman is in labour; if there is no change, make a diagnosis of false labour.

> Diagnose labour only if there has been effacement and dilatation. An incorrect diagnosis of labour in this situation can lead to unnecessary anxiety and interventions.

First stage

Latent phase

- Cervix less than 4 cm dilated.

Active phase

- Cervix between 4 cm and 10 cm dilated
- Rate of cervical dilatation at least 1 cm/hour
- Effacement is usually complete
- Fetal descent through birth canal begins.

Second stage

Early phase (non-expulsive)

- Cervix fully dilated (10 cm)
- Fetal descent continues
- No urge to push.

Late phase (expulsive)

- Fetal presenting part reaches the pelvic floor and the woman has the urge to push
- Typically lasts <1 hour in primigravidae and <30 minutes in multigravidae.

Carry out vaginal examinations at least once every 4 hours in the first stage of labour and plot the findings on the partograph. The partograph is very helpful in monitoring the progress of labour and in the early detection of abnormal labour patterns.

USING THE PARTOGRAPH

1 Record the following patient information:
- Name
- Gravida
- Para
- Hospital number
- Date and time of admission
- Time of ruptured membranes.

2 Assess cervical dilatation. If the cervix is at least 4 cm dilated, mark the dilatation on the Alert line. Use "X" to indicate cervical dilatation. Record the actual time on the X axis, corresponding to this point on the Alert line.

3 Record the following information on the partograph, starting from this point.

Every 30 minutes, record:
- Fetal heart rate
- Contractions:
  - Palpate number of contractions in 10 minutes and shade the corresponding number of boxes
  - Use the following scheme to indicate the duration of contractions:

    Less than 20 seconds

    Between 20 and 40 seconds

    More than 40 seconds

- Oxytocin infusion: record the amount of oxytocin per volume IV fluids in drops per minute when used
- Pulse rate

Every 2 hours, record:
- Temperature

Every 4 hours, record:
- Blood pressure

At every vaginal examination, record:
- Cervical dilatation: use "X"
- Colour of amniotic fluid:
  I = Membranes intact
  C = Membranes ruptured, clear fluid
  M = Meconium stained fluid
  B = Blood stained fluid
- Moulding:
  1 = Sutures apposed
  2 = Sutures overlapped but reducible
  3 = Sutures overlapped and not reducible
- Descent of head by abdominal palpation: assess descent in fifths palpable above the pubic symphysis: record as "O"

Drugs: record drugs given, each time they are given

Urine volume, urine protein and acetone: record every time urine is passed

Figure 11.5

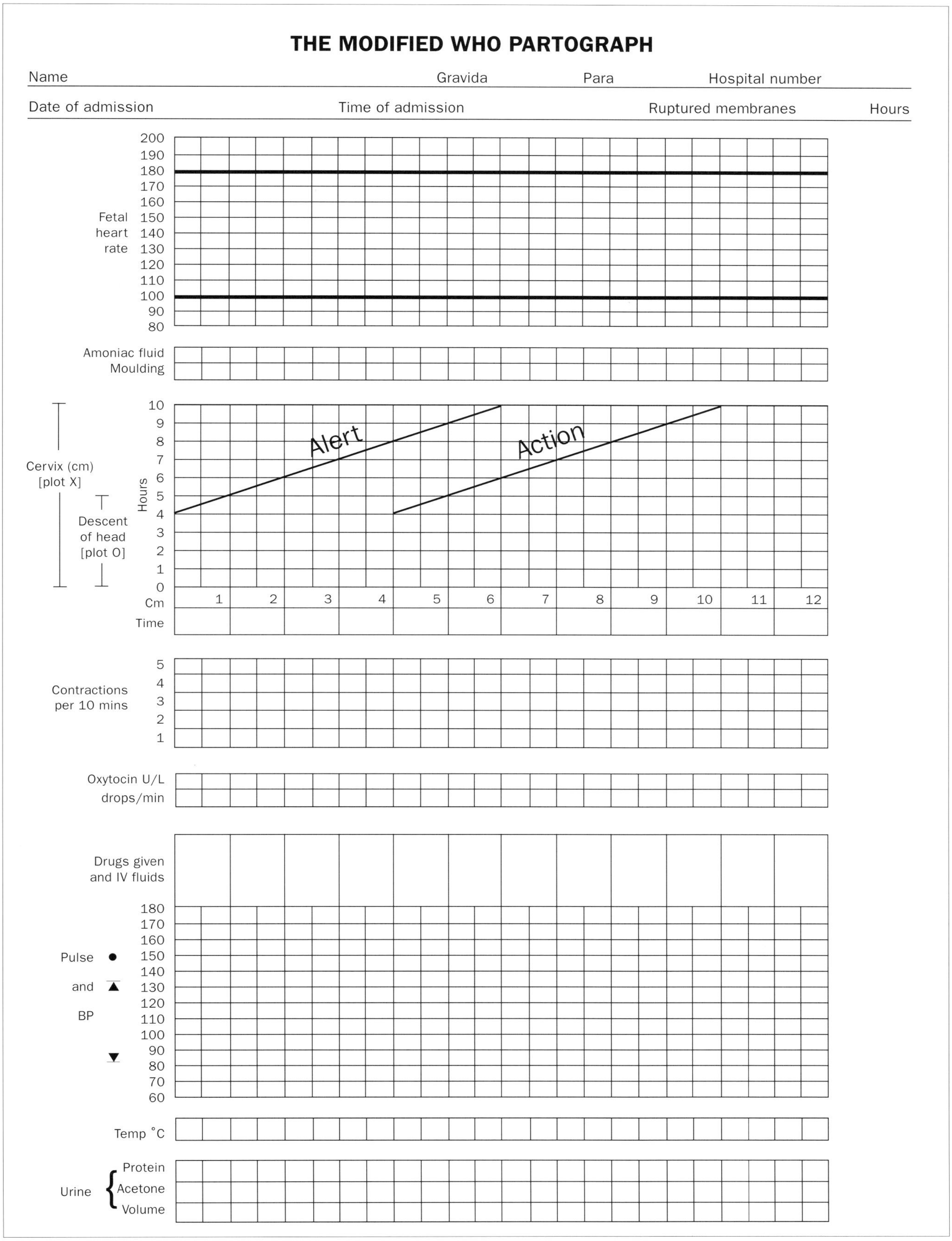
THE MODIFIED WHO PARTOGRAPH
Name
Gravida
Para
Hospital number
Date of admission
Time of admission
Ruptured membranes
Hours
Fetal heart rate
200 190 180 170 160 150 140 130 120 110 100 90 80
Amoniac fluid
Moulding
Cervix (cm) [plot X]
Descent of head [plot O]
Hours
10 9 8 7 6 5 4 3 2 1 0
Alert
Action
Cm
1 2 3 4 5 6 7 8 9 10 11 12
Time
Contractions per 10 mins
5 4 3 2 1
Oxytocin U/L
drops/min
Drugs given and IV fluids
Pulse
and
BP
180 170 160 150 140 130 120 110 100 90 80 70 60
Temp °C
Urine
Protein
Acetone
Volume

Figure 11.5

More frequent vaginal examinations may be required when:
- Membranes rupture
- There is fetal distress
- The woman enters the second stage of labour.

At each vaginal examination, record the following:
- Effacement and dilatation
- Presenting part and station
- Colour and odour of liquor.

Assess progress in labour by:
- Measuring changes in cervical effacement and dilatation in the latent phase
- Measuring the rate of cervical dilatation in the active phase
- Assessing fetal descent in the second stage.

Assess fetal condition by:
- Checking the fetal heart rate during or immediately after a contraction
- Listening in to the fetal heart for one full minute:
  - Every half hour in the active phase
  - After every 5 minutes in the second stage.
- Listening more frequently if an abnormality is detected: while the normal fetal heart rate is between 120 and 180 beats/minute, rates of <100 or >180 are suggestive of fetal intolerance of labour or distress.
- Listening for the fetal heart rate recovery after contractions: repetitive slow recovery indicates fetal distress.

If the membranes are ruptured, check the colour of fluid. Greenish-yellow fluid, blood stained fluid or no fluid are suggestive of placental insufficiency and possibly fetal compromise.

Findings suggestive of satisfactory progress in labour

- Regular contractions of progressively increasing frequency and duration
- Rate of cervical dilatation at least 1 cm/hour in the active phase of labour
- Satisfactory descent with pushing in the expulsive phase
- Cervix closely applied to fetal head.

Findings suggestive of unsatisfactory progress in labour

- Irregular, infrequent and weak contractions
- Cervical dilatation rate slower than 1 cm/hour in the active phase
- No descent with pushing in the expulsive phase
- Presenting part applied loosely to the cervix.

Findings suggestive of risks to the fetus

- Bloodstained amniotic fluid
- Greenish-yellow coloured amniotic fluid
- Fetal heart rate abnormalities, such as decelerations, tachycardias or delayed recovery of fetal heart rate after contraction.

11.3 PROGRESS OF LABOUR

SLOW PROGRESS OF LABOUR ASSOCIATED WITH PROLONGED LATENT PHASE

The diagnosis of a prolonged latent phase is made retrospectively:

- When contractions cease, diagnose as false labour
- When contractions become regular and dilatation progresses beyond 4 cm, diagnose as latent phase.

Mistaking false labour for the latent phase leads to unnecessary induction and unnecessary caesarean section.

The latent phase is prolonged when the cervical dilatation remains less than 4 cm after 8 hours. If a woman has been in the latent phase for more than 8 hours, reassess the situation:

- If there has been no change in cervical effacement or dilatation and there is no fetal distress, review the diagnosis of labour; the woman may not be in labour
- If there has been a change in cervical effacement and dilatation, augment contractions with oxytocin. Artificial rupture of membranes is recommended along with or before augmentation of labour with oxytocin. In areas of high HIV prevalence, however, if elective caesarean section is not the preferred option, try to leave the membranes intact for as long as possible to reduce the risk of transmission of HIV.

Reassess every 4 hours:

- If the woman has not entered the active phase within 8 hours, consider delivery by caesarean section, but be sure the patient is not in false labour
- If membranes are already spontaneously ruptured, induce or augment labour without delay
- In areas of high Group B streptococcal prevalence, give antibiotic prophylaxis starting at 12 hours after rupture of the membranes to help reduce Group B streptococcus infection in the neonate
- If there is any evidence of amnionitis, augment labour immediately and treat with antibiotics.

SLOW PROGRESS OF LABOUR ASSOCIATED WITH PROLONGED ACTIVE PHASE

During active labour, dilatation usually progresses at least 1 cm per hour. Any rate of dilatation slower than this indicates a slow active phase. If the slow active phase is neglected, it can lead to a prolonged active phase. Slow progress of labour in the active phase of labour may be due to one or more of the following causes:

- Inefficient uterine contractions
- Malpresentations and malpositions: e.g. occipito-posterior
- Disproportion between the size of the fetus and the pelvis.

These causes may be interrelated. When the rate of dilatation in the active phase is slower than 1 cm per hour, reassess the mother for poor contractions or malpresentation:

- If there is evidence of obstruction, perform a caesarean section
- If there is no evidence of obstruction, augment labour with amniotomy and oxytocin.

General methods of labour support may improve contractions and accelerate progress:

- Provide emotional support and encouragement
- Encourage walking, sitting and changes of position
- Give abundant fluids either by mouth or IV
- Encourage urination
- Catheterize only as a last resort.

Reassess progress by vaginal examination after 2 hours of good contractions:

- If there is no progress between examinations, deliver by caesarean section
- If there is progress, continue oxytocin and re-examine after 2 hours.

Continue to follow progress carefully.

Inefficient, poor uterine contractions are less common in a multigravida, so make every effort to rule out disproportion before augmenting with oxytocin.

In the active phase of labour, plotting of cervical dilatation will normally remain on, or to the left of the alert line on the partograph. The action line is 4 hours to the right of the alert line. If a woman's labour reaches this line, you will need to make a decision about the cause of the slow progress and take appropriate action.

SLOW PROGRESS OF LABOUR ASSOCIATED WITH PROLONGED EXPULSIVE PHASE

The effective force during delivery of the fetus comes from uterine contractions. Spontaneous maternal "pushing" should be permitted, but the practice of encouraging breath-holding and prolonged effort should be abandoned.

Prolongation of the expulsive phase may also occur for the same reasons as prolongation of the active phase. If malpresentation and obvious obstruction have been excluded, failure of descent in the expulsive stage should also be treated by oxytocin infusion unless contraindicated. If there is no descent even after augmentation with oxytocin, consider assisted delivery.

Assisted vaginal delivery by forceps or ventouse is indicated if the head is engaged (not more than 1/5 of the head is palpable above the pelvic brim) or if the leading bony edge of the fetal head is at 1 cm or more below the level of the ischial spines by vaginal examination.

Caesarean delivery is the preferred option if the head is at a higher level.

SLOW PROGRESS OF LABOUR ASSOCIATED WITH MALPOSITIONS AND MALPRESENTATIONS

Occipito-posterior positions

Spontaneous rotation to the anterior position occurs in 90% of cases. Spontaneous delivery in the posterior position may occur, but labour may be complicated by prolonged first and second stages. Perineal tears and extensions of an episiotomy may complicate delivery.

Arrested labour

Arrested labour may occur when rotation and/or descent of the head does not occur:

- Ensure adequate hydration
- Check maternal and fetal condition
- If there is fetal distress, consider delivery by caesarean section if quick and easy vaginal delivery is not possible
- If there is still no descent after a trial of labour and the head is engaged and at 1 cm or more below the ischial spines, deliver by forceps or ventouse
- If the head is >1/5 palpable on abdominal examination, deliver by caesarean section
- If there is evidence of obstruction or fetal distress at any stage, deliver by caesarean section.

Brow presentation

Spontaneous conversion to either vertex or face presentation may occur, particularly when the fetus is small or when there is fetal death with maceration. It is unusual for spontaneous conversion to occur in an average sized live baby once membranes have ruptured. Arrested labour is usual.

When the fetus is living:

- Deliver by caesarean section.

When the fetus is dead:

- If dilatation is incomplete, deliver by caesarean section
- If dilatation is complete, perform craniotomy or caesarean section.

Do not deliver brow presentation by vacuum extraction, forceps or symphysiotomy.

Face presentation

Prolonged labour is common with face presentation:

- In the chin-anterior position, descent and delivery of the head by flexion may occur
- In the chin-posterior position, the fully extended head is blocked by the sacrum from descent and arrest of labour occurs.

Face presentation, chin anterior, can usually be delivered vaginally. Chin posterior can rarely be delivered vaginally.

- Ensure adequate hydration
- Check maternal and fetal condition
- If there is fetal distress, consider delivery by caesarean section if quick and easy vaginal delivery is not possible
- If the cervix is not fully dilated and it is a chin-anterior position and there is no evidence of obstruction, augment with oxytocin; review progress as with vertex presentation
- If it is a chin-posterior position or there is evidence of obstruction, deliver by caesarean section
- If the cervix is fully dilated *and* it is a chin anterior *and* there is no evidence of obstruction, augment with oxytocin; if descent is satisfactory, deliver by forceps
- If descent is unsatisfactory, deliver by caesarean section
- If the fetus is dead, perform craniotomy or caesarean section.

Do not perform vacuum extraction for face presentation.

Compound presentation (arm prolapsed alongside presenting part)

Spontaneous delivery can occur only when the fetus is very small or dead and macerated. Arrested labour in the expulsive stage is the rule. Replacement of the prolapsed arm is sometimes possible.

1. Place the patient in the knee-chest position. Push the arm above the pelvic brim and hold it there until a contraction pushes the head into the pelvis.
2. Cord prolapse is a risk of this procedure, so be prepared to perform a caesarean section.

Breech presentation

Prolonged labour is an indication for urgent caesarean section in breech presentation (Figures 11.6, 11.7, 11.8). Failure of labour to progress is a sign of possible disproportion.

Transverse lie

Caesarean section is the management of choice, whether the fetus is alive or dead (Figure 11.9).

Delivery through a transverse uterine incision may be difficult, especially if the arm is prolapsed or the fetus is back-down, and often results in extension of the incision with laceration of a uterine artery.

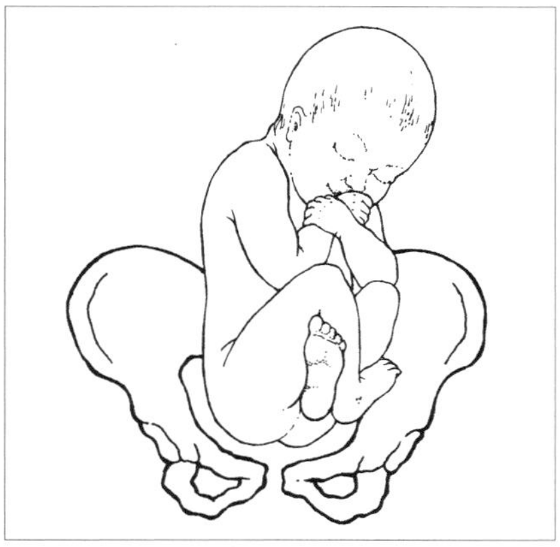

Figure 11.6

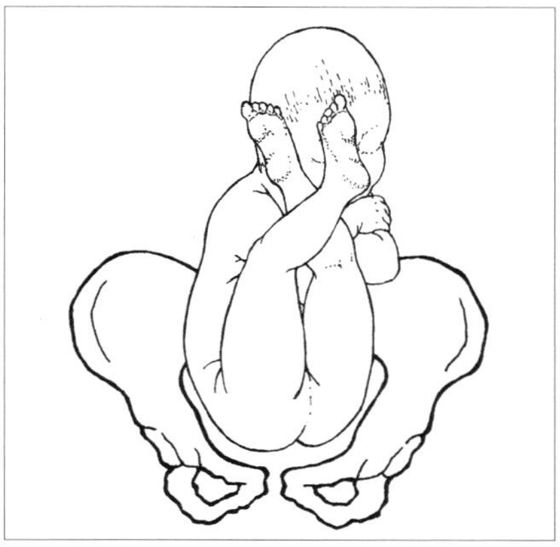

Figure 11.7

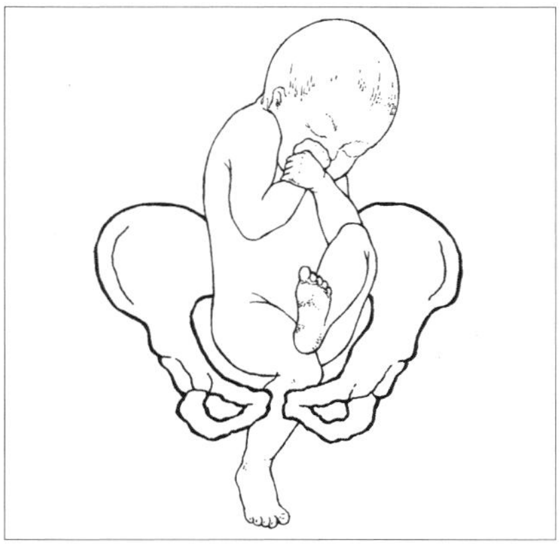

Figure 11.8

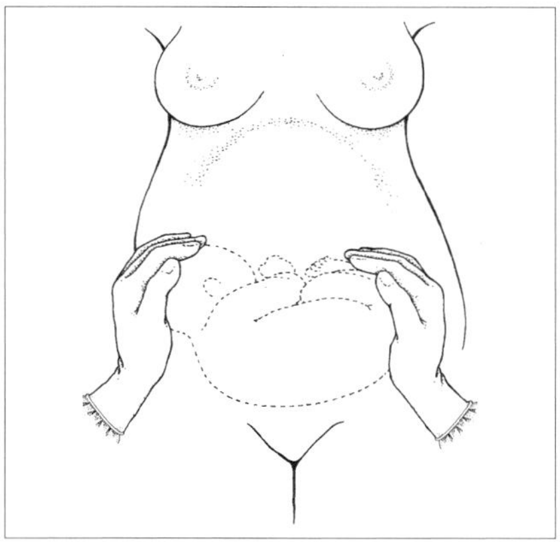

Figure 11.9

11.4 OPERATIVE PROCEDURES

CAESAREAN SECTION

Preparation

1 Review indications. Check fetal presentation and ensure that vaginal delivery is not possible.

2 Obtain consent from the patient after explaining the procedure and the reason for it.

3 Check the patient's haemoglobin concentration, but do not wait for the result if there is fetal or maternal distress or danger. Send the blood sample for type and screen. If the patient is severely anaemic, plan to give two units of blood.

4 Start an IV infusion.

5 Give sodium citrate 30 ml 0.3 molar and/or ranitidine 150 mg orally or 50 mg IV to reduce stomach acidity. Sodium citrate works for 20 minutes only so should be given immediately before induction of anaesthesia if a general anaesthetic is given.

6 Catheterize the bladder and keep a catheter in place during the operation.

11

7 If the baby's head is deep down into the pelvis, as in obstructed labour, prepare the vagina for assistance at caesarean delivery.

8 Roll the patient 15° to her left or place a pillow under her right hip to decrease supine hypotension syndrome.

9 Listen to the fetal heart rate before beginning surgery.

Choice of anaesthesia

In cases of extreme urgency, general anaesthesia can be faster than a spinal and may also be safer if the mother is hypovolaemic or shocked. In lesser degrees of urgency (delivery within 30 minutes required) a well conducted spinal by an experienced anaesthetist minimizes the risk to mother and baby. These issues should be discussed between the surgeon and anaesthetist (see pages 14–12 to 14–14).

Opening the abdomen and making the bladder flap

The abdomen may be opened by a vertical midline skin incision or a transverse skin incision. Caesarean section under local anaesthesia is more difficult to do with the transverse skin incision. The scar following a transverse incision is stronger.

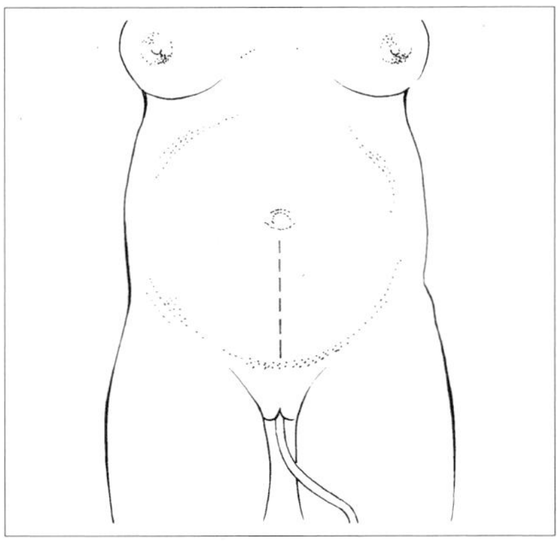
Figure 11.10

Vertical midline incision

1 Make a 2 to 3 cm vertical incision in the fascia (Figure 11.10).

2 Hold the fascial edge with forceps and lengthen the fascial incision up and down, using scissors.

3 Separate the rectus muscles (abdominal wall muscles) with your fingers or scissors.

4 Use your fingers to make a hole in the peritoneum near the umbilicus. Use scissors to lengthen the incision up and down to see the uterus well. Use scissors to separate layers. Open the lower part of the peritoneum carefully to prevent bladder injury.

Transverse incision

1 Make a straight transverse incision in the skin about 3 cm below the line joining the anterior superior iliac spines. The incision should measure 16–18 cm in length.

2 Deepen the incision in the midline about 3–4 cm through the fat down to the rectus sheath.

3 Make a small transverse incision in the rectus sheath. Place the tip of one blade of a partly open scissors under the rectus sheath and the other blade over the rectus sheath and push laterally to cut the sheath.

4 Insert your index finger under the rectus muscle on your side and ask your assistant to do so on the opposite side. Pull the muscles sideways to expose the peritoneum.

5 Open the parietal peritoneum as high as possible with your index finger and enlarge this opening by stretching sideways.

Making the bladder flap

1 Place a bladder retractor over the pubic bone.

2 Using forceps, pick up the loose peritoneum covering the anterior surface of the lower uterine segment and incise with scissors.

3 Extend the incision by placing scissors between the uterus and the loose serosa and cutting about 3 cm on each side in a transverse fashion.

4 Use two fingers to push the bladder downwards off the lower uterine segment. Replace the bladder retractor over the pubic bone and bladder.

Opening the uterus

1 Use a scalpel to make a 3 cm transverse incision in the lower segment of the uterus, about 1 cm below the level where the vesico-uterine serosa was incised to bring the bladder down (Figure 11.11).

2 Widen the incision by placing a finger at each edge, and by pulling up and laterally at the same time. If the lower uterine segment is thick and narrow, extend the incision using scissors instead of fingers in a crescent shape to avoid extension to the uterine vessels.

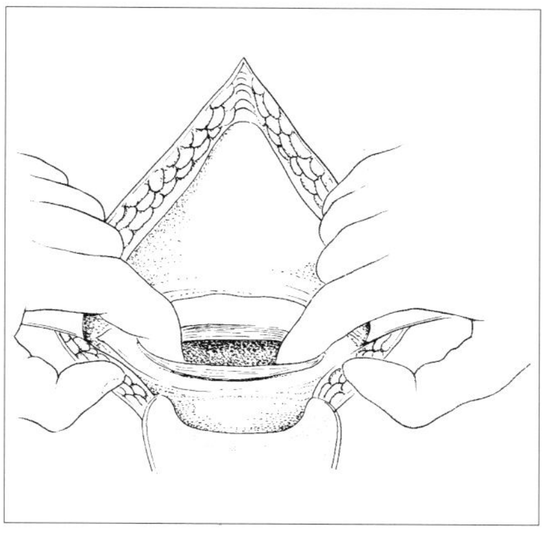

Figure 11.11

Make the uterine incision big enough to deliver the head and body of the baby without tearing the uterine incision.

Delivery of the fetus and placenta

1 To deliver the baby, place one hand inside the uterine cavity between the uterus and the baby's head.

2 Use your fingers to grasp and flex the head.

3 Gently lift the baby's head through the incision, taking care not to extend the incision down towards the cervix (Figure 11.12).

4 With the other hand, gently press on the abdomen over the top of the uterus to help deliver the head.

5 If the baby's head is deep down in the pelvis or vagina, ask an assistant (wearing sterile gloves) to reach under the drapes and push the head up through the vagina. (Figure 11.13).

6 Then lift and deliver the head.

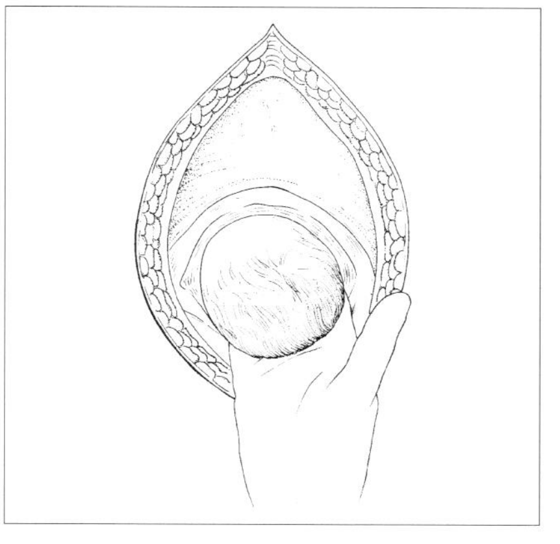

Figure 11.12

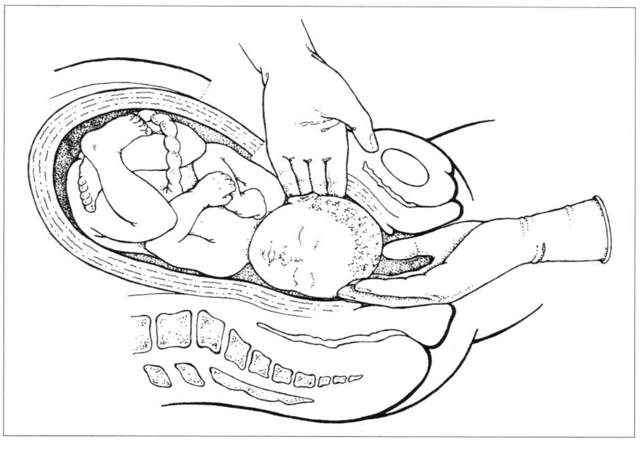

Figure 11.13

7 Suction the baby's mouth and nose when delivered, then deliver the shoulders and body.

8 Give oxytocin 20 units in 1 L IV fluids (normal saline or Ringer's lactate) at 60 drops per minute for 2 hours.

9 Clamp and cut the umbilical cord.

10 Hand the baby to the assistant for initial care.

11 Give a single dose of prophylactic antibiotic after the cord is clamped.

12 If there is foul-smelling liquor, give antibiotics for therapy (see pages 4–10 to 4–11).

13 Keep gentle traction on the cord and massage (rub) the uterus through the abdomen.

14 Deliver the placenta and membranes.

Closing the uterine incision

1 Grasp the corners of the uterine incision with clamps.

2 Grasp the bottom edge of the incision with clamps. Make sure it is separate from the bladder.

3 Look carefully for any extensions of the uterine incision.

4 Repair the incision and any extensions with a continuous locking stitch of 0 chromic non absorbable (or polyglycolic) suture (Figure 11.14).

5 If there is any further bleeding from the incision site, close with figure-of-eight sutures. There is no need for a routine second layer of sutures in the uterine incision.

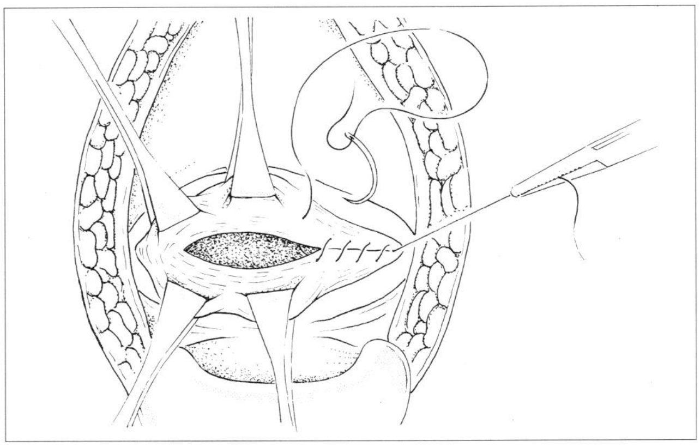

Figure 11.14

Closing the abdomen

Look carefully at the uterine incision before closing the abdomen. Make sure there is no bleeding and that the uterus is firm.

1 Close the fascia with a running stitch of 0 chromic non absorbable (or polyglycolic suture). There is no need to close the peritoneum. Peritoneal closure is not necessary for its healing.

2 If there are signs of infection, pack the subcutaneous tissue with gauze and place loose 0 non absorbable (or polyglycolic) sutures. The skin can be closed with a delayed closure later after the infection has cleared.

3 If there are no signs of infection, close the skin with vertical mattress sutures of 3-0 nylon sutures (or silk) and apply a sterile dressing.

4 Gently push on the abdomen over the uterus to remove clots from the uterus and vagina.

What to do if problems occur

If bleeding is not controlled

1 Massage the uterus.

2 If uterus is atonic, continue to infuse oxytocin and give ergometrine 0.2 mg and prostaglandins, if available (see page 12–7).

3 Transfuse as necessary.

4 Have an assistant press fingers over the aorta to reduce the bleeding until the source of bleeding can be found and stopped.

5 If bleeding is not controlled, perform uterine artery and utero-ovarian artery ligation or a hysterectomy.

Ergometrine is easily destroyed by heat. If logistics are poor, you may need to give what appears to be a very large dose – but beware its use in eclamptic patients as it raises the blood pressure.

When the baby is breech at caesarean section

1 Grasp a foot and deliver it through the incision.

2 Complete the delivery as in a vaginal breech delivery:

- Deliver the legs and body up to the shoulders, then deliver the arms.
- Lay the body on your left forearm. Insert the middle finger of your left hand into the baby's mouth. Place your right palm on the shoulders of the baby. Flex (bend) the head using the fingers of your right hand and deliver it through the incision.

When the baby is transverse (sideways)

1 If the back is up (near the top of the uterus), reach into the uterus and find the baby's ankles. Grasp the ankles and pull gently through the incision to deliver the legs. Complete the delivery as for a breech baby.

2 If the back is down, a high vertical uterine incision may be necessary to deliver the baby. After making the incision, reach into the uterus and grasp the feet. Pull them through the incision and complete the delivery as for a breech baby. To repair the vertical incision, you will need several layers of suture (see below). The patient should not labour with future pregnancies.

In placenta previa

1 If a low anterior placenta is encountered, incise through it and deliver the fetus.

2 If the placenta cannot be detached manually after delivery of the baby, diagnose placenta accreta. This is a common finding at the site of a previous caesarean scar. Perform a hysterectomy.

3 Women with placenta previa are at high risk of postpartum haemorrhage. If there is bleeding at the placental site, under-run the bleeding sites with chromic non absorbable (or polyglycolic) sutures.

4 Watch for bleeding in the immediate postpartum period and take appropriate action.

The high vertical ("classical") incision

1 Open the abdomen through a midline incision skirting the umbilicus:
- Approximately one-third of the incision should be above the umbilicus and two thirds below
- Make the uterine incision in the midline over the fundus of the uterus
- The incision should be approximately 12–15 cm in length
- The lower limit should not extend to the utero-vesical fold of peritoneum.

2 Ask an assistant to apply pressure on the cut edges to control bleeding.

3 Cut down to the level of the membranes and then extend the incision using scissors.

4 After rupturing the membranes, grasp the fetal foot and extract the fetus.

5 Deliver the placenta and membranes.

6 Grasp the edges of the incision with Allis or Green Armytage forceps. Close the incision using at least three layers of suture:
- Close the first layer closest to the cavity, but avoiding the decidua, with a continuous 0 chromic non absorbable (or polyglycolic) suture
- Close the second layer of uterine muscle using interrupted No. 1 chromic non absorbable (or polyglycolic) sutures
- Close the superficial fibres and the serosa using a continuous 0 chromic non absorbable suture (or polyglycolic) suture with an atraumatic needle
- Close the abdomen as for lower segment caesarean section.

Antibiotics

Prophylactic antibiotics in caesarean section decrease post operative infection. They are given after the cord is clamped. Recommended doses are:
- Cefazolin 1 gm IV

Or
- Ampicillin 1–2 g IV: one dose only.

If signs of infection are already present at the time of caesarean section, give
- Ampicillin 1–2 g IV 6 hourly
- *Plus* gentamicin 5 mg/kg/day IV as single daily dose
- *Plus* metronidazole 500 mg 8 hourly until the patient has been afebrile for 24–48 hours.

Tubal sterilization at caesarean section

Tubal ligation may be performed immediately following caesarean section if the woman requested the procedure before labour began.

1 Review for consent of the patient.

2 Grasp the least vascular, middle portion of the tube with a Babcock or Allis forceps.

3 Hold up a loop of tube 2.5 cm in length (Figure 11.15).

4 Crush the base of the loop with artery forceps and ligate it with a 0 plain non absorbable suture (Figure 11.16, 11.17).

5 Excise the loop (a segment of 1 cm in length) through the crushed area (Figure 11.18).

6 Repeat the procedure on the other side.

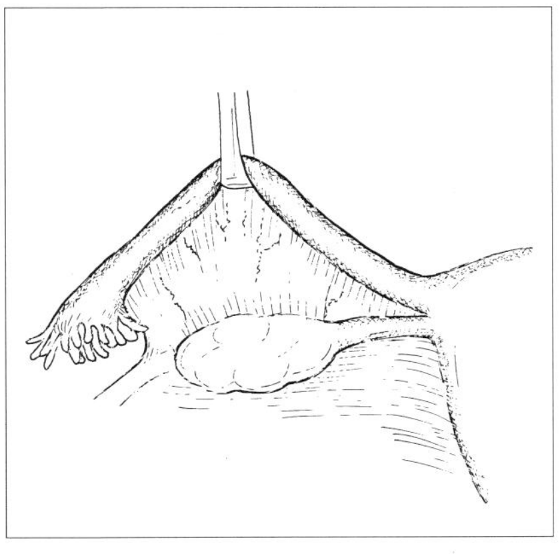

Figure 11.15

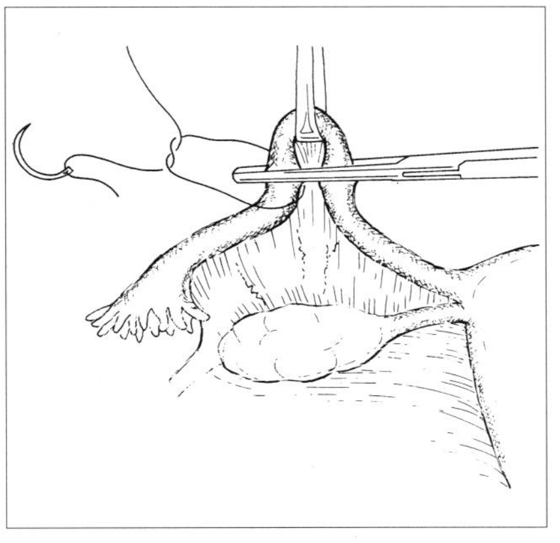

Figure 11.16

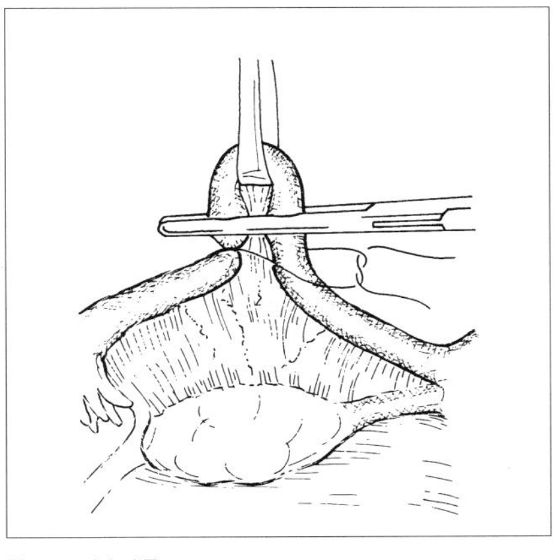

Figure 11.17

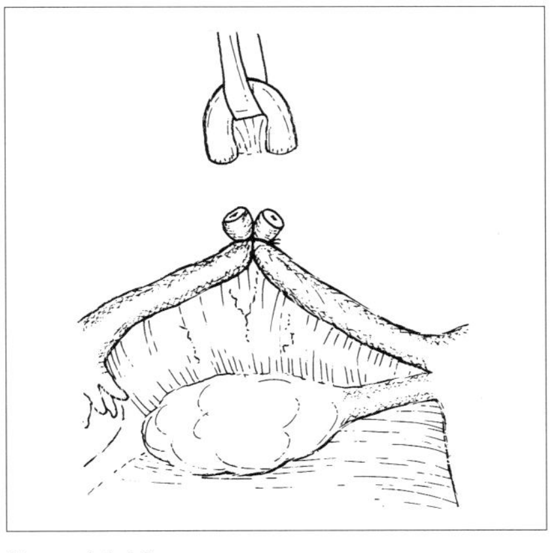

Figure 11.18

Postoperative care after caesarean section

1 Carefully watch and record vital signs, bleeding and urine output. Be prepared to take action if necessary.

2 If bleeding occurs, massage the uterus to expel blood and blood clots. Blood clots in the uterus inhibit uterine contractions.

3 Give:
  - Oxytocin 20 units in 1 L IV fluids (normal saline or Ringer's lactate) at 60 drops per minute
  - Ergometrine 0.2 mg IM
  - Prostaglandins, if available.

4 Use a second IV line to give volume replacement as the above regime only gives an infusion of 4 ml/min which is inadequate in a bleeding patient.

5 If there are signs of infection or the woman currently has fever, give appropriate antimicrobial therapy.

6 Give sufficient analgesic drugs.

7 Give oral fluids the day after surgery. Provide food when the patient is drinking fluids well.

INDUCTION AND AUGMENTATION OF LABOUR

Induction of labour and augmentation of labour are performed for different indications, but the methods are the same.

- Induction of labour: stimulating the uterus to begin labour
- Augmentation of labour: stimulating the uterus during labour to increase the frequency, duration and strength of contractions.

A good contraction pattern is established when there are three contractions in 10 minutes, each lasting more than 40 seconds.

Induction

The success of induction is related to the condition of the cervix at the start of induction:

- Cervix is favourable if it is soft, short and partially dilated
- Cervix is unfavourable if it is firm, long and closed: ripen it using prostaglandin or a Foley catheter before induction.

Prostaglandin E2 is placed high in the posterior fornix of the vagina and may be repeated after 6 hours if required.

If prostaglandin is not available, use a Foley catheter.

1 Gently insert a sterile speculum into the vagina.

2 Hold the catheter with a forceps and introduce it through the cervix. Ensure that the inflatable bulb of the catheter is beyond the internal os.

3 Inflate the bulb with 10 ml of water. Coil the catheter and place in the vagina. Leave the catheter inside until contractions begin, or for at least 12 hours.

4 Deflate the bulb before removing the catheter and then proceed with artificial rupture of membranes (ARM) and oxytocin.

> Do not insert the catheter if there is a history of bleeding or ruptured membranes or obvious vaginal infection.

Artificial rupture of the membranes (ARM)

If the membranes are intact, it is recommended practice in both induction and augmentation to first perform artificial rupture of membranes (ARM). In some cases, this is all that is needed.

Membrane rupture, whether spontaneous or artificial, often sets off the following chain of events:

- Amniotic fluid is expelled.
- Uterine volume is decreased
- Prostaglandins are produced, stimulating labour
- Uterine contractions begin or become stronger.

Technique

1 Review the indications.

2 Listen to and note the fetal heart rate.

3 Ask the patient to lie on her back with legs bent, feet together and knees apart.

4 Wearing sterile gloves, use one hand to examine the cervix. Note and record the consistency, position, effacement and dilatation of the cervix.

5 Use the other hand to insert an amniotic hook or Kocher clamp into the vagina. Guide the hook or clamp towards the membranes along the fingers in the vagina.

6 Place two fingers against the membranes and gently rupture the membranes with the instrument in the other hand. Allow the amniotic fluid to drain slowly around the fingers.

7 Note the colour of the fluid (clear, greenish, bloody). If thick meconium is present, suspect fetal distress.

8 After amniotomy, listen to the fetal heart rate during and after a contraction. If the fetal heart rate is less than 100 or more than 180 beats per minute, suspect fetal distress.

9 If labour is not established 1 hour after ARM, begin oxytocin infusion. If labour is induced because of severe maternal disease (e.g. sepsis or eclampsia), begin oxytocin infusion at the same time as ARM.

In areas of high HIV prevalence, leave the membranes intact for as long as possible to reduce the risk of perinatal transmission of HIV.

Oxytocin stimulation

Use oxytocin with great caution as fetal distress can occur from hyperstimulation and, rarely, uterine rupture can occur. Multiparous women are at higher risk for uterine rupture.

---

1 Record the following observations on a partograph at 30 minute intervals:

- Rate of infusion: changes in the maternal arm position may alter the flow rate

11

- Duration and frequency of contractions
- Fetal heart rate. Listen every 30 minutes, immediately after a contraction. If the fetal heart rate is less than 100 per minute, stop the infusion.

2 Infuse oxytocin 2.5 units in 500 ml of dextrose or normal saline at 10 drops per minute. This is approximately 2.5 mIU/minute.

3 Increase the infusion rate by 10 drops/minute every 30 minutes until a good contraction pattern is established (contractions lasting more than 40 seconds and occurring three times in 10 minutes). The uterus should relax between contractions.

4 Maintain this rate until delivery is completed.

5 If hyperstimulation occurs (any contraction lasts longer than 60 seconds), or there are more than four contractions in 10 minutes, stop the infusion, and relax the uterus using tocolytics (e.g. terbutaline 250 micrograms IV slowly over 5 minutes).

6 If there are not three contractions in 10 minutes, each lasting more than 40 seconds with the infusion rate at 60 drops/minute:
   - Increase the oxytocin concentration to 5 units in 500 ml of dextrose or normal saline and adjust the infusion rate to 30 drops per minute (15 mIU/minute)
   - Increase the infusion rate by 10 drops per minute every 30 minutes until a good contraction pattern is established or the maximum rate of 60 drops per minute is reached.

7 If labour still has not been established using the higher concentration of oxytocin:
   - In multigravida and in women with previous caesarean scars, induction has failed; deliver by caesarean section
   - In primigravida, infuse oxytocin 10 units in 500 ml dextrose or normal saline at 30 drops per minute
   - Increase the infusion rate every half hour by 10 drops per minute every 30 minutes until good contractions are established
   - If good contractions are not established at 60 drops per minute (60 mIU per minute), deliver by caesarean section.

Women receiving oxytocin should never be left alone.

Instrumental delivery

The expulsive forces of labour can be augmented by traction applied to the fetal head. The methods used are:

- Vacuum extraction
- Forceps delivery.

Any trial of instrumental delivery must be treated as a potential caesarean section in terms of preparing for anaesthesia (give ranitidine early) and blood transfusion.

Vacuum extraction (Ventouse)

Figure 11.19 shows the essential elements of a vacuum (Ventouse) extractor.

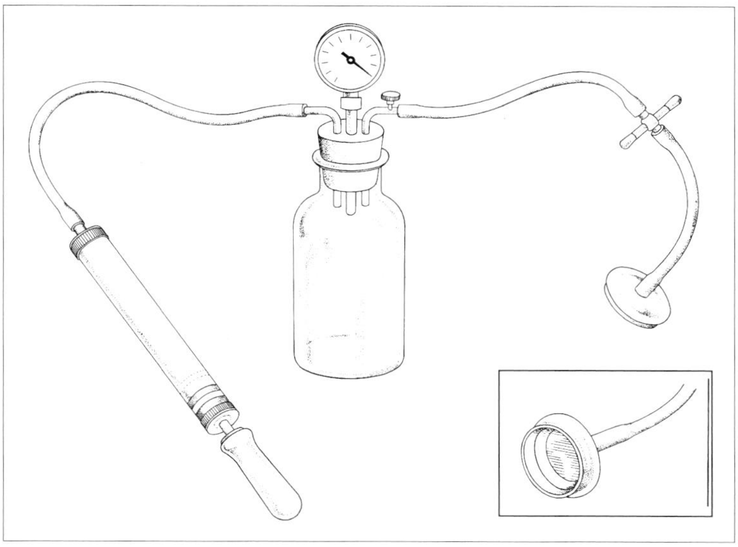

Figure 11.19

1 Review for conditions for vacuum extraction:
- Vertex presentation
- Term fetus
- Cervix fully dilated
- Head at least level with spines and no more than 2/5 above symphysis pubis.

2 Check all connections and test the vacuum on a gloved hand.

3 If necessary, use a pudendal block.

4 Assess the position of the head by feeling the sagittal suture line and the fontanelles. Identify the posterior fontanelle.

5 Apply the largest cup that will fit, with the centre of the cup over the flexion point, 1 cm anterior to the posterior fontanelle. This placement will promote flexion, descent and autorotation with traction (Figure 11.20).

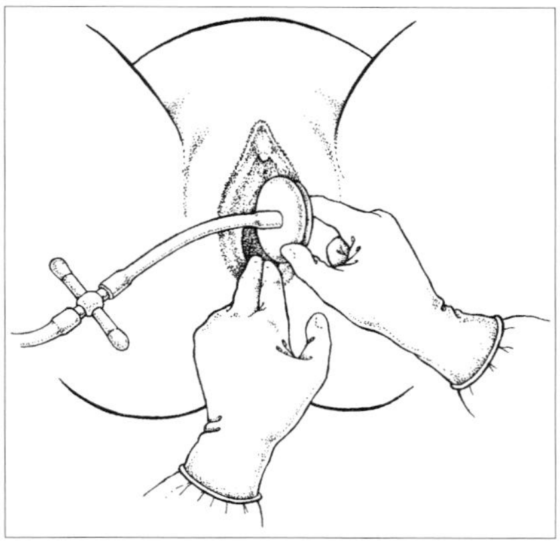

Figure 11.20

6 An episiotomy may be needed for proper placement at this time. If an episiotomy is not necessary for placement, delay the episiotomy until the head is stretching the perineum or the perineum interferes with the axis of traction. This will avoid unnecessary blood loss.

7 Check the application. Ensure there is no maternal soft tissue (cervix or vagina) within the rim.

8 With the pump, create a vacuum of 0.2 kg/cm^2 negative pressure and check the application.

9 Increase the vacuum to 0.8 kg/cm^2 and check the application.

10 After maximum negative pressure, start traction in the line of the pelvic axis and perpendicular to the cup. If the fetal head is tilted to one side or not flexed well, direct traction in a line that will try to correct the tilt or deflexion of the head (i.e. to one side or the other, not necessarily in the midline).

11 With each contraction, apply traction in a line perpendicular to the plane of the cup rim (Figure 11.21).

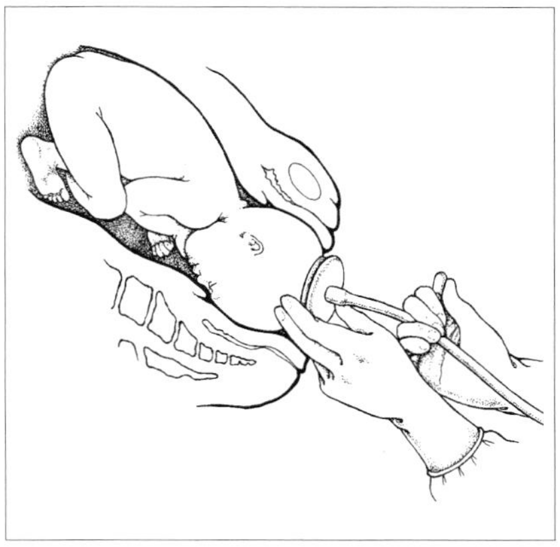

Figure 11.21

11

12 Wearing sterile gloves, place a finger on the scalp next to the cup during traction to assess potential slippage and descent of the vertex.

13 Between contractions:

- Check the fetal heart
- Check the application of the cup.

Using the vacuum extractor

- Never use the cup to actively rotate the baby's head; rotation of the baby's head will occur with traction
- The first pulls help to find the proper direction for pulling
- Do not continue to pull between contractions and expulsive efforts
- With progress, and in the absence of fetal distress, continue the "guiding" pulls for a maximum of 30 minutes.

Vacuum extraction has failed if:

- The head does not advance with each pull
- The fetus is undelivered after three pulls with no descent, or after 30 minutes
- The cup slips off the head twice at the proper direction of pull with a maximum negative pressure.

Every application should be considered a trial of vacuum extraction. Do not persist if there is no descent with every pull. If vacuum extraction fails, perform caesarean section.

Complications

Complications usually result from not observing the conditions of application of traction and from continuing efforts beyond the time limits stated above.

Fetal

- Localized scalp oedema occurs under the vacuum cup; it is harmless and disappears in a few hours
- Cephalhaematoma requires observation and usually will clear in 3–4 weeks
- Intracranial bleeding is rare and requires immediate intensive neonatal care
- Scalp abrasion (common and harmless) and lacerations may occur. Clean and examine lacerations to determine if sutures are necessary. Necrosis is extremely rare.

Maternal

Tears of the genital tract may occur. Examine the woman carefully and repair any tears of the cervix or vagina or repair episiotomy.

Forceps delivery

Review for conditions for forceps delivery:

- Vertex presentation or face presentation with chin anterior

- Cervix fully dilated
- No part of the head is felt on abdominal examination.

The sagittal suture should be in the midline and straight, guaranteeing an occiput anterior (OA) or occiput posterior (OP) position.

Technique

1 Assemble the forceps before application. Ensure that the parts fit together and lock well.

2 Use pudendal block.

3 Lubricate the blades of the forceps.

4 Wearing sterile gloves, insert two fingers of the right hand in the vagina on the side of the fetal head. Slide the left blade gently between the head and the fingers to rest on the side of the head (Figures 11.22, 11.23).

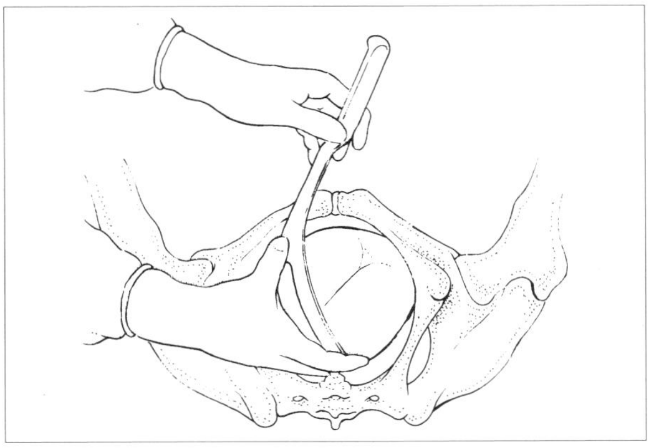

Figure 11.22

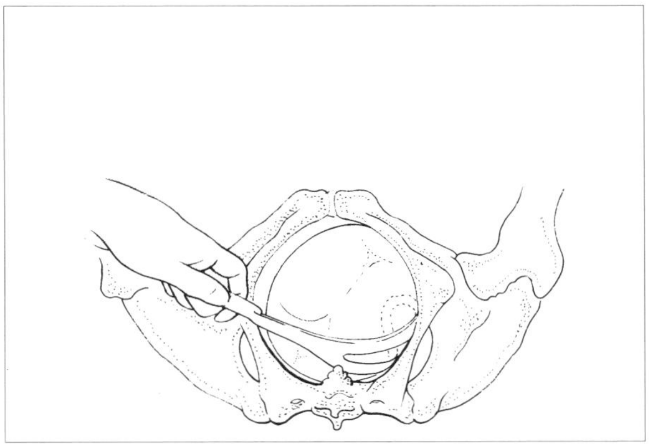

Figure 11.23

5 Repeat the same manoeuvre on the other side using the left hand and the right blade of the forceps (Figure 11.24).

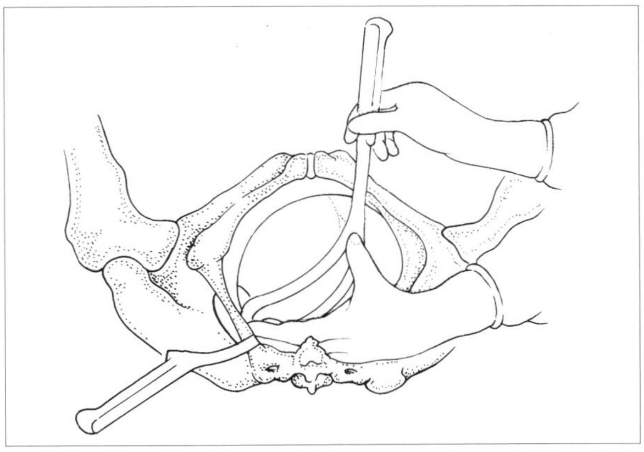

Figure 11.24

6 Depress the handles and lock the forceps. Difficulty in locking usually indicates that the application is incorrect. In this case, remove the blades and recheck the position of the head. Reapply only if rotation is confirmed.

7 After locking, apply steady traction inferiorly and posteriorly with each contraction. The head should descend with each pull. Only two or three pulls should be necessary. (Figures 11.25, 11.26, 11.27, 11.28).

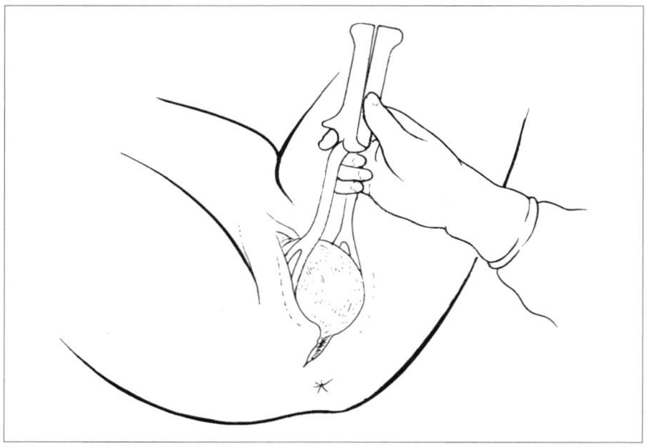

Figure 11.25

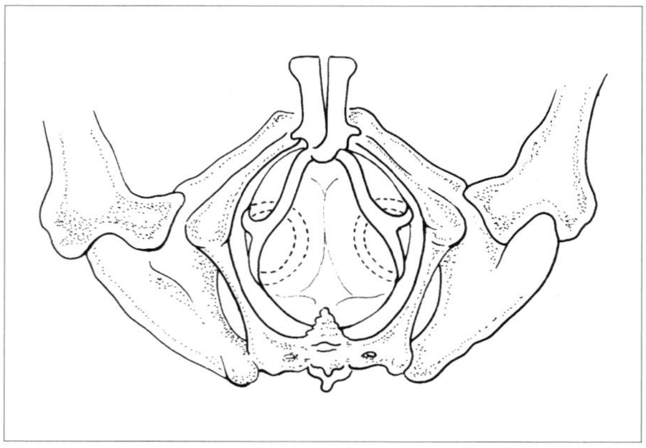

Figure 11.26

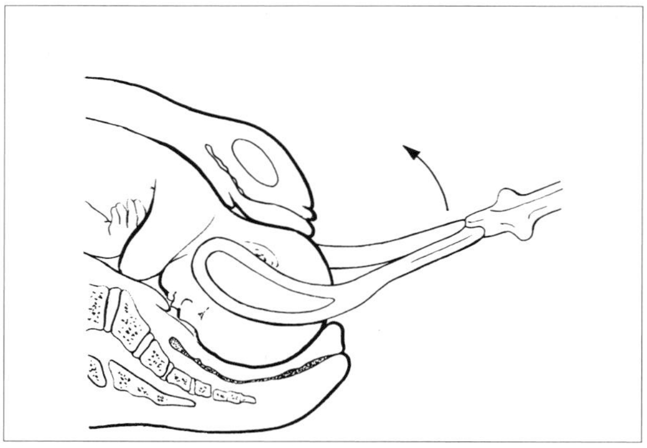

Figure 11.27

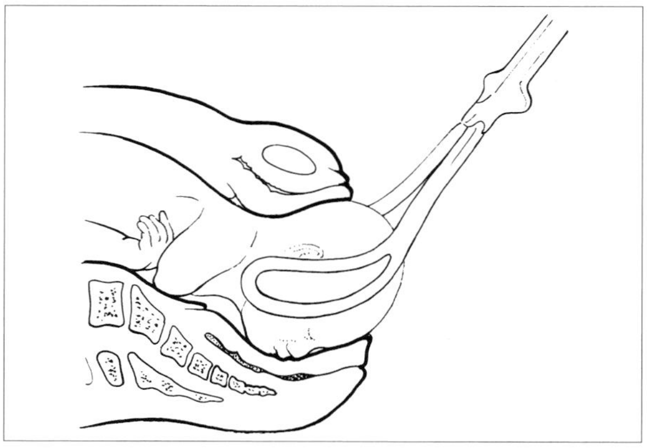

Figure 11.28

8 Between contractions check:
- Fetal heart rate
- Application of forceps.

9 When the head crowns, make a large episiotomy.

10 Lift the head slowly out of the vagina between contractions.

Failure

Forceps delivery has failed if:
- The fetal head does not advance with each pull
- The fetus is undelivered after three pulls.

Every application should be considered a trial of forceps. Do not persist if there is no descent with every pull.

If forceps delivery fails, perform a caesarean section.

Complications

Fetal

- Lacerations of the face and scalp may occur; clean and examine lacerations to determine if sutures are necessary
- Fractures of face and skull require observation
- Injury to facial nerves requires observation. This injury is usually self limiting.

Maternal

- Tears of the genital tract may occur; examine the woman carefully and repair any tears of the cervix or vagina or repair episiotomy
- Uterine rupture may occur and requires immediate treatment.

CRANIOTOMY AND CRANIOCENTESIS

In certain cases of obstructed labour with fetal death, reduction in size of the fetal head by craniotomy makes vaginal delivery possible and avoids the risks associated with caesarean delivery.

Craniocentesis can be performed to reduce the size of a hydrocephalic head to make vaginal delivery possible.

If either procedure is indicated, provide emotional support and encouragement. Explain to the mother and family in advance what has happened and what action you propose.

Give analgesics and possibly diazepam IV slowly or use pudendal block.

Craniotomy (skull perforation)

Perform an episiotomy if required.

In cephalic presentation

1 Make a cruciate (cross shaped) incision on the scalp.
2 Open the cranial vault at the lowest and most central bony point with a craniotome (or a large pointed scissors or a heavy scalpel). In face presentation, perforate the orbits.
3 Insert the craniotome into the fetal cranium and fragment the intracranial contents.
4 Grasp the edges of the skull with several heavy toothed forceps (e.g. Kocher's) and apply traction in the axis of the birth canal.
5 As the head descends, pressure from the bony pelvis will cause the skull to collapse, decreasing the cranial diameter.
6 If the head is not delivered easily, perform a caesarean section.

In breech presentation

1 Make an incision through the skin at the base of the neck.
2 Insert a craniotome (or large pointed scissors or heavy scalpel) through this incision and tunnel subcutaneously to reach the occiput.
3 Perforate the occiput and open the gap as widely as possible.
4 Apply traction on the trunk to cause the skull to collapse as the head descends.

Craniocentesis (skull puncture)

With a dilated cervix

1 Pass a large-bore spinal needle through the dilated cervix and through the sagittal suture line or fontanelles of the fetal skull.

2 Aspirate cerebrospinal fluid until the fetal skull has collapsed and allow normal delivery to proceed.

With a closed cervix

1 Palpate for location of the fetal head.

2 Apply antiseptic solution to the suprapubic skin.

3 Pass a large bore spinal needle through the abdominal and uterine wall and through the hydrocephalic skull.

4 Aspirate the cerebrospinal fluid until the fetal skull has collapsed and allow normal delivery to proceed.

With aftercoming head during breech delivery

1 After the rest of the body has been delivered, insert a large-bore needle through the foramen magnum.

2 Aspirate the cerebrospinal fluid and deliver the aftercoming head as in breech delivery.

During caesarean section

1 Puncture through the uterine wall.

2 Aspirate cerebrospinal fluid prior to making incision.

3 Deliver the baby and placenta as in caesarean section.

Prevention of complications after craniotomy and craniocentesis

1 After delivery, inspect the vagina carefully for laceration and repair any tears or episiotomy.

2 Leave a urinary catheter in place until it is confirmed that there is no bladder injury.

3 Ensure adequate fluid intake and urinary output.

Bleeding in pregnancy and childbirth

12

12.1 BLEEDING

Bleeding is the cause of one in four maternal deaths worldwide. Death may occur in less than two hours after the onset of bleeding associated with childbirth. Anaemia is common in pregnancy and women with anaemia and bleeding are at high risk of death. Appropriate care in pregnancy and labour includes:

- Detection, correction and prevention of anaemia
- Delivery by a skilled attendant
- Active management of the third stage of labour
- Recognition and early management of complications.

Abortions and ectopic pregnancies are associated with bleeding in early pregnancy. In late pregnancy and in labour, bleeding may result from placenta praevia, placental abruption and uterine rupture. Bleeding following childbirth is associated with failure of the uterus to contract (atonic uterus), injuries to the birth canal and retention of placental tissue.

KEY POINTS

- Bleeding causes one in four maternal deaths worldwide
- Prevent anaemia, recognize and treat complications early
- Post partum bleeding is the most common cause of maternal death
- Practise active management of the third stage of labour in all cases to prevent postpartum haemorrhage.

BLEEDING IN EARLY PREGNANCY

Bleeding in early pregnancy is usually related to abortion or miscarriage. Abortion may be of spontaneous onset or induced.

Spontaneous abortion

Spontaneous abortion is the loss of a pregnancy before fetal viability. The stages of spontaneous abortion may include:

- Threatened abortion (pregnancy may continue)
- Inevitable abortion (pregnancy will not continue and will proceed to incomplete/complete abortion)
- Incomplete abortion (products of conception are partially expelled)
- Complete abortion (products of conception are completely expelled).

Induced abortion

Induced abortion is a process by which pregnancy is terminated before fetal viability.

Unsafe abortion

Unsafe abortion is a procedure performed either by persons lacking necessary skills or in an environment lacking minimal medical standards or both.

12

Septic abortion

Septic abortion is an abortion complicated by infection. Sepsis may result from infection if organisms rise from the lower genital tract following either spontaneous or unsafe abortion. Sepsis is more likely to occur if there are retained products of conception and evacuation has been delayed. Sepsis is a frequent complication of unsafe abortion involving instrumentation.

Ectopic pregnancy

An ectopic pregnancy is one in which implantation occurs outside the uterine cavity. The fallopian tube is the site of ectopic implantation in over 90% of cases. As the pregnancy grows, the tube ruptures. Intraperitoneal bleeding can lead to shock. Abdominal pain from rupture of the tube generally *precedes* vaginal bleeding in ectopic pregnancy. In an abortion, abdominal pain usually *follows* vaginal bleeding.

BLEEDING IN LATE PREGNANCY AND LABOUR

Bleeding in late pregnancy and bleeding in labour are usually due to placental abruption or placenta previa.

Placental abruption

Abruption is the detachment of a normally located placenta from the uterus before the fetus is delivered. Fetal distress and fetal death are common when the placenta detaches prematurely. Maternal complications include shock, coagulation failure and renal failure. Immediate delivery is the preferred option.

Placenta previa

Placenta previa is implantation of the placenta at or near the cervix. Recurrent, painless vaginal bleeding in small amounts may occur in late pregnancy. Expectant management is the preferred option unless bleeding is sufficiently severe to cause maternal or fetal distress.

Uterine rupture

Uterine rupture is an important but less common cause of bleeding in late pregnancy and labour. This may occur in obstructed labour and in labour with a scarred uterus. Bleeding from a ruptured uterus may occur vaginally unless the fetal head blocks the pelvis. Bleeding may also occur intra-abdominally. Rupture of the lower uterine segment into the broad ligament, however, will not release blood into the abdominal cavity.

POSTPARTUM HAEMORRHAGE

Postpartum haemorrhage (PPH) is vaginal bleeding in excess of 500 ml after childbirth. The importance of a given volume of blood loss varies with the woman's haemoglobin level. A woman with a normal haemoglobin level will tolerate blood loss that would be fatal for an anaemic woman. Bleeding may occur at a slow rate over several hours and the condition may not be recognized until the woman suddenly enters shock. Risk assessment in the antenatal period does not effectively predict those women who will have PPH.

> Practise active management of the third stage of labour on all women in labour since it reduces the incidence of PPH due to uterine atony.
>
> Closely monitor all postpartum women to determine those that have PPH.

Atonic uterus

Bleeding occurs from the placental site after delivery. Blood vessels in the placental site are surrounded by uterine muscles, which normally contract after delivery and close off the vessels.

> Failure of the uterus to contract (atonic uterus) results in excessive bleeding. This is the commonest cause of bleeding after childbirth.

Other causes of bleeding

Tears in the genital tract may also cause bleeding. Retention of placental tissue and blood clots in the uterine cavity prevent adequate uterine contractions after delivery and are therefore associated with PPH. Infection of retained placental fragments may cause bleeding later in pregnancy.

12.2 DIAGNOSIS AND INITIAL MANAGEMENT

1 Make a rapid evaluation of the general condition of the woman including vital signs (pulse, blood pressure, respiration, temperature).

2 If you suspect shock, immediately begin treatment. Even if signs of shock are not present, keep shock in mind as you evaluate the woman further because her status may worsen rapidly. If shock develops, it is important to begin treatment immediately.

3 Shout for help if the woman is in shock, or is bleeding excessively.

4 Start a rapid IV infusion.

5 Find out if the woman is currently pregnant or has been recently delivered:
- If she is currently pregnant, find out the approximate period of gestation
- If she is currently pregnant and less than 22 weeks, consider abortion and ectopic pregnancy
  – The risk of ectopic pregnancy is greater in any woman with anaemia, pelvic inflammatory disease (PID), threatened abortion or unusual complaints about abdominal pain; if you suspect an ectopic pregnancy, perform bimanual examination gently because an early ectopic pregnancy is easily ruptured

KEY POINTS

Active management of the third stage of labour includes:
- Giving an oxytocic to the mother as soon as the baby is born
- Delivery of the placenta by controlled cord traction
- Uterine massage to ensure that the uterus is contracted.

Diagnosis of vaginal bleeding in early pregnancy

Presenting symptoms and other symptoms and signs typically present	Symptoms and signs sometimes present	Probable diagnosis
• Light[1] bleeding • Closed cervix • Uterus corresponds to dates	• Cramping/lower abdominal pain • Uterus softer than normal	Threatened abortion
• Light bleeding • Abdominal pain • Closed cervix • Uterus slightly larger than normal • Uterus softer than normal	• Fainting • Tender adnexal mass • Amenorrhoea • Cervical motion tenderness	Ectopic pregnancy
• Light bleeding • Closed cervix • Uterus smaller than dates • Uterus softer than normal	• Light cramping/lower abdominal pain • History of expulsion of products of conception	Complete abortion
• Heavy[2] bleeding • Dilated cervix • Uterus corresponds to dates	• Cramping/lower abdominal pain • Tender uterus • No expulsion of products of conception	Inevitable abortion
• Heavy bleeding • Dilated cervix • Uterus smaller than dates	• Cramping/lower abdominal pain • Partial expulsion of products of conception	Incomplete abortion
• Heavy bleeding • Dilated cervix • Uterus larger than dates • Uterus softer than normal • Partial expulsion of products of conception which resemble grapes	• Nausea/vomiting • Spontaneous abortion • Cramping/lower abdominal pain • Ovarian cysts (easily ruptured) • Early onset pre-eclampsia • No evidence of a fetus	Molar pregnancy

[1] Light bleeding: takes longer than 5 minutes for a clean pad or cloth to be soaked

[2] Heavy bleeding: takes less than 5 minutes for a clean pad or cloth to be soaked

  - Consider abortion in any woman of reproductive age who has a missed period (delayed menstrual bleeding with more than a month having passed since her last menstrual period) and has one or more of the following: bleeding, cramping, partial expulsion of products of conception, dilated cervix or smaller uterus than expected. If abortion is a possible diagnosis, identify and treat any complications immediately.
- If she is currently pregnant and more than 22 weeks, consider placenta previa, abruptio placentae and uterine rupture; do not do a vaginal examination at this stage
- If she has been recently delivered, consider postpartum haemorrhage due to atonicity of the uterus first
  - Massage the uterus to expel blood and blood clots; blood clots trapped in the uterus will inhibit effective uterine contractions
  - Give oxytocin 10 units IM

Diagnosis of bleeding in late pregnancy and labour

Presenting symptoms and other symptoms and signs typically present	Symptoms and signs sometimes present	Probable diagnosis
• Bleeding after 22 weeks gestation (may be retained in the uterus) • Intermittent or constant abdominal pain	• Shock • Tense/tender uterus • Decreased/absent fetal sounds • Fetal distress or absent fetal heart sounds	Abruptio placentae
• Bleeding (intra-abdominal and/or vaginal) • Severe abdominal pain (may decrease after rupture)	• Shock • Abdominal distension/free fluid • Abnormal uterine contour • Tender abdomen • Easily palpable fetal parts • Absent fetal movements and fetal heart sounds • Rapid maternal pulse	Ruptured uterus
• Bleeding after 22 weeks gestation	• Shock • Bleeding may be precipitated by intercourse • Relaxed uterus • Fetal presentation not in pelvis/ lower uterine pole feels empty • Normal fetal condition	Placenta previa

Diagnosis of vaginal bleeding after childbirth

Presenting symptoms and other symptoms and signs typically present	Symptoms and signs sometimes present	Probable diagnosis
• Immediate PPH[1] • Uterus soft and not contracted	• Shock	Atonic uterus
• Immediate PPH[1]	• Complete placenta • Uterus contracted	Tears of cervix, vagina or perineum
• Placenta not delivered within 30 minutes after delivery	• Immediate PPH[1] • Uterus contracted	Retained placenta
• Portion of maternal surface of placenta missing or torn membranes with vessels	• Immediate PPH[1] • Uterus contracted	Retained placental fragments
• Uterine fundus not felt on abdominal palpation • Slight or intense pain	• Inverted uterus apparent at vulva • Immediate PPH[1]	Inverted uterus[2]
• Bleeding occurs more than 24 hours after delivery • Uterus softer and larger than expected for elapsed time since delivery	• Bleeding is variable (light or heavy, continuous or irregular) and foul-smelling • Anaemia	Delayed PPH
• Immediate PPH[1] (bleeding is intra-abdominal and/or vaginal) • Severe abdominal pain (may decrease after rupture)	• Shock • Tender abdomen • Rapid maternal pulse	Ruptured uterus

[1] Bleeding may be light if a clot blocks the cervix or if the woman is lying on her back

[2] There may be no bleeding with complete inversion

- Start an IV infusion and infuse IV fluids with 20 units oxytocin in the bag
- Catheterize the bladder.

6 Check to see if the placenta has been expelled and examine the placenta to be certain it is complete.
   - Examine the cervix, vagina and perineum for tears.

12.3 SPECIFIC MANAGEMENT

Diagnosis of the specific condition is made from the symptoms and physical findings.

THREATENED ABORTION

- Medical treatment is usually not necessary
- Advise the woman to avoid strenuous activity and sexual intercourse, but bed rest is not necessary
- If bleeding stops, follow up in antenatal clinic
- Reassess if bleeding recurs
- If bleeding persists, assess for fetal viability or ectopic pregnancy (ultrasound); persistent bleeding, particularly in the presence of a uterus larger than expected, may indicate twins or molar pregnancy
- Do not give medications such as hormones (e.g. oestrogens or progestins) or tocolytic agents (e.g. salbutamol or indomethacin) as they will not prevent miscarriage.

INEVITABLE ABORTION

If pregnancy is less than 16 weeks

1 Plan for evacuation of uterine contents. If evacuation is not immediately possible, give:
   - Ergometrine 0.2 mg IM, repeated after 15 minutes if necessary

   Or

   - Misoprostol 400 mcg by mouth, repeated once after 4 hours if necessary.

2 Arrange for evacuation of the uterus as soon as possible.

If pregnancy is greater than 16 weeks

1 Await spontaneous expulsion of products of conception and then evacuate the uterus to remove any remaining products of conception.

2 If necessary, infuse oxytocin 40 units in 1 L IV fluids (normal saline or Ringer's lactate) at 40 drops per minute to help achieve expulsion of the products of conception.

3 Ensure follow-up of the woman after treatment.

Diagnosis and management of complications of abortion

Symptoms and signs	Complication	Management
• Lower abdominal pain • Rebound tenderness • Tender uterus • Prolonged bleeding • Malaise • Fever • Foul-smelling vaginal discharge • Purulent cervical discharge • Cervical motion tenderness	Infection/sepsis	Begin antibiotics[1] as soon as possible before attempting manual vacuum aspiration
• Cramping abdominal pain • Rebound tenderness • Abdominal distension • Rigid (hard and tense) abdomen • Shoulder pain • Nausea/vomiting • Fever	Uterine, vaginal or bowel injuries	Perform a laparotomy to repair the injury and perform manual vacuum aspiration simultaneously. Seek assistance, if required

[1] Give antibiotics until the woman is fever-free for 48 hours
- Ampicillin 2 g IV every 6 hours
- *Plus* gentamicin 5 mg/kg body weight IV every 24 hours
- *Plus* metronidazole 500 mg IV every 8 hours

INCOMPLETE ABORTION

If bleeding is light to moderate and pregnancy is less than 16 weeks

Use fingers or ring (or sponge) forceps to remove products of conception protruding through the cervix.

If bleeding is heavy and pregnancy is less than 16 weeks

Evacuate the uterus. Manual vacuum aspiration is the preferred method of evacuation. Evacuation by sharp curettage should only be done if manual vacuum aspiration is not available.

If evacuation is not immediately possible, give:
- Ergometrine 0.2 mg IM, repeated after 15 minutes if necessary

Or
- Misoprostol 400 mcg orally (repeated once after 4 hours if necessary).

If pregnancy is greater than 16 weeks

1 Infuse oxytocin 40 units in 1 L IV fluids (normal saline or Ringer's lactate) at 40 drops per minute until expulsion of products of conception occurs.

2 If necessary, give misoprostol 200 mcg vaginally every 4 hours until expulsion, but do not administer more than 800 mcg.
3 Evacuate any remaining products of conception from the uterus.
4 Ensure follow-up of the woman after treatment (see below).

COMPLETE ABORTION

1 Evacuation of the uterus is usually not necessary.
2 Observe for heavy bleeding.
3 Ensure follow-up of the woman after treatment (see below).

ECTOPIC PREGNANCY

Symptoms and signs of ruptured and unruptured ectopic pregnancy

Unruptured ectopic pregnancy	Ruptured ectopic pregnancy
• Symptoms of early pregnancy (irregular spotting or bleeding, nausea, swelling of breasts, bluish discoloration of vagina and cervix, softening of cervix, slight uterine enlargement, increased urinary frequency) • Abdominal and pelvic pain	• Collapse and weakness • Fast, weak pulse (110 per minute or more) • Hypotension • Hypovolaemia • Acute abdominal and pelvic pain • Abdominal distension[1] • Rebound tenderness • Pallor

[1] Distended abdomen with shifting dullness may indicate free blood

Symptoms and signs are extremely variable depending on whether or not the pregnancy has ruptured.

Culdocentesis (cul-de-sac puncture) is an important tool for the diagnosis of ruptured ectopic pregnancy, but is less useful than a serum pregnancy test combined with ultrasonography. If non-clotting blood is obtained, begin treatment at once.

Differential diagnosis

The most common differential diagnosis for ectopic pregnancy is threatened abortion. Others are acute or chronic pelvic infection, ovarian cysts (torsion or rupture) and acute appendicitis.

If available, ultrasound may help to distinguish a threatened abortion or twisted ovarian cyst from an ectopic pregnancy.

Immediate management

1 Order crossmatched blood and arrange for immediate laparotomy.

Do not wait for blood before performing surgery.

2 At surgery, inspect both ovaries and fallopian tubes:
- If there is extensive damage to the tubes, perform salpingectomy (the bleeding tube and the products of conception are excised together): this is the treatment of choice in most cases
- Rarely, if there is little tubal damage, perform salpingostomy (the products of conception can be removed and the tube conserved). This should be done only when the conservation of fertility is very important to the woman, as the risk of another ectopic pregnancy is high.

Autologous blood transfusion

If significant haemorrhage occurs, autologous transfusion can be used if the blood is unquestionably fresh and free from infection (in later stages of pregnancy, blood is contaminated with amniotic fluid, etc. and should not be used for autotransfusion). The blood can be collected after the abdomen is opened.

1 Scoop the blood into a basin and strain through gauze to remove clots.

2 Clean the top portion of a blood donor bag with antiseptic solution and open it with a sterile blade.

3 Pour the woman's blood into the bag and reinfuse it through a filtered set in the usual way.

4 If a donor bag with anticoagulant is not available, add sodium citrate 10 ml to each 90 ml of blood.

For further details of the use of gauze filtration, see *The Clinical Use of Blood* (WHO, 2001, page 275).

ABRUPTIO PLACENTAE

An abruptio placentae (placental abruption, retroplacental bleed) is the detachment of a normally located placenta from the uterus before the fetus is delivered.

1 Assess clotting status using a bedside clotting test. Failure of a clot to form after 7 minutes or a soft clot that breaks down easily suggests coagulopathy.

2 Transfuse as necessary.

3 If bleeding is heavy (evident or hidden), deliver as soon as possible.

4 If the cervix is fully dilated, deliver by vacuum extraction.

5 If vaginal delivery is not imminent, deliver by caesarean section.

In every case of abruptio placentae, be prepared for postpartum haemorrhage.

6 If bleeding is light to moderate (the mother is not in immediate danger), the course of action depends on the fetal heart sounds:

- If fetal heart rate is normal or absent, rupture the membranes with an amniotic hook or a Kocher clamp
- If contractions are poor, augment labour with oxytocin
- If the cervix is unfavourable (firm, thick, closed), perform a caesarean section
- If the fetal heart rate is less than 100 or more than 180 beats per minute:
  - Perform rapid vaginal delivery
  - If vaginal delivery is not possible, deliver by immediate caesarean section.

COAGULOPATHY (CLOTTING FAILURE)

Coagulopathy is both a cause and a result of massive obstetric haemorrhage. It can be triggered by many causes, including:

- Abruption
- Sepsis
- Fetal death
- Eclampsia
- Amniotic fluid embolism.

The clinical picture ranges from major haemorrhage, with or without thrombotic complications, to a clinically stable state that can be detected only by laboratory testing.

> In many cases of acute blood loss, the development of coagulopathy can be prevented if blood volume is restored promptly by infusion of IV fluids.

1 Treat the possible cause of coagulation failure.
2 Use blood products to help control haemorrhage.
3 Give fresh whole blood, if available, to replace coagulation factors and red cells.
4 If fresh whole blood is not available, choose one of the following based on availability:
   - Fresh frozen plasma or cryoprecipitate for replacement of coagulation factors
   - Packed red cells for red cell replacement
   - Platelet concentrates (if bleeding continues and the platelet count is less than 20 000).

For further details refer to *The Clinical Use of Blood* (WHO, 2001, pages 223–224).

RUPTURED UTERUS

Bleeding from a ruptured uterus may occur vaginally unless the fetal head blocks the pelvis. Bleeding may also occur intra-abdominally. Rupture of the lower uterine segment into the broad ligament, however, will not release blood into the abdominal cavity.

1 Restore blood volume by infusing IV fluids (normal saline or Ringer's lactate) before surgery.

2 When stable, immediately perform laparotomy and deliver the baby and placenta.

3 If the uterus can be repaired with less operative risk than hysterectomy would entail and the edges of the tear are not necrotic, repair the uterus. This involves less time and blood loss than hysterectomy.

4 If the uterus cannot be repaired, perform subtotal hysterectomy. If the tear extends through the cervix and vagina, total hysterectomy may be required.

Because there is an increased risk of rupture with subsequent pregnancies, discuss the option of permanent contraception with the woman after the emergency is over.

PLACENTA PREVIA

Placenta previa is implantation of the placenta at or near the cervix (Figure 12.1).

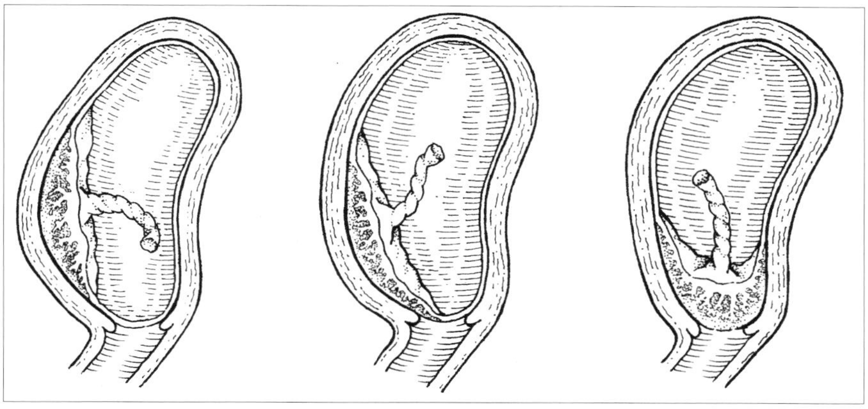

Figure 12.1

If you suspect placenta previa, do not perform a vaginal examination unless preparations have been made for immediate caesarean section.

1 Perform a careful *speculum* examination to rule out other causes of bleeding such as cervicitis, trauma, cervical polyps or cervical malignancy. The presence of these, however, does not rule out placenta previa.

2 Assess the amount of bleeding.

3 Restore blood volume by infusing IV fluids (normal saline or Ringer's lactate).

4 If bleeding is heavy and continuous, arrange for caesarean delivery, irrespective of fetal maturity.

5 If bleeding is light or if it has stopped and the fetus is alive but premature, consider expectant management until delivery or heavy bleeding occurs:

- Keep the woman in the hospital until delivery
- Correct anaemia with oral iron therapy
- Ensure that blood is available for transfusion, if required
- If bleeding recurs, decide management after weighing benefits and risks for the woman and fetus of further expectant management versus delivery.

Confirming the diagnosis

If a reliable ultrasound examination can be performed, localize the placenta. If placenta previa is confirmed and the fetus is mature, plan delivery.

If ultrasound is not available or the report is unreliable and the pregnancy is less than 37 weeks, manage as placenta previa until 37 weeks.

If ultrasound is not available or the report is unreliable and the pregnancy is 37 weeks or more, examine under double set-up to exclude placenta previa, with the woman in the operating theatre with the surgical team present.

The double set-up prepares for either vaginal or caesarean delivery, as follows.

1 Ensure IV lines are running and crossmatched blood is available.

2 Use a sterile vaginal speculum to see the cervix:
   - If the cervix is partly dilated and placental tissue is visible, the diagnosis is confirmed; plan caesarean delivery
   - If the cervix is not dilated, cautiously palpate the vaginal fornices:
     – If you feel spongy tissue, confirm placenta previa and plan caesarean delivery
     – If you feel a firm fetal head, rule out major placenta previa and proceed to deliver by induction
   - If a diagnosis of placenta previa is still in doubt, perform a cautious digital examination:
     – If you feel soft tissue within the cervix, confirm placenta previa and plan delivery (below)
     – If you feel membranes and fetal parts both centrally and marginally, rule out placenta previa and proceed to deliver by induction.

Women with placenta previa are at high risk for postpartum haemorrhage and placenta accreta/increta, a common finding at the site of a previous caesarean scar.

If delivered by caesarean section and there is bleeding from the placental site:

1 Under-run the bleeding sites with sutures.

2 Infuse oxytocin 20 units in 1 L IV fluids (normal saline or Ringer's lactate) at 60 drops per minute.

3 If bleeding occurs during the postpartum period, initiate appropriate management. This may include artery uterine ligation or hysterectomy.

ATONIC UTERUS

An atonic uterus fails to contract after delivery.

1 Continue to massage the uterus.

2 Use oxytocic drugs which can be given together or sequentially.

Use of oxytocic drugs

	Oxytocin	Ergometrine/ methyl-ergometrine	15-methyl prostaglandin F_{2a}
Dose and route	IV: Infuse 20 units in 1 L IV fluids at 60 drops per minute IM: 10 units	IM or IV (slowly): 0.2 mg	IM: 0.25 mg
Continuing dose	IV: Infuse 20 units in 1 L IV fluids at 40 drops per minute	Repeat 0.2 mg IM after 15 minutes If required, give 0.2 mg IM or IV (slowly) every 4 hours	0.25 mg every 15 minutes
Maximum dose	Not more than 3 L of IV fluids containing oxytocin	5 doses (total 1.0 mg)	8 doses (total 2 mg)
Precautions/ contraindications	Do not give as an IV bolus	Pre-eclampsia, hypertension, heart disease	Asthma

Do not give prostaglandins intravenously. They may be fatal.

3 Anticipate the need for blood early and transfuse as necessary.

4 If bleeding continues:
- Check the placenta again for completeness
- If there are signs of retained placental fragments (absence of a portion of maternal surface or torn membranes with vessels), remove remaining placental tissue
- Assess clotting status using a bedside clotting test; failure of a clot to form after 7 minutes or a soft clot that breaks down easily suggests coagulopathy.

5 If bleeding continues in spite of management above:
- Perform bimanual compression of the uterus (Figures 12.2, 12.3) and maintain compression until bleeding is controlled and the uterus contracts

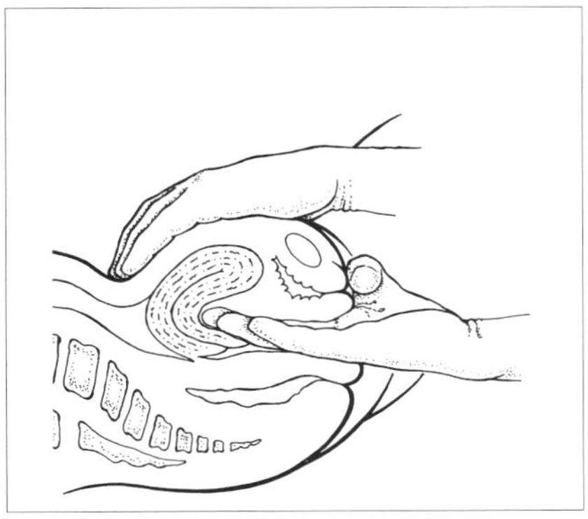

Figure 12.2

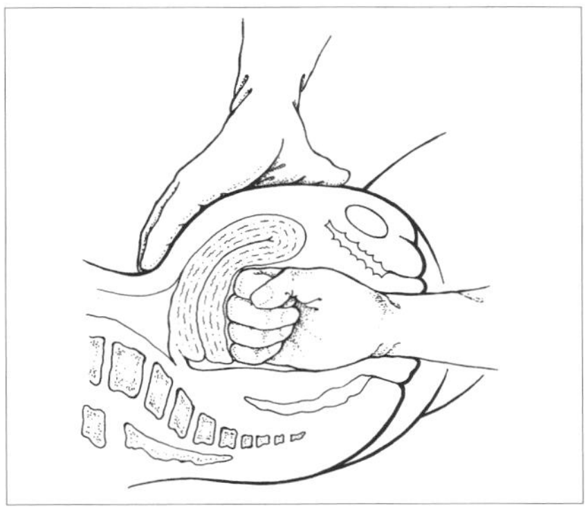

Figure 12.3

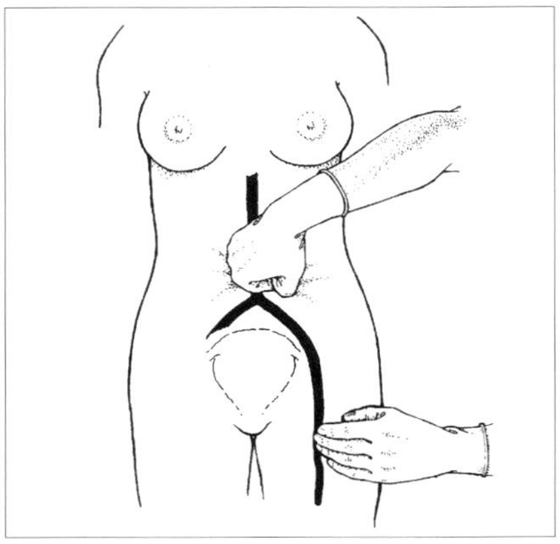
Figure 12.4

- Alternatively, compress the aorta (Figure 12.4).

6 If bleeding continues in spite of compression, perform uterine and utero-ovarian artery ligation; if life-threatening bleeding continues after ligation, perform subtotal hysterectomy.

Packing the uterus is ineffective and wastes precious time.

TEARS OF CERVIX, VAGINA OR PERINEUM

Tears of the birth canal are the second most frequent cause of PPH. Postpartum bleeding with a contracted uterus is usually due to a cervical or vaginal tear, but tears may coexist with atonic uterus.

1 Examine the woman carefully and repair tears of the cervix or vagina and perineum.

2 If bleeding continues, assess clotting status using a bedside clotting test.

RETAINED PLACENTA

1 If you can see the placenta, ask the woman to push it out. If you can feel the placenta in the vagina, remove it.

2 Ensure that the bladder is empty. Catheterize the bladder, if necessary.

3 If the placenta is not expelled, give oxytocin 10 units IM if not already done for active management of the third stage.

4 Do not give ergometrine because it causes tonic uterine contraction, which may delay expulsion.

5 If the placenta is undelivered after 30 minutes of oxytocin stimulation and the uterus is contracted, attempt controlled cord traction.

Avoid forceful cord traction and fundal pressure as they may cause uterine inversion.

6 If controlled cord traction is unsuccessful, attempt manual removal of placenta. Very adherent tissue may be placenta accreta. Efforts to extract a placenta that does not separate easily may result in heavy bleeding or uterine perforation which usually requires hysterectomy.

7 If bleeding continues, assess clotting status using a bedside clotting test. Failure of a clot to form after 7 minutes or a soft clot that breaks down easily suggests coagulopathy.

8 If there are signs of infection (fever, foul-smelling vaginal discharge), give antibiotics as for metritis.

RETAINED PLACENTAL FRAGMENTS

When a portion of the placenta – one or more lobes – is retained, it prevents the uterus from contracting effectively.

1 Feel inside the uterus for placental fragments. Manual exploration of the uterus is similar to the technique described for removal of the retained placenta.

2 Remove placental fragments by hand, ovum forceps or large curette.

3 If bleeding continues, assess coagulation status using a bedside clotting test.

INVERTED UTERUS

The uterus is inverted if it turns inside out during delivery of the placenta.

1 Reposition the uterus immediately. With the passage of time, the constricting ring around the inverted uterus becomes more rigid and the uterus more engorged with blood.

2 If the woman is in severe pain, give pethidine 1 mg/kg *or* morphine 0.1 mg/kg body weight IM or IV slowly.

3 Give a single dose of prophylactic antibiotics after correcting the inverted uterus:

- Ampicillin 2 g IV p*lus* metronidazole 500 mg IV

Or

- Cefazolin 1 g IV *plus* metronidazole 500 mg IV).

4 If there are signs of infection (fever, foul-smelling vaginal discharge), give antibiotics, as for metritis. If necrosis is suspected, perform vaginal hysterectomy. This may require referral to a tertiary care centre.

5 Do not give oxytocic drugs until the inversion is corrected.

DELAYED ("SECONDARY") POSTPARTUM HAEMORRHAGE

1 If anaemia is severe, arrange for a transfusion and provide oral iron and folic acid.

2 If there are signs of infection (fever, foul-smelling vaginal discharge), give antibiotics as for metritis:

- Prolonged or delayed PPH may be a sign of metritis.

3 Give oxytocic drugs.

4 If the cervix is dilated, explore by hand to remove large clots and placental fragments. Manual exploration of the uterus is similar to the technique described for removal of the retained placenta.

5 If the cervix is not dilated, evacuate the uterus to remove placental fragments.

6 Rarely, if bleeding continues, consider uterine and utero-ovarian artery ligation or hysterectomy.

7 Perform histologic examination of curettings or hysterectomy specimen, if possible, to rule out trophoblastic tumour.

12.4 PROCEDURES

MANUAL VACUUM ASPIRATION

1 Provide emotional support and encouragement and give paracetamol 30 minutes before the procedure. Rarely, a paracervical block may be needed.

12

2 Prepare the MVA syringe (for molar pregnancy, when the uterine contents are likely to be copious, have three syringes ready for use):
   - Assemble the syringe
   - Close the pinch valve
   - Pull back on the plunger until the plunger arms lock.

3 Even if bleeding is slight, give oxytocin 10 units IM *or* ergometrine 0.2 mg IM before the procedure to make the myometrium firmer and reduce the risk of perforation.

4 Perform a bimanual pelvic examination to assess the size and position of the uterus and the condition of the fornices.

5 Apply antiseptic solution to the vagina and cervix (especially the os).

6 Check the cervix for tears or protruding products of conception. If products of conception are present in the vagina or cervix, remove them using ring (or sponge) forceps.

7 Gently grasp the anterior lip of the cervix with a vulsellum or single-toothed tenaculum:
   - With incomplete abortion, a ring or sponge forceps is preferable as it is less likely than the tenaculum to tear the cervix with traction and does not require the use of lidocaine for placement.

8 If using a tenaculum to grasp the cervix, first inject 1 ml of 0.5% lidocaine solution into the anterior or posterior lip of the cervix which has been exposed by the speculum (the 10 o'clock or 12 o'clock position is usually used).

9 Dilatation is needed only in cases of missed abortion or when products of conception have remained in the uterus for several days:
   - Gently introduce the widest gauge suction cannula
   - Use graduated dilators only if the cannula will not pass; begin with the smallest dilator and end with the largest dilator (usually 10–12 mm) that ensures adequate dilatation (Figure 12.5)
   - Take care not to tear the cervix or to create a false opening.

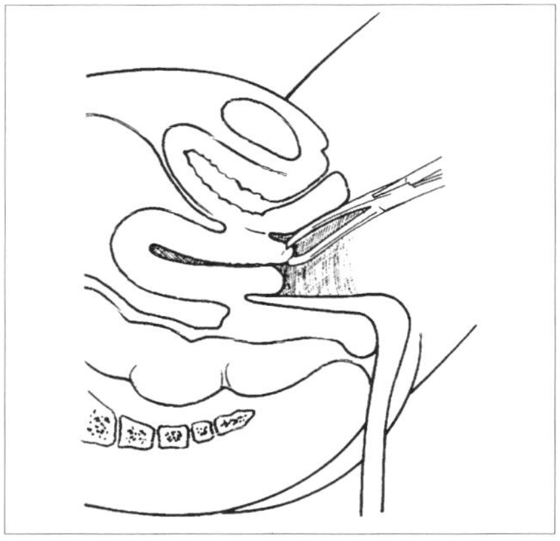

Figure 12.5

10 While gently applying traction to the cervix, insert the cannula through the cervix into the uterine cavity just past the internal os (Figure 12.6). Rotating the cannula while gently applying pressure often helps the tip of the cannula pass through the cervical canal.

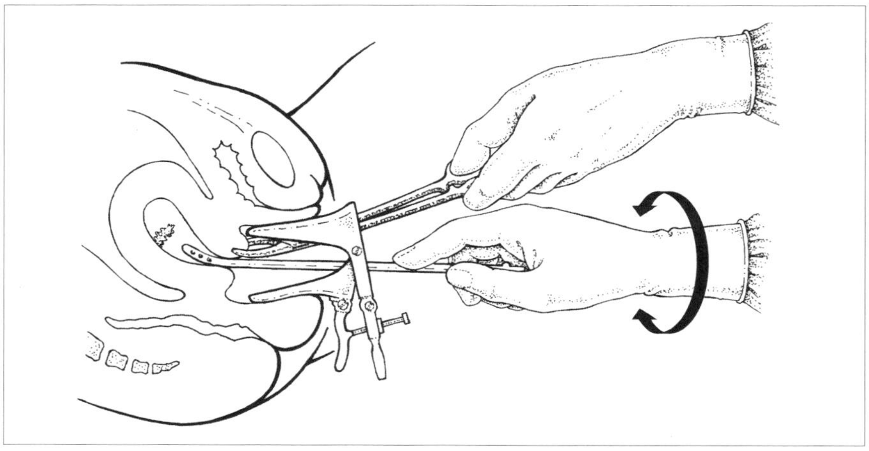

Figure 12.6

11 Slowly push the cannula into the uterine cavity until it touches the fundus, but not more than 10 cm. Measure the depth of the uterus by dots visible on the cannula and then withdraw the cannula slightly.

12 Attach the prepared MVA syringe to the cannula by holding the vulsellum (or tenaculum) and the end of the cannula in one hand and the syringe in the other.

13 Release the pinch valve(s) on the syringe to transfer the vacuum through the cannula to the uterine cavity. Evacuate remaining contents by gently rotating the syringe from side to side (10 to 12 o'clock) and then moving the cannula gently and slowly back and forth within the uterine cavity (Figure 12.7).

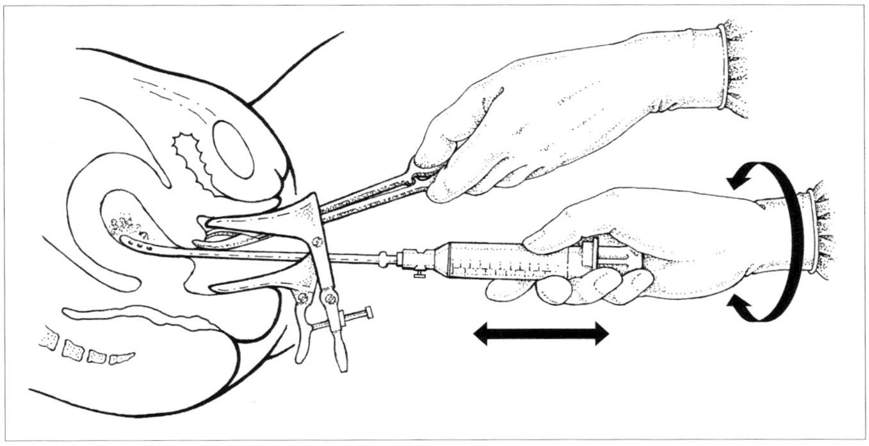

Figure 12.7

14 Check for signs of completion:
- Red or pink foam but no more tissue is seen in the cannula
- A grating sensation is felt as the cannula passes over the surface of the evacuated uterus
- The uterus contracts around (grips) the cannula.

15 Withdraw the cannula. Detach the syringe and place the cannula in decontamination solution. With the valve open, empty the contents of the MVA syringe into a strainer by pushing on the plunger.

16 Perform a bimanual examination to check the size and firmness of the uterus.

17 Quickly inspect the tissue removed from the uterus for quantity and presence of products of conception, to assure complete evacuation and to check for a molar pregnancy (rare). If no products of conception are seen:
- All products of conception may have been passed before the MVA was performed (complete abortion)
- The uterine cavity may appear to be empty but may not have been emptied completely: repeat the evacuation
- The vaginal bleeding may not have been due to an incomplete abortion (e.g. breakthrough bleeding, as may be seen with hormonal contraceptives or uterine fibroids)
- The uterus may be abnormal (e.g. cannula may have been inserted in the nonpregnant side of a double uterus).

18 Absence of products of conception in a woman with symptoms of pregnancy raises the strong possibility of ectopic pregnancy. Gently insert a speculum into the vagina and examine for bleeding. If the uterus is still soft and not smaller or if there is persistent, brisk bleeding, repeat the evacuation.

DILATATION AND CURETTAGE

The preferred method of evacuation of the uterus is by manual vacuum aspiration (see above). Dilatation and curettage should be used only if manual vacuum aspiration is not available.

1 Follow the initial steps as described under Manual Vacuum Aspiration.

2 Gently pass a uterine sound through the cervix to assess the length and direction of the uterus. Gently introduce a large curette. Use graduated dilators only if the curette will not pass. Begin with the smallest dilator and end with the largest dilator that ensures adequate dilatation (usually 10–12 mm) (Figure 12.8). Take care not to tear the cervix or to create a false opening.

3 Evacuate the contents of the uterus with a large curette or ring forceps (Figure 12.9). Gently curette the walls of the uterus until a grating sensation is felt.

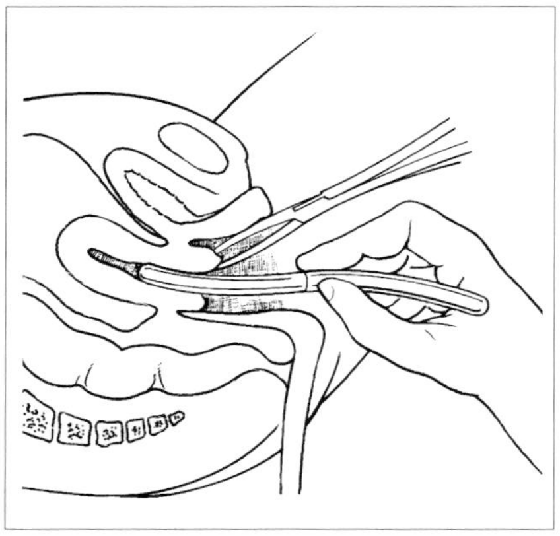

Figure 12.8

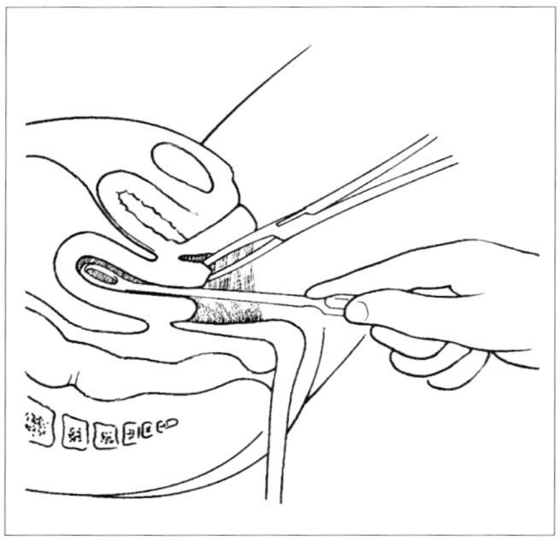

Figure 12.9

4 Perform a bimanual pelvic examination to check the size and firmness of the uterus. Examine the evacuated material. Send material for histopathological examination, if required.

Post-procedure care

1 Give paracetamol 500 mg by mouth as needed.

2 Encourage the woman to eat, drink and walk about as she wishes.

3 Offer other health services, if possible, including tetanus prophylaxis, counselling or a family planning method.

4 Discharge uncomplicated cases in 1–2 hours.

5 Advise the woman to watch for symptoms and signs requiring immediate attention:

- Prolonged cramping (more than a few days)
- Prolonged bleeding (more than 2 weeks)

- Bleeding more than normal menstrual bleeding
- Severe or increased pain
- Fever, rigor, malaise
- Fainting.

CULDOCENTESIS

1 Apply antiseptic solution to the vagina (especially the posterior fornix).

2 Provide emotional support and encouragement. If necessary, use local infiltration with lidocaine.

3 Gently grasp the posterior lip of the cervix with a tenaculum and gently pull to elevate the cervix and expose the posterior vagina.

4 Place a long needle (e.g. spinal needle) on a syringe and insert it through the posterior vagina, just below the posterior lip of the cervix (Figure 12.10).

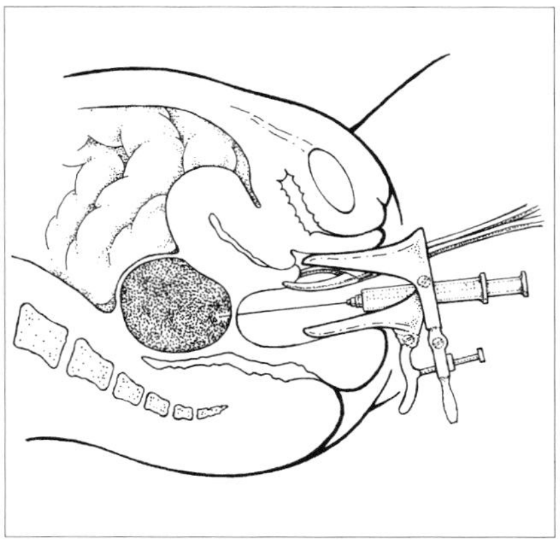

Figure 12.10

5 Pull back on the syringe to aspirate the pouch of Douglas (the space behind the uterus):
   - If non-clotting blood is obtained, suspect ectopic pregnancy
   - If clotting blood is obtained, a vein or artery may have been aspirated; remove the needle, re-insert it and aspirate again
   - If clear or yellow fluid is obtained, there is no blood in the peritoneum; the woman may, however, still have an unruptured ectopic pregnancy and further observations and tests may be needed
   - If no fluid is obtained, remove the needle, reinsert it and aspirate again; if no fluid is obtained, the woman may have an unruptured ectopic pregnancy
   - If pus is obtained, keep the needle in place and proceed to colpotomy.

COLPOTOMY

1 If pus is obtained on culdocentesis, keep the needle in place and make a stab incision at the site of the puncture. Remove the needle and insert blunt forceps or a finger through the incision to break loculi in the abscess cavity (Figure 12.11).

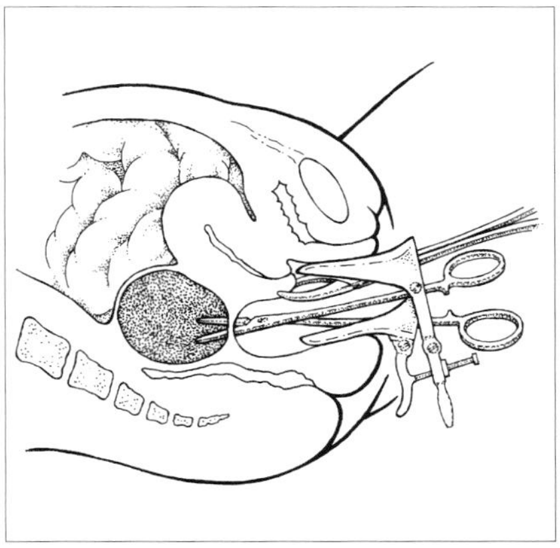

Figure 12.11

2 Allow the pus to drain. Insert a high-level disinfected soft rubber corrugated drain through the incision; if required, use a stitch through the drain to anchor it in the vagina. Remove the drain when there is no more drainage of pus.

3 If no pus is obtained, the abscess may be higher than the pouch of Douglas. A laparotomy will be required for peritoneal lavage (washout).

SALPINGECTOMY FOR ECTOPIC PREGNANCY

1 Give a single dose of prophylactic antibiotics (ampicillin 2 g IV *or* cefazolin 1 g IV).

2 Open the abdomen:
   - Make a midline vertical incision below the umbilicus to the pubic hair, through the skin and to the level of the fascia
   - Make a 2–3 cm vertical incision in the fascia

- Hold the fascial edge with forceps and lengthen the incision up and down using scissors
- Use fingers or scissors to separate the rectus muscles (abdominal wall muscles)
- Use fingers to make an opening in the peritoneum near the umbilicus Use scissors to lengthen the incision up and down in order to see the entire uterus. Carefully, to prevent bladder injury, use scissors to separate layers and open the lower part of the peritoneum
- Place a bladder retractor over the pubic bone and place self-retaining abdominal retractors.

3 Identify and bring to view the fallopian tube with the ectopic gestation and its ovary.

4 Apply traction forceps (e.g. Babcock) to increase exposure and clamp the mesosalpinx to stop haemorrhage.

5 Aspirate blood from the lower abdomen and remove blood clots.

6 Apply gauze moistened with warm saline to pack off the bowel and omentum from the operative field.

7 Divide the mesosalpinx using a series of clamps (Figure 12.12). Apply each clamp close to the tubes to preserve ovarian vasculature.

8 Transfix and tie the divided mesosalpinx with 2-0 chromic non absorbable (or polyglycolic) suture before releasing the clamps.

9 Place a proximal suture around the tube at its isthmic end and excise the tube.

10 Close the abdomen:
- Ensure that there is no bleeding; remove clots using a sponge
- In all cases, check for injury to the bladder and repair it, if found
- Close the fascia with continuous 0 chromic non absorbable (or polyglycolic) suture; there is no need to close the bladder peritoneum or the abdominal peritoneum

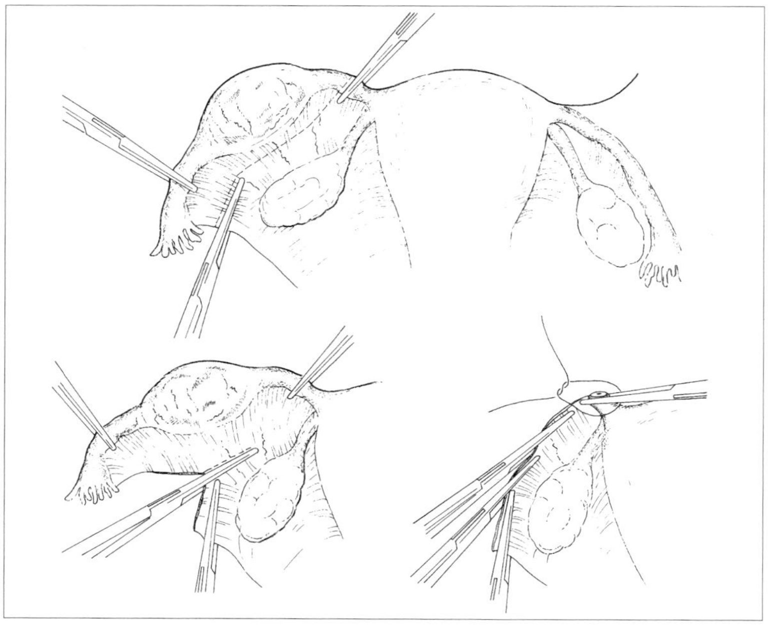

Figure 12.12

- If there are signs of infection, pack the subcutaneous tissue with gauze and place loose 0 non absorbable (or polyglycolic) sutures; close the skin with a delayed closure after the infection has cleared
- If there are no signs of infection, close the skin with vertical mattress sutures of 3-0 nylon (or silk) and apply a sterile dressing.

Salpingostomy

Rarely, when there is little damage to the tube, the gestational sac can be removed and the tube conserved. This should be done only in cases where the conservation of fertility is very important to the woman since she is at risk for another ectopic pregnancy.

1. Open the abdomen and expose the appropriate ovary and fallopian tube.
2. Apply traction forceps (e.g. Babcock) on either side of the unruptured tubal pregnancy and lift to view.
3. Use a scalpel to make a linear incision through the serosa on the side opposite to the mesentery and along the axis of the tube, but do not cut the gestational sac.
4. Use the scalpel handle to slide the gestational sac out of the tube.
5. Ligate bleeding points.
6. Return the ovary and fallopian tube to the pelvic cavity.
7. Close the abdomen.

Post-procedure care

1. If there are signs of infection or the woman currently has fever, give a combination of antibiotics until she is fever-free for 48 hours:
   - Ampicillin 2 g IV every 6 hour *plus* gentamicin 5 mg/kg body weight IV every 24 hours *plus* metronidazole 500 mg IV every 8 hours.
2. Give appropriate analgesic drugs.
3. If salpingostomy was performed, advise the woman of the risk for another ectopic pregnancy and offer family planning.

REPAIR OF RUPTURED UTERUS

1. Give a single dose of prophylactic antibiotics (ampicillin 2 g IV *or* cefazolin 1 g IV).
2. Open the abdomen:
   - Make a midline vertical incision below the umbilicus to the pubic hair, through the skin and to the level of the fascia
   - Make a 2–3 cm vertical incision in the fascia
   - Hold the fascial edge with forceps and lengthen the incision up and down using scissors
   - Use fingers or scissors to separate the rectus muscles (abdominal wall muscles)
   - Use fingers to make an opening in the peritoneum near the umbilicus. Use scissors to lengthen the incision up and down in order to see the

entire uterus. Carefully, to prevent bladder injury, use scissors to separate layers and open the lower part of the peritoneum
- Examine the abdomen and the uterus for site of rupture and remove clots
- Place a bladder retractor over the pubic bone and place self-retaining abdominal retractors.

3 Deliver the baby and placenta.

4 Infuse oxytocin 20 units in 1 L IV fluids (normal saline or Ringer's lactate) at 60 drops per minute until the uterus contracts and then reduce to 20 drops per minute.

5 Lift the uterus out of the pelvis in order to note the extent of the injury.

6 Examine both the front and the back of the uterus.

7 Hold the bleeding edges of the uterus with Green Armytage clamps (or ring forceps).

8 Separate the bladder from the lower uterine segment by sharp or blunt dissection. If the bladder is scarred to the uterus, use fine scissors.

Repairing the uterine tear

1 Repair the tear with a continuous locking stitch of 0 non absorbable (or polyglycolic) suture. If the bleeding points are deep, use figure-of-8 sutures. If bleeding is not controlled or if the rupture is through a previous classical or vertical incision, place a second layer of suture.

2 Ensure that the ureter is identified and exposed to avoid including it in a stitch.

3 If the woman has requested tubal ligation, perform the procedure at this time.

4 If the rupture is too extensive for repair, proceed with hysterectomy. Control bleeding by clamping with long artery forceps and ligating.

Rupture through cervix and vagina

1 If the uterus is torn through the cervix and vagina, mobilize the bladder at least 2 cm below the tear.

2 If possible, place a suture 1 cm below the upper end of the cervical tear and keep traction on the suture to bring the lower end of the tear into view as the repair continues.

Rupture laterally through uterine artery

1 If the rupture extends laterally to damage one or both uterine arteries, ligate the injured artery.

2 Identify the arteries and ureter before ligating the uterine vessels.

Rupture with broad ligament haematoma

1 If the rupture has created a broad ligament haematoma, clamp, cut and tie off the round ligament.

2 Open the anterior leaf of the broad ligament and drain off the haematoma.
3 Inspect the area carefully for injury to the uterine artery or its branches. Ligate any bleeding vessels.

Repair of bladder injury

1 Identify the extent of the injury by grasping each edge of the tear with a clamp and gently stretching. Determine if the injury is close to the bladder trigone (ureters and urethra).
2 Dissect the bladder off the lower uterine segment with fine scissors or with a sponge on a clamp.
3 Free a 2 cm circle of bladder tissue around the tear.
4 Repair the tear in two layers with continuous 3-0 chromic non absorbable (or polyglycolic) suture:
   - Suture the bladder mucosa (thin inner layer) and bladder muscle (outer layer)
   - Invert (fold) the outer layer over the first layer of suture and place another layer of suture
   - Ensure that sutures do not enter the trigone area.
5 Test the repair for leaks:
   - Fill the bladder with sterile saline or water through the catheter
   - If leaks are present, remove the suture, repair and test again.
6 If it is not certain that the repair is well away from the ureters and urethra, complete the repair and refer the woman to a higher-level facility for an intravenous urogram.
7 Keep the bladder catheter in place for at least 7 days and until urine is clear. Continue IV fluids to ensure flushing of the bladder.

Post-procedure care

1 If there are signs of infection or the woman currently has fever, give a combination of antibiotics until she is fever-free for 48 hours:
   - Ampicillin 2 g IV every 6 hours *plus* gentamicin 5 mg/kg body weight IV every 24 hours *plus* metronidazole 500 mg IV every 8 hours.
2 Give appropriate analgesic drugs.
3 If there are no signs of infection, remove the abdominal drain after 48 hours.
4 If tubal ligation was not performed, offer family planning.

If the woman wishes to have more children, advise her to have elective caesarean section for future pregnancies. Because there is an increased risk of rupture with subsequent pregnancies, the option of permanent contraception needs to be discussed with the woman after the emergency is over.

MANUAL REMOVAL OF PLACENTA

1 Provide emotional support and encouragement. Sedation or anaesthesia may be required.

2 Give a single dose of prophylactic antibiotics:
- Ampicillin 2 g IV *plus* metronidazole 500 mg IV
  Or
- Cefazolin 1 g IV *plus* metronidazole 500 mg.

3 Hold the umbilical cord with a clamp. Pull the cord gently until it is parallel to the floor.

4 Wearing sterile gloves, insert a hand into the vagina and up into the uterus along the cord.

5 Let go of the cord and move the hand up over the abdomen in order to support the fundus of the uterus and to provide counter-traction during removal to prevent inversion of the uterus (Figure 12.13). If uterine inversion occurs, reposition the uterus.

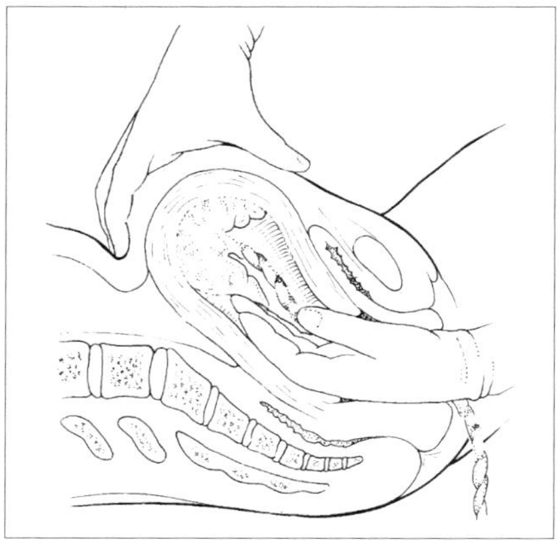

Figure 12.13

6 Move the fingers of the hand laterally until you locate the edge of the placenta.

7 If the cord has been detached previously, insert a hand into the uterine cavity. Explore the entire cavity until a line of cleavage is identified between the placenta and the uterine wall.

8 Detach the placenta from the implantation site by keeping your fingers tightly together and using the edge of your hand to gradually make a space between the placenta and the uterine wall.

9 Proceed slowly all around the placental bed until the whole placenta is detached from the uterine wall.

10 If the placenta does not separate from the uterine surface by gentle lateral movement of the fingertips at the line of cleavage, suspect placenta accreta and proceed to laparotomy and possible subtotal hysterectomy.

11 Hold the placenta and slowly withdraw the hand from the uterus, bringing the placenta with it (Figure 12.14). With the other hand, continue to provide counter-traction to the fundus by pushing it in the opposite direction of the hand that is being withdrawn.

12 Palpate the inside of the uterine cavity to ensure that all placental tissue has been removed.

13 Give oxytocin 20 units in 1 L IV fluids (normal saline or Ringer's lactate) at 60 drops per minute.

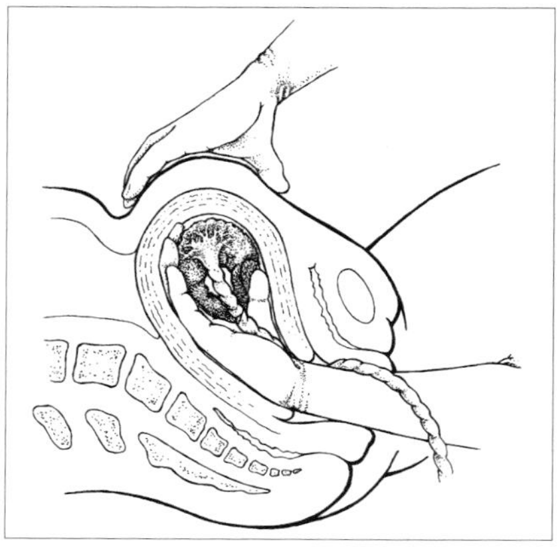

Figure 12.14

14 Have an assistant massage the fundus of the uterus to encourage a tonic uterine contraction.

15 If there is continued heavy bleeding, give ergometrine 0.2 mg IM or prostaglandins.

16 Examine the uterine surface of the placenta to ensure that it is complete. If any placental lobe or tissue is missing, explore the uterine cavity to remove it.

17 Examine the woman carefully and repair any tears of the cervix or vagina, or repair episiotomy.

Problems

If the placenta is retained due to a constriction ring or if hours or days have passed since delivery, it may not be possible to get the entire hand into the uterus. Extract the placenta in fragments using two fingers, ovum forceps or a wide curette.

Post-procedure care

1 Observe the woman closely until the effect of IV sedation has worn off.

2 Monitor the vital signs (pulse, blood pressure, respiration) every 30 minutes for the next 6 hours or until stable.

3 Palpate the uterine fundus to ensure that the uterus remains contracted.

4 Check for excessive lochia.

5 Continue infusion of IV fluids and transfuse as necessary.

REPAIR OF CERVICAL TEARS

1 Apply antiseptic solution to the vagina and cervix.

2 Provide emotional support and encouragement. Anaesthesia is not required for most cervical tears.

3 Ask an assistant to massage the uterus and provide fundal pressure.

4 Gently grasp the cervix with ring or sponge forceps. Apply the forceps on both sides of the tear and gently pull in various directions to see the entire cervix. There may be several tears.

5 Close the cervical tears with continuous 0 chromic non absorbable (or polyglycolic) suture starting at the apex (upper edge of tear), which is often the source of bleeding (Figure 12.15). If a long section of the rim of the cervix is tattered, under-run it with continuous 0 chromic non absorbable (or polyglycolic) suture.

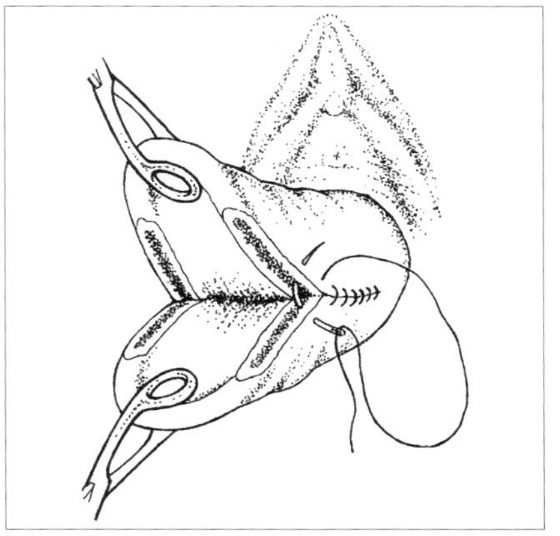

Figure 12.15

6 If the apex is difficult to reach and ligate, it may be possible to grasp it with artery or ring forceps. Leave the forceps in place for 4 hours. Do not persist in attempts to ligate the bleeding points as such attempts may increase the bleeding. Then after 4 hours, open the forceps partially but do not remove.

7 After another 4 hours, if the bleeding has not recurred, remove the forceps completely.

A laparotomy may be required to repair a cervical tear that has extended deep beyond the vaginal vault.

REPAIR OF VAGINAL AND PERINEAL TEARS

Four degrees of tear can occur during delivery:

- First degree — Vaginal mucosa + connective tissue
- Second degree — Vaginal mucosa + connective tissue + muscles
- Third degree — Complete transection of the anal sphincter
- Fourth degree — Rectal mucosa also involved

Repair of first and second degree tears

Most first degree tears close spontaneously without sutures.

1 Use local infiltration with lidocaine. If necessary, use a pudendal block. Anaesthetize early to provide sufficient time for it to take effect.

2 Ask an assistant to massage the uterus and provide fundal pressure.

3 Carefully examine the vagina, perineum and cervix (Figure 12.16). If the tear is long and deep through the perineum, inspect to be sure there is no third or fourth degree tear:
- Place a gloved finger in the anus
- Gently lift the finger and identify the sphincter
- Feel for the tone or tightness of the sphincter
- Change to clean, sterile gloves.

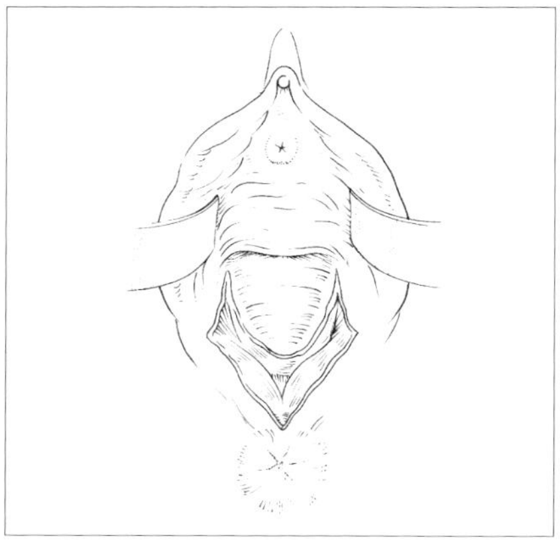

Figure 12.16

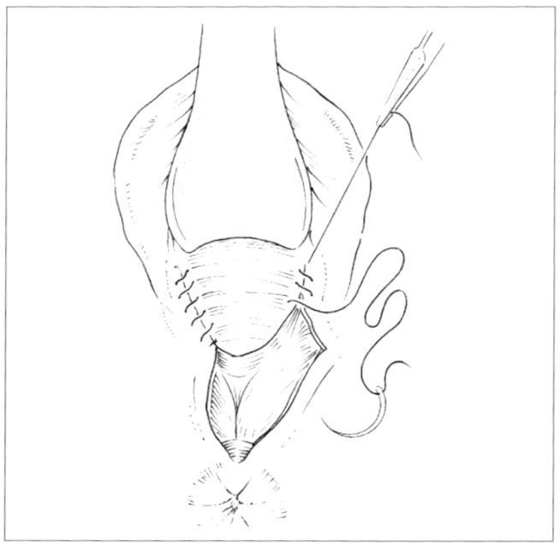

Figure 12.17

4 If the sphincter is injured, see pages 12–27 to 12–28 on the repair of third and fourth degree tears.

5 If the sphincter is not injured, proceed with repair.

6 Repair the vaginal mucosa using a continuous 2-0 suture (Figure 12.17):
- Start the repair about 1 cm above the apex (top) of the vaginal tear, continuing the suture to the level of the vaginal opening

- At the opening of the vagina, bring together the cut edges of the vaginal opening
- Bring the needle under the vaginal opening and out through the perineal tear and tie.

7 Repair the perineal muscles using interrupted 2-0 suture (Figure 12.18). If the tear is deep, place a second layer of the same stitch to close the space.

8 Repair the skin using interrupted (or subcuticular) 2-0 sutures starting at the vaginal opening (Figure 12.19). If the tear was deep, perform a rectal examination. Make sure no stitches are in the rectum.

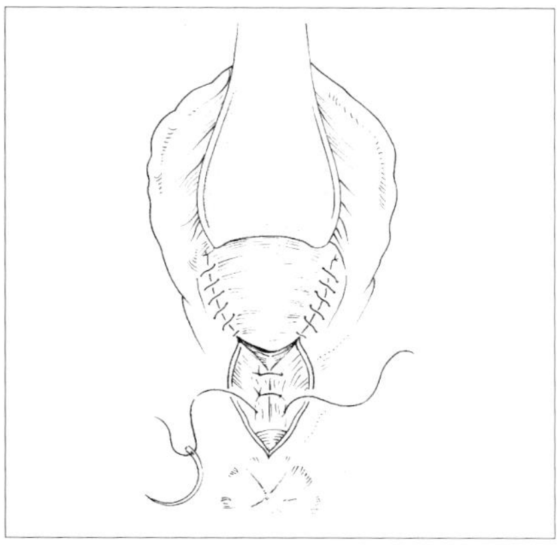

Figure 12.18

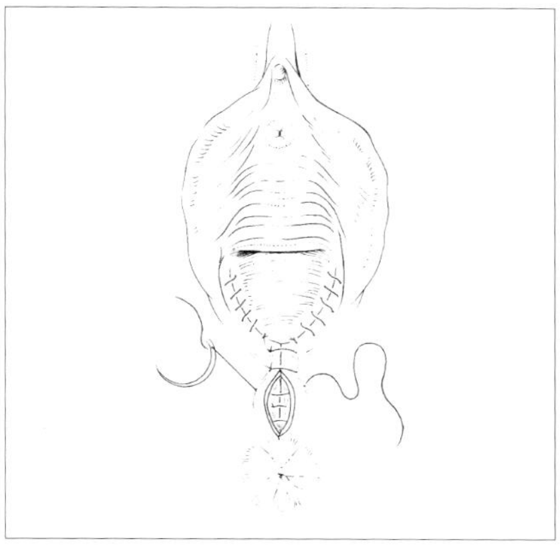

Figure 12.219

Repair of third and fourth degree perineal tears

The woman may suffer loss of control over bowel movements and gas if a torn anal sphincter is not repaired correctly. If a tear in the rectum is not repaired, the woman can suffer from infection and rectovaginal fistula.

Repair the tear in the operating room.

1 If you cannot see all edges of the tear, use regional or general anaesthesia. If you can see all edges of the tear use local infiltration with lidocaine.

2 Ask an assistant to massage the uterus and provide fundal pressure.

3 Examine the vagina, cervix, perineum and rectum. To see if the anal sphincter is torn:
- Place a gloved finger in the anus and lift slightly
- Identify the sphincter, or lack of it
- Feel the surface of the rectum and look carefully for a tear.

4 Change to sterile gloves, apply antiseptic solution to the tear and remove any faecal material, if present.

5 Repair the rectum using interrupted 3-0 or 4-0 sutures 0.5 cm apart to bring together the mucosa (Figure 12.20). Place the suture through the muscularis (not all the way through the mucosa).

6 Cover the muscularis layer by bringing together the fascial layer with interrupted sutures.

7 Apply antiseptic solution to the area frequently.

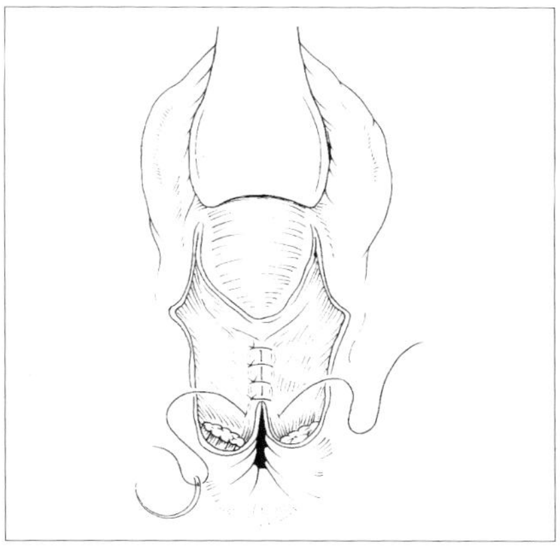

Figure 12.20

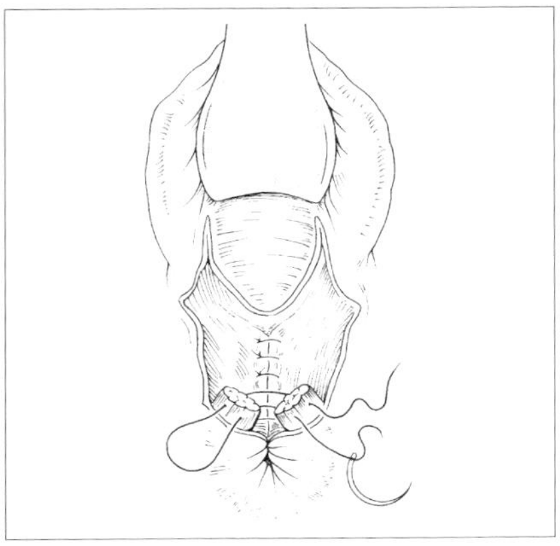

Figure 12.21

8 If the sphincter is torn, grasp each end of the sphincter with an Allis clamp (the sphincter retracts when torn). The sphincter is strong and will not tear when pulling with the clamp. Repair the sphincter with two or three interrupted stitches of 2-0 suture (Figure 12.21).

9 Apply antiseptic solution to the area again. Examine the anus with a gloved finger to ensure the correct repair of the rectum and sphincter. Then change to clean, sterile gloves. Repair the vaginal mucosa, perineal muscles and skin.

Post-procedure care

1 If there is a fourth degree tear, give a single dose of prophylactic antibiotics:
   - Ampicillin 500 mg by mouth *plus* metronidazole 400 mg by mouth.

2 Follow up closely for signs of wound infection.

3 Avoid giving enemas or rectal examinations for 2 weeks.

4 Give stool softener by mouth for 1 week, if possible.

Management of neglected cases

A perineal tear is always contaminated with faecal material. If closure is delayed more than 12 hours, infection is inevitable. Delayed primary closure is indicated in such cases.

- For first and second degree tears, leave the wound open
- For third and fourth degree tears, close the rectal mucosa with some supporting tissue and approximate the fascia of the anal sphincter with 2 or 3 sutures; close the muscle and vaginal mucosa and the perineal skin 6 days later.

Complications

If a haematoma is observed, open and drain it. If there are no signs of infection and the bleeding has stopped, the wound can be reclosed.

If there are signs of infection, open and drain the wound. Remove infected sutures and debride the wound.

If the infection is mild, antibiotics are not required.

If the infection is severe but does not involve deep tissues, give a combination of antibiotics:

- Ampicillin 500 mg by mouth four times per day for 5 days *plus* metronidazole 400 mg by mouth three times per day for 5 days.

If the infection is deep, involves muscles and is causing necrosis (necrotizing fasciitis), give a combination of antibiotics until necrotic tissue has been removed and the woman is fever-free for 48 hours:

- Penicillin G 2 million units IV every 6 hours *plus* gentamicin 5 mg/kg body weight IV every 24 hours *plus* metronidazole 500 mg IV every 8 hours.

12

Once the woman is fever-free for 48 hours, give:

- Ampicillin 500 mg by mouth four times per day for 5 days *plus* metronidazole 400 mg by mouth three times per day for 5 days.

Necrotizing fasciitis requires wide surgical debridement. Perform secondary closure in 2–4 weeks, depending on resolution of infection.

Faecal incontinence may result from complete sphincter transection. Many women are able to maintain control of defaecation by the use of other perineal muscles. When incontinence persists, reconstructive surgery must be undertaken 3 months or more after delivery.

Rectovaginal fistula requires reconstructive surgery three months or more postpartum.

UTERINE INVERSION

1 Start an IV infusion.
2 Give appropriate analgesia and sedation, or if necessary, use general anaesthesia.
3 Thoroughly cleanse the inverted uterus using antiseptic solution.
4 Apply compression to the inverted uterus with a moist, warm sterile towel until ready for the procedure.

Manual correction

1 Wearing sterile gloves, grasp the uterus and push it through the cervix towards the umbilicus to its normal position, using the other hand to support the uterus (Figure 12.22). If the placenta is still attached, perform manual removal after correction.
2 If correction is not achieved, proceed to hydrostatic correction.

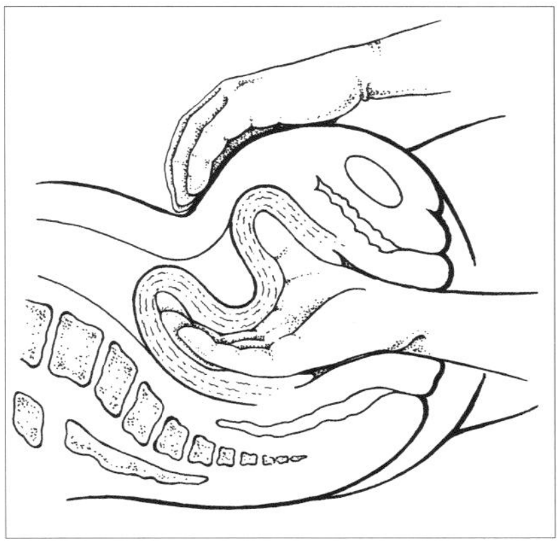
Figure 12.22

It is important that the part of the uterus that came out last (the part closest to the cervix) goes in first.

Hydrostatic correction

1 Place the woman in deep head-down position (head about 0.5 metres below the level of the perineum).
2 Prepare a high-level disinfected douche system with large nozzle and long tubing (2 metres) and a warm water reservoir (3 to 5 L). This can also be done using warmed normal saline and an ordinary IV administration set.
3 Identify the posterior fornix. This is easily done in partial inversion when the inverted uterus is still in the vagina. In other cases, the posterior fornix is recognized by where the rugose vagina becomes the smooth vagina.
4 Place the nozzle of the douche in the posterior fornix.
5 At the same time, with the other hand hold the labia sealed over the nozzle and use the forearm to support the nozzle.

6 Ask an assistant to start the douche with full pressure (raise the water reservoir to at least 2 metres). Water will distend the posterior fornix of the vagina gradually so that it stretches. This causes the circumference of the orifice to increase, relieves cervical constriction and results in correction of the inversion.

Manual correction under general anaesthesia

If hydrostatic correction is not successful, try manual repositioning under general anaesthesia. Halothane is recommended because it relaxes the uterus.

1 Grasp the inverted uterus and push it through the cervix in the direction of the umbilicus to its normal anatomic position.

2 If the placenta is still attached, perform a manual removal after correction.

Combined abdominal-vaginal correction

Abdominal-vaginal correction under general anaesthesia may be required if the above measures fail.

1 Make a midline vertical incision below the umbilicus to the pubic hair, through the skin and to the level of the fascia.

2 Open the abdomen:
- Make a 2–3 cm vertical incision in the fascia.
- Hold the fascial edge with forceps and lengthen the incision up and down using scissors
- Use fingers or scissors to separate the rectus muscles (abdominal wall muscles)
- Use fingers or scissors to make an opening in the peritoneum near the umbilicus. Use scissors to lengthen the incision up and down. Carefully, to prevent bladder injury, use scissors to separate layers and open the lower part of the peritoneum
- Place a bladder retractor over the pubic bone and place self-retaining abdominal retractors.

3 Dilate the constricting cervical ring digitally.

4 Place a tenaculum through the cervical ring and grasp the inverted fundus.

5 Apply gentle continuous traction to the fundus while an assistant attempts manual correction vaginally.

6 If traction fails, incise the constricting cervical ring posteriorly (where the incision is least likely to injure the bladder or uterine vessels) and repeat digital dilatation, tenaculum and traction steps.

7 If correction is successful, close the abdomen:
- Make sure there is no bleeding; use a sponge to remove any clots inside the abdomen
- Close the fascia with continuous 0 chromic non absorbable (or polyglycolic) suture
- If there are signs of infection, pack the subcutaneous tissue with gauze and place loose 0 non absorbable (or polyglycolic) sutures; close the skin with a delayed closure after the infection has cleared

- If there are no signs of infection, close the skin with vertical mattress sutures of 3-0 nylon (or silk) and apply a sterile dressing.

Post-procedure care

1 Once the inversion is corrected, infuse oxytocin 20 units in 500 ml IV fluids (normal saline or Ringer's lactate) at 10 drops per minute:
   - If haemorrhage is suspected, increase the infusion rate to 60 drops per minute
   - If the uterus does not contract after oxytocin, give ergometrine 0.2 mg or prostaglandins IV.

2 Give a single dose of prophylactic antibiotics after correcting the inverted uterus. If there are signs of infection or the woman currently has fever, give a combination of antibiotics until she is fever-free for 48 hours. Give appropriate analgesic drugs.

UTERINE AND UTERO-OVARIAN ARTERY LIGATION

1 Give a single dose of prophylactic antibiotics.

2 Open the abdomen:
   - Make a midline vertical incision below the umbilicus to the pubic hair, through the skin and to the level of the fascia
   - Make a 2–3 cm vertical incision in the fascia; hold the fascial edge with forceps and lengthen the incision up and down using scissors
   - Use fingers or scissors to separate the rectus muscles (abdominal wall muscles)
   - Use fingers to make an opening in the peritoneum near the umbilicus Use scissors to lengthen the incision up and down in order to see the entire uterus. Carefully, to prevent bladder injury, use scissors to separate layers and open the lower part of the peritoneum
   - Place a bladder retractor over the pubic bone and place self-retaining abdominal retractors.

3 Pull on the uterus to expose the lower part of the broad ligament.

4 Feel for pulsations of the uterine artery near the junction of the uterus and cervix.

5 Using 0 chromic non absorbable (or polyglycolic) suture on a large needle, pass the needle around the artery and through 2–3 cm of myometrium (uterine muscle) at the level where a transverse lower uterine segment incision would be made. Tie the suture securely.

6 Place the sutures as close to the uterus as possible, as the ureter is generally only 1 cm lateral to the uterine artery.

7 Repeat on the other side.

8 If the artery has been torn, clamp and tie the bleeding ends.

9 Ligate the utero-ovarian artery just below the point where the ovarian suspensory ligament joins the uterus (Figure 12.23).

10 Repeat on the other side.

11 Observe for continued bleeding or formation of haematoma.

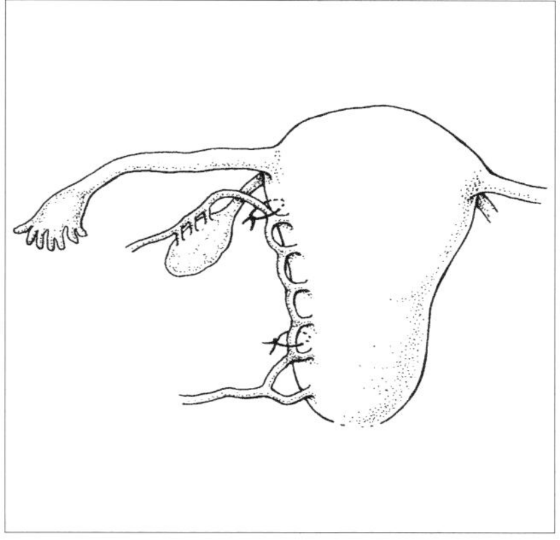

Figure 12.23

12 Close the abdomen. Ensure that there is no bleeding. Remove clots using a sponge. Examine carefully for injuries to the bladder and repair any found.

Post-procedure care

If there are signs of infection or the woman currently has fever, give a combination of antibiotics until she is fever-free for 48 hours. Give appropriate analgesic drugs. If there are no signs of infection, remove the abdominal drain after 48 hours.

POSTPARTUM HYSTERECTOMY

Postpartum hysterectomy can be subtotal unless the cervix and lower uterine segment are involved.

Total hysterectomy may be necessary in the case of a tear of the lower segment that extends into the cervix or bleeding after placenta previa.

1 Give a single dose of prophylactic antibiotics.
2 If there is uncontrollable haemorrhage following vaginal delivery, keep in mind that speed is essential. To open the abdomen:
   - Make a midline vertical incision below the umbilicus to the pubic hair, through the skin and to the level of the fascia
   - Make a 2–3 cm vertical incision in the fascia
   - Hold the fascial edge with forceps and lengthen the incision up and down using scissors
   - Use fingers or scissors to separate the rectus muscles (abdominal wall muscles)
   - Use fingers to make an opening in the peritoneum near the umbilicus. Use scissors to lengthen the incision up and down in order to see the entire uterus. Carefully, to prevent bladder injury, use scissors to separate layers and open the lower part of the peritoneum
   - Place a bladder retractor over the pubic bone and place self-retaining abdominal retractors.
3 If the delivery was by caesarean section, clamp the sites of bleeding along the uterine incision:
4 In case of massive bleeding, have an assistant press fingers over the aorta in the lower abdomen. This will reduce intraperitoneal bleeding;
5 Extend the skin incision, if needed.

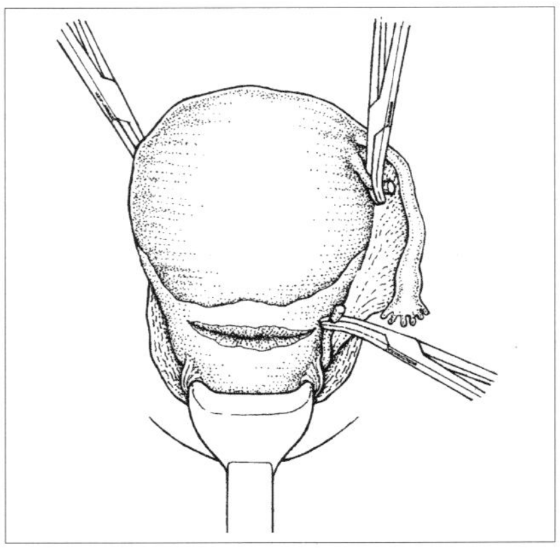

Figure 12.24

Subtotal (supracervical) hysterectomy

1 Lift the uterus out of the abdomen and gently pull to maintain traction.
2 Double-clamp and cut the round ligaments with scissors (Figure 12.24). Clamp and cut the pedicles, but ligate after the uterine arteries are secured to save time.
3 From the edge of the cut round ligament, open the anterior leaf of the broad ligament. Incise to the point where the bladder peritoneum is reflected onto the lower uterine surface in the midline or to the incised peritoneum at a caesarean section.

4 Use two fingers to push the posterior leaf of the broad ligament forward, just under the tube and ovary, near the uterine edge. Make a hole the size of a finger in the broad ligament, using scissors. Doubly clamp and cut the tube, the ovarian ligament and the broad ligament through the hole in the broad ligament (Figures 12.25, 12.26).

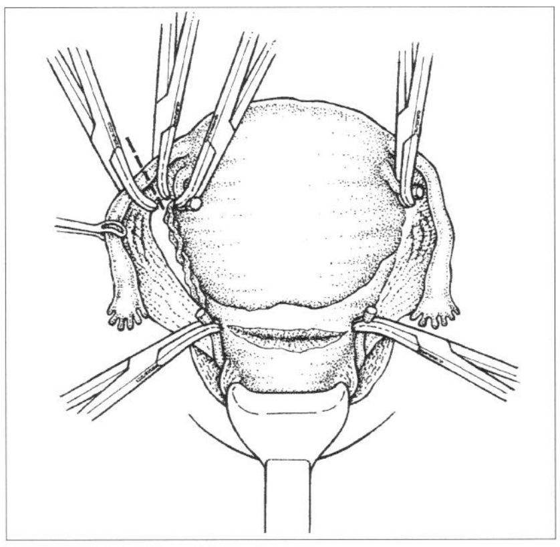

Figure 12.25

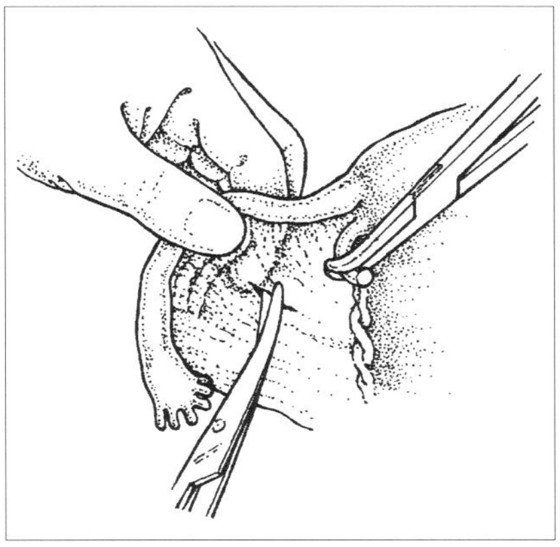

Figure 12.26

The ureters are close to the uterine vessels. The ureter must be identified and exposed to avoid injuring it during surgery or including it in a stitch.

5 Divide the posterior leaf of the broad ligament downwards towards the uterosacral ligaments, using scissors.

6 Grasp the edge of the bladder flap with forceps or a small clamp. Using fingers or scissors, dissect the bladder downwards from the lower uterine segment. Direct the pressure downwards but inwards toward the cervix and the lower uterine segment.

7 Locate the uterine artery and vein on each side of the uterus. Feel for the junction of the uterus and cervix.

8 Doubly clamp across the uterine vessels at a 90° angle on each side of the cervix. Cut and doubly ligate with 0 chromic non absorbable (or polyglycolic) suture (Figure 12.27).

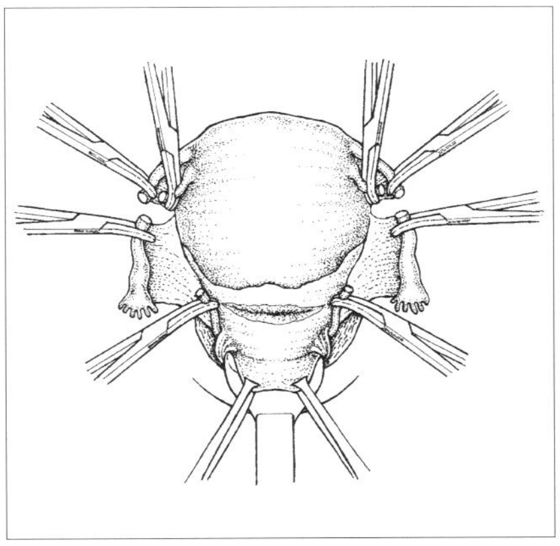

Figure 12.27

12

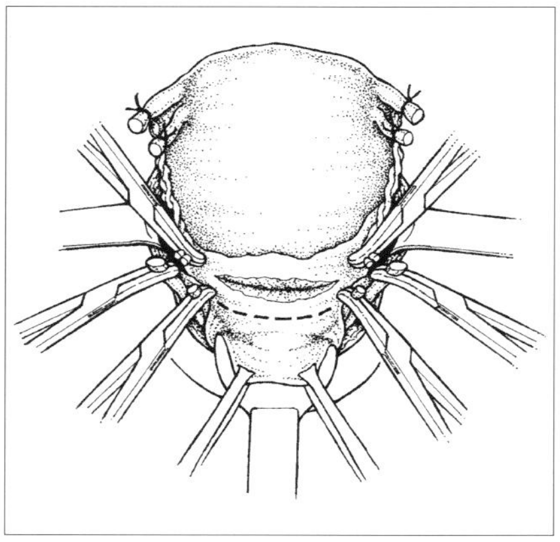

Figure 12.28

9 Observe carefully for any further bleeding. If the uterine arteries are ligated correctly, bleeding should stop and the uterus should look pale.

10 Return to the clamped pedicles of the round ligaments and tubo-ovarian ligaments and ligate them with 0 chromic non absorbable (or polyglycolic) suture.

11 Amputate the uterus above the level where the uterine arteries are ligated, using scissors (Figure 12.28).

12 Close the cervical stump with interrupted 2-0 or 3-0 chromic non absorbable (or polyglycolic) sutures.

13 Carefully inspect the cervical stump, leaves of the broad ligament and other pelvic floor structures for any bleeding.

14 If slight bleeding persists or a clotting disorder is suspected, place a drain through the abdominal wall. Do not place a drain through the cervical stump as this can cause postoperative infection.

15 Ensure that there is no bleeding. Remove clots using a sponge.

16 In all cases, check for injury to the bladder. If a bladder injury is identified, repair the injury.

17 Close the fascia with continuous 0 chromic non absorbable (or polyglycolic) sutures.

Total hysterectomy

The following additional steps are required for total hysterectomy.

1 Push the bladder down to free the top 2 cm of the vagina.

2 Open the posterior leaf of the broad ligament.

3 Clamp, ligate and cut the uterosacral ligaments.

4 Clamp, ligate and cut the cardinal ligaments, which contain the descending branches of the uterine vessels. This is the critical step in the operation:
- Grasp the ligament vertically with a large-toothed clamp (e.g. Kocher)
- Place the clamp 5 mm lateral to the cervix and cut the ligament close to the cervix, leaving a stump medial to the clamp for safety
- If the cervix is long, repeat the step two or three times as needed
- The upper 2 cm of the vagina should now be free of attachments
- Circumcise the vagina as near to the cervix as possible, clamping bleeding points as they appear.

5 Place haemostatic angle sutures, which include round, cardinal and uterosacral ligaments.

6 Place continuous sutures on the vaginal cuff to stop haemorrhage.

7 Close the abdomen (as above) after placing a drain in the extraperitoneal space near the stump of the cervix.

Postoperative care

1 If there are signs of infection or the woman currently has fever, give a combination of antibiotics until she is fever-free for 48 hours.

2 Give appropriate analgesic drugs.

3 If there are no signs of infection, remove the abdominal drain after 48 hours.

12.5 AFTERCARE AND FOLLOW-UP

ABORTION

Tell a woman who has had a spontaneous abortion that spontaneous abortion is common and occurs in at least 15% (one in every seven) of clinically recognized pregnancies. Also reassure the woman that the chances for a subsequent successful pregnancy are good unless there has been sepsis or a cause of the abortion is identified that may have an adverse effect on future pregnancies (this is rare).

Some women may want to become pregnant soon after having an incomplete abortion. The woman should be encouraged to delay the next pregnancy until she is completely recovered.

It is important to counsel women who have had an unsafe abortion. If pregnancy is not desired, certain methods of family planning can be started immediately (within 7 days) provided there are no severe complications requiring further treatment.

Also identify any other reproductive health services that a woman may need. For example, some women may need:

- Tetanus prophylaxis or tetanus booster
- Treatment for sexually transmitted diseases (STDs)
- Cervical cancer screening.

ECTOPIC PREGNANCY

1 Prior to discharge, provide counselling and advice on prognosis for fertility. Given the increased risk of future ectopic pregnancy, family planning counselling and provision of a family planning method, if desired, is especially important.

2 Correct anaemia with oral iron.

3 Schedule a follow-up visit at 4 weeks.

MOLAR PREGNANCY

Recommend a hormonal family planning method for at least 1 year to prevent pregnancy. Voluntary tubal ligation may be offered if the woman has completed her family.

Follow up every 8 weeks for at least 1 year with urine pregnancy tests because of the risk of persistent trophoblastic disease or choriocarcinoma. If the urine pregnancy test is not negative after 8 weeks or becomes positive again within the first year, refer the woman to a tertiary care centre for further follow-up and management

12

BLEEDING IN LATE PREGNANCY AND LABOUR AND POSTPARTUM HAEMORRHAGE

1 Monitor blood loss, vital signs and urine output and treat appropriately. Remember bleeding can recur.

2 After bleeding is controlled (24 hours after bleeding stops), determine haemoglobin or haematocrit to check for anaemia and treat appropriately.

3 Record details or problems and procedures carried out.

4 Inform the woman about these and provide her with a written summary. Provide counselling and advise on prognosis for fertility and childbirth.

5 Schedule a follow-up visit at 4 weeks.

Part 5

Resuscitation and Anaesthesia

Resuscitation and preparation for anaesthesia and surgery

13

13.1 MANAGEMENT OF EMERGENCIES AND CARDIOPULMONARY RESUSCITATION

KEY POINTS

To manage a collapsed patient:

- Keep calm
- Use ABC principles for immediate treatment
- Think about and treat the underlying cause.

The emergency measures that are familiar to most of us are:

A Airway
B Breathing
C Circulation

The necessary ABC steps in cardiopulmonary resuscitation (CPR) learned by health personnel are often not effectively carried out in practice. Panic is the main reason for this.

There is no need to panic, for two reasons:

1 The events that have lead to a sudden collapse have probably been going on for several minutes, if not hours, so you have a few moments more to assess the situation.

2 While thinking about diagnosis and management, you can start simple effective treatments following the ABC routine or, better still, instruct others to do so.

Stay calm when treating a collapsed patient.

The anaesthetist should concentrate on four areas that require immediate action:

- Airway and breathing
- Circulation
- Unconsciousness
- Other immediate problems.

AIRWAY AND BREATHING

Ventilation and intubation

If you are faced with a patient who is not breathing:

1 Open the airway, then ventilate using a self-inflating bag and tight fitting mask, with an oral airway if necessary.

13

2 Unless there is immediate recovery, intubate the trachea and continue ventilation with the bag. Always add oxygen if it is available.

3 If the patient is breathing and has a clear airway, ask yourself if intubation is really needed. The reasons for intubation under these circumstances would be:
   - Need to protect the airway by avoiding aspiration of the stomach contents into the lungs
   - Need to proceed to anaesthesia and surgery for some additional condition that requires immediate attention. For example, a patient with severe facial trauma who is awake, who has a clear airway, is breathing adequately and is not in hypovolaemic shock will need intubation later, when the operating room has been prepared for surgery. This situation is one where you should use the ABC framework to anticipate where problems might occur as treatment proceeds and anaesthesia and surgery are carried out.

The laryngeal mask airway (LMA) is a new device that has an important role in emergency airway management.

Always check that the chest is rising and falling symmetrically with each squeeze of the bag. Note the pressure needed to inflate the lungs: if it is increasing that may indicate a lung problem such as aspiration, bronchospasm or pneumothorax. You must continue with ventilation until the patient starts to breathe adequately or a decision is made to stop CPR.

If a cardiorespiratory arrest occurs during an operation, make sure that the anaesthetic agents have been turned off and you are ventilating with the highest possible percentage of oxygen.

In emergencies: look – feel – listen.

Ten tests of correct tube placement: if in doubt, take it out!

Test	Result	Significance	Reliability/Action
Look with laryngoscope	Tube between cords	Correct tracheal intubation	Certain
Listen/feel	Breathing through tube	Correct tracheal intubation	Probable
Tap sternum	Puff of air from tracheal tube	Correct tracheal intubation	Probable
Inflate with self-inflating bag	Chest rises and falls	Correct tracheal intubation	Probable
Inflate with self-inflating bag	Gurgling noise	Oesophageal intubation	REMOVE TUBE
Pass catheter down tube	Patient coughs (if not paralysed)	Correct tracheal intubation	Probable
Look	Patient remains pink after intubation	Correct tracheal intubation	Probable
Look	Patient becomes cyanosed after intubation	Oesophageal intubation very likely	REMOVE TUBE
Listen with stethoscope	Air entry at apices, axillae and bases	Correct tracheal intubation	Probable
Listen with stethoscope	Air entry over stomach	Oesophageal intubation very likely	REMOVE TUBE

CARDIAC ARREST AND INADEQUATE CIRCULATION

Cardiac arrest exists when there is no detectable heartbeat, major pulse or other sign of cardiac output; the patient is completely unresponsive and breathing stops within a few seconds. Unlike breathing, it is less obvious when there is no blood circulation, especially in patients with dark skins.

You must look for and make the specific diagnosis of circulatory arrest:

- Feel for a pulse in the carotid or femoral artery
- Feel for an apex heartbeat
- Listen at the apex with a stethoscope
- Look for cyanosis or pallor in the tongue.

Having made the diagnosis, the immediate first step must be to do external cardiac massage (ECM). This must start immediately you decide that there is no circulation. Do not hesitate to start ECM if you cannot detect a heartbeat. The action of ECM will alert others more effectively than simply saying "There's a cardiac arrest". It is best to do both.

In cardiac arrest, keep ventilating and continue ECM until there is a response or you decide to stop treatment.

ECM should be performed while positioned well above the patient (Figure 13.1).

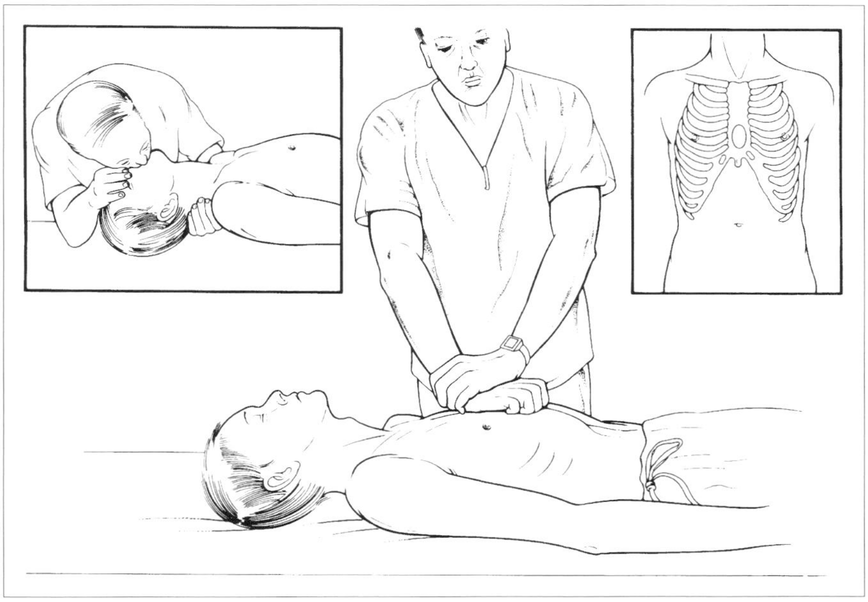

Figure 13.1

At this stage, you are temporarily averting the fatal consequences of cardiopulmonary arrest. The ABC routine is life saving, but only for a few minutes. Some other treatment must be given and normal circulation must be restored if the patient is to survive.

Two people should be assigned duties: ventilation and ECM. They will need relief when they get tired. Assign a third person to feel for the femoral pulse and report to you if it returns.

Your next priority is to diagnose the problem with the circulation and correct it. Your action to achieve this will depend on the facilities you have. You may have no electronic monitoring devices or you may have an ECG and perhaps a defibrillator.

Very often, a device is present in the hospital but does not work when needed or it has to be brought from somewhere else, causing delay. It may be locked in someone's office. You may have an ECG monitor, but have no chest electrodes, or they have dried up through age or are of the wrong type. The mains power lead may have been lost or stolen. The hospital generator may have to be switched on.

There may, therefore, be many reasons why you *think* that you have ECG diagnosis at your hospital whereas in fact you do not. ***Check now*** if, in fact, an ECG monitor is available and if it works when connected to a patient. Remind yourself how to connect it up.

> Do not waste time during a cardiac arrest trying to make an ECG machine work.

When there is no ECG diagnosis

1. Give a chest thump: this is a single blow with the closed fist over the sternum, only done early in a witnessed cardiac arrest, to try and jolt the heart into action.
2. Give epinephrine (adrenaline) 1 mg intravenously.
3. Continue CPR. Pause in CPR every minute or two to feel for pulsations and listen for the heartbeat. If absent, continue CPR.
4. Give atropine 1 mg followed by 2 more doses of epinephrine 1 mg. Effective ECM will carry the epinephrine round into the ventricles and coronary arteries where it will have its effect.
5. During this time, insert an intravenous cannula and start infusion, as below.

> Epinephrine (adrenaline) is life saving in many cases of cardiac arrest. Always use it once the diagnosis is made, even if you do not know the cause of the arrest.

It is usual to abandon CPR if there is no response after 20–30 minutes or if three doses of epinephrine have not produced signs of a heartbeat.

When there is an ECG diagnosis

As you start ECM, call for the ECG monitor. In cardiac arrest, there are three key ECG appearances at cardiac arrest:

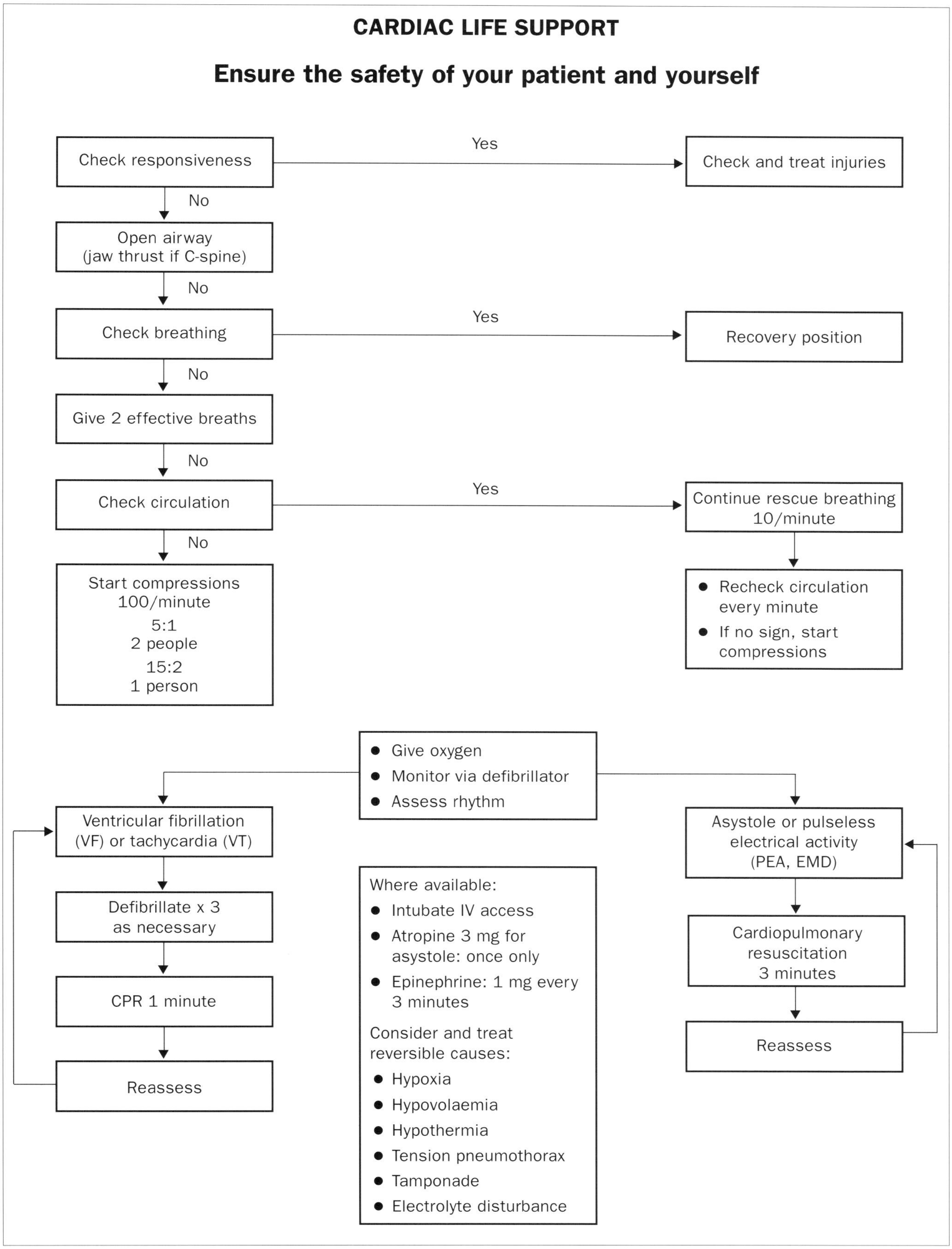
CARDIAC LIFE SUPPORT
Ensure the safety of your patient and yourself
Check responsiveness
Yes
Check and treat injuries
No
Open airway (jaw thrust if C-spine)
No
Check breathing
Yes
Recovery position
No
Give 2 effective breaths
No
Check circulation
Yes
Continue rescue breathing 10/minute
No
Start compressions 100/minute
5:1
2 people
15:2
1 person
• Recheck circulation every minute
• If no sign, start compressions
• Give oxygen
• Monitor via defibrillator
• Assess rhythm
Ventricular fibrillation (VF) or tachycardia (VT)
Defibrillate x 3 as necessary
CPR 1 minute
Reassess
Asystole or pulseless electrical activity (PEA, EMD)
Cardiopulmonary resuscitation 3 minutes
Reassess
Where available:
• Intubate IV access
• Atropine 3 mg for asystole: once only
• Epinephrine: 1 mg every 3 minutes
Consider and treat reversible causes:
• Hypoxia
• Hypovolaemia
• Hypothermia
• Tension pneumothorax
• Tamponade
• Electrolyte disturbance

Figure 13.2

Rhythm	Probable significance
Asystole (straight line)	• Resuscitation and drug treatment needed
Sinus rhythm (but no pulse)	• Hypovolaemia or anaphylaxis • Pulseless electrical activity • Resuscitation and fluids needed
Ventricular fibrillation (Figure 13.3)	• Resuscitation and defibrillation needed

Unless you are familiar with the normal sinus rhythm trace (*and* the benign arrhythmias which do not require immediate treatment), you will not be able to make a decision based on what is shown there.

In order of frequency of occurrence in countries where ischaemic heart disease is rare, the cardiac arrest rhythms are as follows.

Asystole

You will see a straight or smooth wavy line. You may see occasional widened complexes, but no pulse can be felt in the femoral artery. There should always be some electrical activity when ECM is being carried out. A steady straight line may mean the machine is not connected.

Asystole is the terminal event in many severe illnesses, but may be acutely caused by:

- Septicaemia
- Hypoxia
- Excessive vagal tone
- Electrolyte abnormalities
- Severe hypotension.

Treat with epinephrine as above and atropine. The prognosis is very poor.

Pulseless electrical activity (sinus rhythm)

This is also called electromechanical dissociation (EMD). There is a near-normal ECG pattern, but no detectable pulse. There are many causes of this situation and, in the heat of the moment, you have to think clearly. Some of the important causes are:

- Overdose of anaesthetic agent
- Hypovolaemia/blood loss
- Hypoxia (or other ventilation problem)
- Septic or other toxaemia
- Pulmonary embolus
- Cardiac tamponade
- Tension pneumothorax
- Hypothermia.

For the anaesthetist, the first three are the most common.

To treat pulseless electrical activity

Look for a cause. Give epinephrine, if needed.

A glance at the list above should tell you that some of the causes are reversible without drug treatment and that this may not be a true cardiac arrest. If you can withdraw or correct the cause of the arrest (by switching off halothane, increasing intravenous fluids, correcting a problem with the anaesthesia circuit), this will be safer than giving an intravenous bolus of epinephrine.

If there is no detectable circulation after two or three minutes of CPR, even with a diagnosis and corrective measures, give epinephrine as for asystole. The prognosis is good, if the cause can be found.

Ventricular fibrillation

A coarse or fine jagged line denotes chaotic ventricular activity (Figure 13.3). A defibrillator is required.

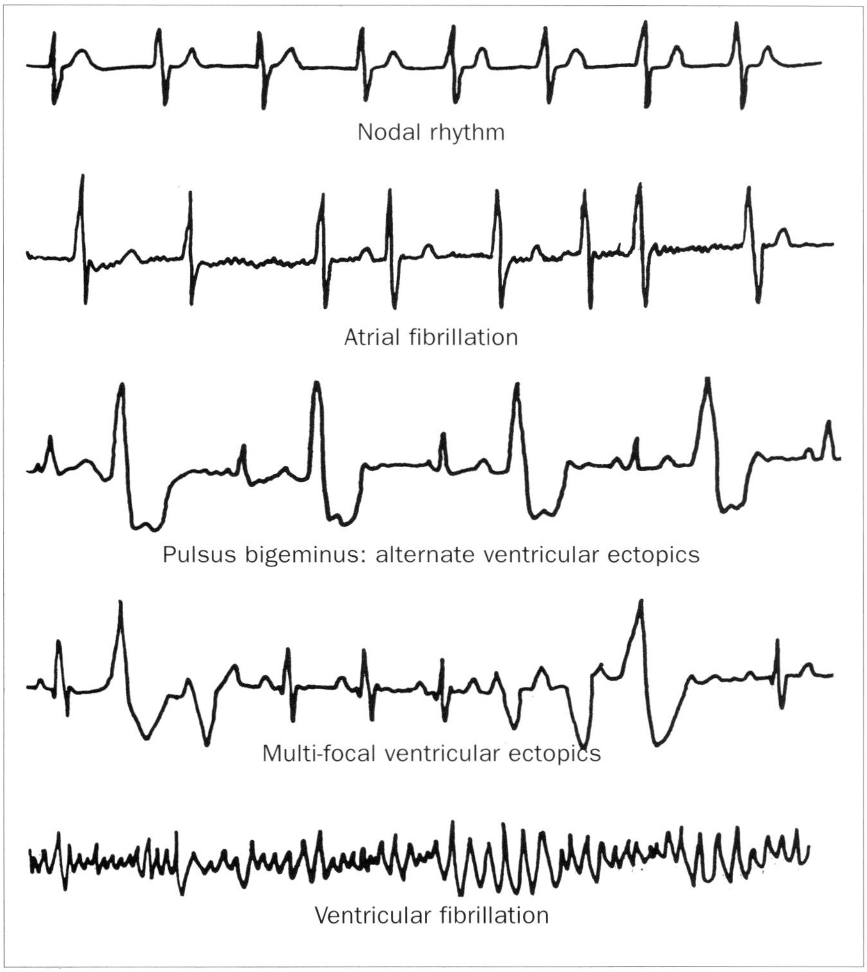

Figure 13.3

To treat, defibrillate. This needs training and experience.

1 Start with 2 x 200 joules DC shock (2 joules/kg body weight) followed by 360 joules if sinus rhythm does not return promptly.
2 Put electrode jelly on the chest, check the orientation of the paddles (labelled "apex" and "sternum") and press them firmly on the chest.

13

3 Tell everyone to stand clear and shock across the heart. No one should be touching the patient or anything that is touching the patient, including the resuscitation bag, as most things conduct electricity.

If you have no defibrillator, a chest thump or epinephrine may produce sinus rhythm.

Prognosis is good, especially if the precipitating cause was halothane and epinephrine interaction or hypoxia.

Haemorrhage

External bleeding can be controlled, usually with pressure. Bleeding into body cavities may be apparent only later; for example, when the circulation has been restored and the rise in blood pressure causes more bleeding and a second fall in blood pressure.

Shock

Shock is a pathological, life threatening condition in which the oxygen supply to the tissues of the body fails. The cause is usually one of the following:

- Hypovolaemia (bleeding)
- Sepsis
- Acute anaphylaxis: from allergy or drug reaction
- Neurogenic (after spinal trauma)
- Heart failure (left ventricular failure).

There may be more than one cause of shock. In surgical patients, look for hypovolaemia and sepsis first.

- In hypovolaemic shock, the circulating volume is reduced by loss of blood or other fluid (e.g. burn transudate). Rapid fluid replacement, starting with normal saline or Hartmann's solution, should restore the circulation towards normal.
- In septic shock, the circulating volume may be normal, but blood pressure is low and tissue circulation is inadequate. Support the circulation with volume infusion, but it may not respond as in hypovolaemic shock.
- In acute anaphylaxis, give epinephrine and intravenous fluids.
- Neurogenic shock follows large neurological injuries: e.g. spinal cord damage. The heart rate is often low and atropine and fluids will be helpful.

Heart failure is beyond the scope of this book. The prognosis is poor when it occurs intra- or postoperatively. Fluids will not help as the circulation is overloaded.

KEY POINTS

Recognize shock by:
- Tachycardia (may be the only sign in a child)
- Thready pulse
- Narrow pulse pressure: e.g. 110/70 becomes 95/75
- Cold hands and feet
- Sweating, anxious patient
- Breathlessness and hyperventilation
- Confusion leading to unconsciousness.

Unconsciousness

Unconsciousness may have many causes including:

- Head injury
- Hypoglycaemia
- Ketoacidosis
- Cerebrovascular event
- Hypoxia
- Hypotension
- Hypertension and eclampsia
- HIV infection
- Drug intoxication.

Assess the response to stimuli, look at the pupils initially and re-examine them later to follow progress. Look for unequal pupils or other localizing signs that may show intracranial haematoma developing.

In many instances, you may attend to and stabilize other systems first and await the return of consciousness as cerebral perfusion and oxygenation improves. After cardiac arrest, a patient who initially had fixed dilated pupils may show smaller pupils after effective CPR. This indicates that a favourable outcome may be possible.

The supine unconscious patient with a full stomach is at grave risk of regurgitation and aspiration due to the unprotected airway. However, if a comatose patient has a clear airway and vital signs are normal:

- Avoid intubation as this will involve drug administration and complicate the subsequent diagnosis
- Nurse the patient in the recovery position
- Monitor the airway and await progress and diagnosis (Figure 13.4).

During CPR, ask yourself: is the patient responding? If not, why not?

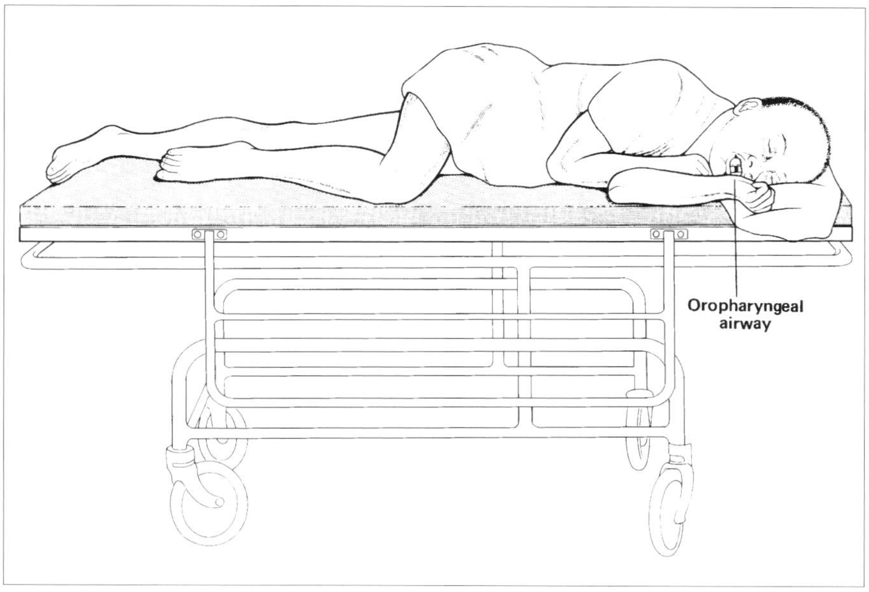

Figure 13.4

13

13.2 OTHER CONDITIONS REQUIRING URGENT ATTENTION

There are some conditions that require immediate treatment as part of resuscitation:

- Sucking chest wound
- Tension pneumothorax
- Cardiac tamponade.

Guidance on further examination and assessment of the trauma patient and on treatment of these conditions is given in the Annex: *Primary Trauma Care Manual.*

ANAEMIA

Anaemia is common in patients scheduled for surgery and often gives rise to disagreements between surgeon and anaesthetist. It is not possible to give any rigid rule on the lowest permissible value of haemoglobin below which transfusion is necessary or surgery cannot be carried out in a particular case. There is general agreement that a patient can tolerate a haemoglobin concentration well below the traditional value of 10 g/dl. A preoperative value of 7 or 8 g/dl is acceptable without the need for transfusion or making a request for blood. The following factors will make a patient *less* tolerant of anaemia than this:

- Significant blood loss anticipated
- Respiratory, cardiovascular disease or obesity
- Old age
- Recent blood loss or surgery.

On the other hand, an emergency, actively bleeding case must go for life saving surgery without delay, no matter what the haemoglobin level. Blood can be crossmatched while anaesthesia and surgery are in progress.

A critical haemoglobin concentration is 4 g/dl, below which significant reduction in oxygen consumption starts to occur. Blood transfusion is mandatory in all such cases.

CONVULSIONS

The convulsing patient presents a difficult acute management problem: the violent jerky movements mean there is little you can do unless a drip has already been put in place through which an anticonvulsant can be given.

Patients do not usually convulse without warning or without a predictable reason. Anticipation and prevention should therefore be possible. Possible causes include:

- Epilepsy
- Neglected pre-eclampsia becoming eclampsia
- Febrile convulsions in children
- Meningitis

- Cerebral irritation: for example, following a period of hypoxia
- Hypoglycaemia
- Encephalopathy or any intracranial lesion such as an abscess or tumour
- HIV
- Cerebral malaria
- Drug poisoning, overdose of local anaesthetic or other toxic state
- Alcohol or narcotic drug withdrawal.

Convulsions are dangerous for the sufferer as there is breath-holding, hypoxia, collapse, biting of tongue or other physical damage. A common problem for the epileptic is falling in a fire. The patient may vomit and aspirate.

Convulsions are usually short lived (although continuous eclamptic fits do occur) and may have stopped by the time an anticonvulsant has been found and given. However, a person who has convulsed once will probably do so again soon and you should take the following preventive measures:

- Well secured drip
- Bolus of diazepam 10 mg IV, repeated 1 or 2 hourly; diazepam 10 mg rectally is safest for children
- Paraldehyde 10 ml IM, where no drip has been put up.

You must urgently look for and treat the cause of the convulsion. Intubation and ventilation is necessary if respiration has ceased.

After a convulsion, most people are disorientated for several minutes or remain in coma.

13.3 INTRAVENOUS ACCESS

Secure intravenous access is needed for all emergency management and should always precede anaesthesia and surgery. With a struggling baby, you may be unable to find a vein. In this case, it may be permissible to give inhalation halothane or intramuscular ketamine.

It is essential that the stomach is empty before starting inhalation induction by mask. This can be done by passing (then removing) a 12–16 FG orogastric tube just before you start. This is a well-tolerated procedure and avoids the catastrophe of regurgitation into an unprotected airway.

KEY POINTS

- Develop the attitude: 'There is a vein in there. I must find it!'
- There is almost no emergency case that can survive without a drip.

HOW TO FIND A VEIN

When access is difficult, make sure you have a good light and an assistant to help you. Ideally, an intravenous cannula should be placed in a vein in the arm that is not over a joint and where fixation is easy, comfortable for the patient and convenient for drug administration and care of the IV site. In shocked patients, such veins may be hard to find.

Often the best veins to use in emergencies are:

- Antecubital fossa
- Femoral vein
- Internal jugular vein.

Do not attempt the subclavian vein as there is a high risk of pleural puncture.

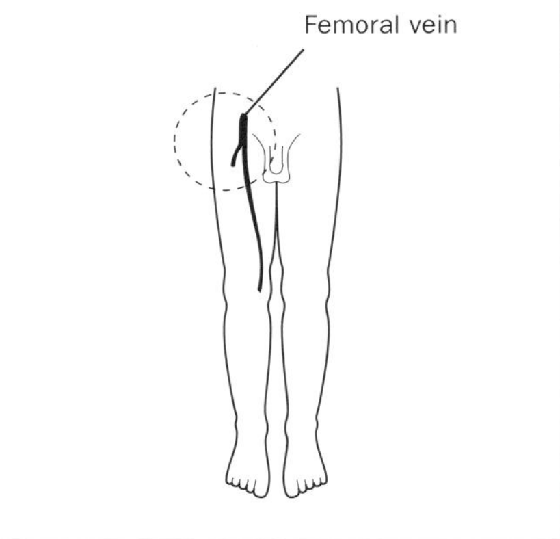

Figure 13.5

Femoral vein

If you are right handed, it is easiest to stand on the patient's right and use your left index and middle fingers to palpate the femoral artery (Figure 13.5). Use a 14, 16 or 18 G (20 G in a child) cannula mounted on a 5 ml syringe.

1 Pointing down at 45 degrees to the skin, puncture at a point on the inguinal skin crease, the thickness of the patient's finger medial to where you feel arterial pulsation.

2 An assistant should apply gentle traction, slight abduction of the leg and prevent flexion at the hip by pressing on the knee.

3 Keeping your left fingers on the artery, probe for the vein while aspirating at each new position. You may feel the point entering the vein or see dark blood fill the syringe, or both. At this moment, you have to decide if the needle tip is in the middle of the vein, just entering or just exiting. Only in the first instance will the cannula slide easily down into the vein.

Often you can aspirate blood, but the cannula will not slide down. ***Do not force it.*** Go further in with the needle fully inserted, take out the needle and connect the syringe directly to the cannula. Aspirate while slowly withdrawing. With skill, you will get the cannula tip in the vein lumen. At this point, it should enter the vein properly when advanced again.

Check for free flow of dark blood with no pressure (that is, it is not in the artery) when the final position has been selected.

4 Tape the cannula securely to the inguinal area, but do not fix the giving set to the leg as it will get pulled out.

KEY POINTS

- Use of the internal jugular vein may be life saving, but serious complications can occur, including air embolism, damage to structures in neck and pneumothorax
- Remove the IV line as soon as an alternative is available.

Internal jugular vein

The internal jugular vein is the most popular vein to choose in severe shock and CPR as well as for elective major surgery.

There must be a clear indication for such an invasive procedure but, provided you follow the rules, complications should be rare.

Two approaches are possible:

- Mid sternomastoid (upper)
- Sternomastoid triangle (lower).

In both cases, the patient should be positioned head down (Trendelenburg position). The ease of successful puncture is directly proportional to the pressure of blood in the internal jugular vein. A patient in hypovolaemic shock should therefore be positioned more head down than one in congestive cardiac failure. The latter may not tolerate a head down position and cannulation can take place on a level bed.

Patients suffering cardiac arrest invariably have distended neck veins and internal jugular vein cannulation is fortunately very easy in these crisis circumstances.

Upper approach

1 With the patient head down, turn the head to the left.

2 On the right sternomastoid muscle, find a point for needle puncture midway between the sternum and the mastoid, on the lateral edge of the muscle. Usually this point will be around the external jugular vein, which should be avoided. According to the circumstances, it may be appropriate to put some local anaesthesia at the puncture point.

3 Use the longest, largest cannula you have (an ordinary IV cannula is only just long enough) 14–18 G, attached to a 5 or 10 ml syringe, and loosen the cannula on the needle to run freely.

4 Holding the plunger between fingertips, puncture the skin and advance the needle at a 45 degrees downward angle, aiming at the right nipple (where it would be in a man). If you are right handed, you must stand well over to the left of the patient's head to get the correct angle (Figure 13.6).

5 Advance with short, sharp stabs while aspirating; after only 2–3 cm depth you should see dark venous blood freely flowing into the syringe. At this point, fix the syringe and needle with the right hand while using your left hand to slide the cannula with a rotating action into the internal jugular vein as far as it will go. It should slide easily.

6 Remove the needle, connect the drip and see if it runs. Flow should be fast although it sometimes pauses when the patient breathes in; this respiratory effect is a sign of hypovolaemia and will stop when you have infused more fluid.

7 Next, drop the bag down below head level and look for dark, undiluted blood running into the set. Do not assume the cannula is correctly placed unless you see this sign. Even then, you should continue to look for swelling in the neck which will indicate that the cannula has come out of the vein.

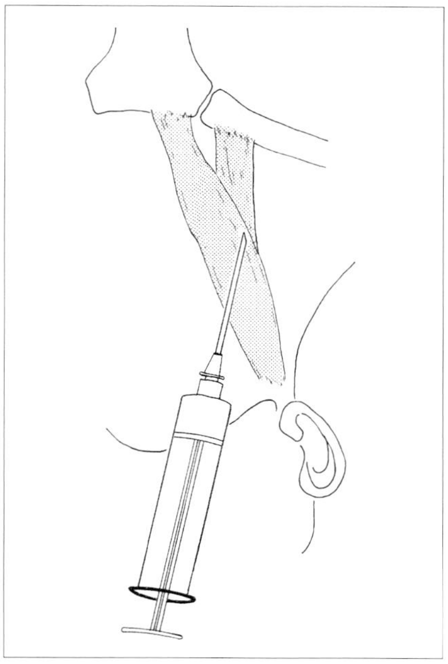

Figure 13.6

Reasons for failure include:

- Not enough head down tilt, especially in a shocked patient
- Needle too far medial (danger of also hitting the thicker walled artery)
- Needle has gone past the vein
- Not aiming at the right nipple.

If the cannula is in an artery, the drip may run at first if the blood pressure is low, but then backs up the giving set with bubbles seen in the bag as the blood pressure returns to normal.

A misplaced cannula may be in the soft tissues, giving a swelling after a few minutes, or in the pleural cavity. In the latter case, it is possible to infuse litres of fluid into the pleural cavity by mistake. For this reason, always lower the IV bag to check for back flow of undiluted blood (not blood stained IV fluid).

Lower approach

The lower approach (Figure 13.7) is easier, especially if there is a lot of muscle tone, but has a much higher risk of pleural puncture. It should be tried only if the upper approach has failed.

Using the same patient positioning as above, identify the triangle made by the sternal and clavicular heads of the sternomastoid muscle, left and right, and the clavicle, below. The internal jugular vein runs downwards just below the skin in this triangle, at the lateral side (below the medial edge of the

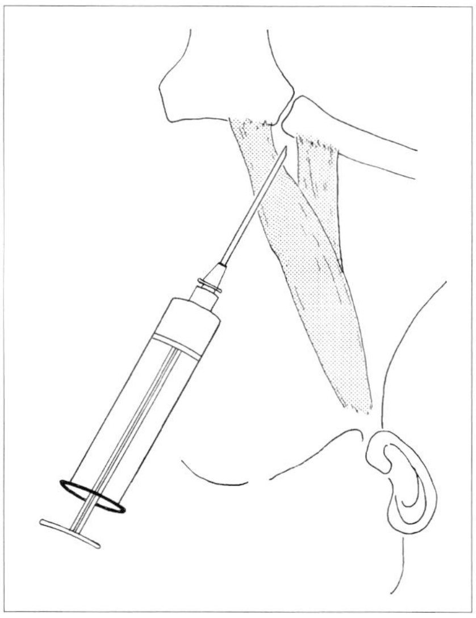

Figure 13.7

clavicular head of the muscle). A cannula can be inserted – *not more than 2 cm deep* – and easily enters the vein at this point. Tests for successful placement are the same as before.

Cannulation of a big central vein is useful for emergencies, but poses more hazards for the patient than a peripheral vein.

Venous cutdown

Venous cutdown (Figures 13.8, 13.9, 13.10) is a useful means of obtaining access to a peripheral vein when percutaneous techniques are insufficient or central lines are not available. The saphenous vein is the most common site of cutdown and can be used in both adults and children.

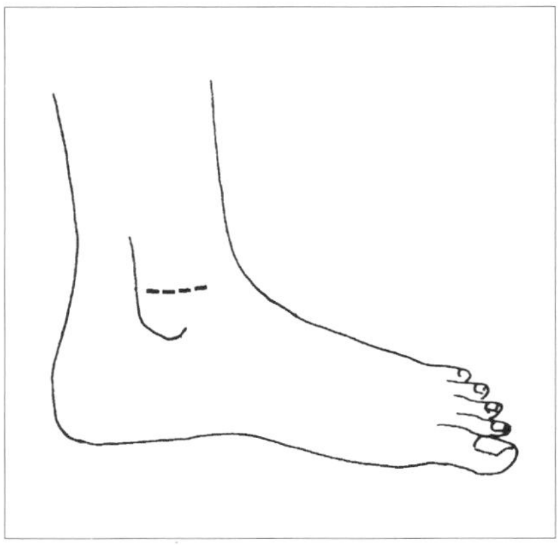

Figure 13.8

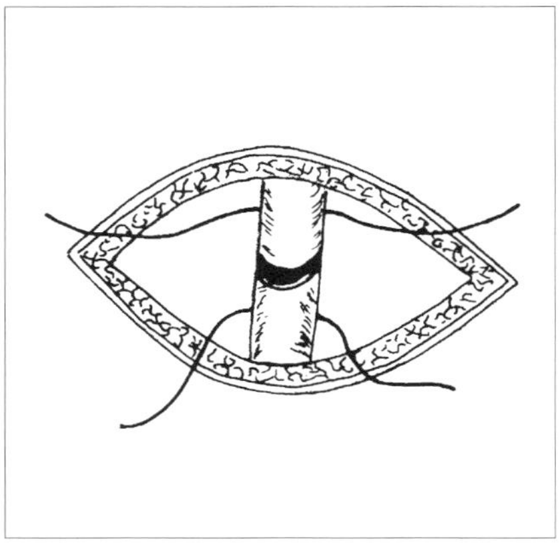

Figure 13.9

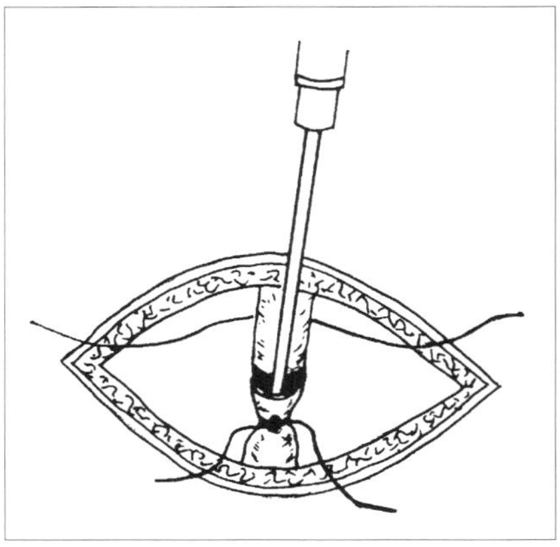

Figure 13.10

No specialized equipment is necessary for this procedure. All that is required is:

- Small scalpel
- Artery forceps
- Scissors
- Wide bore sterile catheter (a sterile infant feeding tube is one alternative).

Make a transverse incision two finger breadths superior and two fingers anterior to the medial malleolus. Use the *patient's* finger breadths to define the incision: this is particularly important in the infant or child. Use the sutures that close the incision to tie the catheter in place. Do not suture the incision closed after catheter removal as the catheter is a foreign body. Allow any gap to heal by secondary intention.

Intraosseous puncture

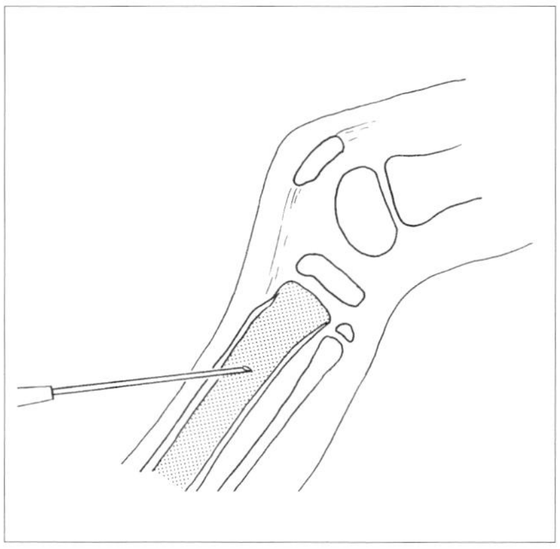

Figure 13.11

Intraosseous puncture (Figure 13.11) can provide the quickest access to the circulation in a shocked child in whom venous cannulation is impossible. Fluids, blood and many drugs may be administered by this route. The intraosseous needle is normally sited in the anterior tibial plateau, 2–3 cm below the tibial tuberosity, thereby avoiding the epiphysial growth plate.

Once the needle has been located in the marrow cavity, fluids may need to be administered under pressure or via a syringe when rapid replacement is required. If purpose-designed intraosseous needles are unavailable, spinal, epidural or bone marrow biopsy needles offer an alternative. The intraosseous route has been used in all age groups, but is generally most successful in children below about six years of age.

Veins in babies and neonates

Finding a vein in a baby can be one of the most difficult technical feats in the entire spectrum of medical practice as well as one of the most distressing for everyone involved.

The anaesthetist usually is called in when everyone else has failed, so there are no easy veins and the child is very distressed by the previous attempts. Intramuscular ketamine, 2–3 mg/kg, is effective in creating the enabling environment for successful venepuncture in calm conditions. It is not a full anaesthetic dose. Wait five minutes before examining the veins.

Preferred approaches are:

- Back of hand (on the ulnar side)
- Scalp
- Ventral surface of wrist (very small veins)
- Femoral vein
- Saphenous vein.

The neonate is not fat and has prominent veins on the forearm and hand. The saphenous vein is also usually easy to find. The saphenous vein is invariably anterior to the medial malleolus, even if it cannot be seen or felt, and a cut down here is possible.

Great vein cannulation is difficult in babies because the large head makes the angle difficult. It is not recommended unless no other veins are available, such as after extensive burns.

Fixing the IV placement on a board or card is essential to immobilize limb joints.

13.4 FLUIDS AND DRUGS

WHAT FLUIDS TO GIVE?

See also *The Clinical Use of Blood* (WHO, 2001).

The initial resuscitating fluid should be either normal saline (0.9% sodium chloride) or Ringer's lactate (also called Hartmann's solution). These fluids are sometimes referred to as crystalloids.

Alternatives are the so-called plasma expanders or colloids. These are starch, gelatin or macro-sugar based solutes dissolved in saline with other electrolytes. They have the osmotic effect of increasing fluid shift from the extravascular into the vascular space (circulating volume), causing a rise in blood pressure.

KEY POINTS

- Always try to calculate the volume and type of fluids lost
- Replace with fluids of a similar volume and composition
- Add the patient's daily maintenance requirements to the fluid needed to replace losses to make the total daily requirement
- Watch carefully for a response to your fluid regime and modify it, if necessary.

13

Colloids also remain in the circulation longer than electrolytes alone and are widely used in the management of hypovolaemic shock, after initial crystalloid infusion.

5% glucose (dextrose) is widely used as a maintenance fluid (a substitute for patients unable to drink water). It has no place in the restoration of circulating volume because it is rapidly distributed throughout the entire body water component of about 40 litres.

HOW MUCH FLUID?

For detailed fluid maintenance regimens, see *The Clinical Use of Blood* (WHO, 2001).

Opinions differ on the volume of crystalloids and colloids that are needed to correct blood and other volume losses from the blood circulation. There are no absolute rules but most authorities agree that you should give about three times the estimated circulation loss as crystalloid fluid. It is far more common for a shocked or dehydrated patient to receive too little intravenous fluid than to receive too much.

More important than any rule on the volume of replacement fluids is to observe the patient's response to volume infusion. The signs that you have given adequate IV fluids and can slow the infusion are:

- Low blood pressure comes up
- Tachycardia slows
- Jugular venous pressure rises
- Urine starts to flow.

Every patient responds differently to fluid therapy. Look for the difference. Avoid fluids containing dextrose during resuscitation.

If, in an adult, the blood pressure has not responded to fluid therapy, or if blood loss is continuing after three or four litres of crystalloid, you may consider changing to a colloid infusion. These solutions usually come in 500 ml polythene containers and up to three (total 1500 ml) are usually given. Give equal volumes of colloid to the estimated blood loss.

After the above fluid therapy the patient will have been haemodiluted and, depending on any continuing blood loss, may also still be in shock. Blood transfusion is an urgent consideration at this stage.

Recent research and experience has shown that a shocked patient with severe anaemia can still have a favourable outcome, provided blood pressure and circulating volume are maintained. Opinion has therefore moved towards giving volume first as crystalloid/colloid and blood transfusion later. In the case of extreme haemodilution (Hb <4 g/dl), there is a risk of heart failure which might then result in a low blood pressure and/or pulmonary congestion with lung crepitations. Using the WHO haemoglobin colour scale will inform you when critically low haemoglobin levels exist.

Whole blood transfusion is the ultimate life saving treatment for haemorrhagic shock.

PAEDIATRIC FLUIDS

In emergency paediatric resuscitation, it is customary to give a fluid bolus of normal saline (20 ml/kg body weight and repeat if needed) as initial therapy as soon as the drip is in place. Meanwhile, make a rapid assessment of the actual deficit based on body weight, dehydration and continuing circulating volume losses. A 3 kg neonate should have 250 ml circulating blood volume, so the initial intravenous fluid load is about 20% of circulating volume.

Subsequent treatment depends on the clinical response. Recent studies of outcome in paediatric emergencies, especially where sepsis is present, have shown that generous fluid regimes giving up to 80 ml/kg in the first 12 hours, using a mixed crystalloid/colloid regimen, have given the best figures for patient survival.

Never use an adult giving set to attach a large bag of IV fluid to a child. If the fluid runs too fast, the whole bag will be given, leading to a fatal overload. Always use a burette giving set; if you do not have a burette, use a syringe to inject measured volumes.

Finally, closely watch the neck veins and the eyes, looking for signs of over-transfusion. If the child was dehydrated with reduced skin turgor, this should have been corrected by fluid therapy. If hourly urine output is needed, insert a urinary catheter or, if there is no catheter, make sure you take account of urinary bladder filling by palpating and percussing the bladder before deciding on further fluid therapy.

When giving blood for replacement in paediatric anaesthesia, the rate of flow is often less than you want, even with a pressure infuser, because the cannula is so small. In this case, a 20 ml syringe and 3-way tap is very useful to draw the blood from the giving set and push it through the small IV cannula. Be careful that all the connections are tight.

Events happen quickly in babies. Monitor closely. See also Unit 3.2: *The Paediatric Patient.*

SPEED OF INTRAVENOUS FLUID THERAPY

As with inadequate volumes of infusion, it is common that shocked patients receive their fluids too slowly.

A slow running drip overnight is the commonest reason for a dead patient in the morning.

13

A general rule for adults is to correct half the estimated deficit in about 30 minutes, then to reassess. If the patient is in shock, you should give fluids as fast as the drip will run until the blood pressure responds, then reassess the rate of flow. If the drip runs too slowly, either a pressure infuser bag may be needed to push it in, or a second drip.

If you are supervising a fast running drip, with a continuous stream through the chamber, you must stay beside the patient until the flow rate can be slowed to a rate that is more usual on a ward with normal nursing supervision. A patient on the ward with a drip will usually be given 3 litres per day as a standard regime. Assume this will happen and make it absolutely clear to ward staff if you want some other regime. Check later that your instructions are being followed.

WHAT BLOOD PRESSURE SHOULD YOU AIM FOR?

Depending on circumstances (such as if the patient is chronically dehydrated or debilitated), it may be preferable to get the blood pressure up to about 90 mmHg systolic over an hour or so before going into the operating room.

On the other hand, an actively bleeding patient (for example, from a ruptured uterus, bleeding peptic ulcer, oesophageal varices, ruptured ectopic pregnancy, severed artery or other severe trauma) should have volume replacement, ketamine anaesthesia, tracheal intubation and surgery all at the same time.

> In severe haemorrhage, control of bleeding is the first priority, whatever the blood pressure or haemoglobin.

If blood is haemorrhaging from one end of a patient, there is little point in pouring fluids in at the other end in the expectation that the blood pressure will come up. The only option is to rush the patient to the operating room and get surgical haemostasis.

13.5 DRUGS IN RESUSCITATION

KEY POINTS

- Always give drugs intravenously during resuscitation
- Most drugs are only helpful once the cause of cardiac arrest has been diagnosed, but epinephrine is an exception and should always be given to patients with circulatory arrest.

While emergency drugs are essential in resuscitation, before giving a drug, the priorities are always:

- Ventilate
- Perform cardiac massage
- Restore circulating volume loss
- Remove any cause, hazard or noxious agent
- Make a diagnosis, if possible.

There are no drugs that will make someone breathe. The only treatment for the non-breathing patient is to inflate the lungs mechanically, preferably with a resuscitation bag and mask or a tracheal tube. If the patient is not relaxed and a tube cannot be passed, a choice arises between:

- Continuing with the bag and mask until improvement or further deterioration (with relaxation) occurs *or*

- Giving a relaxant drug, such as suxamethonium 100 mg, in order to be able to intubate (see pages 14–5 to 14–6).

If you cannot decide whether to give a relaxant to intubate an unstable patient who might deteriorate, think about the other conditions present and talk to the health care personnel looking after these complications to find out the next steps in their management plan.

Ultimately, intubation and oxygenation override all other considerations. You should, however, bear in mind the side effects of suxamethonium, such as hyperkalaemia, a possible contribution to cardiac arrest. A potentially difficult airway (such as after severe facial trauma or soft tissue swelling) will make suxamethonium very hazardous: failure to intubate will mean certain death almost on the end of the needle seconds later.

Drugs in resuscitation (adult doses)

Drug	Indication/action	Dose
Epinephrine (adrenaline)	• Cardiac arrest • Acute anaphylaxis	0.5–1.0 mg IV
Atropine	• Bradycardia • Vagal asystole	0.5–1.0 mg IV
Ephedrine	• Hypotension after spinal anaesthesia (alternatives: phenylephrine or methoxamine)	10–30 mg IV
Calcium chloride	• Inotropic support at cardiac arrest	10 mg in 10 ml IV
Sodium bicarbonate	• Treatment of proven acute acidosis	30–100 mmol
Lidocaine	• Treatment of ventricular arrhythmias	1–2 mg/kg IV
Beta blockers	• Hypertensive crises	Various

Epinephrine (adrenaline)

Epinephrine 1/1000. 1 ml contains 1 mg. This is the standard dose for any cardiac arrest and also where the cause and/or rhythm are unknown. If you have any doubt that the needle or cannula is in the vein, dilute the 1 ml ampoule in 10 ml saline.

For severe hypotension, provided circulating volume has been restored:

- Dilute 1 mg in 10 ml saline
- Give doses of 0.5 ml–1 ml
- Observe the response.

Epinephrine saves lives in cases of acute collapse.

Epinephrine should be given as close to the heart as possible, such as into the internal jugular vein, while external cardiac massage is going on. This is to get the drug to the place where it is going to have an effect: the myocardium. Intra-cardiac epinephrine is not recommended, even as a final measure when all else has failed.

13

Atropine

0.6 – 1 mg (10 – 20 mcg/kg). Give atropine before epinephrine if:
- You see a severe bradycardia
- You suspect excessive vagal tone as a cause (unusual) of asystole.

Vasoconstrictors

Ephedrine 10 – 30 mg for spinal hypotension. Other α receptor agonists such as phenylephrine or methoxamine can be used. Vasoconstrictors are sometimes used in septic shock, but usually with limited effect.

Calcium chloride

10 mg in 10 ml during a cardiac arrest may be used to promote the effects of adrenaline and improve myocardial contractility.

Sodium bicarbonate

Give only when there is a proven acid-base problem.

Lidocaine

1 – 2 mg/kg. Lidocaine has anti-arrhythmic properties. It is not usually needed in CPR.

Beta blockers

Beta blockers have a role in hypertensive crises. Examples are:
- Atenolol
- Propranolol
- Labetolol.

These drugs slow the rate and force of contraction of the heart. They can be used in conjunction with vasodilators such as hydralazine, nitrates and calcium blockers. This type of complex therapy is more likely to be used by a physician in a tertiary hospital.

KEY POINTS

- Always take a history – if the patient cannot tell you, someone else may be able to
- Make a rapid evaluation of a collapsed patient
- Follow this with a full and detailed examination to avoid missing out anything important.

13.6 PREOPERATIVE ASSESSMENT AND INVESTIGATIONS

INITIAL ASSESSMENT

Failure to make a proper assessment of the patient's condition is one of the commonest and most easily avoidable causes of mishaps associated with anaesthesia.

The initial assessment of a patient includes taking a full medical history. The events leading up to admission should be carefully considered: for example, following an accident:

- When did it happen?
- What happened?
- Was the patient a passenger, driver or pedestrian?
- Is there any blood loss?
- How far away did it occur?
- How did the victim get to hospital?
- If unconscious now, was the patient conscious before?

The history is also important with non-trauma emergency surgery but, when there are delays in reaching hospital, perhaps of a week or even a month, the events that started the illness may have been forgotten.

The history of previous surgery is important. In areas of high HIV prevalence for example, peritonitis is a common complication 7–10 days after a caesarean section.

In the case of a child with a breathing difficulty, listen carefully to the history from the parent or guardian. Could there be a foreign body? If there is fever, croup or epiglottitis may be more likely. If a child has a sudden onset of airway obstruction you may learn, on questioning the parents, that the problem has been there intermittently for a longer period, making laryngeal polyps more likely.

In the case of an unconscious patient where there is no cause apparent, the history will usually give the diagnosis.

In the case of a patient needing surgery and anaesthesia, the pathological problem requiring surgery and the proposed operation are also of obvious importance. You will want to know how long the procedure is likely to take. Ask the patient about previous operations and anaesthetics and about any serious medical illnesses in the past.

After listening to the history, you should have some idea of a provisional diagnosis. Before starting the clinical examination, make an "end-of-the-bed" examination of such signs as:

- Breathing pattern (flail segment, asymmetrical or paradoxical movement, tachypnoea, dyspnoea)
- Position of patient (sitting up or lying down)
- Position of arms and legs (showing limb or pelvic fracture)
- Restlessness, such as from pain, hypoxia or shock
- Dehydration (skin turgor, sunken eyes)
- Distended abdomen
- Scars of recent surgery or dressings covering a wound that has not been inspected
- Blood stained clothes.

CLINICAL EXAMINATION

1 Look for general clinical signs before the specific detailed examination:

- Anaemia: look at the tongue, palms, soles of feet, nails and conjunctiva
- Jugular venous pressure: raised in heart failure, low in dehydration and shock

- Skin temperature: compare central with peripheral
- Cyanosis
- Oedema.

Apart from a wasted appearance, the presence of healed herpes zoster scars, scabies pigmentation, enlarged lymph nodes and oral lesions can inform you of the likelihood of HIV infection. Advanced HIV infection gives a poor prognosis after major surgery.

2 Examine the mouth and chin to make an assessment of the ease of tracheal intubation.

CARDIOVASCULAR EXAMINATION

1 Feel the hands:
   - Hot hands indicate a septic state
   - Cold hands may indicate hypovolaemia
   - A febrile torso and cold hands may indicate a septic state or malaria.

2 While holding the patient's hand, feel the pulse:
   - A pulse that is thready or hard to feel indicates inadequate circulation, perhaps hypovolaemia
   - Note the rate: most emergency cases have a fast pulse (tachycardia) from sepsis, hypovolaemia, pain or anxiety
   - Note the rhythm:
     - Regular
     - Irregular: use an ECG monitor to determine the nature of the arrhythmia.

3 Check the blood pressure: is it easy to hear?
   - A thready pulse means difficulty in taking blood pressure and a poor circulation
   - In hypertensive states, such as pre-eclampsia, the blood pressure is sometimes high but hard to detect
   - In shock, the blood pressure is low with a fast pulse.

4 Feel for the apex beat and listen to the heart sounds with the stethoscope.

RESPIRATORY EXAMINATION

1 Ask the patient to cough and listen to the result. You may hear bronchial secretions or wheeze, indicating bronchoconstriction. The patient may be unable to cough in severe respiratory disease.

2 Check that the trachea is central and that both sides of the chest inflate equally on a deep inspiration:
   - Percuss the chest for hyper-resonance (pneumothorax) or dullness (pleural effusion, consolidation or a high liver)
   - Spring the ribs for fractures if there is a history of trauma
   - Listen with the stethoscope all over the chest to elicit areas of reduced breath sounds or added sounds.

An emergency surgical case with concurrent cardiorespiratory disease will need careful postoperative management, oxygen and close monitoring.

ABDOMINAL EXAMINATION

You need to know as much as possible about intra-abdominal pathology. At the very least, this information will tell you about how long surgery will take and whether haemorrhage is likely.

Distended abdomen

If the abdomen is distended, palpation is not informative:

- Acute distension with no history of trauma will usually mean bowel obstruction or ileus from peritonitis
- Abdominal distension after trauma means blood (early) or (later) viscus perforation with peritonitis.

In such cases, urgent laparotomy is indicated with minimal delay.

Ultrasound scan is an important investigation in the management of the non-tympanic distended abdomen.

Soft abdomen

Palpation of a soft abdomen is more informative

- Pain on palpation of a mass and fever suggest inflammation
- A fixed mass, without fever, suggests the possibility of a tumour.

CONSENT AND EXPECTATIONS

Always obtain the consent of the patient before any operation. If the patient is a child, get the parents' consent. Try to find out the expectations of the patient and relatives.

The patient may have been sent to the operating room without explanation. Once you have decided on your anaesthetic technique, explain briefly to the patient what will happen, with reassurance that you will be present all the time to look after breathing and the function of the heart and to make sure that he or she feels no pain. Also explain what to expect on awakening, such as:

- Oxygen
- Intravenous infusion
- Nasogastric tube or surgical drains.

A few minutes of explanation and kindness in your approach will relieve many of the patient's anxieties and make your task as anaesthetist much easier. Once this has been done, it is advisable to ask the patient (or the parents in the case of a child) to confirm by signing that they agree with what you are planning to do.

PREOPERATIVE FASTING AND FLUIDS

For non-emergency patients having general or major conduction anaesthesia, when there is no reason to suspect abnormal gastric or intestinal function, the periods of preoperative fasting which are generally accepted as safe are:

- **Adults**: no solid food for 6 hours; liquids up to 3 hours preoperatively
- **Children**: no solid food for 6 hours; milk up to 4 hours, water up to 2 hours preoperatively.

PREMEDICATION

The majority of anaesthetists do not premedicate their patients unless there is a specific indication. For example, in caesarean section, sodium citrate 0.3 mol/litre 30 ml may be given orally just before anaesthesia to reduce stomach acidity.

Anxiety may be prevented by temazepam 10–20 mg orally 2 hours preoperatively.

AT THE END OF THE ASSESSMENT

At the end of your assessment (history and examination), write down:

- What you have been told
- What you have found on examination
- The action you propose to take.

Make your notes clear to others. Write legibly with the date and time shown. Use medical terminology that other people also use. If you are referring a patient, a clear, legible referral letter is of great importance. Give dates and times, symptoms on admission and describe what treatments have been given so far.

> Before starting any case, ask yourself: "Have I missed anything out?"

INVESTIGATIONS

> Ask: "Will the investigation be useful?"

Routine investigations are frequently requested even when they have no direct bearing on the illness. Such "screening" investigations are expensive and may not be affordable or available in your hospital. Only ask for an investigation if:

- You know why you want it and can interpret the result
- You have a management plan that depends on the result.

We are fortunate in the management of emergencies: most of what we need to know for the safe conduct of anaesthesia can be learned at the bedside from physical signs. We are not as dependent on the laboratory for blood results to the same extent as a general physician. There is only one thing for which the clinician is totally dependent on the laboratory: blood for transfusion.

Blood tests

The following tests may be useful.

Test	Application
Biochemistry	
Potassium	• Renal failure • Deciding on suxamethonium • Diagnosis of cardiac arrhythmias • Fluid therapy
Sodium	• Fluid therapy
Glucose	• Diabetic control
Creatinine or urea	• Renal function
Haematology	
Haemoglobin concentration	• Anaemia
White cell count	• High in the presence of infection • Low in advanced HIV
Platelets	• Bleeding tendency
Blood film	• Malaria parasites[1]

[1] Important in fever, especially postoperatively, as the stress of surgery may provoke a bout of malaria

Blood cultures are useful if a range of antibiotics is available in response.

If an investigation that you would normally ask for is not available, you should still consider it in your management plan; it might become available at another time.

Radiography

The chest X-ray is a useful investigation of any chest trauma patient, especially before a chest drain is placed. Look for:

- Soft tissue swelling outside the ribcage, especially due to air
- Fractured ribs, clavicle or scapula
- Equal lung markings right and left
- Pneumothorax, haemothorax or effusion or consolidation
- Shift of the mediastinum to the right or left or the hemidiaphragms up and down
- Heart abnormalities: size and shape
- Foreign bodies: can sometimes be seen in the bronchi or a coin lodged in the pharynx.

If the X-ray investigation involves taking the patient elsewhere, consider the risks of this unmonitored journey:

- Will oxygen be needed?
- Is resuscitation equipment available?

It is almost impossible to feel a pulse or look for breathing when moving with a patient in a corridor.

If an X-ray is not available, you will have to rely on your clinical skills instead or seek help to improve the diagnosis.

An ultrasound scan is useful for abdominal diagnosis in non-trauma patients.

MANAGEMENT PLAN

After preoperative assessment, make a management plan with the surgical practitioner. The options are:

- Immediate surgery
- Resuscitate and immediate surgery
- Resuscitate and later surgery
- Resuscitate and wait and see if surgery is indicated (and if blood is available).

> Talk to your surgical colleague to make sure you each know what the other will do.

Either of the last two options must be decided on in the case of the "poor risk" patient. Is the patient poor risk or moribund? The distinction between the two is often not clear. The moribund patient cannot be saved, but the treatment should be continued until it is clearly futile.

A poor risk patient is often presented as an "emergency", even though the case may have been neglected for days or weeks. Whether the system failed the patient or the patient failed to use the system, it is still an emergency.

Only your clinical experience, gained over many years, will enable you to manage these cases correctly, balancing the effective use of scarce resources on one side against the best interests of the patient on the other. You should take account of:

- Available resources for the operation, including blood for transfusion
- Available postoperative support
- What will happen if the operation is not carried out.

In anaesthesia, as in most areas of medicine and surgery, you will need at least as much knowledge and skill to make the right choice of technique as you will to implement it. The best anaesthetic in any given situation depends on your training and experience, the range of equipment and drugs available and the clinical situation.

> However strong the indications may seem for using a particular technique, the best anaesthetic technique, especially in an emergency, will normally be one with which you are experienced and confident.

Some of the factors to bear in mind when choosing your anaesthetic technique are:

- Training and experience of the anaesthetist and surgeon
- Availability of drugs and equipment
- Medical condition of the patient

- Time available
- Emergency or elective procedure
- Presence of a full stomach
- Patient's preference.

Not all these factors are of equal importance, but all should be considered, especially when the choice of technique is not obvious.

13.7 ANAESTHETIC ISSUES IN THE EMERGENCY SITUATION

ANAESTHETIC TECHNIQUES

The table below is intended to help you decide what type of anaesthetic might be most suitable for a given surgical procedure.

Suitable anaesthetic techniques for different types of surgery

Type of surgery	Suitable anaesthetic technique
• Major head and neck • Upper abdominal • Intrathoracic • Ear, nose and throat • Endoscopic	General tracheal
• Upper limbs	General tracheal (LMA) *or* Nerve block *or* Intravenous regional
• Lower abdominal • Groin, perineum	General tracheal *or* Spinal
• Lower limbs	General tracheal (LMA) *or* Nerve or field block *or* Combined general and conduction

For minor emergency operations when the patient probably has a full stomach, such as the suture of a wound or manipulation of an arm fracture, conduction (regional) anaesthesia is probably the wisest choice.

For major emergency operations, there is often little difference in safety between conduction and general anaesthesia.

> It is a dangerous mistake to think that conduction anaesthesia is always safe.

When you have come to a decision on the most suitable technique, discuss it with the surgeon and surgical team, who may give you further relevant information. For example, the proposed operation may need more time than can be provided by the technique you have suggested or the patient may need to be placed in an abnormal position. Also check that you have all the drugs and equipment you may need.

KEY POINTS

- Choose a suitable anaesthetic technique that fits in with the patient's condition, the needs of the surgeon and your own experience and skill
- Most cases in district hospitals are full-stomach emergencies, so general anaesthesia will normally require protection of the lungs with a tracheal tube.

You will probably have to decide on one of the following techniques:

- General anaesthesia with drugs given intravenously or by inhalation
- General anaesthesia with intramuscular ketamine
- Spinal anaesthesia
- Nerve block (conduction anaesthesia)
- Infiltration anaesthesia.

There are advantages in combining light general anaesthesia with a conduction block: this technique reduces the amount of general anaesthetic that the patient requires and allows a rapid recovery, with postoperative analgesia being provided by the remaining conduction block.

PLANNING GENERAL ANAESTHESIA

For general anaesthesia, tracheal intubation should be routine, unless there is a specific reason to avoid it (see Figure 13.12 on page 13–29).

Tracheal intubation is the most basic of anaesthetic skills and you should be able to do it confidently whenever necessary. In smaller hospitals, most of the operations are emergencies; the lungs and lives of the patients are in danger if you do not protect them by this manoeuvre.

Remember that all relaxants are contraindicated prior to tracheal intubation if the patient has an abnormality of the jaw or neck or if there is any other reason to think that laryngoscopy and intubation might be difficult (see also *Paediatric emergency anaesthesia*, pages 14–18 to 14–20).

Safety of general and conduction techniques

There are potential risks with all types of anaesthetic. These can be minimized by careful assessment of the patient, thoughtful planning of the anaesthetic technique and skilful performance by the anaesthetist. You should keep records of all the anaesthetics that you give and regularly review complications and morbidity. Some of the possible complications to look for are listed below.

Some complications of general and conduction anaesthesia

General anaesthesia	Conduction anaesthesia
Airway obstruction	Toxicity of drug
Aspiration of gastric contents	Accidental intravascular injection
Allergy or hypersensitivity	Allergic reactions
Hypotension (including supine hypotension in pregnancy)	Massive spread of spinal anaesthetic
Cardiac dysrhythmias	Cardiac depression by local anaesthetic
Trauma to mouth, pharynx, teeth and larynx	Spread of sepsis
Respiratory depression	Depression of the central nervous system and convulsions
Increased intracranial pressure	
Postoperative hypoxia	
Toxic damage to liver or kidneys	

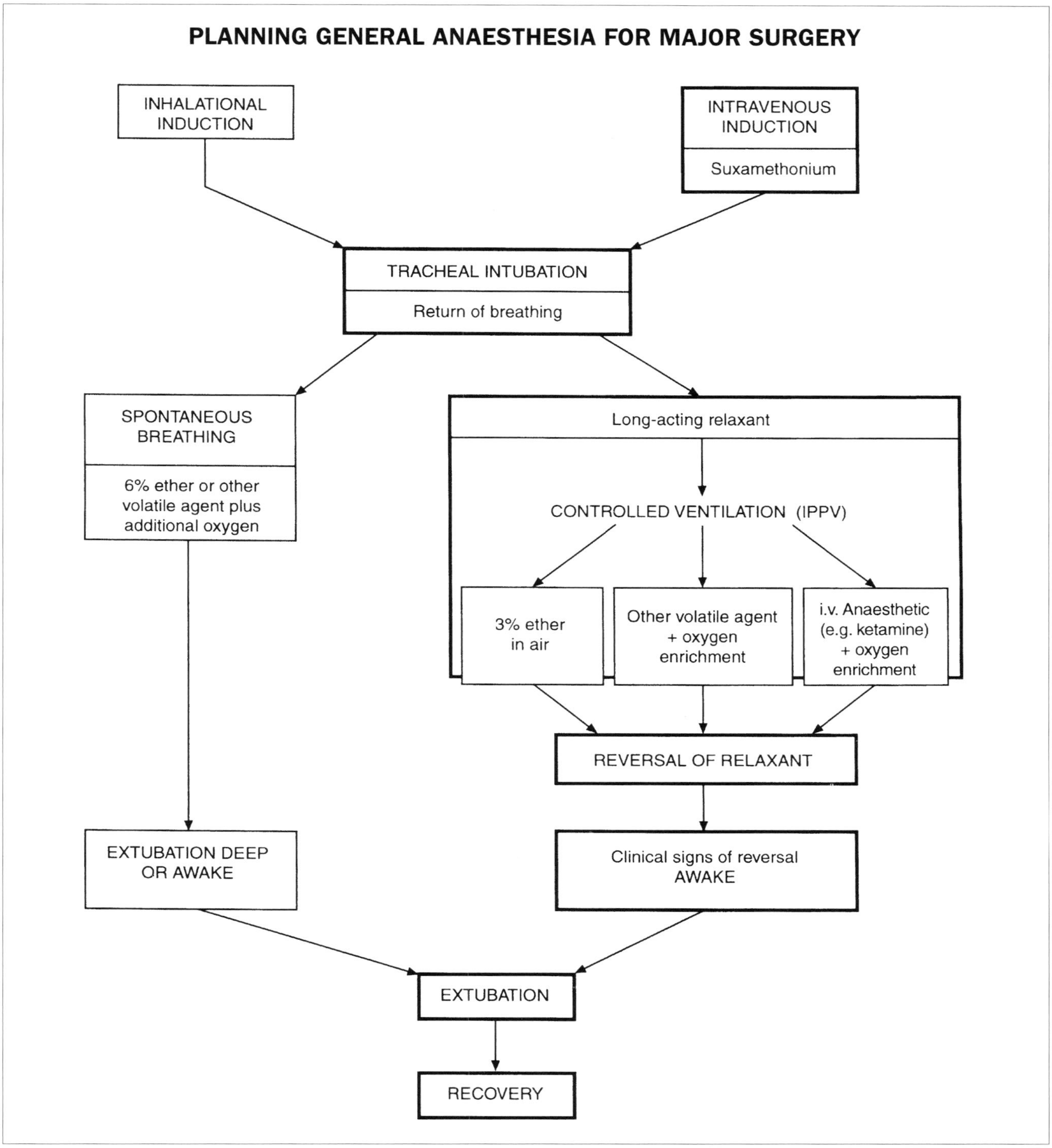

Figure 13.12

CHOICE OF TECHNIQUE IN EMERGENCY ANAESTHESIA

General or regional anaesthesia?

General and regional techniques both have a place in dealing with emergencies. The factors that favour the use of general anaesthesia are:

- Presence of hypovolaemia
- Uncertainty about the diagnosis and length of operation

13

- Unforeseen events
- Lack of time
- Patient distress or confusion.

There are exceptions. For emergency caesarean section, spinal anaesthesia may be better, provided the mother is not shocked, septic or dehydrated. A strangulated inguinal hernia or torsion of the testis occurring in a patient in good general condition can also be performed under spinal anaesthesia.

On the other hand, cord prolapse during labour, shock or severe bleeding indicates general anaesthesia.

In some cases, either general or regional (spinal) anaesthesia may be appropriate:

- Amputations
- Debridement of wounds
- Drainage of abscesses or other septic conditions.

A gunshot wound to the leg, when there is uncertainty about what will be found, would be better explored under general anaesthesia. A few days later, the same patient returning in a stable condition for wound toilet, could have a spinal anaesthetic.

Full stomach and regurgitation risk

As a general rule, all patients must come to the operating room starved (no solids for 6 hours, water allowed up to 2 hours preoperatively). You should assume that the stomach is not empty in injured or severely ill patients, in those that have received an opiate such as pethidine and in pregnant women.

Any method of anaesthesia, including awake techniques, can have an unexpected reaction that can, in theory, lead to unconsciousness, regurgitation and aspiration of stomach contents. You will need to judge each case on its merits, balancing the risk of regurgitation and aspiration against the risks of general or spinal anaesthesia. The general condition of the patient determines the risk of regurgitation more than the choice of technique. If an operation is postponed on the grounds that the patient is not starved, there may be a risk of it not being carried out at all.

Poor risk cases

A typical case where we are unsure of what method to use might be a patient in poor condition whose chronic illness has been neglected. Surgery may give improvement by cleaning, debridement of necrotic tissue or drainage of pus in the hope that healing will take place, suffering will be relieved and the patient will move a step nearer to leaving hospital. Large numbers of such patients are seen every day in hospital operating rooms in any country with a high rate of HIV seroprevalence.

Obstetric sepsis has a high incidence and is the biggest cause of hospital maternal mortality in some countries. Patients frequently develop sepsis up to ten days following septic abortion, ectopic pregnancy and normal or operative delivery. Sometimes, in advanced sepsis, there are disagreements among medical staff about whether to take the case at all.

"Gasping" means a type of respiration with feeble, jerky inspiratory efforts that cause movement of the head in a semiconscious patient. Prognosis is very poor. Predicting the outcome with or without an operation is one of the more difficult judgements in medical practice.

Ketamine is the drug of choice, 1–2 mg/kg IV, according to the condition. Oxygen is mandatory after ketamine because hypoxia usually occurs.

Intubation is recommended for laparotomy. A small abdominal incision and drainage may become a full laparotomy and washout in the intensive care unit. Management with inotropic support is usually needed postoperatively.

A critical moment in the operation is during the initial abdominal exploration and breaking down of adhesions. Endotoxaemia is maximal at this time and sudden death in asystole may occur. Epinephrine should be drawn up ready.

Ketamine is safest for patients who are to have uterine evacuation, where there has been haemorrhage or sepsis.

SPECIAL ANAESTHETIC ISSUES

The solo practitioner giving anaesthesia

Many hospitals in developing countries will have only one person assigned or trained to give anaesthesia. Even so, you should identify and train another person to help you and even take over your duties from time to time. It is quite possible for a single-handed paramedical health worker to have sole responsibility for a major emergency case in a remote location in a developing country that would, elsewhere, have a team of senior experts managing the different requirements of airway, drip, drug administration, ventilation, etc. It is also possible for *you* (if you are a solo, non-specialist practitioner) to do just as good a job as the experts.

However, there are certain things that require the help of a second person:

- Applying cricoid pressure
- Holding a struggling or distressed trauma patient during induction
- Bringing some vital bit of equipment, especially in emergency
- Attending to a problem with the sucker.

It is important for you to identify an *assistant* (not a replacement anaesthetist) who knows the hazards of anaesthesia, how you work and where things are kept. Above all, he or she needs to understand the meaning of acting quickly when things go wrong.

> Never start a case if you are alone with the patient in the operating room.

The full stomach: cricoid pressure

A full stomach is one of the most dangerous situations in the practice of anaesthesia: if a patient aspirates stomach contents into the lungs, the resulting complications mean that the chance of survival will be slight. Aspiration of stomach contents may be one of the most common causes of death on the operating table in developing countries.

Cricoid pressure (pressing on the cricoid cartilage with a pressure of 30 Newtons: 3 kg) is intended to prevent passive regurgitation, but will not stop active vomiting. Active vomiting probably means the patient is awake and has intact protective reflexes; cricoid pressure is therefore not appropriate.

There are two situations where cricoid pressure should normally be applied:

- Anaesthesia for all emergency surgery
- All caesarean sections performed under general anaesthesia.

There are additional dangerous situations where regurgitation is very likely:

- Caesarean section for prolonged obstructed labour, compounded by ruptured uterus, hypovolaemic shock or sepsis, especially where local (herbal) medicines have been given
- Intestinal obstruction
- A patient who has a hiccup
- A patient who coughs, strains or otherwise moves a lot at the moment of attempting to intubate, especially after inhalation induction with no muscle relaxant
- A patient with stomach filled with air during mask inflation of the lungs due to poor mask-holding technique
- Generally debilitated patients with chronic gastrointestinal disease.

Although it has never been subjected to controlled trials to prove its efficacy, properly applied cricoid pressure is believed to be an effective measure to prevent regurgitation.

> If in doubt about the regurgitation risk, apply cricoid pressure – it costs nothing and may save a life.

Spontaneous versus controlled ventilation (IPPV)

Except for neurosurgery, there is no evidence that any operation has a better outcome when controlled ventilation is used instead of allowing the patient to breathe spontaneously. Thoracic procedures involving the open chest cannot, of course, be performed without controlled ventilation as the normal mechanics of breathing requiring negative pressure in the pleural cavity are disrupted.

The shocked patient may suffer a significant reduction in cardiac output if Intermittent Positive Pressure Ventilation (IPPV) is applied, owing to the increased thoracic gas pressure preventing venous return to the heart. Overzealous IPPV, either by hand or ventilator, may be a terminal event in a patient with hypovolaemia.

The use of spontaneous breathing has an additional safety effect of allowing you to monitor cerebral perfusion: breathing will stop if the brain is not being perfused with blood at an adequate pressure. Also, overdose of volatile agent in a spontaneously breathing patient is unlikely.

Where facilities for anaesthesia are limited, ventilators often do not have alarms to warn about disconnection and trained, experienced anaesthetists are not available. Emergency surgery under general anaesthesia in these conditions is safer when performed with the patient breathing spontaneously.

Ventilation in chest and head injuries

The patient with combined chest and other trauma may require intubation as part of general anaesthesia for a laparotomy (such as in cases of a ruptured spleen) or craniotomy (in cases of extradural haematoma). Intermittent Positive Pressure Ventilation (IPPV) is not necessarily part of the early management of chest trauma unless there are specific indications, for example, during cardiopulmonary resuscitation or if hypoxia, respiratory failure or other deterioration occurs.

Rib fractures may cause the lungs to be punctured on sharp ends inside the chest and result in pneumothorax. With further gas being forced into the lungs during ventilation, the pneumothorax may become a tension pneumothorax. A chest drain should be in place.

Lung contusion (consolidation from damage and bleeding) often gets worse in succeeding days so a patient who is comfortably breathing and sitting up with an oxygen mask on the first day post-trauma may later deteriorate and have to be ventilated.

Patients with head injuries can benefit from IPPV in the early stages of admission; it will help to avoid the lethal combination of hypoxia, airway obstruction and hypercarbia, a significant cause of mortality in the immediate period after injury.

However, controlled ventilation itself has not been shown to improve outcome for the head injured patient. There is no point in ventilating a brain dead patient with no prospect of recovery.

Tracheal tube versus laryngeal mask airway

The laryngeal mask airway (LMA) is now commonplace in most countries. It has proved very popular and is far less stimulating to the patient than the tracheal tube. It should not be used to replace intubation for:

- Caesarean section under general anaesthesia
- Laparotomy
- *Any* situation where there is a regurgitation risk (all emergencies).

Insertion can be under deep halothane anaesthesia or, in a paralysed patient or after intravenous induction, with propofol. Do not try LMA insertion after thiopentone as the patient will gag.

Method of insertion

1 With the head extended and mouth open, pass a deflated, lubricated LMA over the tongue and push it up against the soft palate until it comes to rest against the upper oesophageal sphincter and epiglottis. The end point is quite distinct. It must not push the tongue in front of it.

2 Inflate the cuff. A correctly inserted LMA will then move about 5 mm back out of the mouth from its original position.

3 Connect the circuit and check for breathing.

The LMA has been used with success to maintain the airway after failed intubation. This important role of the LMA as an emergency tool in airway management makes it an essential piece of equipment in the operating room in any country in the world.

Mixing drugs

In emergency induction of anaesthesia, it may be convenient to use drugs mixed together in the same syringe for speed and simplicity of administration and increased patient safety. Ketamine and suxamethonium mix well without interaction and give a convenient, reliable one-shot sleep and relaxation effect, of rapid onset, so that you can concentrate on the airway. This is especially valuable if your syringes and needles are of poor quality, are made of glass or have been resterilized. However, many drugs do not mix, notably thiopentone and suxamethonium. Diazepam does not mix well with other drugs.

Pre-oxygenation should be done with one hand holding the mask and the other giving the drugs. If two hands are needed for the drugs, the mask can be held by the patient or an assistant.

Suction

Good suction is of paramount importance in anaesthesia and resuscitation and for all forms of surgery and intensive care. As a resuscitation tool, suction comes second only to a self-inflating bag and mask.

When you need suction, it must be instantly available, right by your hand at all times:

- The sucker must be ready and switched on for any case where a full stomach is suspected or where the airway is being inspected, such as when you are looking for a foreign body or other obstruction
- The sucker must be ready, but can be turned off, for elective procedures.

The power of suction is important. Never believe that a sucker is working until you have raised the tip to your ear and heard its power. Then tuck it under the pillow or mattress ready for use. Make sure the suction tubing will not kink when angled and that the suction motor is protected by a reservoir bottle and a filter.

A foot-operated sucker can be a life saving piece of equipment at a health centre without electricity.

Sucking stimulates the gag reflex and may induce vomiting. Excessive sucking damages the mucosa and causes bleeding. The general rules of suction are:

- Do not suck when going in, especially if you cannot see the sucker tip
- Only suck as much as is needed: that is, when you can hear and see something coming
- Keep the sucker moving and continue sucking on the way out
- When routinely extubating a patient:
  - Always suck both sides of the tube
  - With the tip at the larynx, let the cuff down
  - When the time is right for extubation, re-insert the sucker
  - Remove the tube first then, just afterwards, remove the sucker, sucking all the while.

Use a rigid sucker for emergencies.

Suction in the trachea

A small-bore soft sucker is used for tracheal or bronchial suction. Special precautions are needed if sucking in the trachea: the sucker should be sterile, not the same one as used for the pharynx.

In children, the sucker should not be a tight fit in the small tracheal tube, otherwise the negative pressure may cause lung collapse.

Repeated tracheal suction in the intensive care unit may cause bradycardia and even cardiac arrest, so the ECG monitor must be watched.

Removal of foreign bodies

Removal of foreign bodies is a common job for anaesthetists in developing countries. In a district hospital, it is important that the anaesthetist is able to remove objects in the mouth, airway or pharynx, with or without anaesthesia, using Magill's forceps. Children often hide small coins in their mouths which may slip down into the pharynx.

Have a recent X-ray, if available. After inhalation induction with halothane, a long straight blade laryngoscope is best to go behind the larynx. The child will be apnoeic during pharyngoscopy, so a pulse oximeter should be connected. An object further down in the oesophagus may be out of reach and may require intubation and oesophagoscopy.

An assortment of other items may have been inhaled or become lodged in the upper airway: seeds, fish bones, chicken bones, peanuts, bits of plastic, bottle tops and even leeches. For the airway, there are three general situations:

- Total airway obstruction
- Partial airway obstruction with an object caught at the larynx
- Inhaled smaller foreign body further down in the trachea or bronchi.

The first is obviously very rarely seen in a hospital. If you witness the event, there are two courses of action.

1 The Heimlich manoeuvre. Stand behind the patient, give a sharp upward thrust into the epigastrium (round the front) with both fists to raise intrathoracic pressure and expel the blockage.

2 If that fails, puncture the cricothyroid membrane with a sharp knife and insert a plastic biro tube as a laryngostomy.

The object partly blocking the larynx is often a piece of bone or something flat, irregular and sharp that can be easily removed with Magill's forceps after inhalation induction with halothane and oxygen. There is intense irritation for the patient and stridor may be caused by laryngospasm as well as by the object itself. Inhalation induction may be slow and, if assisted ventilation is easy, it may be permissible to give suxamethonium and IPPV. Though theoretically this may push the object further down, in practice that rarely happens. Do not declare the job complete until you are sure everything has been removed and breathing is comfortable and silent.

Unfortunately, the commonest situation is for a seed or peanut to be inhaled by a child past the cords and into a bronchus. Referral to a centre with a ventilating bronchoscope is mandatory and urgent.

KEY POINTS

- Pre-existing medical problems can have a profound influence on the course of anaesthesia and surgery
- If the patient's condition requires urgent surgery, use your skills to minimize the harmful effects of pre-existing conditions.

13.8 IMPORTANT MEDICAL CONDITIONS FOR THE ANAESTHETIST

ANAEMIA

Severe anaemia interferes with the body's oxygen transport system by reducing the amount of oxygen that can be carried by the blood as oxyhaemoglobin. This means that, to supply the tissues with adequate amounts of oxygen, the heart must pump more blood. This results in the tachycardia, flow murmurs and heart failure sometimes found in severely anaemic patients.

If a severely anaemic patient is to be subjected to surgery, which may cause blood loss, and to anaesthesia, which may interfere with oxygen transport by the blood, all possible steps must be taken to correct the anaemia preoperatively. If time is limited, it may be possible to do this only by transfusion, after consideration of the possible benefits and risks.

There is no absolute haemoglobin concentration below which a patient is "unfit for anaesthesia".

The decision to anaesthetize a patient depends on the circumstances and on the urgency of the need for surgery. Ideally, of course, every patient should have a haemoglobin level "normal" for the community from which he or she comes. However, a patient with a ruptured ectopic pregnancy cannot be sent away with iron tablets or even wait for a preoperative blood transfusion. As a rough guide, most anaesthetists prefer not to anaesthetize a patient whose haemoglobin level is below 8 g/dl if the need for surgery is not urgent, especially if serious blood loss is expected.

Remember that "anaemia" is not a complete diagnosis and may indicate that the patient has another pathological condition that has so far gone undetected. Possibilities include sickle-cell disease, chronic gastrointestinal bleeding from hookworm infection or a duodenal ulcer. The cause of "incidental" anaemia may be far more in need of treatment than the condition requiring surgery. It is therefore important to investigate anaemic patients properly and not to regard anaemia as a "nuisance" for the anaesthetist or to assume that it is necessarily due to parasitic infection.

Emergency surgery

An anaemic patient with an urgent need for surgery has a lower oxygen-carrying capacity of the blood than normal. Avoid drugs and techniques that may worsen the situation by lowering the cardiac output (such as deep halothane anaesthesia) or by allowing respiration to become depressed. Ether and ketamine do not depress cardiac output or respiration significantly.

Oxygen supplementation is desirable for anaemic patients. Blood lost must be replaced with blood, or the haemoglobin concentration will fall further. Ensure that the patient does not become hypoxic during or after the operation.

See also *The Clinical Use of Blood* (WHO, 2001).

HYPERTENSION

Elective surgery

Elective anaesthesia and surgery are contraindicated in any patient with sustained hypertension and blood pressure greater than 180 mmHg (24.0 kPa) systolic or 110 mmHg (14.7 kPa) diastolic. This degree of hypertension will be associated with clinical signs of left ventricular hypertrophy on chest X-rays and electrocardiograms, retinal abnormality and, possibly, renal damage.

Patients whose hypertension has been reasonably well controlled can be safely anaesthetized. It is important not to discontinue any regular treatment with antihypertensive drugs or the patient's blood pressure may go out of control. After a full assessment of the patient, including obtaining a chest X-ray and an electrocardiogram and measuring serum electrolyte concentrations (especially if the patient is taking diuretic drugs), you may carefully use any suitable anaesthetic technique, with the exception of administering ketamine, which tends to raise the blood pressure. If the patient is receiving treatment with beta blockers, the treatment should be continued, but remember that the patient will be unable to compensate for blood loss with a tachycardia, so special attention is needed.

If an elective operation is postponed to allow hypertension to be treated, the patient should normally be allowed a period of 4–6 weeks to stabilize before returning for surgery. It is not safe simply to start antihypertensive drugs the day before an operation.

13

Emergency surgery

In an emergency, the same principles apply to the management of a hypertensive patient as to a patient who has had a recent myocardial infarction. Consider a conduction anaesthetic technique and make every attempt to avoid hypotension, which can precipitate a cerebrovascular accident or myocardial infarction. Severely hypertensive patients whose need for surgery is not urgent should be referred.

RESPIRATORY DISEASES

Tuberculosis is a multisystem disease whose respiratory and other effects may present problems for the anaesthetist. There are, firstly, the problems of anaesthetizing a patient with a severe systemic illness, who may have nutritional problems and abnormal fluid losses from fever combined with a poor oral intake of fluid and water and a high metabolic rate requiring a greater supply of oxygen than normal.

Local problems in the lung – the production of sputum, chronic cough and haemoptysis – may lead to segmental or lobar collapse, resulting in inadequate ventilation and oxygenation. Tracheal tubes may quickly become blocked with secretions, so frequent suction may be necessary. In sick patients who cannot cough effectively, a nasotracheal tube may be left in place after surgery or a tracheostomy performed to allow for aspiration of secretions.

Contamination of anaesthetic equipment with infected secretions must also be considered. If you have to anaesthetize a patient with tuberculosis, use either a disposable tracheal tube, which you can then throw away, or a red rubber tube which, after thorough cleaning with soap and water, can be autoclaved. The patient's breathing valve and anaesthetic tubing will also need to be sterilized. Black antistatic breathing hose can be autoclaved. It is unlikely that the self-inflating bag (SIB) in a draw-over system will be contaminated but, if you sterilize an SIB, be careful, as many of these are damaged by autoclaving. If you use a Magill breathing system on a Boyle's machine, the whole system should be autoclaved, as the patient can breathe directly into the bag. If you cannot see how to overcome contamination problems with inhalational anaesthesia, use ketamine or a conduction technique instead.

ASTHMA AND CHRONIC BRONCHITIS

Elective surgery

For elective anaesthesia and surgery in a patient with a history of asthma, the asthmatic condition should be under control and the patient should have had no recent infections or severe wheezing attacks. If the patient takes drugs regularly, treatment must not be discontinued. Special inquiry must be made about any former use of steroids, systemically or by inhaler. Any patient who has previously been admitted to hospital for an asthmatic attack should be referred for assessment.

The patient with chronic bronchitis has some degree of irreversible airway obstruction. In taking a history, you should ask about exercise tolerance, smoking and sputum production. The patient must be told to give up smoking completely at least four weeks before the operation. Simple clinical tests of lung function may be valuable; healthy people can blow out a lighted match 20 cm from the mouth without pursing their lips and can count aloud in a normal voice from 1 to 40 without pausing to draw breath. The nature of the operation is of great importance; elective surgery on the upper abdomen is contraindicated, since respiratory failure in the postoperative period is likely. Patients needing such surgery must be referred to a hospital where their lungs can be ventilated artificially for 1–2 days postoperatively if necessary.

Conduction anaesthesia combined with intravenous sedation with small doses of diazepam may be a better choice of technique than conduction anaesthesia alone or general anaesthesia. If general anaesthesia is necessary, premedication with an antihistamine such as promethazine, together with 100 mg of hydrocortisone, is advisable. It is important to avoid laryngoscopy and intubation during light anaesthesia, as this is likely to lead to severe bronchospasm. Ketamine is quite suitable for intravenous induction because of its bronchodilator properties.

For short procedures:

- Avoid intubation
- Use 30% oxygen or more.

Ether and halothane are both good bronchodilators, but ether has the advantage that, should bronchospasm develop, epinephrine (0.5 mg subcutaneously) can safely be given. This would be very dangerous with halothane which sensitizes the heart to the dysrhythmic effects of catecholamines. Aminophylline (up to 250 mg for an adult by slow intravenous injection) can be used as an alternative to epinephrine if bronchospasm develops; it is compatible with any inhalational agent.

At the end of any procedure that includes tracheal intubation, extubate with the patient in the lateral position and still deeply anaesthetized; the laryngeal stimulation might otherwise again provoke intense bronchospasm.

Emergency surgery

For emergency surgery, use a technique with intubation and IPPV with added oxygen. Postoperatively, give oxygen at not more than 1 litre/minute via a nasal catheter. Be careful with opiates, as the patient may be unusually sensitive to respiratory depression.

DIABETES

When a diabetic patient needs surgery, it is important to remember that he or she is more likely to be harmed by neglect of the long term complications of diabetes than from the short term control of blood glucose levels. Make a full preoperative assessment, looking especially for symptoms and signs of peripheral vascular, cerebrovascular and coronary disease, all of which are common in patients with diabetes, as is chronic renal failure.

KEY POINTS

- Look for medical complications in the diabetic patient
- Low blood sugar is the main intraoperative risk from diabetes
- Monitor blood sugar levels and treat, as necessary.

Elective surgery

The diabetic patient who needs elective surgery is not difficult to handle. In the short term, the only major theoretical risk is that undetected hypoglycaemia might occur during anaesthesia. Most general anaesthetics, including ether, halothane and ketamine, cause a small and harmless rise in the blood sugar concentration and are therefore safe to use. Thiopental and nitrous oxide have little effect on the blood sugar concentration; no anaesthetic causes blood sugar to fall.

Diabetic patients may be classified according to whether their diabetes is controlled with insulin (insulin-dependent diabetes or Type I) or by diet and/ or oral hypoglycaemic drugs (non-insulin dependent diabetes or Type II).

Insulin-dependent diabetes

For insulin-dependent patients, ensure that the diabetes is under reasonably good control:

- On the morning of the operation, do not give the patient food or insulin; this will ensure a normal or slightly elevated blood sugar concentration, which will tend to rise slowly
- Measure the blood sugar concentration shortly before anaesthesia; it will probably be 7–12 mmol/litre but, if it is higher than 12 mmol/ litre:
  - Give 2–4 International Units of soluble insulin intravenously or subcutaneously
  - Measure the blood sugar again in an hour.
  - Give further doses of insulin as necessary.

As an alternative, if frequent blood sugar measurements are impossible:

- Put 10 International Units of soluble insulin into 500 ml of 10% glucose to which 1 g of potassium chloride (13 mmol) has been added
- Infuse this solution intravenously at 100 ml/hour for a normal-sized adult
- Continue with this regimen until the patient can eat again and then return to normal antidiabetic treatment.

This scheme is simple and will maintain blood glucose levels in most diabetic patients in the range 5–14 mmol/litre. However, make regular checks of blood glucose concentration and change the regimen, if necessary. Note that, if glass infusion bottles are used, the dose of insulin will need to be increased by about 30%, as the glass adsorbs insulin.

Where several patients are due to undergo surgery on a given day, diabetic patients should be first on the list, since this makes the timing and control of their insulin regimen much easier.

Non-insulin dependent diabetes

If the patient's diabetes is controlled by diet alone, you can normally use an unmodified standard anaesthetic technique suitable for the patient's condition and the nature of the operation.

Patients with non-insulin dependent diabetes controlled with oral hypoglycaemic drugs should not take their drugs on the morning of anaesthesia. Because certain drugs (notably chlorpropamide) have a very long duration of action, there is some risk of hypoglycaemia, so the blood sugar concentration should be checked every few hours until the patient is able to eat again.

If difficulties arise with these patients, it may be simpler to switch them temporarily to control with insulin, using the glucose plus insulin infusion regimen described above.

Emergency surgery

The diabetic patient requiring emergency surgery is rather different. If the diabetes is out of control, there is danger from both diabetes and the condition requiring surgery. The patient may well have:

- Severe volume depletion
- Acidosis
- Hyperglycaemia
- Severe potassium depletion
- Hyperosmolality
- Acute gastric dilatation.

In these circumstances, medical resuscitation usually has priority over surgical need, since any kind of anaesthesia attempted before correction of the metabolic upset could rapidly prove fatal.

Resuscitation will require large volumes of saline with potassium supplementation (under careful laboratory control). There is no point in giving much more than 4 International Units of insulin per hour, but levels must be maintained either by hourly intramuscular injections or by continuous intravenous infusion. The patient will need a nasogastric tube and a urinary catheter.

If the need for surgery is urgent, use a conduction anaesthetic technique once the circulating volume has been fully restored. Before a general anaesthetic can be given, the potassium deficit and acidosis must also have been corrected, or life-threatening dysrhythmias are likely. The level of blood sugar is much less important; it is better left on the high side of normal.

OBESITY

Obese patients (who may also be diabetic) face a number of problems when anaesthesia is necessary. Obesity is often associated with hypertension – though with a very fat arm the blood pressure is difficult to measure and may appear high when in fact it is not. Because of the extra body mass, the cardiac output is greater than in a non-obese person; more work is also required during exertion, which places greater stress on the heart. The association of smoking, obesity and hypertension is often a fatal one, with or without anaesthesia.

Because of the mass of fat in the abdomen, diaphragmatic breathing is restricted and the chest wall may also be abnormally rigid because of fatty infiltration. Breathing becomes even more inefficient when the patient is lying down, so IPPV during anaesthesia is recommended, with oxygen enrichment if possible.

Extra technical problems are found in obese patients. A fat neck makes airway control and intubation difficult and excess subcutaneous fat leads to difficulty with venepuncture and conduction anaesthesia. Do not give drugs on a weight basis, as this will result in an overdose. For most drugs given intravenously, a 120 kg patient needs only about 130% of the normal dose for an adult of 60–70 kg. For general anaesthesia in the obese patient, a technique based on tracheal intubation with IPPV using relaxants is recommended.

PREVENTION OF BLOOD-SPREAD INFECTIONS DURING ANAESTHESIA AND SURGERY

Because of the risk of infection, blood transfusion must be used only when medically necessary and when the potential benefits outweigh the risks. The decision to transfuse should be based on both the patient's condition and the local availability and safety of blood supplies. Where blood supplies are scarce or unsafe, it may be possible to use pre-donation by the patient in elective cases or to use autologous transfusion in emergencies.

Minimize the risk of transmission of infection:

- Never leave syringes attached to needles that have been used on a patient
- For intravenous injections, use plastic infusion cannulae with injection ports that do not require the use of a needle, wherever possible
- Ensure that blood spills are immediately and safely dealt with
- Use gloves for all procedures where blood or other body fluids may be spilled
- Where blood spillage is likely, use waterproof aprons or gowns and eye protection.

Practical anaesthesia

14

14.1 GENERAL ANAESTHESIA

KEY POINTS

- Have a clear plan before starting anaesthesia
- Never use an unfamiliar anaesthetic technique in an emergency
- Always check your equipment
- Make sure you have an assistant before starting.

Several different types of drug produce anaesthesia. The aim is to provide a pleasant induction and lack of awareness for the patient, using a technique that is safe and that provides good operating conditions. Unfortunately, the ideal anaesthetic drug with all the desired qualities does not exist. It is common practice, therefore, to combine several drugs, each of which provides a single component of anaesthesia. This can be represented diagrammatically as a triangle whose corners represent sleep (unconsciousness), muscular relaxation, and analgesia (lack of response to painful stimulation) (Figure 14.1).

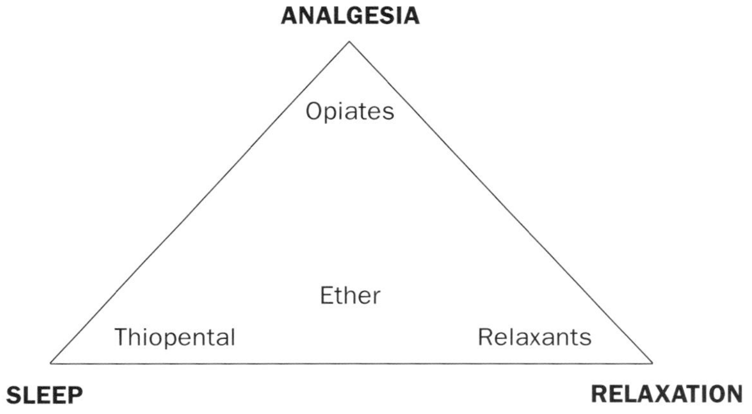

Figure 14.1

Certain drugs, such as thiopental, produce unconsciousness without relaxation or analgesia and are suitable only for inducing anaesthesia. In contrast, ether produces a mixture of sleep, analgesia and relaxation but, because of its pungent smell and high solubility in blood, it is rather inconvenient and slow (though safe) for induction of anaesthesia.

The muscle relaxants produce muscular relaxation alone and may therefore be used to provide good surgical relaxation during light anaesthesia, allowing the patient to recover rapidly at the end of anaesthesia.

Opiate drugs, such as morphine and pethidine, produce analgesia with little change in muscle tone or level of consciousness. The choice of the most suitable combination for any given patient and operation calls for careful thought and planning.

14

PREPARATION FOR GENERAL ANAESTHESIA

> Make sure that an experienced and trained assistant is available to help you with induction. Never induce anaesthesia when alone with the patient.

Before starting, check that you have the *correct patient* scheduled for the *correct operation* on the *correct side*. The responsibility for this check belongs to both the anaesthetist and surgeon. The surgeon should mark the operation site with an indelible marker before the patient comes to the operating room.

Check that the patient has been properly prepared for the operation and has had no food or drink for the appropriate period of time. It is normal to withhold solid food for six hours preoperatively, but a milk feed can be given to babies up to three hours preoperatively. Clear fluids are regarded as safe up to two hours preoperatively if gastric function is normal.

Measure the patient's pulse and blood pressure, and try to make him or her as relaxed and comfortable as possible.

> Induction of anaesthesia is a critical moment. Before inducing anaesthesia – *check*.

Before you start, check the patient's progress through the hospital up to this moment. Then check that your actions will be the right ones. It is also vital to check your equipment before you give an anaesthetic. The patient's life may depend on it.

Make sure that:

- All the apparatus you intend to use, or might need, is available and working
- If you are using compressed gases, there is enough gas and a reserve oxygen cylinder
- The anaesthetic vaporizers are connected
- The breathing system that delivers gas to the patient is securely and correctly assembled
- Breathing circuits are clean
- Resuscitation apparatus is present and working
- Laryngoscope, tracheal tubes and suction apparatus are ready and have been decontaminated
- Needles and syringes are sterile: never use the same syringe or needle for more than one patient
- Drugs you intend to use are drawn up into labelled syringes
- Any other drugs you might need are in the room.

> Always begin your anaesthetic with the patient lying on a table or trolley that can be rapidly tilted into a head-down position in case of sudden hypotension or vomiting.

Before inducing anaesthesia, always ensure adequate intravenous access by inserting an indwelling needle or cannula in a large vein, unless this is impossible.

The choice of technique for induction of anaesthesia lies between:

- Intravenous injection of a barbiturate, ketamine or propofol
- Intramuscular injection of ketamine
- Inhalational induction ("gas induction").

INTRAVENOUS INDUCTION

Intravenous induction is pleasant for the patient and easy for the anaesthetist. It will be the technique of choice in many cases, but care is always needed as it is relatively easy to give an overdose or to stop the patient from breathing. If breathing stops, the patient may die unless you can easily ventilate the lungs with a face mask or tracheal tube.

The first rule of intravenous induction is that it must *never* be used in a patient whose airway is likely to be difficult to manage. For such a patient, inhalational induction is inherently much safer. Alternatively, the patient should be intubated while still awake. Intravenous induction will also suddenly reveal any pre-existing dehydration, hypovolaemia or hypotension. These conditions must be corrected preoperatively or there will be a dangerous fall in blood pressure on injection of the drug.

Thiopental

Thiopental is presented as ampoules of yellow powder that must be dissolved before use in sterile distilled water or saline to make a solution of 2.5% (25 mg/ml). Higher concentrations are dangerous, especially if accidentally injected outside a vein, and should not be used.

The normal practice is to give a "sleep" dose, by injecting the drug slowly, until the patient becomes unconscious and loses the eyelash reflex. The average sleep dose in a healthy adult is 5 mg/kg of body weight, but much less (2 mg/kg) is needed in sick patients. An overdose of thiopental will cause:

- Hypotension
- Respiratory arrest.

Injection of thiopental is almost always painless. If the patient reports pain, stop injecting immediately because the needle is probably outside the vein and may even have entered an artery. Avoid injection into the elbow, if possible, because it is easy to enter the brachial artery by mistake.

Thiopental is cumulative in the body and slowly metabolized. It is therefore not suitable for the maintenance of anaesthesia.

Propofol

Propofol is a recently introduced, intravenous anaesthetic that can be used for induction of anaesthesia. It is a white emulsion which, like thiopental,

14

Drugs used in anaesthesia

Drug	Average dose	Route of administration	Special precautions, side effects
Induction agents			
Thiopental	4–5 mg/kg	IV	Cardiorespiratory depression, loss of airway
Propofol	1.5–2.5 mg/kg	IV	Cardiorespiratory depression, apnoea, loss of airway
Ketamine	1–3 mg/kg 6–8 mg/kg	IV IM	Hypertension, avoid in pre-eclampsia and head injury
Inhaled anaesthetics			
Halothane	1–2%	Inhalation	Hypotension, cardiac arrhythmias
Ether	3–8%	Inhalation	Respiratory irritation, flammable agent, slow recovery
Nitrous oxide	50–70%	Inhalation	Awareness, hypoxic mixtures
Relaxants			
Suxamethonium	1 mg/kg	IV/IM	Anaphylactoid reactions, malignant hyperthermia (very rare) Drug degrades in hot climates
Vecuronium	0.2 mg/kg	IV	Use only if you have reversal drugs
Opiate analgesics			
Morphine	0.2 mg/kg	IV/IM	Respiratory depression
Pethidine	1 mg/kg	IV/IM	Respiratory depression
Benzodiazepines			
Diazepam	0.1–0.15 mg/kg	IV	Respiratory depression, loss of consciousness, adverse effects on fetus if given before delivery
Local anaesthetics	**Maximum dose**		
Lidocaine plain	4 mg/kg	IV/inf/ spinal/ topical	CNS and cardiovascular depression, convulsions
Lidocaine with epinephrine (adrenaline)	7 mg/kg	As lidocaine	CNS and cardiovascular depression, convulsions
Bupivacaine	2.0 mg/kg	As lidocaine but **not** IV	CNS depression, cardiac arrest
Vasoconstrictors			
Ephedrine	5–10 mg bolus (adult)	IV	Essential drug for spinal anaesthesia
Drugs used in resuscitation			
Epinephrine (adrenaline)	0.5–1 mg	IV/IM (adult) for anaphylaxis	
Atropine		0.6 mg bolus IV/IM (up to 3 mg for organophosphate poisoning)	

produces unconsciousness in one arm to brain circulation. Its depressant effects on respiration and blood pressure are greater than those of thiopental, especially if it is injected quickly and, after injection, there is often a respiratory arrest requiring manual inflation of the patient's lungs. Injection is often painful unless a small amount of lidocaine (20 mg of lidocaine in 200 mg of propofol) is added just before injection.

The chief advantage of propofol is in the quality of recovery. Patients are much less drowsy postoperatively; this is an advantage if they have to leave hospital the same day.

The normal induction dose of propofol is 2–2.5 mg/kg of body weight. At present, it is much more expensive than thiopental. To avoid bacterial contamination, ampoules must be used immediately after being opened.

Ketamine

Induction with ketamine is similar in principle to induction with thiopental and the same precautions apply. The average induction dose is 1–2 mg/kg of body weight. The standard formulations are:

- 50 mg/ml
- 100 mg/ml.

Be sure to check which formulation of ketamine you have.

The patient's appearance as he or she loses consciousness is different from when barbiturates are used and the patient may not appear to be "asleep". The eyes may remain open, but the patient will no longer respond to your voice or command or to painful stimuli. If you try to insert an oropharyngeal airway at this stage, the patient will probably spit it out. Muscle tone in the jaw is usually well maintained after ketamine has been given, as is the cough reflex. A safe airway is not guaranteed since, if regurgitation or vomiting of gastric contents occurs, there is still severe danger of aspiration into the lungs.

After induction with ketamine, you may choose to proceed to a conventional inhalational anaesthetic, with or without relaxants and intubation. For short procedures, increments of ketamine may be given intravenously or intramuscularly every few minutes to prevent the patient responding to painful stimulation. This method of anaesthesia is simple, but produces no muscular relaxation. Ketamine is also not a cheap drug. If your supplies are limited, try to reserve ketamine for cases where there are few suitable alternatives; for example, for short procedures in children when access to the airway may be difficult.

Suxamethonium

Suxamethonium is a depolarizing, short-acting muscle relaxant which is widely used to facilitate intubation, especially for emergencies. The dose is 1–2 mg/kg or 100 mg for a full size adult or a woman having a caesarean section under general anaesthesia. It gives a rapid onset of total paralysis when given intravenously. Intramuscular suxamethonium is also effective within 2–4 minutes.

There are circumstances when suxamethonium should never be given; commonly encountered contraindications are:

- Potential or established airway obstruction: for example, after facial trauma
- Serum potassium level that is already high, such as in renal failure, or that might rise, such as in severe burns
- Allergy to the drug or a family history of malignant hyperthermia.

Other non-depolarizing relaxants have a longer duration of action and generally require specialist skills to be safe. They are beyond the scope of this book.

INTRAMUSCULAR INDUCTION

Ketamine may also be given by intramuscular injection to induce anaesthesia. With a dose of 6–8 mg/kg of body weight, induction occurs within a few minutes, followed by 10–15 minutes of surgical anaesthesia. At 8 mg/kg of body weight, ketamine produces a marked increase in salivary secretions. If you use intramuscular ketamine, give atropine (which can be mixed with the ketamine) to prevent excessive salivation.

Further doses of ketamine can be given intramuscularly or intravenously, as required. Intramuscular doses last longer and wear off more slowly. If ketamine is used as the sole anaesthetic agent, patients sometimes complain afterwards of vivid dreams and hallucinations; giving diazepam either before or at the end of anaesthesia can reduce these. They do not occur if ketamine is used only for induction and is followed by a conventional anaesthetic.

INHALATIONAL INDUCTION

Inhalational anaesthesia forms the basis of most general anaesthetic techniques in common use, although intravenous techniques are an alternative. There are two different systems available for delivering anaesthetic gases and vapours to the patient:

- Draw-over system: uses air as the carrier gas with added volatile agents or compressed medical gases
- Continuous-flow system: compressed medical gases (which must have a minimum of 30% oxygen) pass through flow meters and vaporizers to supply anaesthetic to the patient.

Draw-over systems can be used with either cylinders or oxygen concentrators as their oxygen source; Boyle's machines function only if cylinders are available. The draw-over system is capable of producing first-class anaesthetic and surgical conditions. Modern draw-over apparatus has proved extremely reliable, easy to understand and maintain and economical in use. However, some small hospitals, and many larger ones, are equipped with continuous-flow machines. Detailed descriptions of both systems are found in *Anaesthesia at the District Hospital* (WHO, 2001).

Inhalation (gas) induction is the technique of choice for inducing anaesthesia when the patient's airway is difficult to manage. If you use an intravenous induction for such a patient and "lose" the airway, the patient may die of hypoxia if you are unable to ventilate the lungs. In contrast, inhalational induction can proceed only if the patient has a clear airway down which the anaesthetic can pass. If the airway becomes obstructed, the patient will stop taking up further anaesthetic and redistribution of the drug in the body will lighten the anaesthesia. As this happens, the patient will clear the obstruction. Inhalational induction is also preferred by some children who may object to needles.

Inhalational induction is an important technique. Practise regularly; it is simple and requires only patience, care and observation. Either draw-over or continuous-flow apparatus can be used for inhalational induction (Figure 14.2) but slightly differing techniques are needed.

Using draw-over apparatus

The best agents to use are ether (for example from the EMO or PAC vaporizer) and halothane (for example from the PAC or Oxford Miniature Vaporizer (OMV)). If oxygen is available (1 litre/minute), it should be added with a T-piece.

For a smooth induction:

1 Gently apply a well fitting face mask and begin induction with halothane. Halothane is preferable because, unlike ether, it is not an irritant.

   Gradually increase the concentration until the patient is asleep (maximum 2–3% halothane).

2 Then, slowly turn on the supply of ether and increase the concentration by 1% every five breaths. If the patient coughs or holds his or her breath, reduce the ether concentration immediately by a third of its setting and try again.

3 When you reach 8% ether, turn off the halothane. You may then proceed to laryngoscopy and intubation after further deepening the anaesthesia by increasing the ether concentration to about 15%.

   Watch for the onset of paralysis of the lower intercostal muscles to show that the anaesthesia is deep enough. The addition of oxygen is desirable at least until after intubation. At high altitude, you will need more oxygen supplement.

4 If your attempt at intubation does not succeed, reapply the face mask and deepen the anaesthesia again for a second attempt:
   - If intubation is still impossible, *but* you can maintain a clear airway using a face mask, you may proceed to give anaesthetic with the face mask, using ether at 7–10% to provide relaxation if required
   - If relaxation is not required, reduce the ether concentration to 6%. With ether at this concentration your patient can, if necessary, manage without oxygen supplementation, provided that he or she is not very young, old, ill or anaemic.

Take special care if halothane is used as an alternative to ether; it depresses the heart and respiration. Give additional oxygen if at all possible and use a tracheal tube and controlled ventilation for all but brief operations.

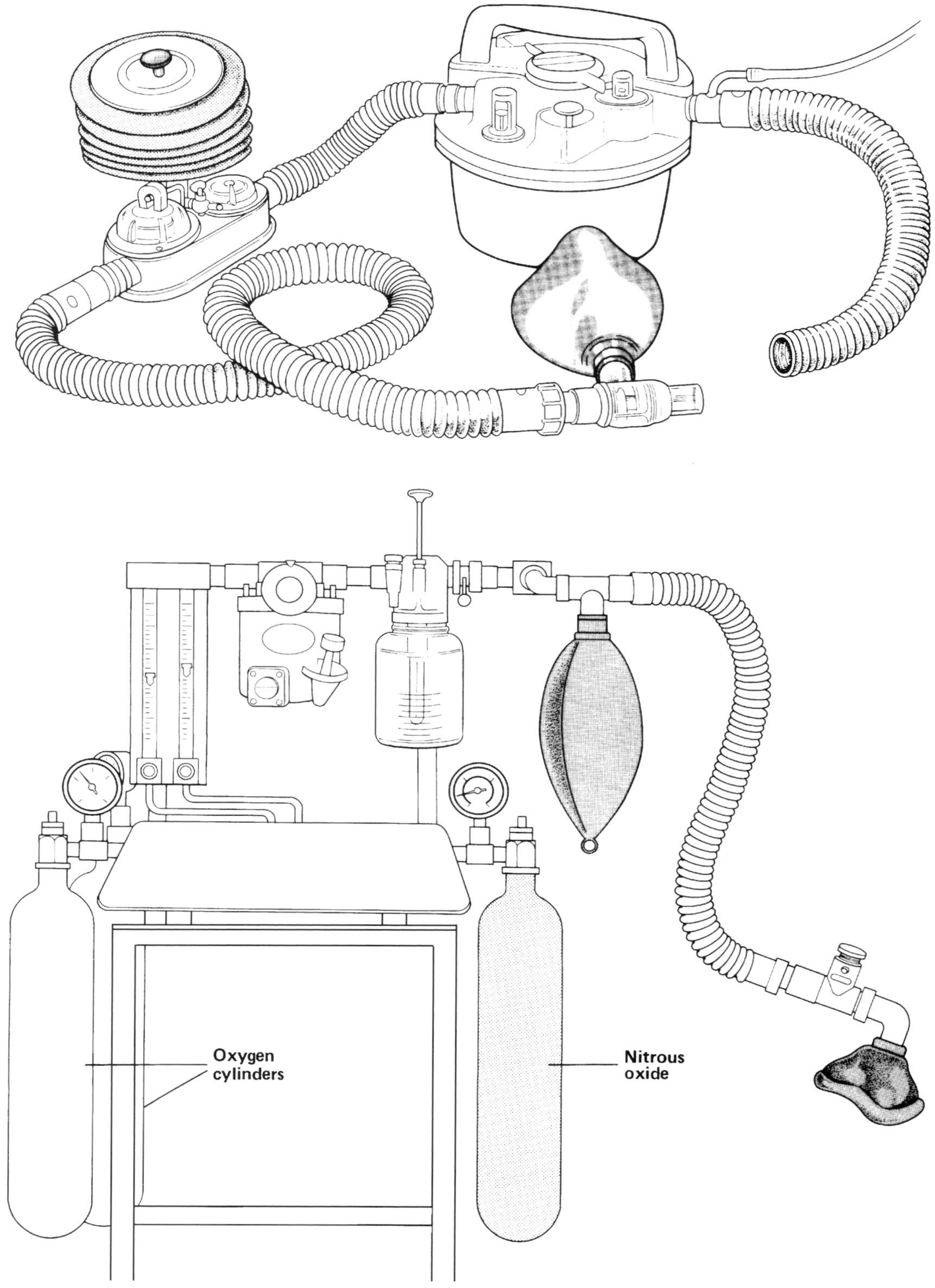

Figure 14.2

Using a compressed gas machine

1 Check your machine, making sure that you have adequate supplies of gas for the duration of anaesthesia:
- *Oxygen should be used at a concentration of not less than 30%* to allow for any leaks or inaccuracy of the flow meters
- Use an oxygen analyser at the gas outlet, if possible
- If you are using a one-way breathing valve at the patient end of the circuit, set the total gas flow (oxygen or oxygen plus nitrous oxide) higher than the patient's minute volume.

2 If you are using halothane as your main anaesthetic agent, place the face mask on the patient's face and gradually increase the halothane concentration up to a maximum of 3%, reducing it to 1.5% after the patient has settled or after intubation.

3 If you are using ether (without halothane) as your volatile agent:
- Turn on the supply of ether from the Boyle's bottle with the face mask held about 30 cm above the patient's face
- Gradually lower the mask over the next minute to slowly increase the ether concentration in the inspired gas; this is usually well tolerated
- Once the mask is in contact with the face, slowly increase the ether concentration over a few minutes
- The patient will be ready for intubation when you can see paradoxical (inward) movement of the lower ribs during inspiration.

MAINTENANCE OF ANAESTHESIA

All anaesthetics are constantly being eliminated from the body, either by being breathed out, metabolized or excreted by the kidney, so it is necessary to continue to give more drug throughout anaesthesia. There is no formula for calculating the amount you need to give. Only by monitoring the patient's physiology and responses can you decide if you need to increase, reduce or maintain the rate of administration

Anaesthesia too light

Check the patient is breathing adequately; retained carbon dioxide may be the cause. Signs that anaesthesia may be too light include:
- Patient moves
- Rising pulse and blood pressure
- Sweating, tears.

Anaesthesia too deep

- Falling pulse and blood pressure
- Depressed breathing.

In addition to monitoring the cardiovascular, respiratory and nervous systems, make regular checks of your equipment. The commonest cause of awareness during anaesthesia is the vaporizer running dry.

14

Waking the patient up

There is no antidote for anaesthesia:

- Whenever you give a drug, you must have an idea of how long its effect will last
- Different drugs wear off at different rates; be prepared to continue to support the patient's breathing and airway for as long as necessary at the end of the case
- Remove the tracheal tube only if the patient is either deeply anaesthetized (to avoid laryngeal spasm) or is awake.

Give extra oxygen before and after the end of the anaesthetic. Continue to monitor the patient just as carefully after you have turned the anaesthetic off until he or she is fully awake.

KEY POINTS

- If you plan to intubate, always have a backup plan in case of failure
- Don't persist with multiple attempts just to prove you can do it.

FAILED INTUBATION

Don't panic. Have a plan.

Expected difficult intubation

Before every intubation, but especially if you expect difficulties, have ready (or know the location of) emergency tools, such as:

- Intubating stylet
- Long bougie
- Laryngeal mask airway (LMA).

The LMA can often be passed to maintain the airway when intubation is impossible. If the stomach is full, as is often the case in emergencies, you will have to balance the risk of regurgitation with the LMA in place against the same risk during further attempts at intubation, or complete failure to intubate.

Unexpected difficult intubation

If you cannot see the larynx clearly enough to get the tube in, possible remedies include:

- Reposition the head – try a pillow under the head
- Pass an intubating bougie or use a stylet to make the tube more curved
- Hold the laryngoscope to give *upward* traction
- Reposition the blade if the tongue is blocking the view
- Change the blade:
  - If it is too big, you look down the oesophagus
  - If it is too small, you cannot lift the epiglottis
- Give further relaxant or deeper halothane anaesthesia to abolish reflexes.

Only if you can remedy one or more of the above problems should you try again, but remember to:

- Call for help
- Stay calm
- Re-oxygenate (mask and airway) and watch the oximeter
- Maintain cricoid pressure, if needed
- Consider the need for more atropine.

If intubation still fails, stop any further attempts at intubation. Remember that it is an abuse of the patient to have several people lining up to try their skills at this "interesting" case.

There are then the following two possible courses of action.

1 If the operation must now go ahead under general anaesthesia, for example, in haemorrhage, ruptured uterus, long standing intestinal obstruction:
   - Try inserting an LMA
   - If LMA insertion is not possible, try an oral airway and inhalation anaesthesia with a face mask
   - If neither of the above are possible, give ketamine with oxygen by face mask
   - Maintain cricoid pressure if there is a regurgitation risk.

2 If the operation can be postponed:
   - Allow the patient to wake up, while maintaining oxygenation and ventilation as best you can
   - Use regional or spinal anaesthesia or abandon the procedure and refer the patient.

Do not make your ability to intubate more important than the patient's life.

Endotracheal tube in the oesophagus

Apply the ten tests of correct tube placement on page 13–2. If in doubt, remove the tube and follow the steps above.

No ventilation of the lungs

If you thought intubation was successful, but you cannot ventilate the lungs, think of the following:

- Oesophageal tube
- Tube is blocked
- Patient circuit wrongly connected or configured
- Obstruction in the trachea
- Tube is against the wall of the trachea or tube cuff has herniated: *let down the cuff.*

Only if you have tested and eliminated the above, consider:

- Severe bronchospasm
- Wrong drug administration: e.g. neostigmine
- Aspiration of gastric contents

14

- Tension pneumothorax
- Pulmonary oedema
- Infection, such as bronchitis or pneumonia.

Vomiting and regurgitation

Seeing stomach contents in the unprotected airway of an unconscious patient is probably the worst thing that can happen in the practice of anaesthesia. Do not let this happen to you.

Aspiration of stomach contents into the lungs is often a terminal event for the patient. However, regurgitation is both predictable and avoidable.

This is the moment when you must act with the greatest speed. Options are:

- Tilt the bed head down, continue cricoid pressure (or put it on) and suck away the vomitus with the biggest, most powerful rigid sucker you can find
- Turn the patient on to the side and suck.

The choice will depend on which can be done fastest, according to the workings of the table, the available manpower and size of the patient. In either case, intubation is recommended as soon as possible to protect the airway and also to suck down the trachea, both for diagnostic and therapeutic reasons.

Give steroids, antibiotics and bronchodilators if aspiration is suspected. The pulse oximeter may show desaturation and the lungs may become stiff to inflate.

KEY POINTS

- If using general anaesthesia in an eclamptic patient, there may be a huge rise in blood pressure at intubation
- Prevent this with a bolus of 2–3 G magnesium sulfate before intubation.

14.2 ANAESTHESIA DURING PREGNANCY AND FOR OPERATIVE DELIVERY

Caesarean section is the commonest major operation in many areas of the developing world. Most cases present as emergencies in labour. Management of emergency caesarean section is the everyday activity of all anaesthetists.

Mothers may present *in extremis* in obstructed labour or with ruptured uterus, haemorrhage, sepsis or anaemia of several days' duration. The primary reason for performing caesarean section in these circumstances is to save a mother's life. Both general and spinal anaesthesia can be used. Epidural is less common owing to the time, expense and expertise required for use of the technique.

Several changes occurring in pregnancy are relevant for anaesthesia:

- Blood volume begins to rise
- Cardiac output begins to rise
- There is less increase in the number of red cells, so the haemoglobin concentration falls
- As the uterus enlarges, respiration comes to depend more on thoracic than diaphragmatic movement
- Gastric emptying becomes less efficient.

In late pregnancy:

- The uterus presses back on the inferior vena cava when the patient lies on her back, causing a fall in cardiac output
- There may also be a severe fall in blood pressure – the "supine hypotensive syndrome" – but most non-anaesthetized patients are able to maintain their blood pressure by widespread vasoconstriction
- During general or spinal anaesthesia, the capacity for vasoconstriction is lost; this is likely to result in a severe fall in blood pressure to levels that are dangerous for both mother and baby.

Supine hypotension can be prevented merely by ensuring that the mother is never fully supine.

A pillow or sandbag must always be placed under one hip to tilt the uterus slightly to one side; this is perfectly simple to do even with the patient in the lithotomy position. *This simple precaution must always be carried out in obstetric patients receiving either general or spinal/epidural anaesthesia.*

When you anaesthetize a pregnant woman for delivery, there are two patients to deal with: mother and child. Most drugs cross the placenta quickly. This is a problem, since the aim is to anaesthetize the mother, but to allow the baby to be born without any drug-induced depression of body functions, especially of respiration. For this reason, drugs that can cause depression of the fetus, such as sedative premedication, should not be given.

Don't be so concerned about the baby that you fail to give the mother a sufficient dose of anaesthetic.

A suitable general anaesthetic technique is outlined below. Spinal anaesthesia is often as good or better, and is described on pages 14–23 to 14–25.

1 Before inducing anaesthesia, give a 30 ml dose of a liquid antacid, such as sodium citrate 0.3 mol/litre (77.4 g/litre), to neutralize excess gastric acid.

2 Insert a wedge or cushion under one hip to tilt the uterus off the inferior vena cava:
   - Never induce anaesthesia with the patient in the lithotomy position
   - If she is already in that position, her legs must be lowered for induction to avoid regurgitation of gastric contents.

3 Set up a fast-flowing infusion of an appropriate fluid into a large vein and preoxygenate the patient.

4 Induce anaesthesia as for an emergency:
   - Preoxygenate
   - Apply cricoid pressure
   - Administer a previously calculated dose of thiopental or ketamine
   - Intubate the patient after giving suxamethonium
   - Give IPPV.

For a full account of managing the full stomach, see page 13–32.

14

Laryngoscopy in the pregnant woman is sometimes more difficult than usual. Always prepare a spare tube of a small size (5–6 mm) in case the patient has laryngeal oedema secondary to pre-eclampsia.

Avoid high concentrations of ether or halothane, as these will reduce the uterine tone and increase bleeding. However, in a spontaneously breathing patient, you will not be able to maintain adequate anaesthesia (the mother will push) at ether concentrations below about 8–10% or halothane below 1.5%. You may give opiates intravenously once the umbilical cord is clamped and then reduce the concentration of the volatile agent.

Be prepared to give an oxytocic drug intravenously when requested by the surgeon, but never give ergometrine to a woman with pre-eclampsia as it may cause a hypertensive crisis. Syntocinon causes hypotension and should be given in two divided doses of 5 mg IV.

The average blood loss from caesarean section is 600–700 ml, so make sure that you give enough fluid replacement. You may need to transfuse blood.

In addition to looking after the mother, you may have to resuscitate the baby, so be prepared with infant resuscitation equipment and a separate oxygen supply.

If mother and child are both critically ill, it is your clear duty to attend to the mother first.

Always try to have a trained assistant with you for these cases. At the end of anaesthesia, remember that the mother still has a full stomach; remove the tracheal tube with her in the lateral position.

KEY POINTS

- For children under 15 kg, differences in anatomy and physiology mean you will have to significantly modify your anaesthetic technique
- Pay special attention to fluid and heat losses in children.

14.3 PAEDIATRIC ANAESTHESIA

PRINCIPLES

Most of the general principles of anaesthesia can be applied to children, but there are some significant anatomical and physiological differences between children and adults that can cause problems, especially in neonates and children weighing less than about 15 kg.

Airway

Children have a large head in relation to body size and you must therefore position them differently from an adult, sometimes with a pillow under the shoulders rather than the head, to clear the airway or to perform laryngoscopy.

The larynx of a child also differs from that of an adult. In the adult, the narrowest part of the air passage is at the level of the vocal cords; in the child the narrowest part is below this, at the level of the cricoid cartilage:

- The airway is circular in cross–section, so a correct fit can usually be obtained with a plain (not cuffed) tracheal tube

- A small air leak should usually be present around the tube, but if a completely airtight fit is required, pack the pharynx with gauze moistened with water or saline; never use liquid paraffin (mineral oil), as this causes lung damage
- It is acceptable to use a cuffed tube of less than 6.0 mm, but do not inflate the cuff.

Because the airway of a child is narrow, a small amount of oedema can produce severe obstruction (Figure 14.3).

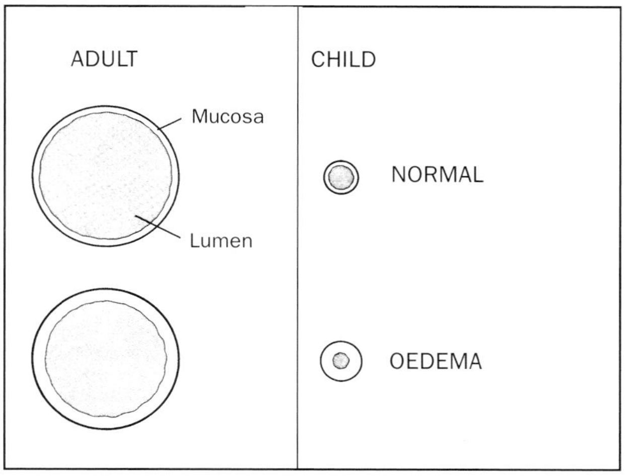

Figure 14.3

Oedema can easily be caused by forcing in a tracheal tube that is too tight, so if you suspect that your tube is too large, change it immediately. Damage is most likely from a tube that is both too large and left in the trachea too long.

As a rough guide for normally nourished children more than about 2 years old, use the following formula to calculate the internal diameter of the tube likely to be of the correct size.

Internal diameter of tube (mm) = (age in years + 4.5) ÷ 4

Other rough indicators of the correct size of tube are:

- Diameter the same as the child's little finger
- Most neonates will need a tube of 3 mm internal diameter
- For premature infants, a 2.5 mm tube may be necessary
- To estimate the length of tube needed, double the distance from the corner of the child's mouth to the ear canal
- To check, look at the child's head from the side while holding the upper end of the tube level with the mouth to give you an idea of how far into the chest the tube will go.

Always have one tube a size larger and one a size smaller ready in case you need to change.

For infants, use a small straight laryngoscope blade. If one is not available, use the tip of a Macintosh blade designed for adults as it is only slightly curved. After intubation, always listen over both lungs to make sure that the tube has not entered a bronchus.

Abdomen

A child's abdomen is more protuberant than an adult's and it contains the greater part of the viscera. (Many of the viscera of an adult are situated in the relatively larger pelvic cavity). The diaphragm is therefore less efficient in a child. The rib cage is also less rigid than an adult's. These factors mean that abdominal distension can very easily give rise to respiratory difficulty.

Metabolic rate

The metabolic rate is higher in children than in adults, while the lungs are less efficient and smaller in relation to oxygen requirements. For this reason, children have higher respiratory rates than adults and their lungs must be ventilated more rapidly. Obstruction or apnoea leads to a very rapid onset of cyanosis.

Heart rate

The normal heart rate at birth is about 140 per minute, but it may swing widely in response to stress.

A child's heart rate is higher than that of an adult, but the resting sympathetic tone is low, so reflex vagal stimulation can lead to severe bradycardia: e.g during laryngoscopy or surgery. For this reason, atropine (0.015 mg/kg of body weight) is almost always included in premedication for infants.

Hypothermia can occur very rapidly in an infant because of the high surface-to-volume ratio of the body; it may result in a severe metabolic disturbance.

Hypoglycaemia

Hypoglycaemia may be a problem in babies:

- Babies do not need to be starved for more than three hours preoperatively and should be fed as soon as possible after the operation
- Use glucose infusions during anaesthesia:
  - To help to maintain the blood sugar level
  - Infuse glucose instead of physiological saline to avoid a sodium load that the baby's kidneys are unable to excrete
  - For most paediatric operations, other than minor ones, give glucose 5% (or glucose 4% with saline 0.18%) at a rate of 5 ml/kg of body weight per hour in addition to replacing the measured fluid losses.

Blood volume

The neonate has a proportionately higher blood volume (90 ml/kg of body weight) than the adult (70 ml/kg) but, even so, what appears to be a small blood loss may have serious effects:

- Measure blood losses during the operation as accurately as possible; if suction apparatus is in use, a simple method is to use a measuring cylinder in the suction line rather than the usual large container
- If blood loss amounts to more than 5% of blood volume, an intravenous infusion is necessary
- If blood loss exceeds 10–20% of blood volume, consider blood transfusion.

PAEDIATRIC ELECTIVE ANAESTHESIA

Most children weighing more than 15 kg can be anaesthetized by using the techniques described in this book for adult patients, but with the dosage reduced in relation to weight.

In children below 15 kg, the anatomical and physiological differences described above become more important and inhalational apparatus must be adapted, although ketamine can be used without any modifications in technique. "Adult" breathing systems give rise to problems in small children because the valves have too large a dead space. In addition, vaporizers of the draw-over type do not work effectively at the low minute/volumes and flows generated by an infant's lungs. These problems can be overcome in a number of ways:

- Replace the adult-size breathing valve with an infant-size valve that has a smaller internal volume and dead space
- If possible, replace the adult-size bag with a small one
- You must use intubation and controlled ventilation for infants under 10 kg; the flow you generate into the bellows during IPPV will be enough to allow the vaporizer to work reasonably accurately.

If oxygen is available, you can convert a draw-over system to a continuous-flow mode.

1 Connect a flow of oxygen from a cylinder or concentrator (or oxygen plus nitrous oxide) to the side arm of your oxygen-enrichment T-piece and close off the open end with a bung.

2 Set the fresh gas flow to 300 ml/kg of body weight per minute with a minimum of 3 litres/minute.

3 Intubate and ventilate the patient or allow spontaneous breathing using an Ayre's T-piece system, as described below. Use a T-piece system (Ayre's T-piece) instead of the Magill breathing system usually used for adults. The valveless T-piece system requires a relatively high gas flow, but is suitable for both spontaneous and controlled ventilation.

Spontaneous breathing can be monitored by watching the slight movement of the open-ended reservoir bag. To change to controlled ventilation:

1 Hold the bag in your hand with your thumb towards the patient.

2 Partly occlude the outlet by curling your little finger round it (this needs practice) and squeeze the bag in the palm of your hand to inflate the lungs.

3 Then release the bag to allow the expired gas to escape.

Continuous monitoring of heart rate and respiration is essential in small children. A precordial or oesophageal stethoscope is invaluable for this.

- Use an infant-sized cuff to measure the blood pressure
- Palpate the arterial pulses and check the colour and perfusion of the extremities
- Monitor the urine flow if a urinary catheter is in place; a good urine output (0.5 ml/hour per kg of body weight) is reassuring
- At the end of the operation, check the temperature to ensure that the patient has not become hypothermic.

PAEDIATRIC EMERGENCY ANAESTHESIA

The techniques in emergency neonatal and paediatric anaesthesia are not very different from those required in elective paediatric anaesthesia. Few major paediatric surgical cases are performed at the district hospital level. Here the common requirement is for ketamine or inhalation anaesthesia with halothane for incision and drainage of abscess or removal of foreign body.

Anaesthesia management for foreign body removal is given on pages 14–32 to 14–34. Other emergency airway problems in children include:

- Croup
- Epiglottitis
- Retropharyngeal abscess
- Laryngeal polyps.

Croup, tracheobronchitis and epiglottitis

Croup is the name for laryngo-tracheitis and describes the characteristic cough. Conservative treatment is usually possible: avoid over-stimulation of the child and give:

- Humidified oxygen
- Nebulized epinephrine
- Antibiotics
- Steroids: dexamethasone 0.15 mg/kg intravenously daily.

Epiglottitis (and severe croup that is not responding to treatment) can make the epiglottis and larynx so swollen that the airway is almost blocked. The child is very unwilling to lie down and copious secretions run out of the mouth because swallowing is painful. The child is also febrile, distressed, toxic and cyanosed so careful handling is essential. Do not attempt to put up an intravenous infusion while the child is awake as this will cause deterioration. A lateral X-ray shows the “thumb print” sign of the enlarged epiglottis.

Do not send a child in respiratory distress to the X-ray department. Urgent management is needed.

Take the child to the operating room and prepare every available aid to intubation:

- Smaller size tracheal tubes with pre-inserted, lubricated stylets
- Spare laryngoscopes with different blades
- Emergency cricothyroid puncture kit or intravenous cannula, if available.

Without any delay, with suction ready:

1 Hold the child firmly in the sitting position and give inhalation induction with halothane and oxygen until asleep.

2 Continue for as long as possible (usually the airway will become obstructed at some stage) then transfer to the supine position and intubate as quickly as you can:
   - Be prepared for distorted anatomy
   - A small tracheal tube with introducer is essential
   - Make sure the surgeon is prepared for an emergency cricothyroid puncture if you cannot intubate and cardiorespiratory arrest is about to occur.

3 Keep the child intubated for at least 24 hours in an intensive care location with constant nursing, suction, oxygen and high dose antibiotics.

Ensure that the nurses understand the need to prevent the tube becoming blocked with dried secretions.

Retropharyngeal abscess

Retropharyngeal abscess is quite common in younger babies. In areas of high HIV prevalence, it can occur in any age group. The cry is characteristic of obstruction just above the larynx. Feel the swollen neck and examine the oropharynx with a wooden spatula or your finger and the presence of a fluctuant retropharyngeal abscess should be very obvious. A wide bore needle aspiration confirms the diagnosis.

There are two ways to manage the case.

1 Inhalation induction with oxygen and halothane, tracheal intubation and incision and drainage with a rigid sucker to completely evacuate the cavity,

   Or

2 In very young babies before dentition, avoid any anaesthesia, puncture the abscess with a pair of forceps while the patient is awake, then immediately turn the baby face-down so the pus runs out.

The first method allows better access for suction and complete evacuation of the retropharyngeal space.

Laryngeal polyps or papillomata

Laryngeal polyps are a problem in children of all ages. Acute airway obstruction can occur, so patients sometimes present as emergencies:

- Induce deep inhalational anaesthesia
- Gently remove as many papillomata as you can with Magill's forceps, avoiding damage to the cords from where the papillomata are arising

- Have good suction ready and wear a pair of goggles
- Have a small endotracheal tube with introducer ready at all times.

The polyps can recur for years and semi-permanent tracheostomy is sometimes required.

Other paediatric emergencies

Typical major emergency cases presenting at a referral hospital might be laparotomy (for colostomy in cases of imperforate anus, Hirschsprung's disease or other intestinal obstruction), peritonitis or surgery for major trauma.

PREPARATIONS BEFORE INDUCTION

- Intravenous infusion:
  - Always use a paediatric burette and avoid, if at all possible, connecting a neonate or infant to a 1 litre bag via a normal adult giving set (see page 13–17)
  - Add 10 ml 50% dextrose to 100 ml in the burette
- Endotracheal tube sizes: have available all the sizes from 3.0 to 6.5 mm
- Empty a full stomach:
  - Just before starting anaesthesia, pass a wide bore orogastric tube into the stomach to empty it
  - Apply gentle suction while moving the tube around then remove it.

Temperature

Most patients undergoing emergency surgery and anaesthesia will become hypothermic during the procedure, particularly during a long operation. This is especially true of babies and neonates. There are various measures that will minimize hypothermia:

- Warm the operating room
- Use an electric heating blanket, but check the control and beware of overheating, burns and electric shock
- Wrap the baby in warm, dry towels
- Reduce the time that skin is uncovered during induction and preparation of the skin
- Warm blood and IV fluids: see *The Clinical Use of Blood* (WHO, 2001, pages 120–121)
- Use heated IV fluid bags near the patient; again, beware burns
- Transfer the patient from the incubator to the operating table at the latest possible moment
- Use an overhead radiant heater during induction and postoperatively in ICU.

Hypothermia down to 33–34 °C causes:

- Respiratory depression
- Shivering
- General circulatory collapse with vasoconstriction.

Hypothermia does not itself cause any harm and the patient may be allowed to warm up with the assistance of an overhead heater, if available, provided that:

- Ventilation is supported for a few hours postoperatively
- Oxygenation is maintained
- Cardiovascular indices are maintained, such as urine output and blood pressure.

As the temperature rises, vasodilatation will cause a fall in blood pressure which must be corrected with volume replacement.

Atropine is well known to exacerbate hyperthermia and tachycardia and may even precipitate febrile convulsions. It should be avoided in a febrile child.

14.4 CONDUCTION ANAESTHESIA

Practical conduction anaesthesia cannot be learned from a book, but only by working with an experienced practitioner. For a detailed description of some common techniques, see *Anaesthesia at the District Hospital* (WHO, 2001).

Techniques of conduction (regional) anaesthesia use locally acting drugs to block nerve impulses before they reach the central nervous system.

Local anaesthetic drugs depress the electrical excitability of tissues. When injected close to nerves, they block the passage of the depolarization wave necessary for the transmission of nerve impulses.

TOXICITY AND SAFETY OF LOCAL ANAESTHETIC DRUGS

All local anaesthetic drugs:

- Are potentially toxic
- May depress the central nervous system
- May cause drowsiness, which may progress to unconsciousness with twitching and possibly convulsions
- May cause hypotension related either to extensive sympathetic blockade, (for example, after "high" spinal anaesthesia) or to direct depression of cardiac function from high blood levels of the drug.

These reactions are most likely to occur if the drug is accidentally injected into a vein or if an overdose is given by using either too high a concentration or too large a volume of drug.

Toxic effects – usually cardiac dysrhythmias – may also occur after intravascular injection or rapid absorption of a vasoconstrictor drug, such as epinephrine, which is frequently mixed with local anaesthetic to prolong the latter's action. Occasionally, patients have a true allergic reaction to the local anaesthetic drug, but this is unusual.

If a severe toxic reaction occurs, prompt resuscitation is needed:

- Give oxygen and IPPV if there is severe respiratory depression
- Give a dose of suxamethonium and ventilate the lungs for the initial treatment of convulsions, when associated with hypoxia

KEY POINTS

- Local anaesthetic drugs can be toxic – you must know the maximum safe dose
- Avoid spinal anaesthesia in patients who are shocked or not fully resuscitated.

- If the convulsions persist, you may need to give anticonvulsant drugs such as diazepam or thiopental intravenously, but do not give them as first-line treatment to a patient who may be hypotensive.

It follows from the above that full facilities for resuscitation should be available whenever you use conduction anaesthesia, just as they should when you use general anaesthesia.

As with all drugs, the maximum safe dose is related to the size and condition of the patient. Avoid toxicity by using the most dilute solution that will do the job, for example:

- 1% lidocaine or 0.25% bupivacaine for most nerve blocks
- 0.5% lidocaine or prilocaine for simple infiltration.

The rate of absorption of the drug can also be reduced by injecting it together with a vasoconstrictor drug, such as epinephrine, which is most often used in a dilution of 5 mg/ml (1:200 000); for infiltration, 2.5 mg/ml (1:400 000) is enough. Pre-mixed ampoules of local anaesthetic and epinephrine are often available but, if they are not, you can easily mix your own.

To make a 1:200000 dilution of epinephrine (adrenaline), add 0.1 ml of 1:1000 epinephrine to 20 ml of local anaesthetic solution.

The addition of epinephrine has two useful effects:

- It reduces the rate at which local anaesthetic is absorbed from the injection site, by causing vasoconstriction, and therefore allows a larger dose of local anaesthetic to be used without toxic effects
- Since local anaesthetic is removed from the injection site more slowly, the duration of anaesthesia increases by up to 50%.

When injecting local anaesthetic, use a small gauge needle:

- 21 or 23 gauge for nerve blocks
- 23 or 25 gauge for infiltration.

This reduces the risk of toxicity; it is easy to inject an excessive dose through a large-bore needle.

The maximum safe doses of various local anaesthetic drugs are shown in the following table.

Drug	Maximum dose mg/kg	Maximum dose mg/60 kg adult
Lidocaine 1%	4	240
Lidocaine 1% + epinephrine 1:200 000	7	420
Bupivacaine 0.25%/0.5%	2	120

Contraindications and precautions

It is a common misconception that general anaesthesia is more dangerous than conduction anaesthesia. In fact, for major surgery, there is no evidence of any difference in morbidity and mortality between patients undergoing good-quality general anaesthesia and those undergoing conduction anaesthesia.

Certain specific contraindications to conduction anaesthesia exist, including:

- True allergy to local anaesthetic drugs
- Sepsis at the intended site of injection
- Inability to guarantee sterile equipment for injection
- Systemic treatment of the patient with anticoagulant drugs.

General precautions and basic equipment:

- Ensure that the patient has been properly prepared and fasted, as for general anaesthesia
- Ensure that apparatus for resuscitation is at hand in case there is an adverse reaction
- Insert an IV cannula and, for major operations, set up an intravenous infusion of an appropriate fluid.

Sedation during conduction anaesthesia

Patients undergoing surgery under conduction anaesthesia often need some sedation to reduce anxiety or to help them to lie still. This is best achieved by oral premedication – drugs taken orally are safer and less expensive. A small additional dose of intravenous sedative is sometimes necessary, but do not use this to "cover up" an inadequate conduction technique.

> Do not let "sedation" drift into unconsciousness with an uncontrolled airway. A sedated patient should still be able to talk to you.

SPINAL ANAESTHESIA

Spinal anaesthesia is a technique commonly used for caesarean section (CS). When given by an experienced anaesthetist for an elective caesarean section, it can be safe and very effective. Nevertheless, it represents a major physiological disturbance and may be dangerous or even fatal when used in emergency for a patient who is dehydrated, hypovolaemic or shocked.

For sick patients undergoing emergency caesarean section, the recommended techniques are:

- General anaesthesia with ketamine
- General inhalational anaesthesia
- Local infiltration techniques.

Management of a high or total spinal

Do not ignore signs that your spinal anaesthetic is progressing higher than the maximum permissible level of T4 (the nipple line). As soon you have given the spinal and positioned the patient, observe the effects. These commence faster with lidocaine than with bupivacaine. The onset of the spinal block at the correct height should make the mother comfortable because the pains of labour are abolished. Signs of respiratory distress and hypotension include:

- Restlessness
- Difficulty in breathing
- Complains of nausea or vomits
- Cannot speak
- Rolls head from side to side
- Loses consciousness
- Hypoxia.

These are very serious warning signs. Additionally, you may find the blood pressure and heart rate have fallen unacceptably (below 80 mmHg systolic and less than 50–60 beats/minute). Ask the patient to squeeze your hand: if she cannot, she may be unconscious or paralysed. It is usually not possible to know precisely if the patient is unresponsive because of hypotension (reduced cerebral blood flow) or because the spinal solution has spread too high.

Act immediately to treat the unresponsive patient, whether the cause is hypotension or a high spinal.

Managing unexpected effects of a spinal anaesthetic

To treat hypotension:

1. Increase the rate of fluid infusion as fast as possible, using a pressure bag, if needed.
2. Tilt the table to the left, if not already tilted.
3. Give a vasopressor: ephedrine 10 mg, repeated as necessary.

To treat the respiratory difficulty, give oxygen and IPPV, using an anaesthetic face mask and self-inflating bag or bellows, or the anaesthetic machine patient circuit.

At this point, it is possible that the situation will resolve itself: the heart rate and blood pressure may rise again, the patient breathes unassisted and you continue with spinal anaesthesia.

Equally, however, the high spinal may progress further, or even become a "total spinal". In this condition, there is no detectable cardiopulmonary activity. Start the following emergency measures without delay, as for any cardiopulmonary resuscitation:

- Intubation
- Ventilation with oxygen
- Intravenous epinephrine.

The question often arises: how should you intubate a mother who is clearly unable to breathe (and when inflation by mask is insufficient) but who is still conscious? Do you need to give thiopental and suxamethonium?

In the presence of hypotension:

- Avoid thiopental: give 10 mg of diazepam instead

- Judge the need for suxamethonium to intubate on the basis of the patient's the state of relaxation
- Give 0.2–0.5 mg of epinephrine intravenously if the blood pressure does not respond to ephedrine.

A high or total spinal is a "pharmacological" cardiopulmonary arrest occurring in a healthy person. Every case should make a complete recovery. Death or cerebral damage from delayed recognition of the signs or poor management is inexcusable.

A death or complication after spinal anaesthesia is usually due to neglect of vital signs.

14.5 SPECIMEN ANAESTHETIC TECHNIQUES

KETAMINE ANAESTHESIA

Ketamine as the sole method of anaesthesia is widely used without any safeguards of the airway. However, it cannot be recommended as a completely safe method in the presence of a full stomach due to the risk of regurgitation and aspiration.

Ketamine anaesthesia is suitable:

- When muscle relaxation is not required, especially in children
- As a "fall-back" technique if your inhalational apparatus, or gas supply for a Boyle's machine, fails
- If you have to give general anaesthesia without inhalational apparatus, for example at an accident to release a trapped casualty.

Unsupplemented ketamine

1 Give a sedative drug and atropine as premedication.

2 Insert an indwelling intravenous needle or cannula. In a struggling child, it is more convenient to delay this until after ketamine has been given intramuscularly.

3 Give ketamine 6–8 mg/kg of body weight intramuscularly or 1–2 mg/kg intravenously (mixed with an appropriate dose of atropine, if not already given in premedication).

4 After intravenous injection of ketamine, the patient will be ready for surgery in 2–3 minutes, and after intramuscular injection in 3–5 minutes.

5 Give supplementary doses of ketamine if the patient responds to painful stimuli. Use half the original intravenous dose or a quarter of the original intramuscular dose.

GENERAL ANAESTHESIA WITH INTUBATION

This technique is suitable as a universal method of giving anaesthesia to an adult for any major surgery, including caesarean section, or if intubation is specifically indicated: for example, for protection of the airway.

KEY POINTS

- Ketamine is a full general anaesthetic; do not neglect routine precautions
- General anaesthesia with intubation and controlled ventilation is effectively a universal technique – although relatively time-consuming for short cases, there is almost no procedure for which it is unsuitable.

It is contraindicated when difficult intubation is anticipated. See page 14–32.

Normally it is expected that spontaneous breathing will return after the initial muscle relaxation required for intubation has worn off, but it cannot be assumed that this will happen or that breathing will be adequate for every patient. Some patients will have adequate spontaneous respiration throughout the procedure; others will not.

The following will make it *less* likely that a patient will have adequate spontaneous breathing under anaesthesia:

- Exaggerated reflex response from intubation: for example, abdominal straining, rise in blood pressure
- Strong surgical stimulation
- Obesity or any cause of diminished respiratory function
- Head down position
- Unusually muscular patient
- Surgery around, or movement of, the head, neck or tracheal tube
- Upper abdominal surgery
- Use of halothane without analgesic supplement
- Small size tracheal tube.

An open thoracic procedure cannot, of course, be conducted with spontaneous breathing. See page 14–38 for how to monitor for adequacy of respiration.

Unless contraindicated, it is important that you give an analgesic supplement (for example, pethidine 1 mg/kg intravenously at induction) if halothane is to be the sole agent for maintenance of anaesthesia.

1 Preoxygenate the patient by giving:
   - High concentration of oxygen to breathe for at least 3 minutes

   Or
   - 10 breaths of pure oxygen at a flow of 10 litres/minute from a closely fitting anaesthetic face mask.

   Loading the lungs with oxygen in this way allows the patient to remain well oxygenated even if tracheal intubation takes several minutes.

2 If there is a risk of regurgitation of stomach contents, apply cricoid pressure from the time of injection of anaesthetic until the trachea has been successfully intubated with a cuffed tracheal tube.

3 Induce anaesthesia with a sleep dose of thiopental, usually 5 mg/kg of body weight for an adult, injected intravenously over 30–45 seconds.

4 Intubate the trachea after producing muscle relaxation with suxamethonium (1 mg/kg of body weight).

5 Ventilate either with 10% ether or 1.5% halothane for 3 minutes to establish inhalational anaesthesia.

6 When the effect of suxamethonium wears off, usually after 3–5 minutes, await the return of spontaneous breathing. Oxygen supplementation is mandatory if halothane is used and is strongly advised for ether. Do not allow surgical diathermy if you are using ether.

7 If spontaneous breathing is inadequate, you must support the respiration by manual assistance or by mechanical ventilation. With the latter, you may additionally give a long acting (non-depolarizing) muscle relaxant. The detailed description of this technique is beyond the scope of this book.

8 At the end of surgery, turn off the inhalational anaesthetic agent and give as much oxygen as possible. As the anaesthetic wears off, respiration will become irregular and breath-holding will occur.

9 Monitor or continue to assist breathing until the patient breathes deeply and regularly and the mucous membranes are pink.

10 If there is a regurgitation risk (for example, in caesarean section) turn the patient into the lateral position and extubate when he or she is awake, after careful suction of secretions from the mouth and pharynx. If you cannot turn the patient, ensure that the stomach is empty before extubation by, for instance, passing an orogastric tube. Breath-holding may occur if extubation is carried out before regular respiration has returned. This is a critical moment and experience is required to know the right moment at which to extubate.

11 Continue to give as much oxygen as possible using a tight-fitting face mask, looking closely for adequate respiration and pink colour of mucous membranes while maintaining a clear airway, with jaw thrust if needed.

Inhalational technique without intubation

Use this technique only if the patient's stomach is known to be empty.

1 Induce anaesthesia by any safe and convenient technique.

2 Ensure that the jaw muscles are relaxed.

3 Insert an oropharyngeal or laryngeal mask airway.

4 Connect the breathing system either to an anaesthetic face mask or laryngeal mask.

5 Beware of leaks around the cuff of the face mask or laryngeal mask.

Remember that this technique provides no protection against regurgitation or aspiration of gastric contents. It should not be used where there is any risk of this occurring and is not therefore suitable for emergencies or obstetric cases, among others.

TOTAL INTRAVENOUS ANAESTHESIA

In some countries, increasing use is being made of total intravenous anaesthesia (TIVA) in which all anaesthetic drugs, including drugs such as relaxants and analgesics, are given by intravenous infusion at a rate precisely controlled by an electronic syringe pump that effectively eliminates the need for a vaporizer.

At present, the drugs most suitable for such techniques – such as propofol, midazolam and ketamine – may be too expensive for widespread use. It is not possible to substitute cheaper drugs such as thiopental, as they accumulate to very high levels during continuous infusion. If a suitable range of short-acting drugs becomes available at reasonable prices, TIVA may become more widely accepted and used at the district hospital level. The following technique, using TIVA with ketamine, is however suitable, economical and widely used.

TIVA with ketamine

1 After premedication with atropine and pre-oxygenation, induce anaesthesia with a fast-running ketamine infusion containing 1 mg/ml (average adult dose 50–100 ml).

2 Give suxamethonium and intubate the trachea.

3 Maintain anaesthesia with ketamine 1–2 mg/minute (more if the patient has not received premedication). After breathing returns, give a non-depolarizing relaxant.

4 Ventilate with air, enriched with oxygen if available.

5 At the end of surgery, reverse the muscle relaxation and extubate with the patient awake, as after inhalational anaesthesia.

SPECIMEN SPINAL TECHNIQUE FOR ELECTIVE CAESAREAN SECTION

1 Preload the patient with 500–1000 ml of normal saline or Hartmann's solution.

2 Perform a lumbar puncture in the lateral or sitting position. Use strict asepsis. To prevent post-spinal technique headaches, always use a fine gauge spinal needle: 25 or 27 gauge.

3 Inject about 1.5–2ml of 5% "heavy" lidocaine or 2 ml bupivacaine with the patient in the lateral position
   - Heavy lidocaine 5% with 7.5% dextrose is commonly used, as it is inexpensive; unfortunately, it lasts only 45–60 minutes, so the surgeon should be experienced and the caesarean section a straightforward one without adhesions
   - Where available, 0.5% isobaric or hyperbaric bupivacaine is preferable to lidocaine.

4 Immediately after injecting the spinal dose of drug, turn the mother into the horizontal position, but with the pelvis wedged so that the gravid uterus leans substantially to the left side. Make sure the mother's position is secure and that she cannot fall.

5 Be extra vigilant, and actively treat any fall in systolic blood pressure to below 90 mmHg (12.0 kPa). Hypotension can harm both fetus and mother. Initial treatment of hypotension is to give up to 1000 ml of colloid or crystalloid solution rapidly, within 5 minutes or less.

6 If the pressure remains low, give:
   - Vasoconstrictor, such as ephedrine, in 5–10 mg increments
   - Consider using a continuous ephedrine infusion: 30 mg in 500 ml
   - If this is not available, give a diluted solution of 0.5 mg adrenaline diluted in 20 ml normal saline intravenously, 1 ml at a time; this is effective, though rather abrupt in onset and offset.

7 Always give oxygen to the mother during the operation.

The ideal height of block is between the xiphisternum (T5/6) and nipple line (T4). Remember that in pregnant women at term, the block very easily goes high. Give a dose reduced by 0.5 ml compared with the dose you would give to a non-pregnant woman of the same size. For example:

- Small woman: 1.2 ml heavy lidocaine
- Medium height woman: 1.5 ml heavy lidocaine
- Large woman: 2 ml heavy lidocaine.

If using isobaric (non-glucose containing) solutions, *increase* the dose by 0.5 ml. For example, a small woman having a first time caesarean section, with easy surgery and short duration of operation expected, would receive 1.2 ml heavy lidocaine. A large woman having her third caesarean section would be better given 2.5 ml of isobaric bupivacaine because obesity and adhesions will mean a longer operation.

Bupivacaine appears to require 0.5 ml more than lidocaine. Plain lidocaine 2% can be used, but the block is not so good and 2.5 ml will be needed in a mother where 1.5 ml of 5% lidocaine would have been used.

If surgery is prolonged and the patient starts to feel pain, give IV analgesics such as opiates or low dose ketamine.

CAESAREAN SECTION IN PRE-ECLAMPSIA AND ECLAMPSIA

In all degrees of pre-eclampsia, spinal anaesthesia is preferable to general anaesthesia because:

- It causes vasodilatation
- There is no hypertensive response to intubation
- There is no need to manage a difficult airway.

Clotting studies may not be available but, if there are no reasons to suspect abnormal clotting, the carefully executed spinal using a 25G needle is the method of choice in a cooperative patient.

Methods of general anaesthesia for caesarean section in pre-eclampsia vary. Halothane is traditional. Ether releases adrenaline which, in theory, exacerbates the condition but does not seem to do so in practice. As ether is generally preferable to halothane for caesarean section, it is a good choice for general anaesthesia in pre-eclampsia.

Never give ketamine in pre-eclampsia.

Potential problems with the induction of anaesthesia

- Conscious level: sedative drugs may require a reduction in the dose of induction agent
- Difficult airway due to oedema
- Hypertensive response to intubation
- Difficult intubation due to laryngeal oedema
- Difficulties measuring blood pressure due to the low volume state and vasoconstriction.

14

Patients should be monitored in the intensive care unit postoperatively, with special emphasis on:

- Blood pressure
- Urine output
- Fluid balance
- Conscious level
- Airway oedema.

After eclampsia (fits), the management is similar to the above but general anaesthesia must be used if the mother is unconscious. Pulmonary oedema may be a problem, necessitating controlled ventilation. Eclamptic fits must be controlled postoperatively. A bitten tongue may cause difficult intubation.

After prolonged eclampsia, mothers are unconscious and in very poor condition. Some surgeons opt for local infiltration anaesthesia of the abdominal wall to perform caesarean section. This should not be allowed for two reasons.

1. Often the analgesia is insufficient and the pain, even in an unconscious patient, puts the blood pressure even higher.
2. Hypoxia during the procedure is very likely and should be prevented with intubation and ventilation with oxygen.

ANAESTHESIA FOR EVACUATION OF RETAINED PRODUCTS OF CONCEPTION (ERPC)

Removal of retained products in the uterus is a semi-urgent procedure because puerperal sepsis rapidly takes hold, with potentially fatal consequences. In a busy maternity unit, there are often many cases to deal with each day: women who have aborted, often with established infection, and mothers with retained products.

Ideally, the method of anaesthesia should avoid the use of volatile agents, because they may produce uterine relaxation and excessive bleeding. This is especially true when evacuations are performed in septic cases, when the uterus is bulky or when the patient has bled a lot already:

- A total intravenous anaesthetic technique (TIVA) is ideal, using ketamine 2–4 mg/kg; this drug also has oxytocic properties
- Give diazepam 5–10 mg intravenously pre-induction to settle the patient and to avoid hallucinations postoperatively
- Alternative TIVA methods are:
  - Pethidine 50 mg IV followed by increments of thiopental 2.5% up to a maximum dose of 500 mg

  Or
  - Incremental propofol, 20–30 ml.

Oxytocin may be required by infusion postoperatively, 20–40 units in 1 litre normal saline.

Clinical circumstances may lead to evacuations being done with diazepam (10 mg) and pethidine (50 mg), but many patients will not tolerate this method and the consequent movements mean that an incomplete evacuation is carried out. To avoid this situation, ketamine is the method of choice.

EMERGENCY LAPAROTOMY

In many hospitals, emergency laparotomy for peritonitis, bowel obstruction or abdominal trauma is second in frequency only to caesarean section as a major intervention. Without surgery, death is certain. Good anaesthetic management determines the outcome in equal measure to good surgery.

After initial resuscitation, the overall aims are to intubate, ventilate and maintain the blood pressure. The following actions to achieve this are important.

1 Put a large bore cannula (16 gauge) in place and have a stock of IV fluids (normal saline or Ringer's lactate) available. Run the drip fast, but watch for overfilling of the internal jugular vein.
2 Check blood pressure every few minutes and oxygen saturation, if you have an oximeter.
3 Insert a nasogastric tube and suck on the tube or use gravity to empty the stomach as much as possible just before induction. Be sure the tube is not blocked.
4 Have the sucker switched on and a large Yankauer sucker ready under the pillow.
5 Preoxygenate and use cricoid pressure: regurgitation is common.
6 Check the airway and the position of the head to make sure intubation will not be difficult.
7 Give a cardiostable induction. If in doubt about the circulating volume, use ketamine 1–2 mg/kg. Otherwise, thiopental is quite acceptable; give a reduced dose (2 mg/kg) if the patient is in poor condition or the blood pressure is low.
8 Give suxamethonium 100 mg as soon as possible after the induction agent. Run the drip fast during the injection.
9 Intubate as quickly as possible and inflate the cuff.
10 Ventilate and check the position of the tube.
11 Check blood pressure and oxygenation again before starting ether or halothane. If the blood pressure is still low, you may wish to continue with ketamine and oxygen alone.

Ventilation with or without a relaxant may be needed, although many patients will have adequate spontaneous respiration. If the abdomen is distended, assist ventilation by hand.

Use a non-depolarising muscle relaxant such as vecuronium only if there is a mechanical ventilator in the operating room and if postoperative ventilatory support is available.

Intensive care management is advised, where available, with particular attention to intravenous fluids and urine output. Continuing hypovolaemia, sepsis and hypotension are the main causes of death in the first 24 hours postoperatively.

EMERGENCY CASE WITH A COMPLICATED AIRWAY

The complicated airway means obstruction: either existing already in the awake patient or waiting to happen as soon as consciousness is lost.

Causes of obstruction include:
- Vomit
- Oedema
- Blood
- Abscess or tissue infection
- Slough
- Pus
- Abnormal anatomy
- Debris
- Foreign body
- Tumour
- Tissue damage.

The obstruction might be at the mouth, inside the mouth, in or around the neck. With a foreign body, there may be obstruction further down in the airway, in the trachea. It may be related to the proposed surgery or be unrelated in origin and an unwelcome surprise.

There are so many different causes and scenarios relating to a blocked airway that detailed management protocols are impossible to give. If you are presented with a complicated airway, remember that the patient was breathing when he came to you, otherwise he would have died somewhere on the way. Good management depends on:
- Preserving the airway for as long as possible
- Increasing the oxygen reserve in the lungs
- Inducing anaesthesia
- Securing the airway, under controlled conditions, by passing a tracheal tube.

Principles for induction of anaesthesia in obstructed airway

1 Assess the need to hurry. Have a diagnosis and a plan before starting. If possible, have a more experienced anaesthetist in the operating room or nearby.

2 Gather everything you might need for a difficult airway. Some or all of the following may be useful:
- Intubating bougies
- Laryngoscope: two, if possible, with different blades
- Stylets
- Different sizes of endotracheal tubes: put a lubricated stylet in the smallest tube
- Laryngeal mask airway
- Different size oropharyngeal and nasopharyngeal airways
- Different shaped masks
- Emergency laryngotomy puncture set.

3 Use a little head-up tilt of the table, which usually assists the airway. A child can sit on the table or even on your knee for the induction and then be laid horizontally when asleep.

4 Have the sucker switched on with a Yankauer fitted and soft catheters ready.

5 Assess the regurgitation risk, especially if the patient has also swallowed a lot of blood. Assign a person to give cricoid pressure.

6 Use the pulse oximeter.

7 Have a drip running, with intravenous induction drugs ready drawn up.

8 Be well protected: patients with airway trauma may cough blood at you. Gloves are essential; a mask and glasses will prevent blood getting in your eyes or mouth.

9 Do not examine any wound or lift any dressing around the airway until everything is in place: this action may cause the patient to cough and the airway may be lost or haemorrhage may start.

10 Try to fit a mask to the airway and give oxygen. Observe the pulse oximeter and the movement of the bag or bellows. This will tell you the effectiveness of pre-oxygenation and how easy inhalation induction will be.

11 Induce anaesthesia. Never give any intravenous anaesthetic drug, especially suxamethonium, unless you are sure that you can ventilate by mask and that endotracheal intubation will be possible or an LMA can be passed.

Giving an intravenous drug will cause loss of the airway and stop the breathing. Can you handle that? If not, do not give an intravenous drug.

With facial trauma, the destruction of bone and tissue makes holding the mask and pre-oxygenation more difficult, but intubation after suctioning may be easier. In extreme cases of neck trauma (such as assault by knife), the trachea can be intubated through the neck wound.

The classical method is to use inhalation anaesthesia with halothane when faced with a potentially obstructed airway. In practice, this is not always successful: induction takes a long time if ventilation is poor or obstructed. Struggling or coughing may make things worse, increase bleeding and result in total airway obstruction. You may start with one method and find yourself forced to use another or a combined intravenous plus inhalation technique.

Always have an alternative plan, which takes into account the patient's condition, your own skills and the resources available. Be flexible, be prepared for your plan to go wrong and do not get fixed on one choice of anaesthesia.

Postoperative airway management is likely to be more complicated than the preoperative status because of:

- Tissue swelling
- Residual narcosis
- Postoperative ("reactive") haemorrhage
- Haematoma formation.

Therefore, before doing anything to the airway, check what airway management facilities will be available postoperatively. Avoid managing a patient with a persistent obstructed airway in a district hospital operating room, with nowhere except an ordinary ward to send him or her postoperatively. You may choose to refer such a patient to the central hospital with an intensive care unit and avoid any procedures on the airway. Alternatively, you could intubate at your hospital and travel with the patient to the referral centre.

KEY POINTS

- The most important monitors are the eyes, ears, hands and brain of the anaesthetist
- Keep your attention focused on the patient first, then on the monitoring devices.

14.6 MONITORING THE ANAESTHETIZED PATIENT

A person who is unconscious, whether because of injury or illness or because of the influence of general anaesthetic drugs, lacks many vital and protective reflexes and depends on other people for protection and maintenance of vital functions. It is the duty of the health staff to ensure that the patient is protected during this critical period. One person must never act as both anaesthetist and surgeon at the same time; a trained person must always be available specifically to look after the airway, monitor the patient and care for all vital functions.

CARE OF UNCONSCIOUS PATIENTS

Position

Always induce anaesthesia with the patient on a table or trolley that can rapidly be tilted into a steep, head-down position to deal with any sudden onset of hypotension or, should the patient vomit, to allow the vomit to drain out of the mouth instead of into the lungs.

Once anaesthetized, the patient should not be put into an abnormal position that could cause damage to joints or muscles. If the lithotomy position is to be used, two assistants should lift both legs at the same time, and place them in the stirrups, to avoid damage to the sacro-iliac joint.

Eyes

The eyes should be fully closed during general anaesthesia or the cornea may become dry and ulcerated. If the lids do not close "naturally", use a small piece of tape to hold them. They should always be taped in this way if the head is to be draped and additional protective padding is advisable. If the patient is to be placed in the prone position, take special care to prevent pressure on the eyes, which could permanently damage vision.

Teeth

Teeth are at risk from artificial airways and laryngoscopy, especially if they are loose, decayed or irregularly spaced. Damage from oral airways most often occurs during recovery from anaesthesia, when an increase in muscle tone causes the patient to bite. Laryngoscopy may damage teeth, particularly the upper front incisors, if they are used as a fulcrum on which to lever the laryngoscope. It is safer to remove a loose tooth deliberately because, if dislodged by accident, it may be inhaled and result in a lung abscess.

Peripheral nerves

Certain peripheral nerves, such as the ulnar nerve at the elbow, may be damaged by prolonged pressure. Others, such as the brachial plexus, may be damaged by traction. Careful attention to the patient's position and the use of soft padding over bony prominences can avoid these problems. Tourniquets, if used, must be carefully applied with padding and must never be left inflated for more than 90 minutes as ischaemic nerve damage may occur.

Respiration

Unrestricted breathing is essential for the unconscious patient. Make sure that the surgeon or assistant is not leaning on the chest wall or upper abdomen. Steep, head-down positions restrict movement of the diaphragm, especially in obese patients, and controlled ventilation may therefore be necessary.

If a patient is placed in the prone position, insert pillows under the upper chest and pelvis to allow free movement of the abdominal wall during respiration.

> Handle patients gently at all times, whether they are awake or unconscious.

Burns

Protect the anaesthetized patient from being burned accidentally. Beware of inflammable skin cleaning solutions that can be ignited by surgical diathermy. To prevent diathermy burns, apply the neutral diathermy electrode firmly and evenly to a large area of skin over the back, buttock or thigh. If other electrical apparatus is in use, beware of the risk of electrocuting or electrically burning the patient.

Hypothermia

Keep unconscious patients as warm as possible by covering them and keeping them out of draughts. Most general and regional anaesthetics cause skin vasodilatation, which increases heat loss from the body. Although the skin feels warm, the patient's core temperature may be falling rapidly. Hypothermia during anaesthesia has two harmful effects:

- It increases and prolongs the effects of certain drugs, such as muscle relaxants
- By causing the patient to shiver during the recovery period, it increases oxygen demand, leading to hypoxia.

MONITORING

A monitor is, strictly speaking, a device that warns or alerts you to an abnormal event, such as low blood pressure, by sounding an alarm. A manual blood pressure cuff will not warn you of anything – it simply measures blood pressure – and you have to know something is wrong. The term "monitoring" has been extended to mean "actively looking for abnormal patient events". In other words, the major part of this job lies with the person doing the measurement who must actively seek the information.

14

> Monitoring means *looking* at the patient.

In the past 20 years, more technological progress has been made in the field of monitoring during resuscitation and anaesthesia than in most other fields of medicine. These developments have made it possible to conduct a case almost without laying a hand on the patient, yet remain informed of the pulse, blood pressure, respiration, oxygen saturation, skin temperature or other physiological change.

However, the prohibitive training and equipment costs involved (both in capital outlay and maintenance) to sustain this advanced technology mean that anaesthetists in the developing world will usually not have more than the basic traditional monitoring tools (blood pressure cuff and stethoscope) with perhaps the chance of a pulse oximeter if they are lucky. Thus, the sensory system of the anaesthetist him/herself becomes the most important monitoring device. The only maintenance it requires is to use it.

> It is a fundamental rule in anaesthesia that you must never leave your patient unattended.

The five senses are: hearing, smell, sight, touch and taste. Only the last one is of little use to the alert anaesthetist. The first four are essential. Unfortunately, the word 'alert' is often changed to the overused word 'vigilant' and after being declared very important, is then, in practice, disregarded.

The non-alert anaesthetist does not observe the things going around him or her and does not recognize a change in the patient's condition. Such a person fails to act logically to react to changes, and is undoubtedly the greatest hazard for the patient under anaesthesia.

Sophisticated monitoring devices sometimes act as a distraction to an anaesthetist who would do a better job with a manual blood pressure cuff and a finger on the pulse.

> It is usually more important to look at the patient than the equipment but the alert anaesthetist pays constant attention to both.

Imagine your own "zone of interaction", that is a physical space around you. Events occurring in this zone may affect your work and are your concern. Expand this space outward so that it meets and interacts with the equivalent zones of other people in the operating room and you communicate with them.

Sometimes two or more anaesthetists organise themselves into a "group anaesthetist" to conduct anaesthesia, perhaps for a difficult case. This can be very dangerous for the patient because, firstly, no one person is in charge and, secondly, communications within the group may be poor. It is often necessary to have one or more assistants for a case, but remember that there must always be only one person in charge of anaesthesia. That person delegates a specific task to an assistant, such as "take the blood pressure" and the assistant then reports back the result to the anaesthetist in charge of the case. If, for example, the blood pressure is found to be low and halothane is on 3%, the person taking the blood pressure should inform the anaesthetist in charge who then decides what to do about it, rather like the captain of a ship who ultimately has responsibility for that ship.

If the person in charge goes off duty while the patient is still on the table, he or she must hand over to another person in charge.

Observe the general operating room surroundings.

Reduce unnecessary noise. Noises may distract you from hearing important things going wrong with your patient or that some equipment is malfunctioning. For example:

- An oxygen concentrator may be making a noise it was not making yesterday – ask why
- The patient's breathing may have become noisy, or changed in frequency; possibly there is airway obstruction or inadequate anaesthesia
- The ventilator may be making an unusual sound, perhaps indicating a leak or disconnection.

Excessive operating room background noise from music or too many people talking at once is a distraction. Ventilators and monitoring devices cannot be heard.

Operating room chatter means not thinking about the patient.

Smells may indicate:

- Dirty suction machine, operating table or mattress
- Abdominal or other sepsis
- Leaking anaesthetic agent or wrongly filled vaporizer
- Overheating motor or electric plug
- Blocked operating room drain.

Check whether the temperature of the room is too hot for the staff or too cold for the patient and assess whether a warming blanket is needed.

Observe the operating table. How does it work? Is it too high, too low, tilted, braked?

Check the location of important equipment and drugs.

If there are wires and tubes on or around the patient or the operating table, make sure that they are not tangled up, knotted, twisted, kinked or lying on the floor. Check that the sucker tube will reach the patient.

Most important of all, monitor the oxygen flow to the anaesthesia machine or patient circuit (perhaps by feeling the flow of gas against your face). Ensure you can generate a positive pressure with the bag or bellows to inflate the lungs.

Observe the patient immediately before anaesthesia.

In addition to making a preoperative assessment on the ward, just before anaesthesia, observe the awake patient on the table from the psychological viewpoint. The patient's expectations of treatment and reaction to being in this strange environment will affect the changes in blood pressure and other autonomic functions during anaesthesia and the need for postoperative analgesia.

Monitoring spontaneous respiration

You should monitor respiration movements in spontaneously breathing patients under anaesthesia. During spontaneous breathing, observe the respiratory rate and tidal volume by looking first at chest and abdomen, then at your anaesthesia apparatus, that is the movement of the bag or bellows or the movement of, and noise from, the breathing valve, such as an Ambu valve. Smooth, regular, spontaneous breathing is itself a useful sign that all is well. If hypotension from unsuspected (or unreported) operative haemorrhage occurs, the reduced cerebral blood flow means there will also be a change in the breathing pattern or breathing may cease altogether.

General anaesthesia with spontaneous breathing, therefore, used widely in developing countries, has valuable inherent safety aspects.

However, as always, *you must check.* Every few minutes, squeeze the bag or depress the bellows and make sure there is a satisfactory corresponding movement of the chest or abdomen. A problem with a partially blocked or kinked endotracheal tube, or one that has moved down and entered the right main bronchus will be detected this way.

Monitoring the depth and rate of breathing also informs you about the level of anaesthesia. Different anaesthetic agents will produce different characteristics in the breathing pattern:

- Halothane anaesthesia produces fairly rapid, shallow breathing
- Ether anaesthesia produces increased minute volume with increased rate and depth of respiration which usually does not need assistance from the anaesthetist, although it will take longer to reach this steady state
- Ketamine anaesthesia may give an irregular breathing pattern.

If you cannot see the chest or abdomen, rearrange the drapes so that you can.

Whatever the method of maintaining anaesthesia, it is a general rule that more anaesthesia will reduce respiration (both in the rate and tidal volume) so, again, spontaneous breathing has the safety feature that even if the anaesthetist is not monitoring the movements of respiration at all, the patient breathing a volatile agent will regulate the depth of anaesthesia automatically and will not get an overdose.

Monitoring respiration with IPPV

IPPV means Intermittent Positive Pressure Ventilation. If you have a ventilator you also must have the monitoring apparatus to make it safe. The anaesthetized patient connected to a mechanical ventilator can far more easily receive an overdose than one breathing spontaneously. Pay constant attention to the blood pressure and heart rate.

The commonest way to give a fatal overdose of anaesthetic is by mechanical ventilation (IPPV).

Other essential respiratory monitoring of ventilated patients includes:

- Listening to the noise of the ventilator: a noise of escaping gas with each ventilator breath or the weight and arm falling down too quickly usually means a disconnection
- Observation of the rise and fall of the chest and or abdomen: no movement means disconnection or a blocked tube
- Movement of the airway pressure gauge on the ventilator:
  - No movement means disconnection
  - Increased movement means a blocked or kinked endotracheal tube.

The normal upper limit for airway pressure (AWP) is 30 cm water. A low AWP (10–15) means compliant lungs and normal function. AWP above 30 may mean:

- Partial obstruction with mucus or foreign material
- Endobronchial intubation
- Bronchospasm
- Abdominal muscles pushing the diaphragm
- Pulmonary oedema
- Consolidation of the lungs
- Pneumothorax.

If the airway pressure is getting higher and higher as the operation proceeds, think of these things. Recognize that you will have problems with getting the patient to breathe spontaneously postoperatively. You may need to plan postoperative ventilation in the intensive care unit.

If you have an old ventilator with no alarms, you must be especially vigilant. You are the alarms.

No matter what ventilator you have, when connecting it to the patient for the first time, check that the inspiratory/expiration phases of the ventilator correspond to the rise and fall of the chest and abdomen.

Monitoring the cardiovascular system

The cardiovascular system is a close second behind the respiratory system in order of monitoring, though equal in importance.

Feel the pulse rate, heart rhythm and pulse volume and compare them with the preoperative values. The best place to feel the pulse is at the wrist, palpating the radial artery. Other convenient sites are the temporal artery or brachial artery.

Pulse rate

The pulse or heart rate varies greatly with age, method of anaesthesia and pathology. Neonates and babies should have a heart rate between 100 and 150. Older patients do not tolerate tachycardia well and adults ideally should not have a heart rate much above 100. However, heart rate is increased by:

- Pain
- Light anaesthesia
- Fever
- Raised carbon dioxide levels
- Sepsis
- Toxaemia
- Volume depletion.

A mixed picture emerges which the alert anaesthetist must observe and interpret, adjusting the methods of patient management so that dangerous abnormalities or changes in the cardiovascular system are returned towards normal.

In general, a spontaneously breathing patient on a higher dose of volatile agent as the sole anaesthetic, with no opiate given, will have a heart rate higher (90–120) than one being ventilated, having been given a muscle relaxant and mixed volatile agent/opiate anaesthesia (70–90). The latter is called a balanced technique.

A low heart rate is less easy to interpret and may have many causes. It may be normal, for example in a sportsman, or due to excessive vagal tone such as in organophosphate poisoning. A heart rate persistently below 50 in an adult and below 90 in a neonate should be treated.

Never allow yourself to be denied access to monitoring of respiration, pulse and blood pressure.

Heart rhythm

The heart rhythm is more difficult to monitor. The presence of an arrhythmia can be detected by feeling an irregular pulse at the wrist. The actual diagnosis of the arrhythmia – and, therefore, the decision on correct management – usually requires an ECG monitor. Fortunately, because ischaemic heart disease is rare in developing countries, serious abnormalities of rhythm are uncommon. Many arrhythmias occur under anaesthesia, are not detected by anyone and resolve spontaneously after recovery causing no harm.

If you detect some abnormality in feeling the pulse that is worrying or new, or you see it on the ECG screen, consider the following options.

1 Increase the ventilation with IPPV and check the corresponding chest movements.

2 Check that oxygen is flowing and *reaching* the patient and he or she is not hypoxic.

3 Check the blood pressure: if it is high, increase the depth of anaesthesia by increasing the ventilation and percentage of volatile agent – add an opiate.

4 Consider halothane as a possible cause and change to another agent.

5 Consider an electrolyte abnormality, such as hypokalaemia.

6 Check whether epinephrine has been given by the surgeon without your knowledge.

7 Consider lidocaine 100 mg IV bolus (1.5 mg/kg).

Pulse volume

Pulse volume means the fullness of the pulse. A good volume pulse may slowly become weak and thready during an operation where blood loss is not being corrected by replacement, even if blood pressure itself is maintained.

Blood pressure

Blood pressure is the single most important thing to measure, after feeling the pulse. While non-invasive blood pressure machines (NIBP) are widely used, a manual aneroid or mercury sphygmomanometer gives just as good a result. If you have an NIBP machine, find out how it works and remember to look at it. Set the reading interval to 3–5 minutes.

For manual checks, it is customary to use only the fingers (not the stethoscope) to get a value for blood pressure during anaesthesia because:

- It is quicker
- The systolic pressure gives the information you need about myocardial function
- Changes in blood pressure, rather than absolute values, are more important.

If the blood pressure goes down, consider:

- Decompensation in hypovolaemia
- Haemorrhage
- Overdose of volatile agent
- Excessive intrathoracic pressure: faulty breathing system or pneumothorax
- Caval compression in pregnancy: supine hypotensive syndrome
- Recent drug administration
- Spinal anaesthesia going too high
- Surgical compression of a vessel or the heart
- Intrinsic cardiac problem
- Hypoxia
- Endotoxaemia.

If the blood pressure goes up, consider:

- Carbon dioxide retention: patient not ventilating adequately
- Insufficient depth of anaesthesia
- Response to intubation in a hypertensive patient
- Inotropic drug administration
- Endogenous hormones: thyrotoxicosis or (rarely) phaeochromocytoma.

Using the stethoscope

Using the stethoscope on the chest to monitor breath sounds and heart sounds should not replace your senses as an input device: it should only add information. It must not be allowed to cause your "zone of interaction" to shrink. For example, many anaesthetists will tape the stethoscope to the chest, put both earpieces in place and devote their entire monitoring attention, very vigilantly, to the sounds of the heart and respiration. They then fail to notice other important complications of the procedure, such as falling blood pressure, haemorrhage, patient waking up, surgical crisis, hypoxia, hypothermia, drip running out or alarming monitors.

While everyone has a different way of using the stethoscope as a monitoring tool in anaesthesia, it is suggested that it should stay round your neck for occasional use all over the chest, rather than be fixed on the chest *and* fixed in your ears.

The weighted stethoscope plus earpiece is a better continuous monitoring tool than the ordinary stethoscope. This device has a heavy metal cylinder that sits on the chest and is connected via a long, lightweight tube to a comfortable single foam earpiece. It allows more freedom of movement, although the sounds are very faint compared to those from the usual stethoscope. Thermoplastic shaped earpieces can be individually made.

Monitoring after a spinal anaesthetic

Since the patient who has received spinal anaesthesia is awake, there is often an erroneous assumption that no monitoring is necessary. In fact, spinal anaesthesia may be associated with just as many complications as general anaesthesia, as the figures below show. Monitoring of blood pressure and respiration is, if anything, *more* important after spinal than after general anaesthesia. Check that cardiopulmonary resuscitation equipment is available and working and monitor cerebral perfusion by regularly talking to the patient and observing facial expression.

In many district hospitals, there is a high rate of complications of spinal anaesthesia, including severe hypotension (10%) and respiratory arrest (3%) These can easily occur when spinal anaesthesia is treated as an action to be performed rather than a process to be monitored. The result of such neglect can be a dead patient.

> Monitor your patient very closely immediately after giving a spinal anaesthetic. One of the best ways to monitor such a patient is to talk to them throughout anaesthesia.

Depth of anaesthesia

Only in the worst-risk cases, where the condition of the patient is so poor that even light anaesthesia is life threatening, should you accept a very light plane of anaesthesia that unavoidably carries the risk of awareness. In most emergencies, you have sufficient control of the cardiovascular system to enable an adequate, non-aware state of anaesthesia to be maintained. The complication of awareness is generally confined to the paralysed patient who cannot show that anaesthesia is too light by moving.

When you give an intravenous hypnotic drug, ask yourself: are you sure you gave it? Where did it go? When turning on a vaporizer, check it is full.

Depth of anaesthesia can be monitored by looking at:

- Cardiovascular signs: few patients with normal heart rate and blood pressure will be aware, although beta blockers may prevent a tachycardia
- Pupils: they should be small and non-reactive, although ether may give a large pupil due to its sympathomimetic effects; a reactive pupil probably means the patient can hear you and may feel pain
- Sweating and tears: these signs mean the patient is too "light".

In all the above, you must also consider carbon dioxide retention due to hypoventilation. Check the ventilation urgently.

> If a patient seems to be too 'light', check the ventilation first: the signs may be due to hypercarbia.

Urine output

A catheterized patient should have a bag connected so that you can check the *urine output* during the operation. If there is no urine, check the bladder to make sure there is no obstruction. Aim for a minimum output of 0.5 ml/kg per hour.

Electronic monitoring

Modern monitors often have multiple functions of oximetry, ECG, carbon dioxide, NIBP and temperature all together in one monitor.

Pulse oximeter

The pulse oximeter is simple to use. It informs about heart rate and especially oxygenation. Its greatest value is in diagnosing hypoxia during induction of anaesthesia in healthy patients.

Unfortunately, in emergency cases with circulatory collapse, when oxygenation information is most needed, the oximeter often cannot read the capillary pulse. In such cases, when the oximeter suddenly fails to read, it is a sign that deterioration is taking place. On the other hand, when the reading returns, it means the blood pressure has come up and your resuscitation efforts are perhaps being successful.

> If the pulse oximeter will not give a reading, it usually means that something is wrong with the circulation.

Never believe the oximeter if the indicated pulse rate does not agree with the real one felt at the wrist. Readings from a pulse oximeter are often unreliable in infants and neonates with poor circulation. If an adult probe is used, there may be a 10% saturation difference between readings on the toe and the finger in babies.

Every case under anaesthesia should have the pulse oximeter in place, especially:

- For induction
- At the end of anaesthesia
- In recovery.

Remember, however, that when things go wrong, except in hypoxia, the pulse oximeter is almost useless.

Other monitors

Electrocardiograph (ECG)

- Useful to show changes in heart rate and rhythm
- Needs a supply of patient electrodes (disposable)
- Gives no indication of cardiac output
- Less useful than an oximeter
- Best used in poor risk patients or when dysrhythmias are expected.

Capnograph

- Measures carbon dioxide in expired air
- Can be used to confirm correct position of tracheal tube
- Can indicate changes in ventilation and cardiac output
- Can indicate disconnections and respiratory arrest

Monitoring events

Make regular checks of the volume in the sucker. During caesarean section, it is important to differentiate between aspirated liquor and blood. The amount of losses must be added to the blood in the swabs and compared to the patient's estimated circulating volume in order to give appropriate replacement fluids or blood.

Change of plan or operation

In places where diagnostic facilities are limited, there is more uncertainty about what will be found during surgery. The operation may turn out to be longer or shorter than expected – more usually the former. Pay attention to what is going on and adapt your anaesthesia to the changed circumstances.

Patient positioning

If head up or down tilt is needed this will affect cerebral perfusion (head up) or respiration (head down).

Watch the surgeon

Be prepared for the following:

- There may be sudden or unexpected bleeding
- Traction on visceral structures can produce a severe bradycardia
- If adrenaline is injected (to reduce bleeding) during halothane anaesthesia, cardiac arrhythmias can result. Be prepared.

14.7 POSTOPERATIVE MANAGEMENT

IN RECOVERY

Recovery should be a well staffed, warm, well lit area of the operating room with oxygen, suction and resuscitation equipment available to treat complications.

If the patient is restless, something is wrong.

Look out for the following in recovery:

- Airway obstruction
- Hypoxia
- Haemorrhage: internal or external
- Hypotension and/or hypertension
- Postoperative pain
- Shivering, hypothermia
- Vomiting, aspiration
- Falling on the floor
- Residual narcosis.

The recovering patient is fit for the ward when:

- Awake, opens eyes
- Extubated
- Blood pressure and pulse are satisfactory
- Can lift head on command
- Not hypoxic
- Breathing quietly and comfortably
- Appropriate analgesia has been prescribed and is safely established.

POSTOPERATIVE EXTUBATION

Some patients are extubated on the table, others in recovery and still others in the intensive care unit, sometimes even after several days. If you expect that a prolonged period of intubation will follow postoperatively, select a suitable non-irritant tube for starting the case.

In general, it is better to extubate the patient yourself at the end of surgery, on the table when he or she is fully awake, with good suction and oxygenation and under controlled conditions. You can also monitor the airway, breathing and vital reflexes in the immediate post-extubation period. If you have a pulse

KEY POINTS

The three events that probably contribute most to mortality in the postoperative period are:

- Non-running drip
- Postoperative hypotension
- Respiratory failure.

oximeter connected, it must not be removed until the patient has been extubated and remains well oxygenated on room air.

Self extubation by the patient might cause some damage to the larynx as the cuff will not be deflated and there may also be secretions in the pharynx that normally would have been sucked away. However, self extubation is usually a harmless event and shows at least that the patient is awake and has good muscle power. The LMA is sometimes taken out in theatre with suction or sometimes left for the patient himself to pull out when fully awake.

When to leave the endotracheal tube in place

Always bear in mind that an tracheal tube left in place for several hours has the potential to become blocked. This will happen more quickly if the tube is small, there are secretions, pus or blood in the lungs or if nursing care is inadequate. As a general rule, you can expect any tracheal tube to become blocked within 24 hours.

> A blocked tracheal tube = a dead patient.

Situations when you should leave the tracheal tube in place or delay extubation include:

- Airway problems
  - Patients with potential airway problems such as major maxillofacial surgery or trauma, large thyroidectomies or other swelling in the airway may sometimes be left intubated for the first overnight period in case there is swelling that might cause airway obstruction
  - Decide in advance whether to leave the tube in and give a sedative and opiate analgesic so that it is tolerated otherwise the patient's coughing or attempts to self-extubate will cause more difficulties than intubation solves
- Haemodynamically unstable patients: very sick patients from haemorrhage or sepsis who:
  - Do not fully recover
  - Might need ventilation
  - Suffer cardiovascular collapse in the postoperative period
- Hypoxic patients who might need ventilation
- Patients who do not wake up as planned:
  - In general, do not extubate an unconscious patient after surgery or one who shows no cough reflex when moving the tube in the trachea
  - Wait until the patient is breathing (not breath-holding or biting the tube) and shows a gag reflex and, ideally, opens his or her eyes.

Nasogastric/orogastric tube

All emergency cases have potentially full stomachs. At the end of surgery, there should be a nasogastric tube in place; the stomach may, in any case, have been emptied during the operation. An orogastric tube is very easy to pass under anaesthesia, but further intestinal contents reflux into the stomach and may regurgitate at extubation.

Neonates

Neonates are at special risk for apnoeic attacks in the hours and days post-operation. A neonatal ventilator and the necessary postoperative care are unlikely to be available. The anaesthetist may choose to leave the neonate intubated so that the nursing staff can hand ventilate when required. On the other hand, it is common in a neonatal emergency for there to be secretions in the chest which will thicken in the postoperative period and block a size 3 tube very easily. The choice is not easy.

PAIN MANAGEMENT AND TECHNIQUES

Effective analgesia is an essential part of postoperative management.

The important injectable drugs for pain are the opiate analgesics. Nonsteroidal anti-inflammatory drugs (NSAIDs), such as diclofenac (1 mg/kg) and ibuprofen can also be given orally and rectally, as can paracetamol (15 mg/kg).

There are three situations where an opiate might be given:

- Preoperatively
- Intraoperatively
- Postoperatively.

Opiate premedication is rarely indicated, although an injured patient in pain may have been given an opiate before coming to the operating room. Opiates given pre- or intraoperatively have important effects in the postoperative period since there may be delayed recovery and respiratory depression, even necessitating mechanical ventilation. The short acting opiate fentanyl is used intra-operatively to avoid this prolonged effect.

Naloxone antagonizes (reverses) all opiates, but its effect quickly wears off.

The commonly available inexpensive opiates are pethidine and morphine. Morphine has about ten times the potency and a longer duration of action than pethidine.

The ideal way to give analgesia postoperatively is to:

- Give a small intravenous bolus of about a quarter or a third of the maximum dose (e.g. 25 mg pethidine or 2.5 mg morphine for an average adult)
- Wait for 5–10 minutes to observe the effect: the desired effect is analgesia, but retained consciousness
- Estimate the correct total dose (e.g. 75 mg pethidine or 7.5 mg morphine) and give the balance intramuscularly.

With this method, the patient receives analgesia quickly and the correct dose is given.

If opiate analgesia is needed on the ward, it is most usual to give an intramuscular regimen:

- Morphine:
  - Age 1 year to adult: 0.1–0.2 mg/kg
  - Age 3 months to 1 year: 0.05–0.1 mg/kg
- Pethidine: give 7–10 times the above doses if using pethidine.

Opiate analgesics should be given cautiously if the age is less than 1 year. They are not recommended for babies aged less than 3 months unless *very close monitoring* in a neonatal intensive care unit is available.

If a good level of monitoring by ward nurses exists, a system of regular pain scoring (assessment) combined with intramuscular opiates can be effective for controlling severe pain.

The use of **regular** oral or rectal paracetamol as a routine for postoperative patients improves pain control and reduces the need for opiates. NSAIDS can be used with paracetamol, or as an alternative.

Because of individual patient (and sociocultural) variations, the dose needed to achieve the right effect is often not precisely known. Excessive sedation or respiratory depression may result. Morphine and pethidine are legally controlled because of their addiction potential. However, addiction following the medical use of opiates is very rare and fear of it should not prevent the use of these effective drugs to treat severe pain.

Opiates are generally cardiostable; if the blood pressure is low, it is more logical to increase the intravenous fluids *and* give the analgesic if the patient is in pain.

A common misconception is that sedatives and analgesics are the same thing: they are not. *Diazepam is not an analgesic.*

The condition of the patient will largely determine the need for analgesia: you must judge what is required. In general, the severely ill or debilitated patient with sepsis, bowel obstruction or other metabolic derangement should not receive opiate analgesia in the immediate postoperative period. On the other hand, an otherwise fit trauma patient will need postoperative analgesia. Children after orthopaedic procedures are usually in particular need. Thoracotomy, chest trauma and chest drains can be very painful: the pain restricts breathing and causes hypoxia and postoperative chest problems.

Patients with head injury and those after intracranial surgery traditionally receive codeine phosphate 30–60 mg because of the sedating and respiratory depressant effects of morphine. Hypercarbia from respiratory depression is particularly dangerous in a spontaneously breathing patient with brain trauma.

Postoperative pain usually increases the blood pressure and this can be harmful, especially if the patient was hypertensive preoperatively.

You may have used a volatile agent, such as halothane, as the sole method of maintaining anaesthesia for an operation. When this has worn off at the end of the operation, you must check if the patient is suffering pain and give appropriate analgesia.

When using halothane as the sole anaesthetic in a fit patient, give an opiate analgesic with the induction agent.

It is widespread and very bad practice among inexperienced anaesthetists to withhold analgesia in order to have a robustly screaming patient going along the theatre corridor back to the ward.

Good practice is to balance the amount of analgesia given, so that adequate pain relief is provided while respiratory depression is avoided.

Prescribe regular analgesia. In practice, "On demand" often means "Not given".

POSTOPERATIVE FLUID MANAGEMENT

Postoperative management, especially in emergency cases, poses a complex problem in finding the right fluid balance. Not all the volumes that have been lost and replaced will be known.

In terms of input and output, consider:

- Replacement of the preoperative deficit:
  - The patient may have been dehydrated for several days
  - The longer the history of illness before operation, the more fluids you should give postoperatively
  - This may result in a 5–10 litre positive fluid balance in the first 24 hours postoperatively
- Replacement of losses during the operation plus other fluids given in the course of anaesthesia; again, input will greatly exceed output, resulting in a positive fluid balance
- Expected further losses: e.g. from nasogastric drainage, other drains, bleeding
- Hypothermic patient warming up: as the peripheries become warm, more circulating volume is needed
- Normal maintenance requirement.

Your decision on how to give the fluid will be determined by three factors:

- The need to correct a residual deficit from the preoperative state – as estimated above: this should ideally be given fast as a fluid bolus, under your direct supervision
- A maintenance schedule
- The patient's response, including:
  - Slowing of tachycardia
  - Urine output
  - Increased blood pressure
  - Rising jugular venous pressure
  - Return of skin turgor to normal
  - Sunken eyes returning to normal.

Maintenance fluids

- Give 3 litres a day to an adult (125 ml/hour); rotate 1 litre bags over 8 hours
- With normal body electrolytes, give normal saline followed by 5% dextrose (glucose) followed by Ringer's lactate; 5% glucose is suitable only as replacement for water in patients who cannot drink
- Replace other fluid losses with solutions containing sodium: normal saline or Hartmann's solution, with added potassium 20 mmol/litre, if necessary.

When deciding on your fluid regime, use all the variables above to enable you to write down what must be given. If you are unsure how much to give, write up a regime for the next hour only, and then come back and check the patient's response.

It is useful to have laboratory estimations of sodium and potassium after a few days of fluid therapy to adjust the input accordingly. Normal values are:

- Sodium: 125–145 mmol/litre
- Potassium: 3.5–5.5 mmol/litre
  - Additional potassium supplements may be required if hypokalaemia is demonstrated (K+ less than 3.5 mmol/litre)
  - Potassium must be diluted and given slowly at not more than 20 mmol/hour
  - The average adult will need about 100 mmol to increase plasma levels by 1 mmol/litre.

See also *The Clinical Use of Blood* (WHO, 2000) for further information on fluid regimens.

Blood

Only give blood if absolutely necessary because of the risk of acute or delayed reactions and of transfusion-transmissible infection.

Fluid balance chart

The fluid balance chart measures the patient's hourly fluid intake and output over a 24 hour period. At the end of 24 hours, the total measured output (urine, drains, nasogastric drainage) is subtracted from the total measured intake (intravenous infusion, oral intake). The result is called the fluid balance.

A "positive" fluid balance means that there is more intake than output: that is, the patient is accumulating water. In fact, a positive fluid balance is not really positive because there are certain outputs that are not measured very accurately (e.g. faeces) and others that are not possible to measure at all (in sweat and respiration – so called "insensible" losses). Thus a normal healthy adult will appear to have a positive fluid balance of about 1–1.5 litres a day.

For these reasons, in the first 24 hours, the fluid balance chart will usually show a big positive balance, perhaps as high as 10 litres. In succeeding days, fluid balance should revert to the normal 1–1.5 litre positive per day.

In general, if a severely ill patient, such as a septic surgical case, shows a persistent positive fluid balance each day, it means an ongoing illness that is not resolving.

Care of the infusion site

Postoperative infusions are life saving. Loss of the drip and failure to correct hypotension is the commonest cause of death during the first postoperative night after major surgery.

All patients having major surgery will need a postoperative infusion to correct any deficit and for maintenance. Secure placement of the intravenous cannula is very important:

- Use a vein in a position that will last a long time in the wards
- Secure the cannula and giving set carefully; you should be able to lift the arm with the giving set
- Use tape that sticks to the skin and use the wings or other large part of the IV cannula for attachment.

INTENSIVE CARE UNIT

It is often difficult to know for certain whether a particular patient needs to be nursed postoperatively in the intensive care unit (ICU), if one exists in your hospital. The person making the decision, whether surgeon or anaesthetist, has to balance the risk of the patient dying from an avoidable cause on the ordinary ward against the waste of expensive resources if a patient is admitted to ICU for no good reason.

Intensive monitoring is generally required in the following cases:

- Cranial neurosurgery
- Head injuries with airway obstruction
- Intubated patients, including tracheostomy
- After surgery for major trauma
- Abdominal surgery for a condition neglected for more than 24 hours
- Chest drain in the first 24 hours
- Ventilation difficulties
- Airway difficulties, potential or established: e.g. post-thyroidectomy, removal of a large goitre
- Unstable pulse or blood pressure, high or low
- Anuria or oliguria
- Severe pre-eclampsia or eclampsia
- Surgical sepsis
- Complications during anaesthesia or surgery, especially unexpected haemorrhage
- Hypothermia
- Hypoxia
- Neonates, after any surgery.

Postoperative ventilation

Mechanical ventilation (IPPV) may be a planned part of postoperative management for a major operation or decided on at the end of surgery because circumstances demand it. IPPV should be continued postoperatively under the following circumstances:

- Respiratory depression or oxygen saturation <80%
- Deteriorating general condition
- Severely distended abdomen
- Severe chest trauma
- Head injury or after intracranial surgery.

Avoid giving long acting muscle relaxants to facilitate IPPV. If the patient is "fighting" the ventilator, ask why? Is he/she hypercarbic? In pain? Hypertensive? Treat these needs first before giving a relaxant.

There are non-surgical reasons for ventilation, including organophosphate poisoning, snakebite, tetanus and some head injuries, but probably only if the patient is breathing on admission.

Usually the decision to ventilate is quite easily made from the above observations. *But, if in doubt, ventilate.*

With no ventilator, a patient in respiratory failure will rapidly die of hypoxia and hypercarbia. Many people die purely for lack of a short period of ventilation in the postoperative period or after trauma.

Discharge from the ICU

The decision to discharge the patient from the ICU very much depends on the quality of care to be found on the ward to which the patient is being transferred. The following conditions should be met before discharging the patient from ICU:

- Conscious
- Good airway, extubated and stable for several hours after extubation
- Breathing comfortably
- Stable blood pressure and urine output.
- Haemoglobin >6 g/dl or blood transfusion in progress
- Minimal nasogastric drainage and has bowel sounds, abdomen not distended
- Afebrile
- Looks better, sitting up, not confused.

Pressure for beds to treat more urgent cases may mean that these guidelines have to be modified. If a patient dies after discharge from ICU, try to find out why the death took place and to learn from it, especially if it appears that the death was avoidable.

Try to put a system in place where patients discharged from ICU are followed up for a week. Find out what happened to them.

Anaesthetic infrastructure and supplies

15

15.1 EQUIPMENT AND SUPPLIES FOR DIFFERENT LEVEL HOSPITALS

However well trained you are as an anaesthetist, your ability to provide safe anaesthesia is completely dependent on the availability of the drugs, oxygen supply and equipment in your hospital. Drugs and oxygen must be correctly ordered and stored and equipment kept in safe working order by regular cleaning, maintenance and checks. Hospitals that do not follow these basic requirements will soon fail to provide safe anaesthesia.

The items of equipment listed in the tables on pages 15–2 to 15–4 are those necessary for provision of a service of resuscitation, acute care and emergency anaesthesia, at three levels, in a country with a limited health budget.

General medical or surgical equipment items are not included. Items in square brackets are alternatives or optional extras. "IVI (intravenous infusion) equipment" means everything needed to put up a drip and give an intravenous drug, including:

- Syringes
- Needles
- Butterflies
- Cannulae
- Giving sets (solution and blood, where appropriate)
- Fluids: normal saline or Ringer's lactate
- Adhesive tape in all sizes.

KEY POINTS

- Different levels of hospital require different personnel, equipment and drugs
- Drugs must be correctly ordered and stored
- Hospitals with an intensive care unit may need additional equipment and supplies.

THE INTENSIVE CARE UNIT

Referral hospitals usually have an intensive care unit (ICU). However, facilities for intensive care should be available in every hospital where surgery and anaesthesia are performed.

At the simplest level, the ICU is a ward that has a better standard of nursing and is better equipped than a general ward. While both medical and surgical cases will be admitted there, the ICU is particularly important for the postoperative care of major or complicated surgical cases and is usually located near the operating room. If facilities allow, full monitoring and ventilation may continue after the operation, but for a much longer period. In most hospitals, over 70% of ICU admissions will be postoperative surgical patients.

15

Level 1: Small hospital or health centre

- Rural hospital or health centre with a small number of beds and a sparsely equipped operating room for minor procedures
- Provides emergency measures in the treatment of 90–95% of trauma and obstetrics cases (excluding caesarean section)
- Referral of other patients (for example, obstructed labour, bowel obstruction) for further management at a higher level

Procedures

- Normal delivery
- Uterine evacuation
- Circumcision
- Hydrocoele reduction, incision and drainage
- Wound suturing
- Control of haemorrhage with pressure dressings
- Debridement and dressing of wounds
- Temporary reduction
- Cleaning or stabilization of open and closed fractures
- Chest drainage (possibly)

Personnel

- Paramedical staff without formal anaesthesia training
- Nurse-midwife

Drugs

- Ketamine 50 mg/ml injection, 10 ml
- Lidocaine 1% or 2%
- [Diazepam 5 mg/ml injection, 2 ml]
- [Pethidine 50 mg/ml injection, 2 ml]
- [Epinephrine (adrenaline)] 1 mg injection
- [Atropine 0.6 mg/ml]

Equipment: capital outlay

- Adult and paediatric resuscitators
- Foot sucker
- [Oxygen concentrator]

Equipment: disposable

- IVI equipment
- Suction catheters size 16 FG
- Examination gloves

Level 2: District/provincial hospital

- District or provincial hospital with 100–300 beds and adequately equipped major and minor operating theatres
- Short term treatment of 95–99% of the major life threatening conditions

Procedures

Same as Level 1 with the following additions:

- Caesarean section
- Laparotomy (usually not for bowel obstruction)
- Amputation
- Hernia repair
- Tubal ligation
- Closed fracture treatment and application of plaster of Paris
- Eye operations, including cataract extraction
- Removal of foreign bodies: for example, in the airway
- Emergency ventilation and airway management for referred patients such as those with chest and head injuries

Personnel

- One [two] trained anaesthetists
- District medical officers, senior clinical officers, nurses, midwives
- Visiting specialists or resident surgeon and/or obstetrician/gynaecologist

Drugs

Same as Level 1, but also:

- Thiopental 500 mg or 1 g powder
- Suxamethonium bromide 500 mg powder
- Atropine 0.5 mg injection
- Epinephrine (adrenaline) 1 mg injection
- Diazepam 10 mg injection
- Halothane 250 ml inhalation
- [Ether 500 ml inhalation]
- Lidocaine 5% heavy spinal solution 2 ml
- [Bupivacaine 0.5% heavy or plain, 4 ml]
- Pethidine 50 mg injection
- [Hydralazine 20 mg injection]
- Frusemide 20 mg injection
- Dextrose 50% 20 ml injection
- Aminophylline 250 mg injection
- Ephedrine 30/50 mg ampoules

Equipment: capital outlay

- Complete anaesthesia, resuscitation and airway management system consisting of:
  - Oxygen source
  - Vaporizer(s)
  - Hoses
  - Valves
  - Bellows or bag to inflate lungs
  - Face masks (sizes 00–5)
  - Work surface and storage
  - Paediatric anaesthesia system
  - Adult and paediatric resuscitator sets
- [Pulse oximeter]
- Laryngoscope Macintosh blades 1–3 [4]
- Oxygen concentrator[s] [cylinder]
- Foot sucker [electric]
- IV pressure infusor bag
- Adult and paediatric resuscitator sets
- Magills forceps (adult and child), intubation stylet and/or bougie

Equipment: disposable

- IVI equipment (minimum fluids normal saline, Ringer's lactate and dextrose 5%)
- Suction catheters size 16 FG
- Examination gloves
- Sterile gloves sizes 6–8
- Nasogastric tubes sizes 10–16 FG
- Oral airways sizes 000–4
- Tracheal tubes sizes 3–8.5
- Spinal needles sizes 22 G and 25 G
- Batteries size C

15

Level 3: Referral hospital

A referral hospital of 300–1000 or more beds with basic intensive care facilities. Treatment aims are the same as for Level 2, with the addition of:

- Ventilation in operating room and ICU
- Prolonged endotracheal intubation
- Thoracic trauma care
- Haemodynamic and inotropic treatment
- Basic ICU patient management and monitoring for up to 1 week: all types of cases, but with limited or no provision for:
  - Multi-organ system failure
  - Haemodialysis
  - Complex neurological and cardiac surgery
  - Prolonged respiratory failure
  - Metabolic care or monitoring

Procedures

Same as Level 2 with the following additions:

- Facial and intracranial surgery
- Bowel surgery
- Paediatric and neonatal surgery
- Thoracic surgery
- Major eye surgery
- Major gynaecological surgery, for example, vesico-vaginal repair

Personnel

Clinical officers and specialists in anaesthesia and surgery

Drugs

Same as Level 2 with the following additions:

- Vecuronium 10 mg powder
- [Pancuronium 4 mg injection]
- Neostigmine 2.5 mg injection
- [Trichloroethylene 500 ml inhalation]
- Calcium chloride 10% 10 ml injection
- Potassium chloride 20% 10 ml injection for infusion

Equipment: capital outlay

Same as Level 2 with the following additions (one of each per operating room or per ICU bed, except where stated):

- Pulse oximeter, spare probes, adult and paediatric*
- ECG (electrocardiogram) monitor*
- Anaesthesia ventilator, electric power source with manual override
- Infusion pumps (2 per bed)
- Pressure bag for IVI
- Electric sucker
- Defibrillator (one per operating room/ICU)
- [Automatic blood pressure machine*]
- [Capnograph*]
- [Oxygen analyzer*]
- Thermometer [temperature probe*]
- Electric warming blanket
- Electric overhead heater
- Infant incubator
- Laryngeal mask airways sizes 2, 3, 4 (3 sets per operating room)
- Intubating bougies, adult and child (1 set per operating room)

* It is preferable to buy combined modalities all in one unit

Equipment: disposable

Same as Level 2 with the following additions:

- ECG dots
- Ventilator circuits
- Giving sets for IVI pumps
- Yankauer suckers
- Disposables for suction machines
- Disposables for capnography, oxygen analyzer, in accordance with manufacturers' specifications:
  - Sampling lines
  - Water traps
  - Connectors
  - Filters
  - Fuel cells

Equipment for the ICU

The ICU does not necessarily need to have ventilators or other expensive machines. An ICU might be a ward where:

- Oxygen is available
- Drips are kept running overnight
- At least hourly measurements and observations are made of:
  - Blood pressure
  - Pulse rate
  - Urine output
  - Oxygenation
  - Conscious level
  - Other general observations of the patient.

The monitoring of the patient *all night long* is the deciding factor in the success or failure of the ICU. Another important feature is whether staff take action when the measurements or observations show that something is wrong.

The provision of one or more simple, reliable electric ventilators (not gas or oxygen dependent) will double the usefulness of a basic ICU. Small, portable mains/battery ventilators with integral compressors are available, although they are relatively expensive.

The pulse oximeter

The pulse oximeter is the most widely used physiological monitoring device. It is especially useful in clinical anaesthesia and in the ICU and is simple to use. Unfortunately, capital costs are still very high, and sustainability is poor because of electronic failures and the short life span and high cost of new finger probes. The expected lifetime is probably only 3–4 years and many probes will need to be replaced during this time.

> The pulse oximeter should be the minimum standard of monitoring in every operating room where regular major surgery is carried out.

15.2 ANAESTHESIA AND OXYGEN

A high concentration of oxygen is needed during and after anaesthesia:

- If the patient is very young, old, sick, or anaemic
- If agents that cause cardiorespiratory depression, such as halothane, are used.

Air already contains 20.9% oxygen, so oxygen enrichment with a draw-over system is a very economical method of providing oxygen. Adding only 1 litre per minute may increase the oxygen concentration in the inspired gas to 35–40%. With oxygen enrichment at 5 litres per minute, a concentration of 80% may be achieved. Industrial-grade oxygen, such as that used for welding, is perfectly acceptable for the enrichment of a draw-over system and has been widely used for this purpose.

KEY POINTS

- A reliable oxygen supply is essential for anaesthesia and for any seriously ill patients
- In many places, oxygen concentrators are the most suitable and economical way of providing oxygen, with a few backup cylinders in case of electricity failure
- Whatever your source of oxygen, you need an effective system for maintenance and spares
- Clinical staff need to be trained how to use oxygen safely, effectively and economically.

15

To add oxygen to a draw-over system, use a T-piece and reservoir tube at the vaporizer inlet (Figure 15.1).

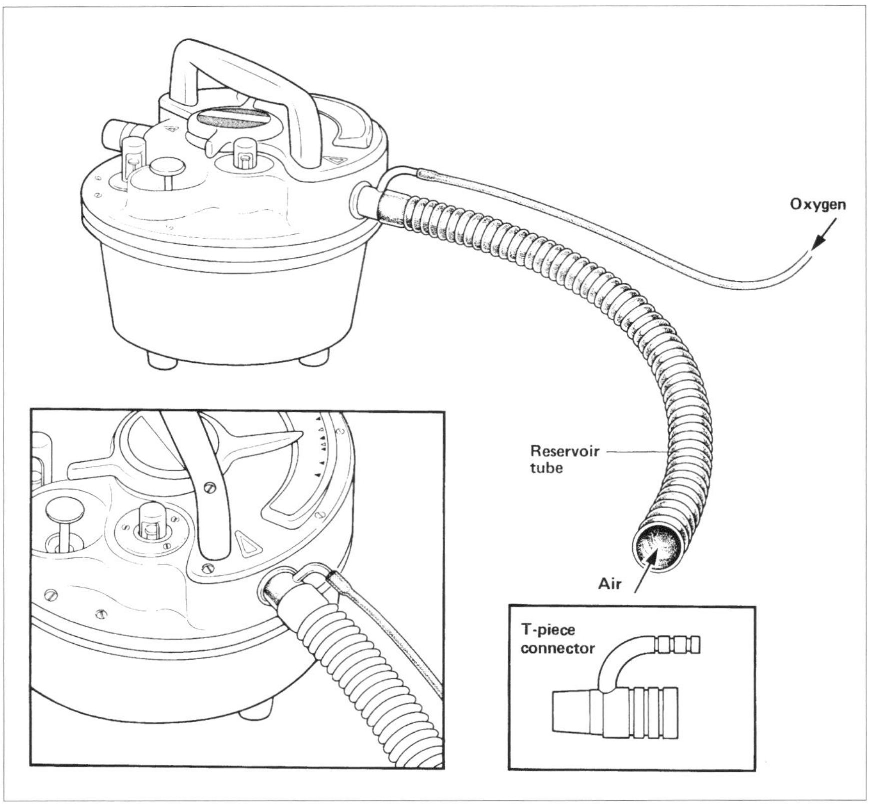

Figure 15.1

If a ready-made T-piece with reservoir is unavailable, you can easily make an improvised alternative using a small-bore oxygen tube threaded into a large-bore tube. Connect the T-piece and reservoir tube (or your improvised version) to the vaporizer inlet and turn on the oxygen supply. By doing this, the oxygen that flows from the cylinder during expiration is not wasted, but is stored in the reservoir tube for the next inspiration. The reservoir tubing should, of course, be open to the atmosphere at its free end to allow the entry of air and it should be at least 30 cm long.

OXYGEN SOURCES

In practice, there are two possible sources of oxygen for medical purposes:

- Cylinders: derived from liquid oxygen
- Concentrators: which separate oxygen from air.

For remote hospitals that cannot obtain oxygen cylinders on a regular basis, there is a strong case for introducing concentrators. However, cylinders can be used to supply oxygen during power cuts and concentrators cannot. Without electricity, the flow of oxygen from a concentrator will stop within a few minutes.

The ideal oxygen supply system is one based primarily on concentrators, but with a back-up supply from cylinders.

Cylinder system	Concentrator system
• Inexpensive to buy	• More expensive to buy
• Expensive to operate	• Inexpensive to operate
• Needs year-round supply of cylinders	• Needs only electricity
• Training and maintenance needed	• Training and maintenance needed
• Can store oxygen oxygen	• Cannot store oxygen: provides only when power supply is on

Details of the necessary apparatus for such a system, designed to supply oxygen reliably to up to four children or two adults, are available from the Department of Blood Safety and Clinical Technology, World Health Organization and from the Procurement Office, UNICEF. For details, contact:

Department of Blood Safety and Clinical Technology
World Health Organization
1211 Geneva 27
Switzerland
Fax: +41 22 791 4836   E-mail: bct@who.int
http://www.who.int/bct/dct

Procurement Office
UNICEF
3 United Nations Plaza
NY 10017, USA

OXYGEN CYLINDERS

Cylinders of oxygen are produced by a relatively expensive industrial process. An oxygen cylinder needs a special valve (regulator) to release the oxygen in a controlled way and a flow meter to control the flow. Without a flow meter, the use of oxygen from cylinders is very wasteful; without a regulator it is also extremely dangerous.

Not all oxygen cylinders are the same; there are at least five different kinds of cylinder in use in different countries. A regulator will fit only one type of oxygen cylinder. Precise information on the type of oxygen cylinder in use should be obtained from the local oxygen supplier *before* ordering regulators. This should be confirmed by someone with technical knowledge who works in the hospital, such as an anaesthetist, chest physician or fully trained hospital technician.

An international standard exists for the identification of oxygen cylinders, which specifies that they should be painted white. Unfortunately, the standard is widely ignored. Medical oxygen cylinders originating in the USA are normally green, while those originating in Commonwealth countries are usually black with white shoulders. Cylinders of industrial oxygen should also be identified clearly, but this is not always the case. Never use any cylinder to supply gas to a patient unless you are sure of its contents.

Getting oxygen to patients requires more than simply having oxygen cylinders available. You must have in place an entire functioning system, comprising not only the apparatus for oxygen delivery, but also people who have been trained to operate it and a system for maintenance, repair and supply of spare parts.

A complete system for using oxygen in cylinders requires:

- Reliable source of oxygen supply in cylinders
- Transport to get the cylinders to the hospital
- Procedures to ensure that the hospital orders the appropriate amount of oxygen
- Apparatus to deliver oxygen from the cylinder to the patient:
  - Suitable regulator
  - Flow meter
  - Oxygen delivery tubing
  - Humidifier
  - Tube to carry oxygen to the patient's face
  - Nasal catheter (or mask) to deliver the oxygen to the patient's airway
- Person with clinical training to give the correct amount of oxygen, in the correct manner, to the patients who need it
- Person with technical training to inspect the apparatus, maintain it in good condition and repair it when necessary
- Adequate budget to ensure the consistent availability of the oxygen supply.

Safe use of oxygen cylinders

The oxygen supply from a cylinder must be connected through a suitable pressure-reducing valve (regulator). For larger cylinders, this valve is incorporated into the cylinder's pressure gauge; on a Boyle's machine both the gauge and the pressure-reducing valve are part of the machine.

Using oxygen from cylinders without a regulator is extremely dangerous.

When connecting a cylinder to the anaesthetic apparatus, make sure that the connectors are free from dust or foreign bodies that might cause the valves to stick. Never apply grease or oil, as it could catch fire in pure oxygen, especially at high pressure. Remember that an oxygen cylinder contains compressed oxygen in gaseous form and that the reading on the cylinder pressure gauge will therefore fall proportionately as the contents are used. A full oxygen cylinder normally has a pressure of around 13 400 kPa (132 atmospheres, 2000 p.s.i.). It should always be replaced if the internal pressure is less than 800 kPa (8 atmospheres, 120 p.s.i.) as failure is then imminent.

> Oxygen cylinders are dangerous objects. If they fall over, they may injure or even kill.

Make sure that cylinders are safely stored and mounted. In storage, they should lie horizontally. In use, they should be securely fixed in the vertical position to a wall or be kept standing secured with a restraining strap or chain.

Supplies, equipment and maintenance

Compressed oxygen is expensive and using it may pose logistical and cost problems for small or remote hospitals. In the United Republic of Tanzania, for example, a recent survey showed that 75% of district hospitals had an oxygen supply for less than 25% of the year. A reliable system for cylinder oxygen depends on a good source of supply and reliable year-round transportation. In many countries, oxygen cylinders must be bought rather than rented and frequent losses of cylinders in transit impose additional costs.

Fortunately, since oxygen is needed for a variety of industrial as well as medical applications, it is widely available. Because cylinders of "industrial" oxygen and of "medical" oxygen are produced by the same process (the fractional distillation of air), good-quality industrial oxygen is perfectly safe for medical use. It may also be easier to obtain and less expensive, since a price premium is often levied for "medical-grade" oxygen. However, if you obtain oxygen from an unorthodox source, you must check it for purity before use (a portable analyzer may be used).

Efficient and economical use of oxygen – while still ensuring that the patient receives the maximum benefit – is important. If properly understood, oxygen supplies can be used quite economically. The oxygen concentration of air (21%) generally needs to be increased only to about 40% in order to bring great benefit to the majority of patients who need extra oxygen.

OXYGEN CONCENTRATORS

Oxygen concentrators are suitable for use in all levels of hospital. They provide oxygen more cheaply than cylinders, as well as making oxygen available in hospitals where a regular supply of cylinders is difficult to obtain. It is strongly recommended that only those models listed by the World Health Organization as suitable should be purchased for use in district hospitals. An up-to-date list of suitable concentrators currently known to meet the recommended performance standard is available from the Department of Blood Safety and Clinical Technology, World Health Organization and UNICEF supplies concentrators meeting the Performance Standard at a very economical price (see page 15–7).

Oxygen concentrators designed for use with individual patients normally give a flow rate of up to 4 litres per minute of near-pure oxygen at relatively low pressure. This oxygen can be used in exactly the same way as oxygen from a cylinder:

- As the supply for T-piece enrichment into a draw-over system
- For use with a nasal catheter, prongs or face mask to give postoperative or ward oxygen.

The oxygen from a concentrator is at relatively low pressure and therefore cannot be used in a compressed gas (Boyle's) anaesthetic machine.

If there is an electrical power failure, the oxygen flow from a concentrator will continue for about a minute only, so make sure you have a back-up system for use in such emergencies – either a generator to maintain electrical supply, or a cylinder of compressed oxygen.

Oxygen concentrators have been installed in many hospitals where cylinders are not consistently available. Concentrators ensure a more reliable and lower-cost supply of oxygen than cylinders. An oxygen concentrator uses zeolite to separate oxygen from nitrogen in air. The oxygen produced by concentrators is at least 90% pure and can be used in the same way as oxygen from cylinders, with the same beneficial effects.

Oxygen concentrators require much less energy than fractional distillation and have the additional advantage that oxygen is easily produced in the operating room or at the patient's bedside, provided that there is an electricity supply (a small concentrator uses about 350 W). The purchase price of a concentrator is about half the cost of a year's supply of oxygen from cylinders and running costs for electricity and spare parts are low.

A complete system for oxygen delivery based on concentrators, requires:

- Manufacturer and supplier of concentrators
- Electricity in the hospital: either mains electricity or a generator
- System to ensure that a sufficient supply of major spare parts is purchased and stored centrally and an adequate supply of minor spare parts, such as air intake filters, is available at each hospital
- Apparatus to deliver oxygen from the concentrator to the patient, which includes:
  - Flow meter (included in every concentrator)
  - Oxygen delivery tubing
  - Humidifier
  - Tube to carry oxygen to the patient's face
  - Nasal catheter (or mask) to deliver the oxygen to the patient's airway
- Person with clinical training to give the correct amount of oxygen, in the correct manner, to the patients who need it
- Person with technical training to maintain the apparatus in good condition and to repair it when necessary
- Adequate budget to ensure the consistent availability of the oxygen supply.

For successful use in a district hospital, a concentrator must:

- Be capable of functioning in adverse circumstances:
  - Ambient temperature up to 40 °C
  - Relative humidity up to 100%
  - Unstable mains voltage
  - Extremely dusty environment
- Be incapable of delivering an oxygen concentration of less than 70% oxygen

- Have a comprehensive service manual
- Have a supply of spare parts for two years' use.

A hospital planning to use oxygen concentrators should consider buying at least two. Remember that no piece of equipment will last for ever, especially if it is neglected. Hospitals need to plan for regular maintenance – usually after every 5000 hours of use. Servicing the machines is not complicated and can, if necessary, be carried out by the user after simple training.

15.3 FIRES, EXPLOSIONS AND OTHER RISKS

All operating room staff should be aware of the risks of fire or explosion as a result of the use of anaesthetic vapours. It is important to distinguish between gas mixtures that can burn and those that are explosive. Explosions are much more dangerous to both staff and patients. Of the inhalational anaesthetics mentioned in this book, only ether is flammable or explosive in clinical concentrations:

- Mixtures of ether and air in the concentrations used for anaesthesia are flammable
- Mixtures of ether and air (whatever the concentration) are not explosive
- Mixtures of ether with oxygen or nitrous oxide are explosive
- Other substances used in the operating room, such as alcoholic skin preparations, also present a risk of fire or even explosion in the presence of high concentrations of oxygen.

There is no site within the draw-over apparatus or breathing system where a fire or explosion could start. The point of risk is therefore the place where the patient's expired gas enters the room – or at any point where anaesthetic gas accidentally leaks into the room from the apparatus. If you are using 3–5% ether as an anaesthetic in combination with a muscle relaxant, it is likely that the ether concentration in the patient's expired gas will be less than the lowest flammable concentration (2%).

If ether is used on a compressed gas machine (Boyle's machine), the gases are always explosive.

When flammable gases are in use, the most likely sources of combustion in the operating theatre are the surgical diathermy machine and other electrical apparatus. Static electricity is unlikely to start a fire, but may trigger an explosion if an oxygen-rich gas mixture is present.

To minimize the risk of explosion, never allow the simultaneous use of diathermy on a patient anaesthetized with ether. If one of these techniques must be used for the benefit of the patient, the other must not be allowed.

15

If possible, your operating room and equipment should be of the antistatic type. This is important in a dry climate, but less so in a humid one where a natural coating of moisture on objects prevents the buildup of static.

Electrical sockets and switches should either be spark-proof or be situated at least 1 metre above floor level. The patient's expired gases should be carried away from the expiratory valve down wide-bore tubing at least to the floor (ether is heavier than air) or out of the operating room. Make sure that no-one stands on the hose and that there is nothing that could trigger combustion near the end of the tubing. If you use oxygen enrichment during induction, but not surgery, the patient's expired gas will cease to be explosive within 3 minutes of stopping the addition of oxygen.

No potential cause of combustion or source of sparking should be allowed within 30 cm of any expiratory valve through which a potentially flammable or explosive mixture is escaping.

15.4 CARE AND MAINTENANCE OF EQUIPMENT

The important principles of care and maintenance are:

- The anaesthetist working alone in a small hospital must understand and take responsibility for the upkeep of apparatus as well as for the care of patients
- All equipment requires regular inspection, maintenance and repair to prevent it from rapidly deteriorating and becoming dangerous
- Make a detailed list or inventory of the equipment you have to enable you to identify any extra items needed
- As well as basic equipment, list spare parts, batteries and other consumables that will be needed and find out in advance how you can obtain them
- Try to estimate when new parts will be required and order spares well in advance, before the machine breaks down and leaves you in difficulty
- Ensure that all types of apparatus are kept in a clean and dust-free environment, away from extremes of temperature and covered when not in use
- Ensure that vaporizers are drained of anaesthetic if they are unlikely to be used for a week or more
- Put a cork or spigot in the end of any gas port or tubing during storage to prevent the entry of insects.

A detailed description of the types of anaesthetic equipment likely to be found in a district hospital appears in *Anaesthesia at the District Hospital* (WHO, 2001).

For technical advice about simple maintenance, see *Maintenance and Repair of Laboratory, Diagnostic Imaging and Hospital Equipment* (WHO, 1994) and *Care and Safe Use of Hospital Equipment* (Skeet and Fear, VSO Publications).

Part 6

Traumatology and Orthopaedics

Acute trauma management

16

16.1 TRAUMA IN PERSPECTIVE

Violence is a leading public health problem. Each year more than two million people die as a result of injuries caused by violence. Many more survive their injuries, but remain permanently disabled. Among people aged 15–44 years, interpersonal violence is the third most common cause of death, suicide the fourth and war the sixth. In addition to injuries and death, violence can result in a wide variety of health problems. These include profound mental health problems, sexually transmitted diseases, unwanted pregnancies as well as behavioural problems.

Throughout the world, injuries have become a major public health problem. In industrialized countries, intentional and unintentional (accidental) injuries have become the third most common cause of overall mortality and a main cause of death among the 18–40 year old age group. Trauma, including injuries resulting from road traffic accidents, is the second most common cause of death after AIDS in the 18–25 age group. This has a huge impact on financial stability in any society.

Trauma prevention is the most important aspect of trauma care management. Medical and nursing teams are in a unique position to educate patients and health workers about effective ways of preventing injury.

KEY POINTS

- Correct management within the first few hours after the injury is vital
- Your hospital should have a trauma system, such as Primary Trauma Care, to ensure that life-threatening conditions can be quickly identified and treated
- Hospital staff should be trained in acute trauma care, which requires effective teamwork.

TRAUMA CARE SYSTEMS AND TRAINING

The Annex contains the *Primary Trauma Care Manual: Trauma Management in District and Remote Locations* which can be used for quick reference and also to teach the basic knowledge and skills needed to identify traumatized patients who require rapid assessment, resuscitation and stabilization of their injuries.

The *Primary Trauma Care Manual* provides a foundation on which doctors and nurses can build the necessary knowledge and skills for trauma management with minimal equipment and without sophisticated technological requirements.

Factors given special consideration in the *Primary Trauma Care Manual* include:

- The great distances over which patients may have to be transported to reach hospital
- The time taken for them to reach hospital
- Possible absence of high-technology equipment and supplies
- Possible lack of specialists in trauma care at district hospitals.

16

> The prevention of trauma is by far the least expensive and most effective way of reducing the injuries and deaths caused by trauma.

Preventive strategies include:
- Improvements in road safety
- Better driver training
- Pedestrian and cyclist awareness
- Wearing of seat belts in cars or helmets for motor cyclists
- Preventing drivers from drinking alcohol
- Limiting civil and urban unrest.

These strategies are not easy to implement and success in trauma prevention in an area depends on many factors, including:
- Culture
- Availability of personnel
- Politics
- Health budget
- Training.

16.2 PRINCIPLES OF PRIMARY TRAUMA CARE MANAGEMENT

AIMS IN MANAGING THE INJURED PATIENT

1 Examine, diagnose and treat life-threatening complications of trauma as soon as the patient arrives in the hospital.

2 Use the simplest treatment possible to stabilize the patient's condition.

3 Perform a complete, thorough examination of the patient to ensure that no other injuries are missed.

4 Constantly reassess the patient for response to treatment; if the patient's condition deteriorates, reassess the patient.

5 Start definitive treatment only after the patient is stable.

6 When definitive treatment is not available locally, have a plan for the safe transfer of the patient to another centre.

Trauma deaths

Trauma deaths occur in three time periods.

Immediate deaths

Patients who do not reach the hospital alive die from overwhelming injuries, including:
- Rupture of the heart or pulmonary artery
- Overwhelming haemorrhage
- Massive destruction of brain or other neural tissue.

Such deaths can be reduced only by preventive strategies in the community.

Early deaths

Patients who arrive alive at the hospital need immediate resuscitation to survive. Many deaths in the early time period are preventable with appropriate early diagnosis and treatment of severe life-threatening injuries such as:

- Pneumothorax
- Flail chest
- Abdominal haemorrhage
- Pelvic and long bone injuries.

Late deaths

Late deaths occur as a result of:

- Infection
- Multiple organ failure.

Appropriate initial care can prevent late complications and death.

> However long since the injury, trauma care must start immediately the patient arrives. If you do this, you can save lives and prevent complications and disability.

16.3 SIX PHASES OF PRIMARY TRAUMA CARE MANAGEMENT

The successful management of severe trauma is dependent on the following six steps.

1 Triage
2 Primary survey
3 Secondary survey
4 Stabilization
5 Transfer
6 Definitive care.

The sequence of PTC is illustrated in Figure 16.1 (page 16–4):

- Start resuscitation at the same time as making the primary survey
- Do not start the secondary survey until you have completed the primary survey
- Do not start definitive treatment until the secondary survey is complete.

TRIAGE

Triage means sorting and treating patients according to priority, which is usually determined by:

- Medical need
- Personnel available
- Resources available.

16

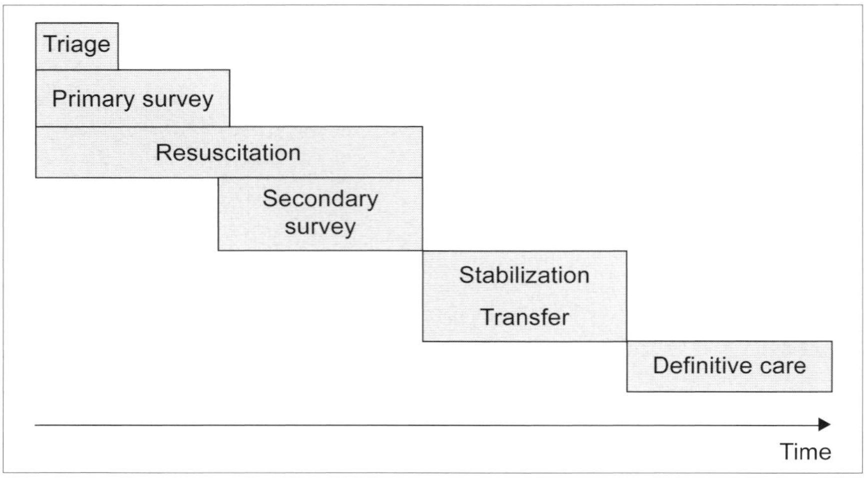

Figure 16.1

Patients are routinely sorted according to priority:
- In the clerking of patients
- Setting the order of operating lists
- In emergency rooms
- In disaster areas.

PRIMARY SURVEY

This section is covered at length in the Annex: *Primary Trauma Care Manual.*

Make a full primary and secondary survey of any patient who is injured, especially patients who have:
- History of:
  - A fall >3 metres
  - Road traffic accident: net speed >30 km/hour
  - Thrown from a vehicle or trapped in a vehicle
  - Pedestrian or cyclist hit by a car
  - Unrestrained occupant of a vehicle
  - Death of a person in the same accident or from assault
  - Injury from high or low velocity weapon
- And/or on examination:
  - Airway or respiratory distress
  - Blood pressure <100 mmHg
  - Glasgow Coma Scale <13/15 (see Annex, page PCTM–23)
  - Penetrating injury
  - >1 area injured.

The importance of ABCDE

ABCDE is a simple way of remembering the essentials of the primary survey. This is the first survey of PTC; it is also something you must return to whenever the patient's condition becomes worse – whether this occurs 5 minutes or 5 days after the patient arrives.

A is for Airway

No oxygen can reach the tissues if the airway is obstructed; the commonest cause of obstruction is unconsciousness combined with the supine position, which causes the tongue to fall back and the pharynx to collapse. Other causes include neck trauma and foreign bodies.

B is for Breathing

Even with an open airway, no oxygen reaches the lungs unless the patient is breathing or someone provides artificial ventilation of the lungs. Breathing may stop because of severe head injury, hypoxia, mechanical or circulatory arrest.

C is for Circulation

Oxygen in the lungs cannot reach the tissues unless the heart is working; common reasons for inadequate circulation include blood loss (shock) and increased pressure on the heart from pneumothorax or haemopericardium. Shock and low blood pressure are dangerous for all patients, but especially for patients with head injury, as the blood supply to the brain will be further reduced. This causes a vicious circle in which hypoxia causes further brain swelling which, in turn, reduces the flow of blood to the brain.

D is for Disability and neurological Damage (brain and spinal cord)

Checking for neurological damage is a vital part of the primary survey. Do not make a full neurological examination at this stage. Grade the patient's initial level of consciousness using a simple classification such as:

- A Alert
- V Verbal response
- P Resonance to Pain
- U Unresponsive.

Complete the examination within 30 seconds.

E is for Exposure

Remove the patient's clothing and examine the whole patient, front and back, but do not allow the patient to get cold. Examining the whole patient is the only way to be sure that you have not missed other injuries.

Immediately treat any life-threatening problems, such as bleeding, pneumothorax or obstructed airway, that you find during the ABCDE primary survey. Less urgent problems, such as an arm fracture, must wait until the patient is stable; they will be picked up in the secondary survey and should be treated appropriately in the definitive care phase.

The ABCDE is easy to remember in English. If you are reading this in another language, try to find a simple way of remembering these points in the right order in your own language. In an emergency, a simple aid such as this is useful to help you remember the six phases of Primary Trauma Care Management, but it does not replace the need to think carefully about each patient.

Resuscitation skills

There are a small number of practical skills that are essential for the initial resuscitation of injured patients. The only way to learn them is by gaining practical experience under the supervision of a person who is skilled in their use. An experienced anaesthetist or trauma surgeon will also be able to help you gain practice and experience.

The skills you need include:

- Making a rapid examination to diagnose and treat life-threatening injuries, including the possible need for cardiopulmonary resuscitation
- Airway skills: simple manoeuvres, artificial airway use, tracheal intubation and tracheostomy, if needed
- Reliably siting an intravenous cannula in any available vein
- Management of shock
- Patient handling: care of spinal injuries, in-line traction and log rolling
- Insertion of a chest drain.

These techniques, and other procedures such as tracheostomy, are covered in the Annex: *Primary Trauma Care Manual* and on pages 16–8 to 16–13.

SECONDARY SURVEY

The purpose of the secondary survey is to make sure you examine all systems and parts of the body to ensure that nothing important is missed. During the secondary survey, you should identify all the injuries and start to think about your treatment plan. An X-ray examination, if available, is part of the secondary survey.

> If there is any unexplained deterioration at any time, you must repeat the primary survey.

During the secondary survey, look in detail at:

- Head, neck and spine
- Nervous system: now you can do a more extensive neurological examination
- Thorax
- Abdomen: if you suspect intra-abdominal bleeding consider diagnostic peritoneal lavage; even if this is negative, you may need to do an urgent laparotomy
- Pelvis and limb injuries

After the secondary survey, fully document your findings, including:

- Detailed history of the injury
- Previous medical history
- Medication
- Drug allergies
- Findings during examination of primary and secondary survey:
  - Results of any special investigations
  - Details of treatment given and the patient's response.

STABILIZATION AND TRANSFER

You have examined the patient, treated life-threatening conditions and made a second examination to detect any other injuries. The management plan of the patient should now be clear.

When documentation has been completed, analgesia administered, laboratory investigations sent and any fractures immobilized, you can then decide on the best treatment option:

- Transfer to the ward
- Transfer to the operating room
- Transfer to the X-ray department
- Transfer to another hospital.

Before referring a patient:

- Remember that referral is not a form of medical treatment
- Make contact with the referral centre to ensure that they can help
- Anticipate what else may go wrong on the road and be prepared for it
- Provide pain relief for the journey
- Arrange for a trained person to go with the patient.

For more details on transfer, see pages 1–15 and 3–3.

DEFINITIVE CARE

Once the patient has been resuscitated, stabilized and transferred, the planned correction of the injury can proceed.

In order to save the patient's life, it may be necessary to carry out an immediate surgical procedure as part of the initial primary survey and early resuscitation. The decision whether to rush the patient to the operating room needs careful consultation and good communication between the surgeon and anaesthetist.

Special patients and special situations

Be aware of special patients and special situations. Children and pregnant women, for example, have special needs and may need different treatment because their anatomy and physiology vary from that of a non-pregnant adult. Details of the differences are given in Unit 3.2: *The Paediatric Patient*, Unit 14.3: *Paediatric Anaesthesia* and the Annex: *Primary Trauma Care Manual*.

16.3 PROCEDURES

The remainder of this Unit contains details of procedures which, although not described in detail in the Annex: *Primary Trauma Care Manual*, may be needed in the management of severely injured patients.

16

INSERTION OF CHEST DRAIN AND UNDERWATER SEAL DRAINAGE

Indications for underwater-seal chest drainage are:

- Pneumothorax
- Haemothorax
- Haemopneumothorax
- Acute empyema.

Technique

1 Prepare the skin with antiseptic and infiltrate the skin, muscle and pleura with 1% lidocaine at the appropriate intercostal space, usually the fifth or sixth, in the midaxillary line (Figure 16.2). Note the length of needle needed to enter the pleural cavity; this information may be useful later when you are inserting the drain.

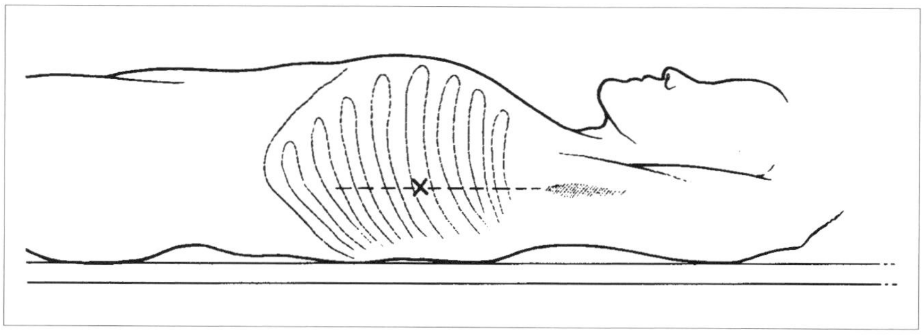

Figure 16.2

2 Aspirate fluid from the chest cavity to confirm your diagnosis (Figure 16.3).

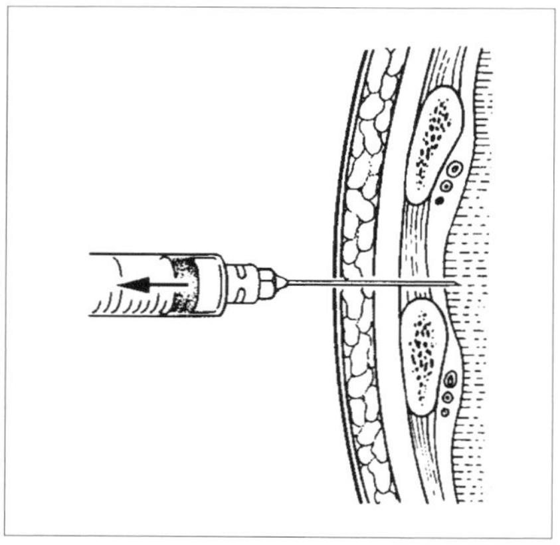

Figure 16.3

3 Make a small transverse incision just above the rib to avoid damaging the vessels under the lower part of the rib (Figures 16.4, 16.5). In children, it is advisable to keep strictly to the middle of the intercostal space.

4 Using a pair of large, curved artery forceps, penetrate the pleura and enlarge the opening (Figures 16.6, 16.7). Use the same forceps to grasp the tube at its tip and introduce it into the chest (Figures 16.8, 16.9).

5 Close the incision with interrupted skin sutures, using one stitch to anchor the tube. Leave an additional suture untied adjacent to the tube for closing the wound after the tube is removed. Apply a gauze dressing.

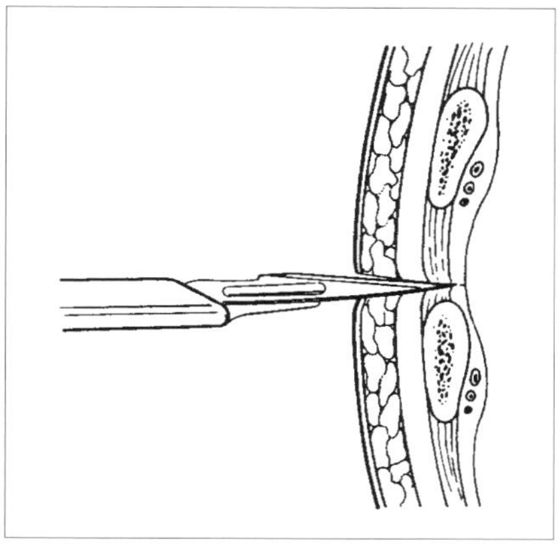

Figure 16.4

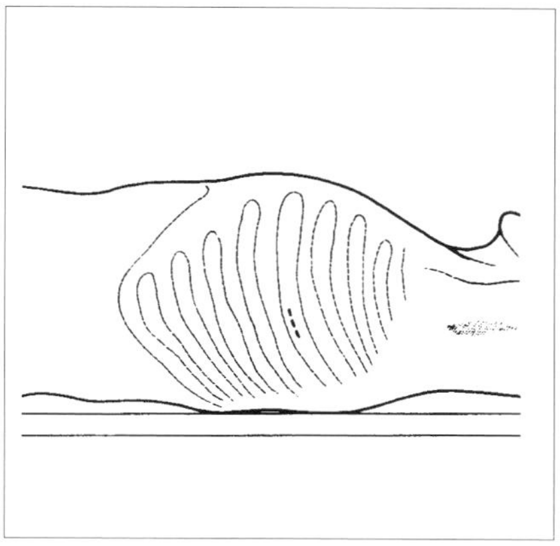

Figure 16.5

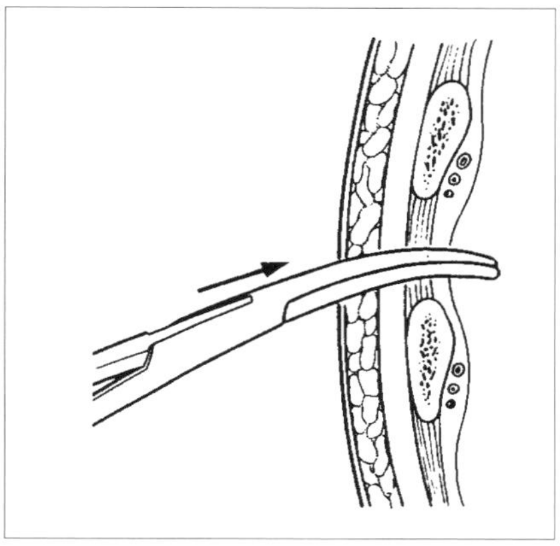

Figure 16.6

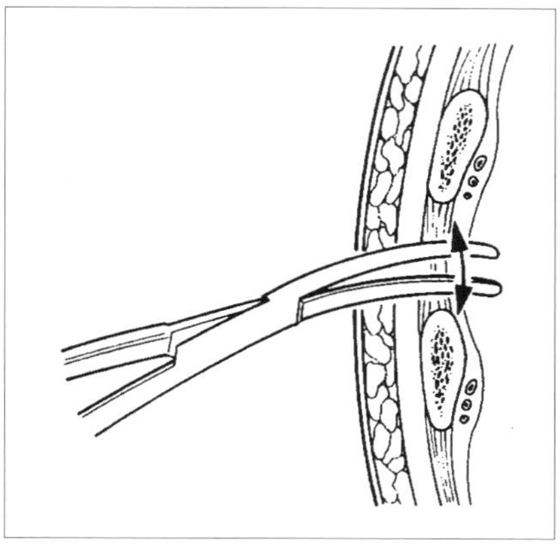

Figure 16.7

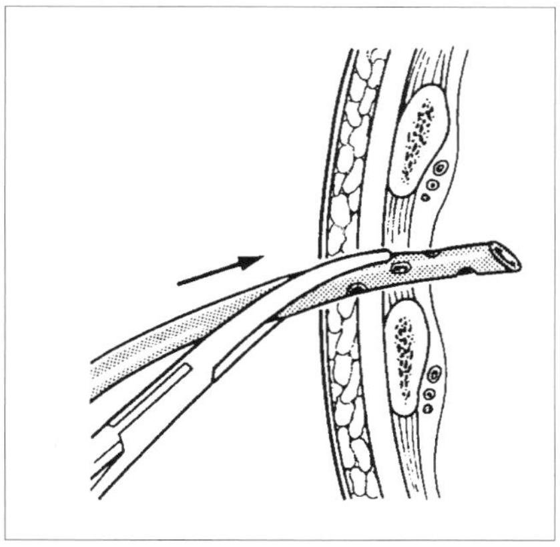

Figure 16.8

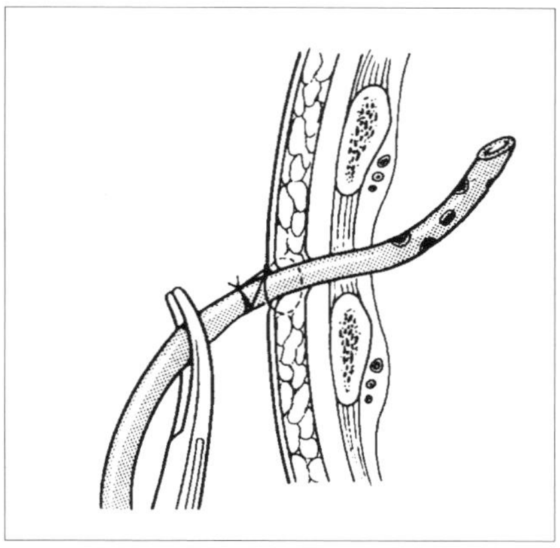

Figure 16.9

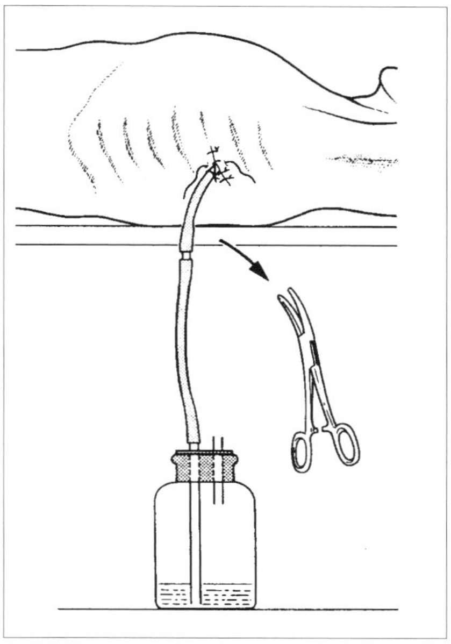

Figure 16.10

6 Connect the tube to the underwater-seal drainage system and mark the initial level of fluid in the drainage bottle (Figure 16.10).

Aftercare

Place a pair of large artery forceps by the bedside for clamping the tube when changing the bottle. The drainage system is patent if the fluid level swings freely with changes in the intrapleural pressure. Persistent bubbling over several days suggests a bronchopleural fistula and is an indication for referral.

Change the connecting tube and the bottle at least once every 48 hours, replacing them with sterile equivalents. Wash and disinfect the used equipment to remove all residue before it is resterilized.

If there is no drainage for 12 hours, despite your "milking" the tube, clamp the tube for a further 6 hours and X-ray the chest. If the lung is satisfactorily expanded, the clamped tube can then be removed.

To remove the tube, first sedate the patient and then remove the dressing. Clean the skin with antiseptic. Hold the edges of the wound together with fingers and thumb over gauze while cutting the skin stitch that is anchoring the tube. Withdraw the tube rapidly as an assistant ties the previously loose stitch.

TRACHEOSTOMY

The indications for tracheostomy are:

- Anticipated difficulty in managing the airway
- Need to transport an unconscious patient.

The surgical management of an acute airway obstruction is an emergency cricothyroidotomy (see the Annex: *Primary Trauma Care Manual*, pages PCTM–5 and 6.

Technique for elective tracheostomy

1 Place the patient supine on a table or bed. Extend the neck by placing a sandbag (or a rolled towel for infants and children) under the shoulders (Figure 16.11).

2 Prepare the skin with antiseptic and infiltrate local anaesthetic into the skin from the suprasternal notch along the midline to the thyroid cartilage (Figure 16.12).

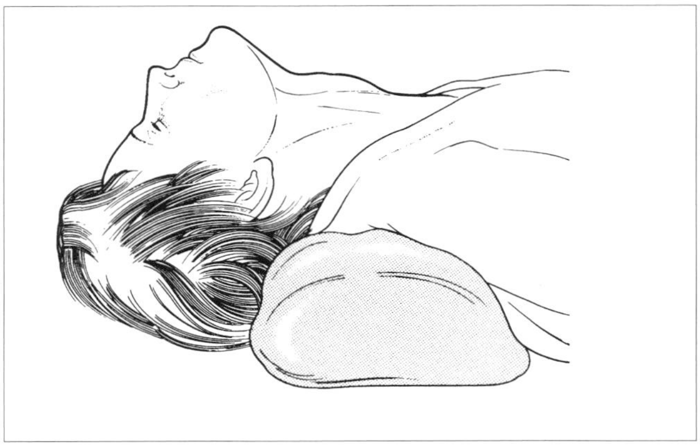

Figure 16.11

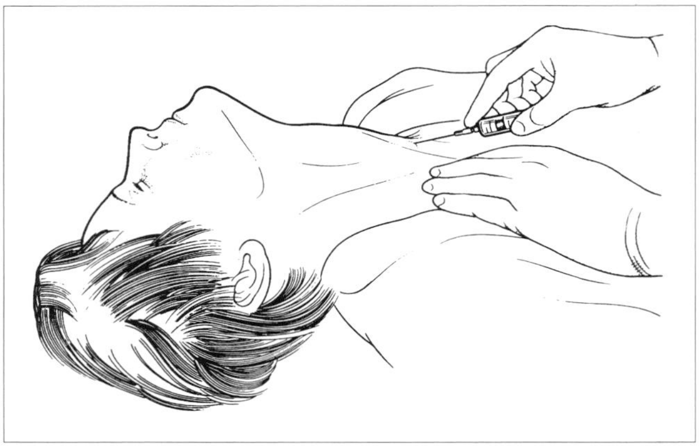

Figure 16.12

3 Palpate the cricoid cartilage to ascertain its position (Figure 16.13) and make a midline incision between its inferior border and the superior margin of the suprasternal notch (Figures 16.14, 16.15).

16

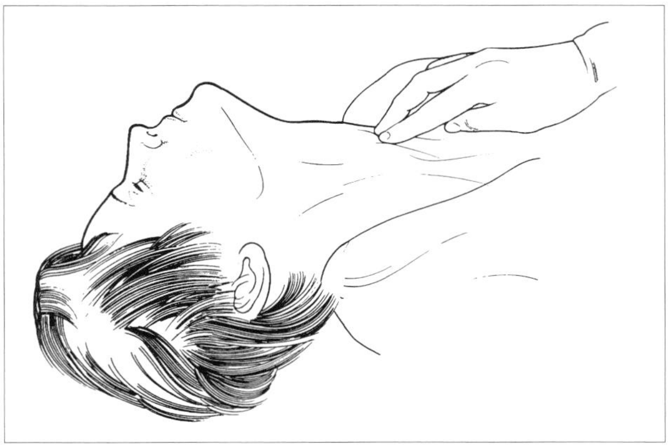

Figure 16.13

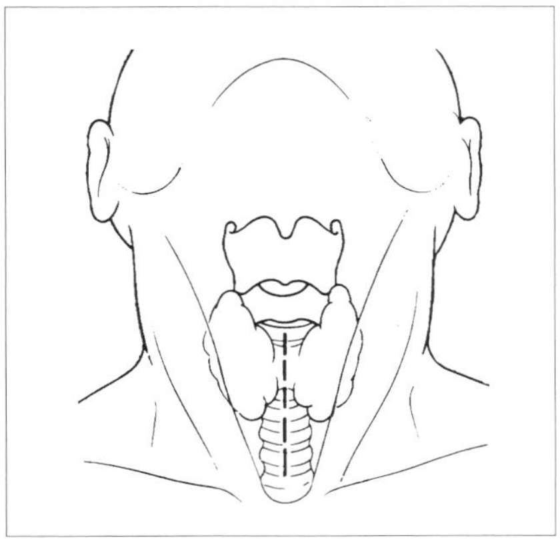

Figure 16.14

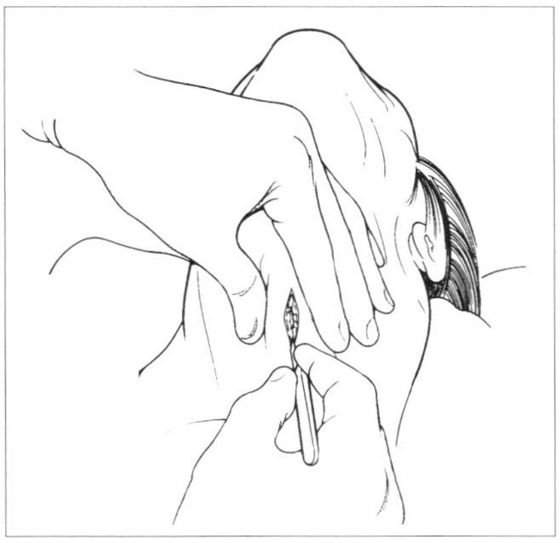

Figure 16.15

4 Separate the strap muscles from the midline by blunt dissection (Figure 16.16) to expose the trachea with the thyroid isthmus lying anterior to it. Retract the isthmus either upwards or downwards, or divide it between artery forceps and ligate the ends (Figures 16.17, 16.18). Divide and retract the pretracheal fascia (Figure 16.19) to expose the second and third tracheal cartilages. Then lift and steady the trachea with small skin-hook retractors.

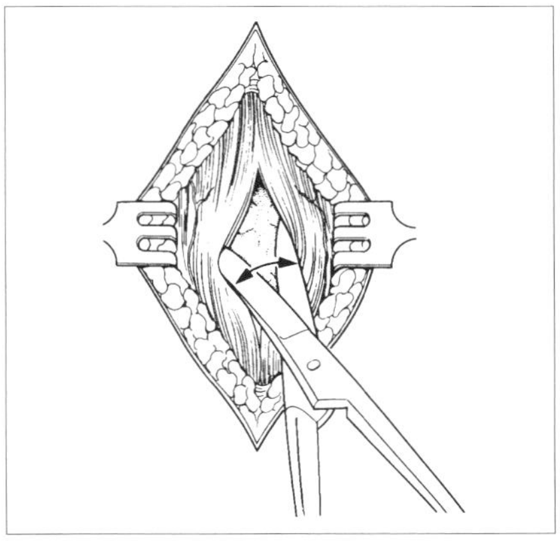

Figure 16.16

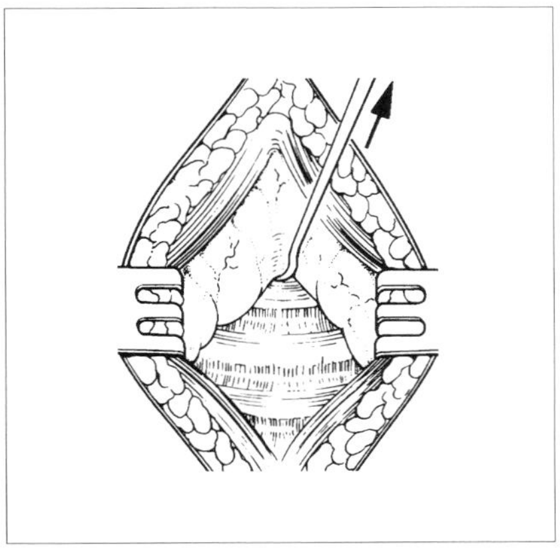

Figure 16.17

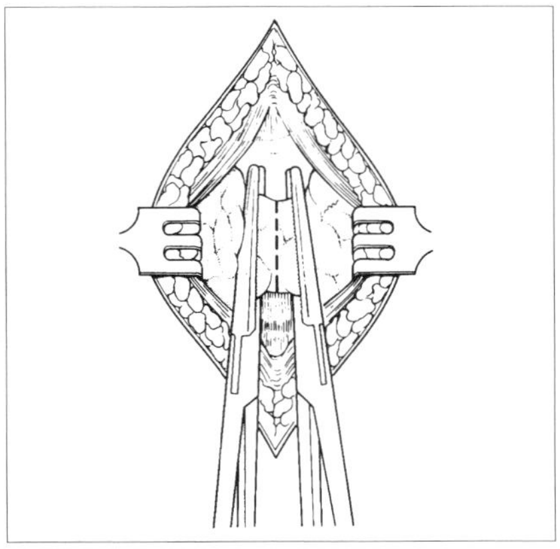

Figure 16.18

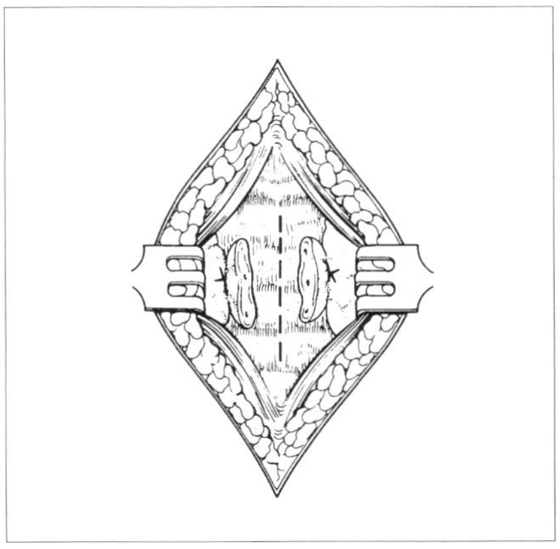

Figure 16.19

16

- In infants and children, make a transverse intercartilaginous incision between the second and third rings (Figure 16.20). Avoid excising a piece of the trachea. The incision will open further as you extend the neck over the rolled towel.

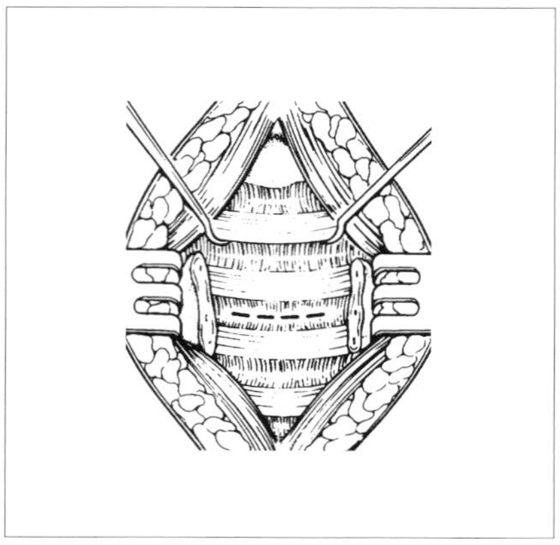

Figure 16.20

- In adults, excise a small rounded segment of the trachea (Figure 16.21). The size of the resulting hole should conform to that of the tracheostomy tube.

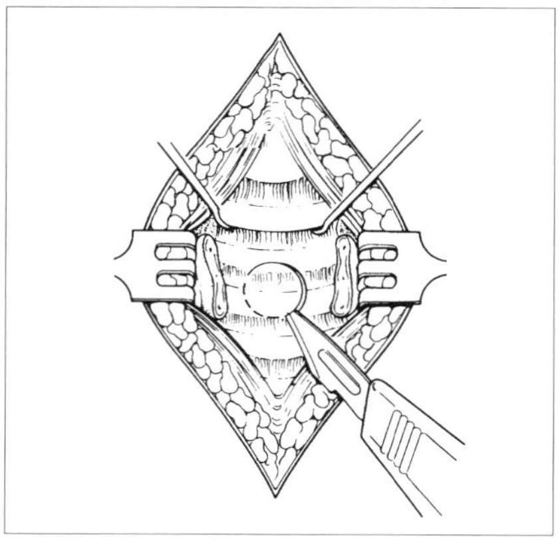

Figure 16.21

5 Aspirate secretions from the trachea at this stage (Figure 16.22) and again after insertion of the tube.

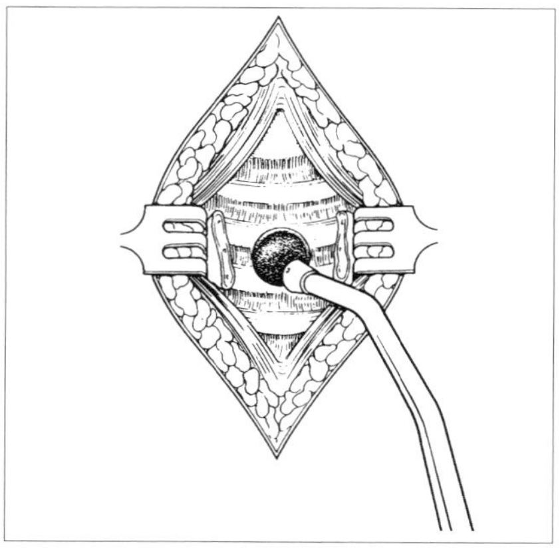

Figure 16.22

6 Insert the tracheostomy tube set, remove the obturator and loosely stitch the skin with interrupted 2-0 thread (Figures 16.23, 16.24):

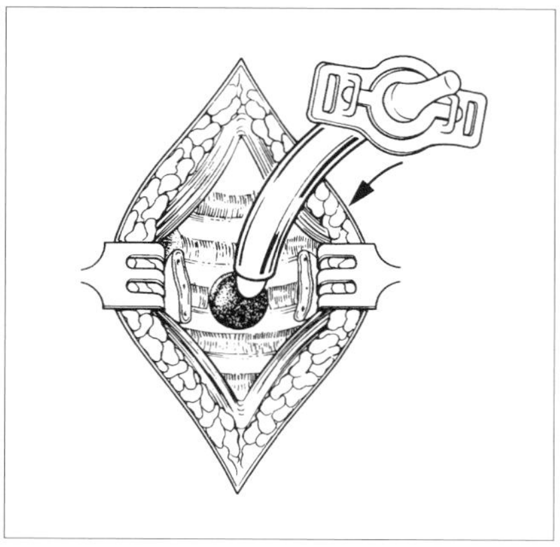

Figure 16.23

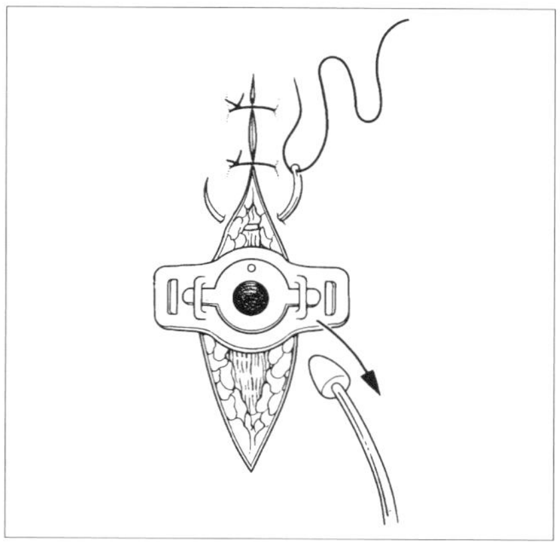

Figure 16.24

- In children, remove the rolled towel from under the shoulders before stitching the skin; a linen tape can be passed behind the neck to join the wings of the tube and hold it in place (Figure 16.25).

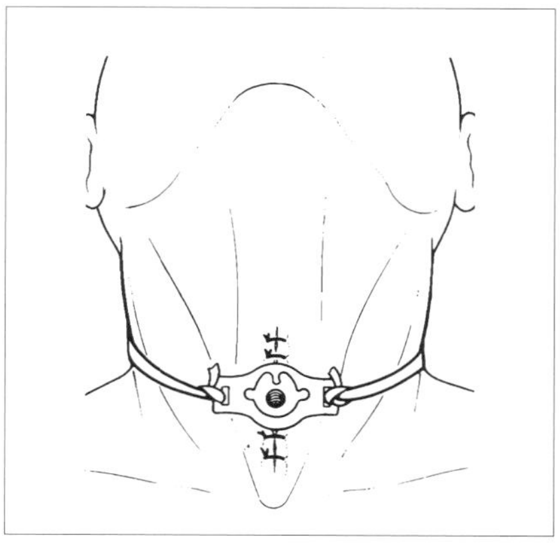

Figure 16.25

7 When placing the tracheostomy tube in the trachea, ensure that it enters the lumen accurately and completely. If the patient has been intubated, ensure that the tracheostomy tube is below the endotracheal tube; if necessary, withdraw the endotracheal tube to make this possible. Assess and confirm the patency of the inserted tracheostomy tube using the bell attachment of a stethoscope. If there is a normal flow of air through the tube, a loud blast will be heard with each expiration. With incomplete obstruction, the noise will be softer and shorter, accompanied by a wheeze or whistle. If the tube has been placed pretracheally or if it is completely blocked with secretions, no sound will be heard. Remove and replace the tube if you have any doubts about its position or patency.

Aftercare

Aspirate secretions from the tracheobronchial tree regularly, using a sterile catheter passed down through the tracheostomy tube. Avoid irritating the bronchi, which could stimulate coughing.

The air around the patient should be kept warm and humid by means of a humidifier. When necessary, instil small amounts of sterile physiological saline into the bronchi to soften the mucus.

Change the inner tracheostomy tube at regular intervals. If the outer tube becomes dislodged, reinsert it immediately and check its position both by clinical examination and chest radiography. Always have a spare tube available.

Refer the patient for further treatment, if necessary.

Complications

Complications include:

- Early postoperative bleeding
- Infection
- Surgical emphysema
- Atelectasis
- Crust formation.

Stenosis of the trachea is a possible late complication.

FASCIOTOMY

See Unit 18: Orthopaedic Trauma (18.8: Complications).

BURR HOLES

See Unit 17: Orthopaedic Techniques (17.6: Cranial Burr Holes).

Orthopaedic techniques

17

17.1 TRACTION

SKIN TRACTION

Skin traction requires pressure on the skin to maintain the pulling force across the bone. A maximum of 5 kg of weight may be applied using this method. More than 5 kg of weight will result in the skin becoming excoriated with blister formation and pressure sores caused by slipping of the tightly wrapped strapping. Wrapping the straps more tightly to prevent slipping increases the risk of creating a compartment syndrome in the injured extremity.

If more than 5 kg of weight is needed to control the fracture, use skeletal traction instead.

> Do not apply traction to skin with abrasions, lacerations, surgical wounds, ulcers, loss of sensation or peripheral vascular disease.

Technique

1 Clean the limb with soap and water and dry it. If available, use a commercial traction set, which will contain adhesive tapes, traction cords, spreader bar and foam protection for the malleoli. This is usually not available, so improvise the apparatus as described below.

2 Measure the appropriate length of adhesive strapping and place it on a level surface with the adhesive side up. Ask the patient about adhesive tape allergy before applying.

3 Place a square wooden spreader of about 7.5 cm (with a central hole) in the middle of the adhesive strapping (Figure 17.1).

4 Gently elevate the limb off the bed while applying longitudinal traction. Apply the strapping to the medial and lateral sides of the limb, allowing the spreader to project 15 cm below the sole of the foot (Figure 17.2).

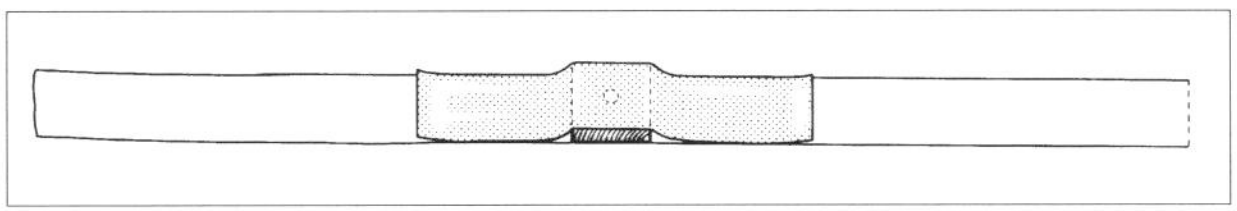

Figure 17.1

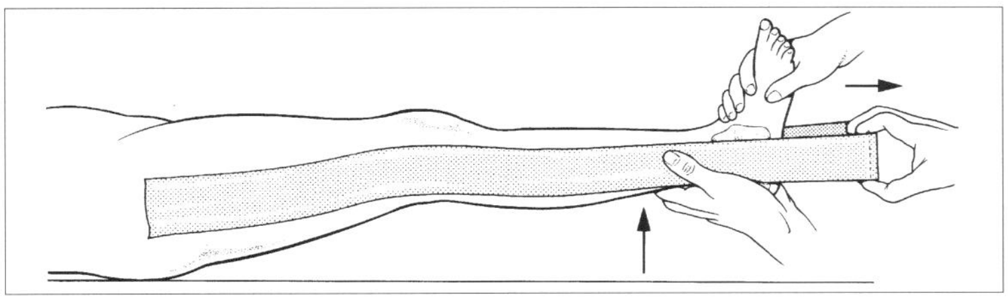

Figure 17.2

KEY POINTS

- Use an appropriate method of traction to treat fractures of the extremities and cervical spine
- Apply extremity traction to the skin or to the skeleton using a pin inserted through the bone distal to the fracture
- Apply traction to the cervical spine using a head halter chin sling or skull tongs
- The weight applied through the traction system counteracts the muscle force pulling across the fracture, keeping the bone in proper alignment and length.

17

5 Pad bony areas with felt or cotton-wool. Wrap crepe or ordinary gauze bandage firmly over the strapping (Figure 17.3).

6 Elevate the end of the bed, and attach a traction cord through the spreader with the required weight (Figure 17.4). The weight should not exceed 5 kg.

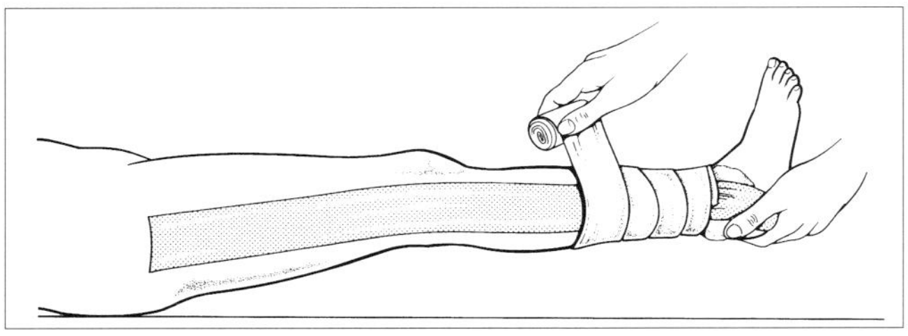

Figure 17.3

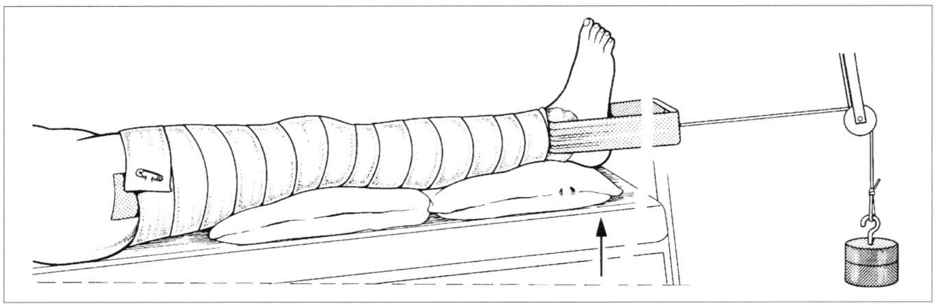

Figure 17.4

Complications

- Allergic reactions from the adhesive material
- Blister formation and pressure sores from slipping straps
- Compartment syndrome from over-tight wrap
- Peroneal nerve palsy from wraps about the knee.

SKELETAL TRACTION

Apply skeletal traction by placing a metal pin through the metaphyseal portion of the bone and apply weight to the pin. It is important to place the pin correctly to avoid injury to vessels, nerves, joints and growth plates. The amount of weight to be used depends on the fracture but, generally, between 1/10 and 1/7 of body weight is safe and adequate for most fractures.

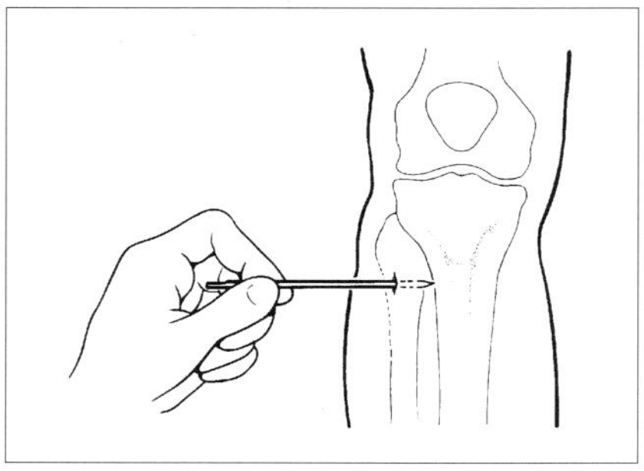

Figure 17.5

Technique

1 Wash the skin with antiseptic solution and cover the surrounding area with sterile drapes. Infiltrate the skin and soft tissues down to the bone with 1% lidocaine on both the entrance and exit sides.

2 Make a small stab incision in the skin and introduce the pin through the incision horizontally and at right angles to the long axis of the limb. Proceed until the point of the pin strikes the underlying bone (Figure 17.5). Ideally, the pin should pass through the skin and subcutaneous tissue, but not through muscles.

3 Insert the pins with a T-handle or hand drill (Figure 17.6). Advance the pin until it stretches the skin of the opposite side and make a small release incision over its point (Figure 17.7).

4 Dress the skin wounds separately with sterile gauze. Attach a stirrup to the pin, cover the pin ends with guards and apply traction (Figure 17.8).

5 Apply counter-traction by elevating the appropriate end of the bed or by placing a splint against the root of the limb.

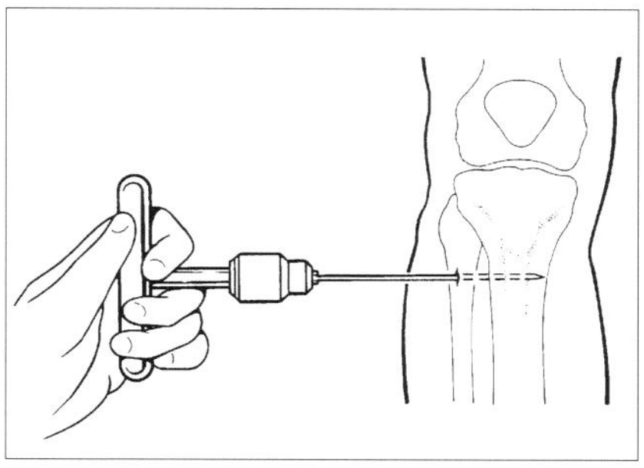

Figure 17.6

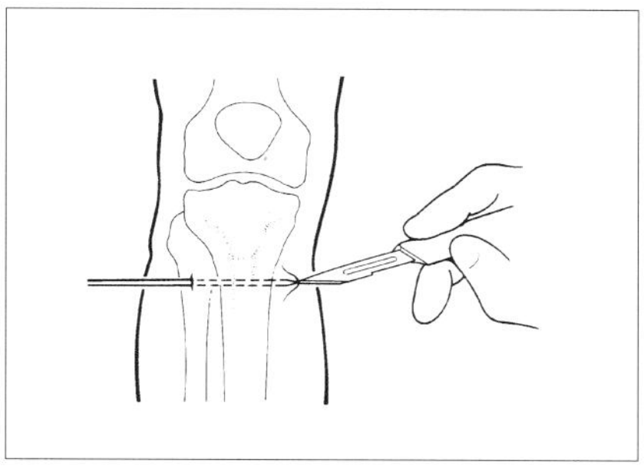

Figure 17.7

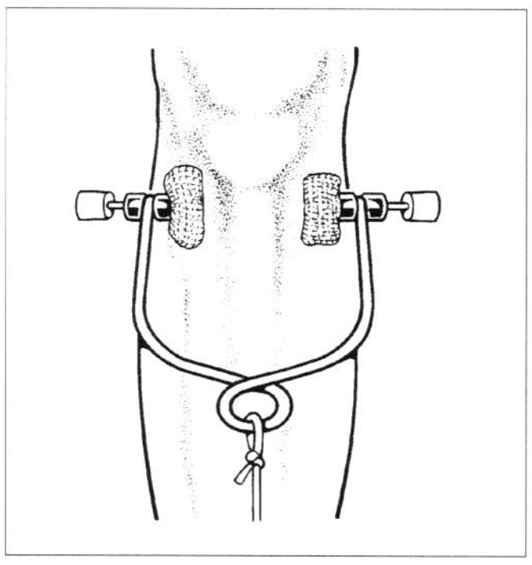

Figure 17.8

Sites of pin placement

Proximal tibia

Insert the pin 2 cm distal to the tibial tubercle and 2 cm behind the anterior border of the tibia (Figure 17.5). Begin on the lateral side to avoid the common peroneal nerve.

Calcaneus

Insert the pin 4.5 cm inferior and 4 cm posterior to the tip of the medial malleolus (Figure 17.9). Begin on the medial side to avoid damage to the posterior tibial artery and nerve and to avoid entering the subtalar joint.

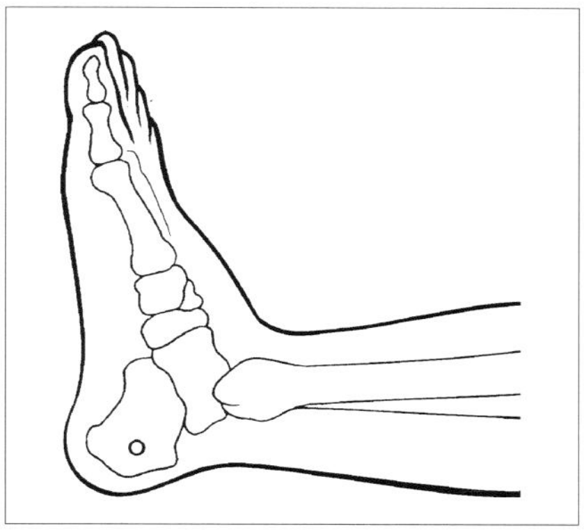

Figure 17.9

Distal femur

Insert the pin from the medial side, in the mid-portion of the bone, at the level of the proximal pole of the patella. This should be just proximal to the flare of the femoral condyles and posterior to the synovial pouch of the knee joint.

Olecranon

Insert the pin from the medial side of the ulna 2 cm from the tip of the olecranon and 1 cm anterior to the posterior cortex. This should avoid the ulnar nerve which passes through the groove inferior to the medial epicondyle of the humerus (Figure 17.10).

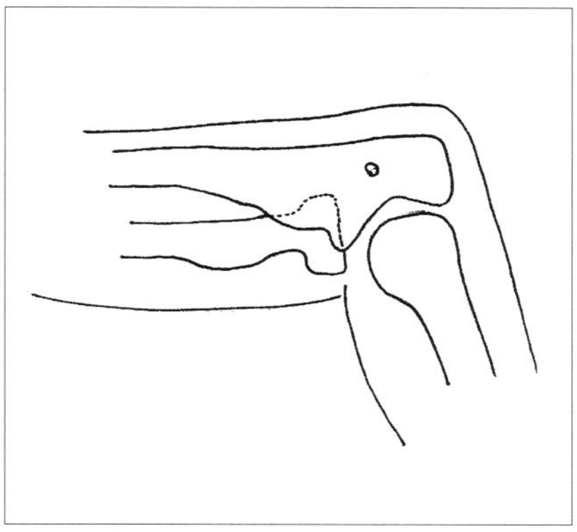

Figure 17.10

Complications

- Pin tract infection is common:
  - The skin will look inflamed with drainage about the pin; the pin will eventually loosen
  - Control the infection with wound cleansing, dressing changes and antibiotics
  - If this fails, place a new pin at a different site or discontinue traction
- Joint stiffness is prevented by active and active-assisted exercise.

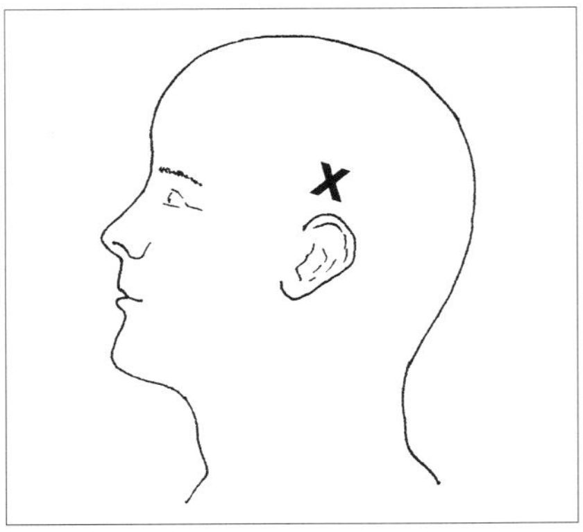

Figure 17.11

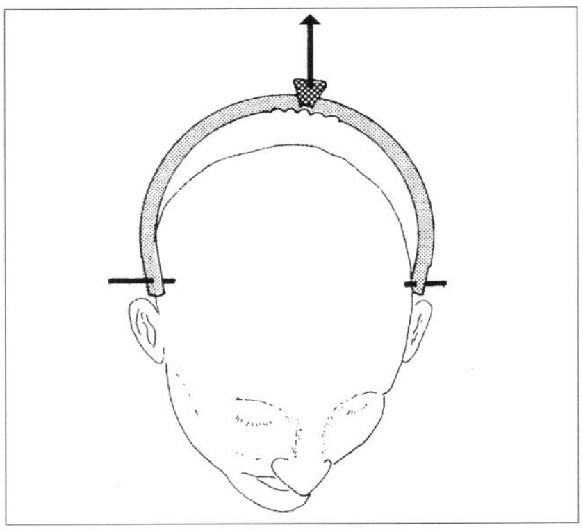

Figure 17.12

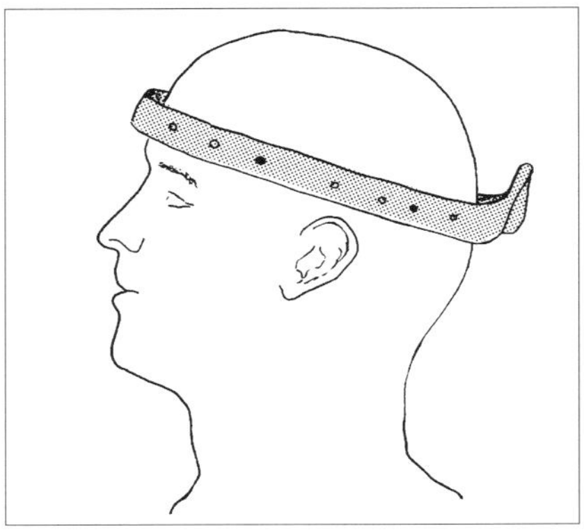

Figure 17.13

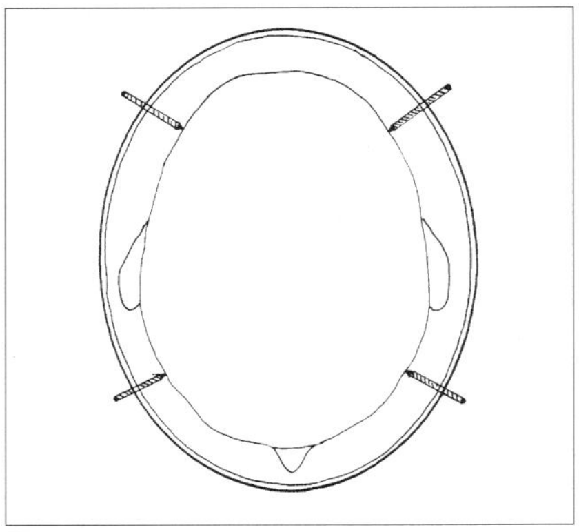

Figure 17.14

SKULL TRACTION

Use skull traction for traumatic and infectious conditions in the cervical spine. Apply it to the skin using head halter traction or to the skull bones using Gardner-Wells tongs or a halo device.

Technique: Gardner-Wells tongs

1 Place the pins below the brim of the skull in line with the external auditory meatus, 2–3 cm above the top of the pinna (Figures 17.11 and 17.12).

2 Prepare the patient's scalp by shaving the hair and washing the skin with an antiseptic solution.

3 Position the tongs correctly and mark the pin entrance points.

4 Infiltrate the pin sites with 1% lidocaine and make stab wounds through the skin and down to the bone. Insert the pins by alternately tightening one side and then the other, until 3.6 kg of torque is applied. Determine the tightness with a special torque screwdriver or by tightening the pins, using two fingers only to grip the screwdriver.

5 Dress the wounds with sterile gauze and apply the appropriate traction weight. Tighten the pins again once on the following day, then leave them alone unless they are loose.

Technique: halo traction

1 Determine the ring size by measuring the head circumference or by trial. The clearance should be 1–2 cm at all points.

2 Carefully place the patient's head off the end of the bed and hold it with a special headholder, or with an assistant. The halo should be just above the eyebrows and ears (Figure 17.13).

3 Use two pins posterior-laterally and two in the lateral third of the forehead. These may be placed as far back as the hairline for cosmetic reasons, but should be anterior to the temporal muscle (Figure 17.14).

4 Shave the hair under the selected sites for the pin holes, wash the skin with antiseptic solution and infiltrate with 1% lidocaine through the four holes selected.

5 Advance the pins to finger tightness while keeping the halo placement symmetrical. Ask the patient to keep his/her eyes closed during the procedure to avoid pulling the skin upward and preventing eye closure once the pins are tight.

6 Next, tighten the pins sequentially across the diagonals. If a torque screwdriver is available, tighten the screws to 34–45 cm/kg. If not, twist the screws tight while holding the screwdriver with two fingers.

7 Tighten the screws once after 1–2 days and thereafter only if loose. Traction can now be applied or the patient can be placed in a halo jacket.

EXTREMITY TRACTION

The following are examples of traction arrangements for the upper and lower extremities.

17

Figure 17.15: Dunlap's traction
Figure 17.16: Olecranon traction
Figure 17.17: Perkin's traction
Figure 17.18: Perkin's traction
Figure 17.19: Russell's traction
Figure 17.20: 90/90 balance suspension

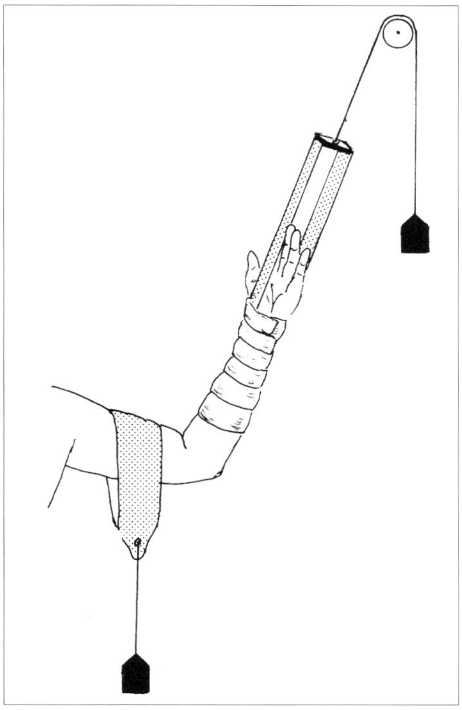

Figure 17.15

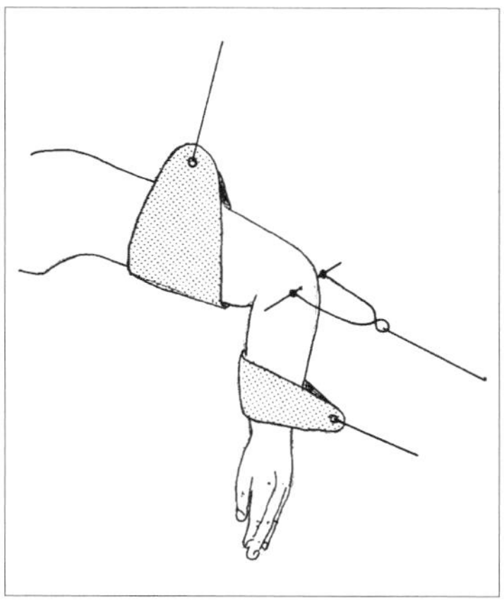

Figure 17.16

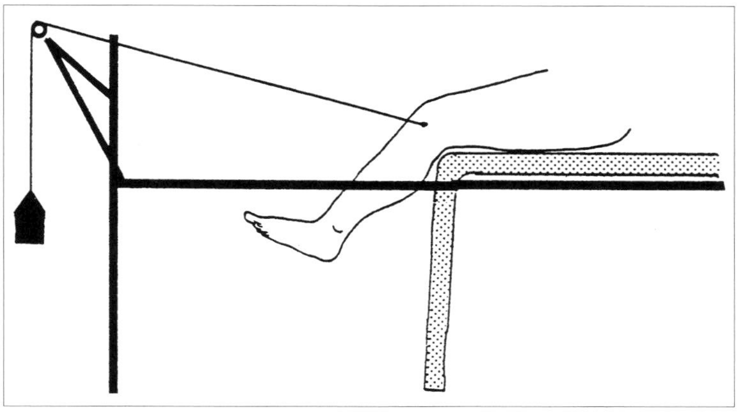

Figure 17.17

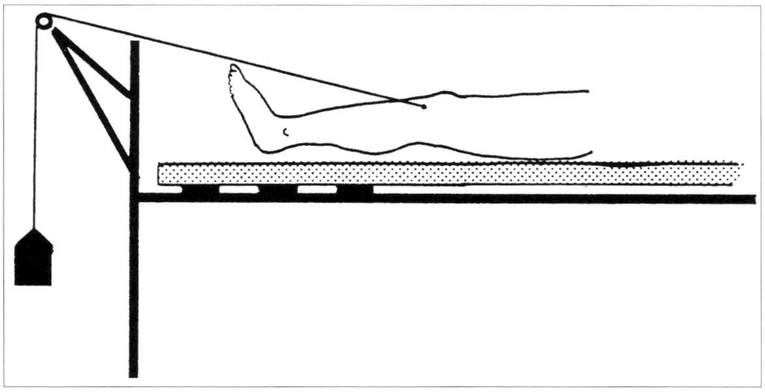

Figure 17.18

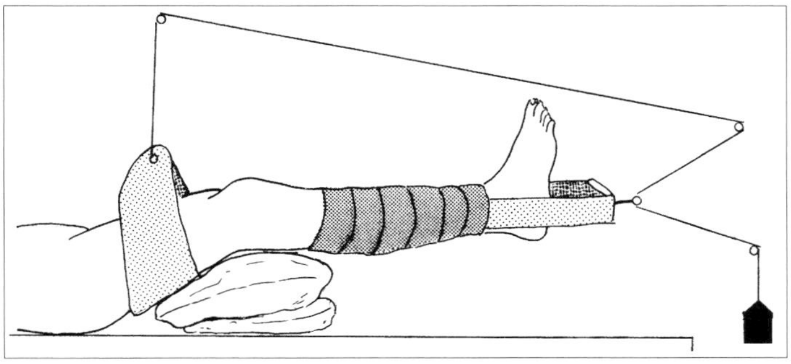

Figure 17.19

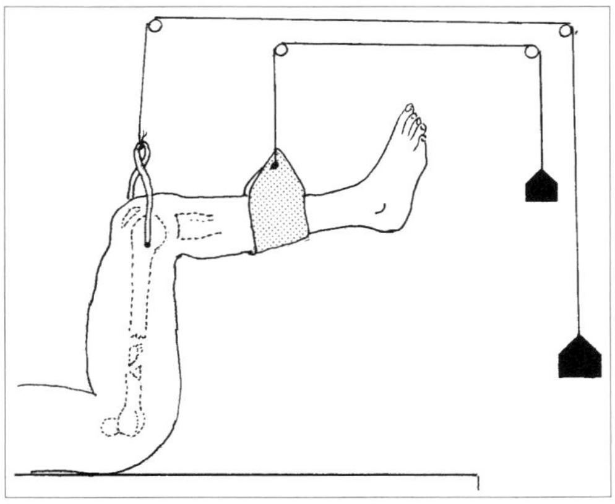

Figure 17.20

KEY POINTS

- Casts and splints provide immobilization of the extremities or spine following injuries, or in cases of other abnormalities of bone or soft tissues
- Use plaster or fibreglass to construct casts and splints
- If necessary, wood and cardboard will serve as temporary splints
- Casts are wrapped circumferentially around the extremity, providing more rigid fixation than splints
- Use a splint for acute injuries to allow room for swelling.

17.2 CASTS AND SPLINTS

MATERIALS

Plaster of Paris bandage

Plaster of Paris bandage is available in a ready-made form or is prepared locally.

To prepare plaster of Paris bandage, use dry cotton gauze (muslin) bandage, 500 cm long and 15 cm wide. Unroll a portion of the bandage on a dry table with a smooth top and apply plaster powder (anhydrous calcium sulfate or gypsum) evenly to the surface (Figure 17.21).

Gently but firmly rub the powder into the mesh of the cotton and carefully roll up the powdered portion. Begin the same process with the next section until the entire roll has been powdered. The plaster bandage can be used immediately or stored in a dry place for future use.

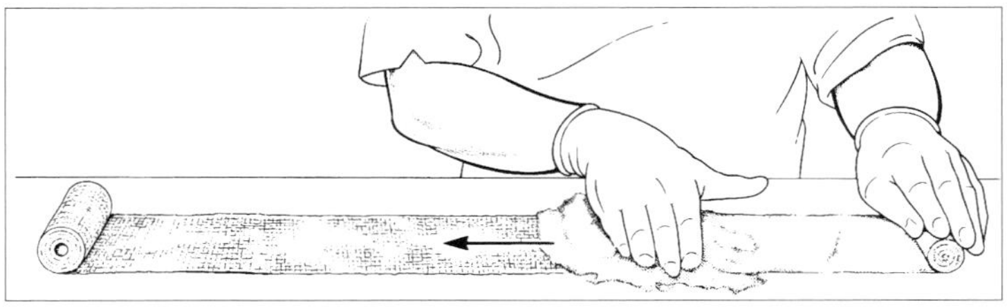

Figure 17.21

Fibreglass

Fibreglass cast and splint material is available from suppliers in ready-made rolls. It is lighter than plaster and resistant to water, but is more difficult to remove and is more expensive.

CAST APPLICATION

1 Clean the skin and apply dressings to any wounds. If available, apply stockinet to the extremity, avoiding wrinkles. Next, apply a uniform thickness of cotton padding over the stockinet and put extra padding over any bony prominence such as the patella, the elbow or the ankle (Figure 17.22).

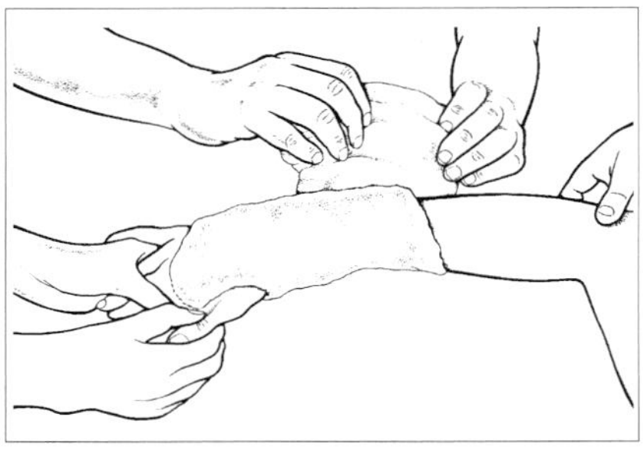

Figure 17.22

2 Soak the plaster roll in a pail containing water at room temperature. Do not use warm water as the heat given off by the plaster as it sets may burn the patient. Leave the plaster in the water until it is completely soaked and the air bubbles cease to rise.

3 Gently pick up the ends of the bandage with both hands and lightly squeeze it, pushing the ends together without twisting or wringing (Figure 17.23).

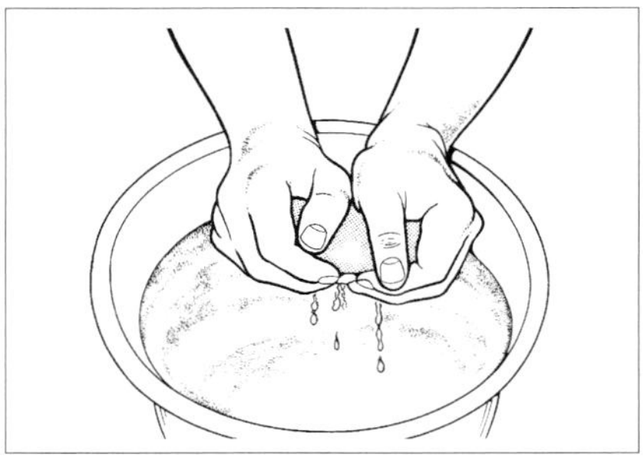

Figure 17.23

4 While applying the plaster, hold the relevant part of the body steady in the correct position. Movement will cause ridges to form on the inside of the plaster. Work rapidly and without interruption, rubbing each layer firmly with the palm so that the plaster forms a homogenous mass rather than discrete layers.

5 Apply the plaster by unrolling the bandage as it rests on the limb. Do not lift it up from the patient or apply tension to the roll. Overlap the previous layer of plaster by about half the width of the roll (Figure 17.24).

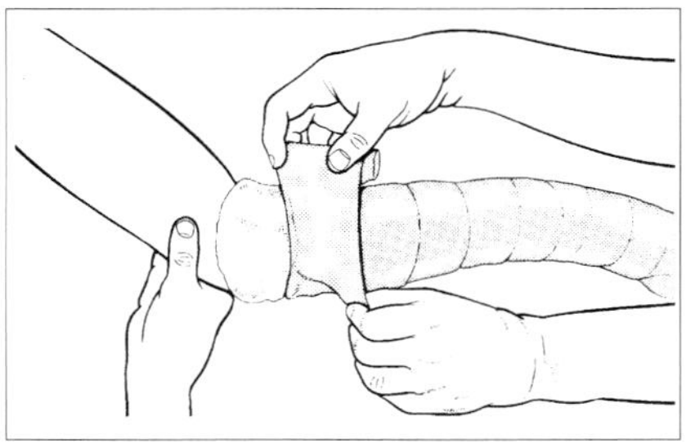

Figure 17.24

6 Mould the plaster evenly around the bony prominences and contours. Leave 3 cm of padding at the upper and lower margins of the cast to protect the skin from irritation by the edge of the cast. This can be folded back over the edge and incorporated in the last layer of plaster to provide a smooth edge (Figure 17.25).

7 Mould the cast until the plaster sets and becomes firm. Complete drying takes 24 hours so advise the patient to take care not to dent the cast or apply weight to it during this time.

8 The technique for application of a fibreglass cast is similar, but the fibreglass is slightly elastic and will contour to the body more easily. It sets firmly in about 30 minutes and will not be affected by water after that time.

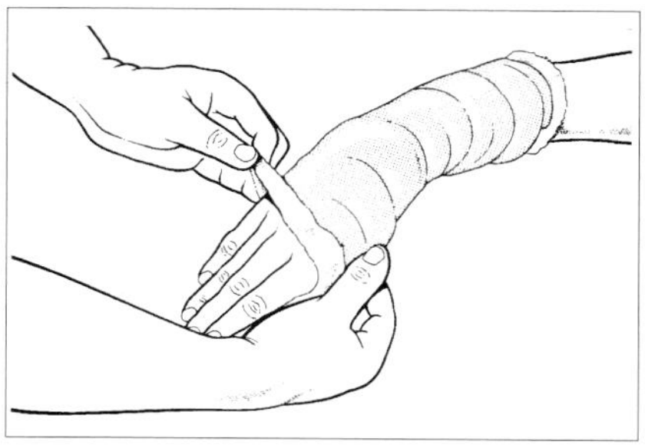

Figure 17.25

SPLINT APPLICATION

1 Measure the length of material needed to secure the limb. Place 3–5 layers of the measured padding on a flat surface and unroll 5–10 layers of plaster on to the padding (Figure 17.26).

2 Grasp the plaster layer at each end, dip into the water and gently squeeze together without twisting. Place the wet plaster on the padding and smooth with the palm into a homogeneous layer.

3 Place the splint on the extremity, with the padding side toward the patient, mould it to the limb contours and secure with an elastic bandage or gauze wrap (Figure 17.27).

4 An alternative method is to split a circular cast lengthwise, remove the anterior half and secure it similarly with an elastic bandage.

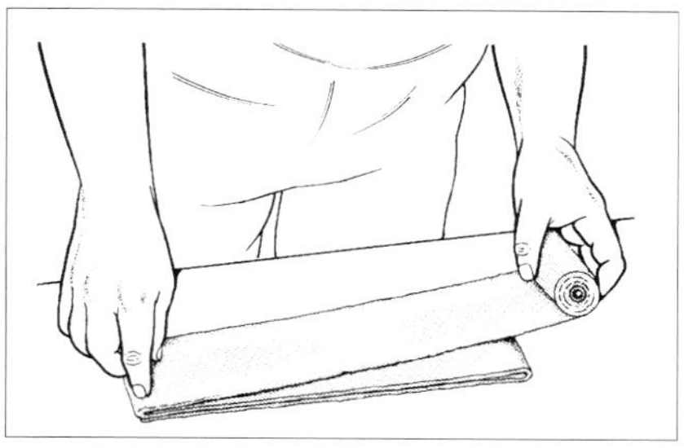

Figure 17.26

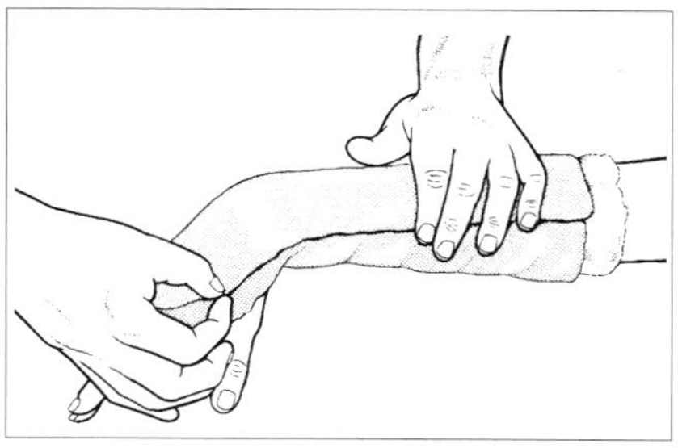

Figure 17.27

Patient instructions

Give oral and written instructions to the patient and/or to accompanying relatives or other attendants. Give the instructions in non-technical language that the patient can understand, as in the example below.

Caring for a cast or splint

- Keep the cast or splint dry at all times
- Do not try to scratch your skin under the cast or splint with a sharp or blunt object
- Allow the cast to dry for 24 hours before putting weight on it or resting it on a hard surface
- For acute injuries, elevate the injured part for 24–48 hours and wiggle your fingers or toes frequently
- Return to the health clinic immediately if:
  - Your cast or splint gets wet or becomes soft or broken
  - You have increasing pain
  - You experience numbness or tingling, or have difficulty moving your fingers or toes
  - You see a change in skin colour of the extremity
  - Your cast or splint has a foul odour.

17

REMOVING A CAST

Remove the cast with an oscillating electric cast saw, if available, or with plaster shears (Figure 17.28).

1 Make two cuts along opposing surfaces of the cast, avoiding areas where the bone is prominent. Begin cutting at an edge, then loosen the cast with a plaster spreader (Figure 17.29).

2 Complete the division of the plaster and the padding with plaster scissors, being careful not to injure the underlying skin (Figure 17.30).

3 Under difficult conditions, or if the patient is a child, soften the plaster by soaking it in water, or water with vinegar added, for 10–15 minutes and then remove it like a bandage.

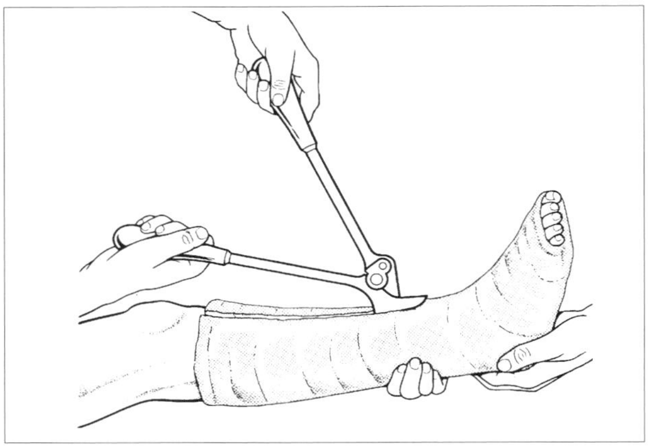

Figure 17.28

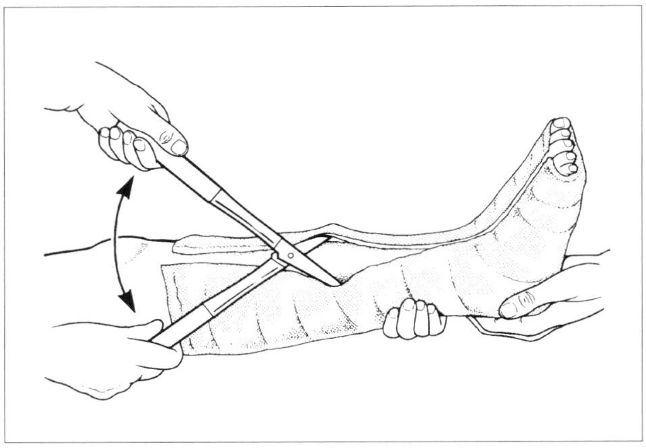

Figure 17.29

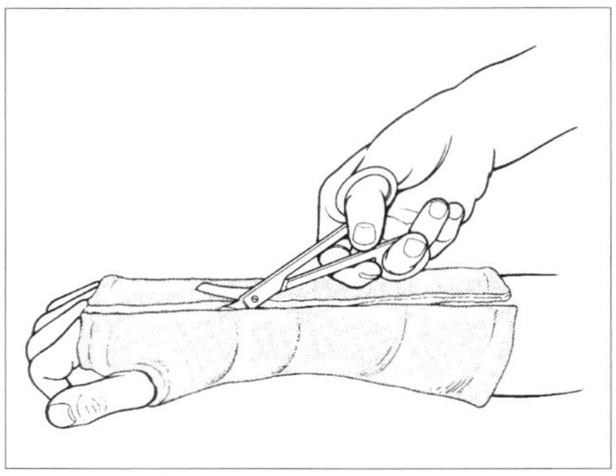

Figure 17.30

Complications

Most problems are caused by improper initial application of the cast.

Pressure sores

Pressure sores result from skin necrosis caused by localized pressure from the inner aspect of the cast. They occur over prominent bony areas, from ridges formed in the plaster during improper application and from foreign bodies placed under the cast. Common sites are:

- Anterior superior iliac spine
- Sacrum
- Ankle
- Dorsum of the foot
- Distal ulna at the wrist.

Areas under pressure begin as painful spots but, if ignored, the underlying skin becomes anaesthetic as an open wound develops. Drainage on the cast follows, often with a foul smelling odour. Treat pressure sores as follows.

1 Put on a new cast or cut a window in the plaster at the suspected site (Figure 17.31). If there is ulceration, clean the wound and treat with dressing changes.

2 Fill the hole in the cast with padding and replace the plaster window. Hold the plaster in place with a firm bandage (Figure 17.32).

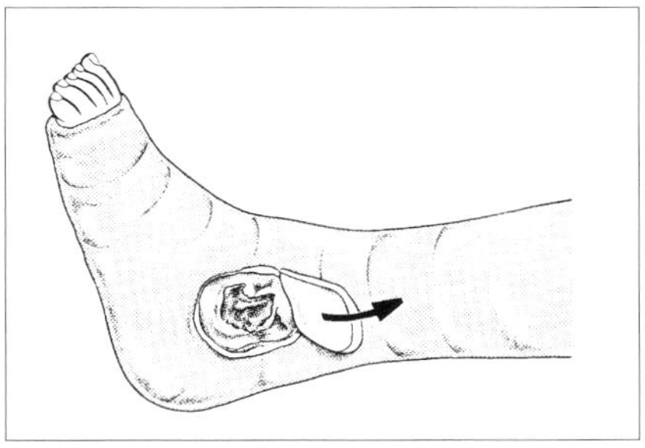

Figure 17.31

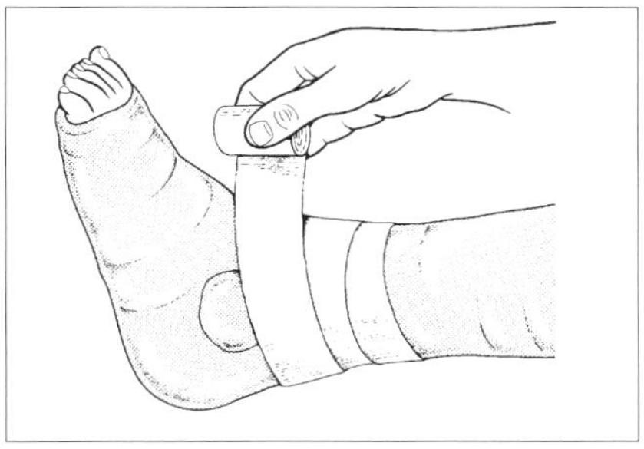

Figure 17.32

Skin blistering

The skin under the plaster becomes dry and scaly because the discarded epithelium is not washed off. Rarely, the skin is susceptible to plaster or fibreglass allergy and dermatitis develops. In hot weather, staphylococcal infection of the hair follicles and sweat glands can lead to a severe painful and purulent dermatitis.

Antihistamines, systemic antibiotics and elevation of the limb should relieve the symptoms within 48 hours. In severe cases, or if there is no improvement, use another method to treat the fracture.

Typical casts and splints

- Figure 17.33: Short arm thumb spica cast
- Figure 17.34: Long arm cast
- Figure 17.35: Short leg patella tendon bearing cast
- Figure 17.36: Cylinder cast

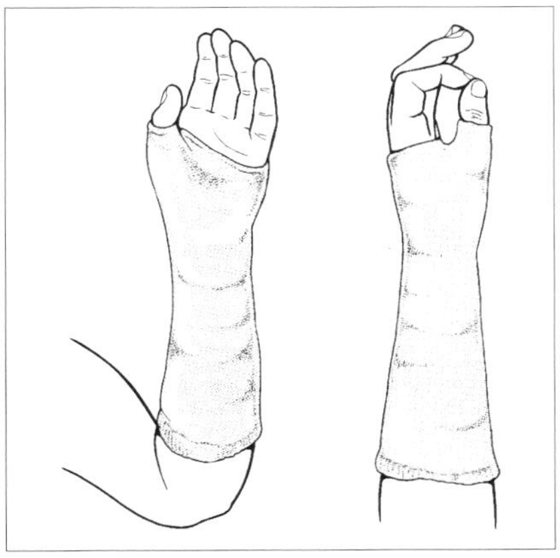

Figure 17.33

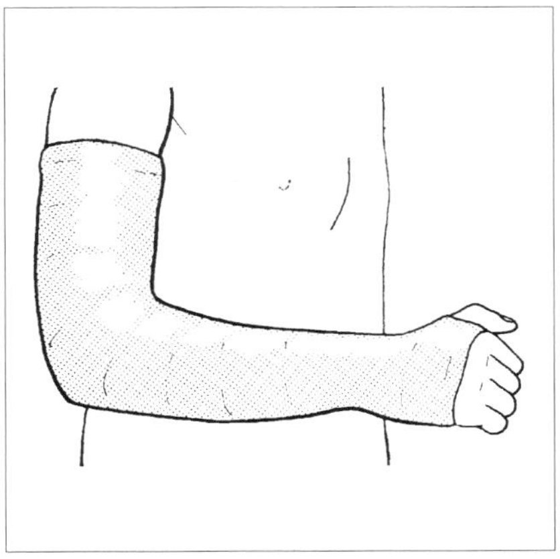

Figure 17.34

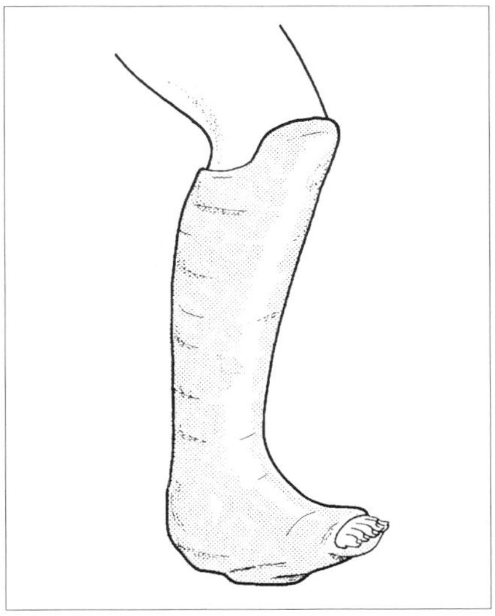

Figure 17.35

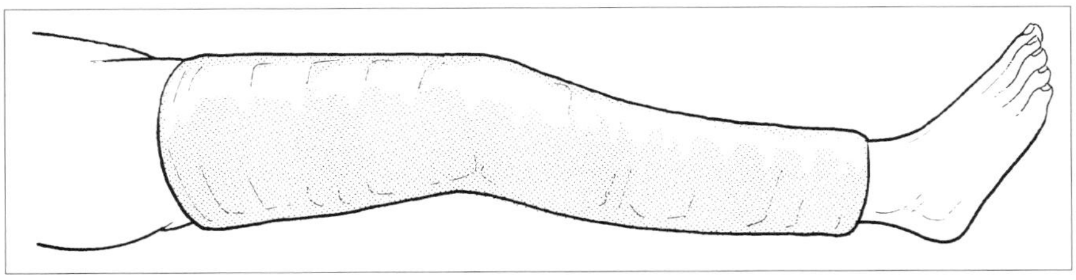

Figure 17.36

17

- Figure 17.37: Hip spica cast
- Figure 17.38: Minerva jacket
- Figure 17.39: Sugartong splint
- Figure 17.40: 3-way ankle splint

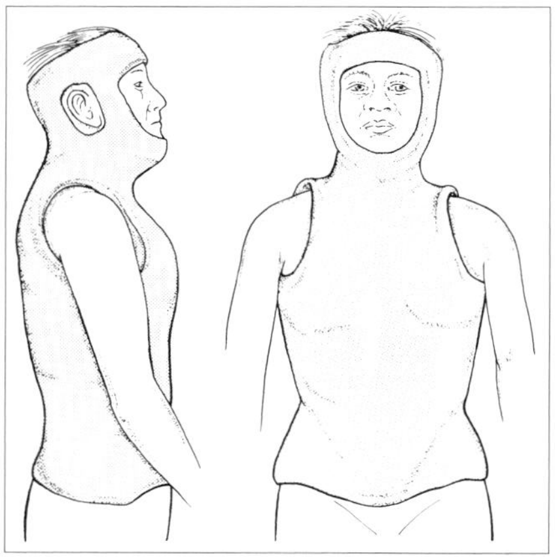

Figure 17.38

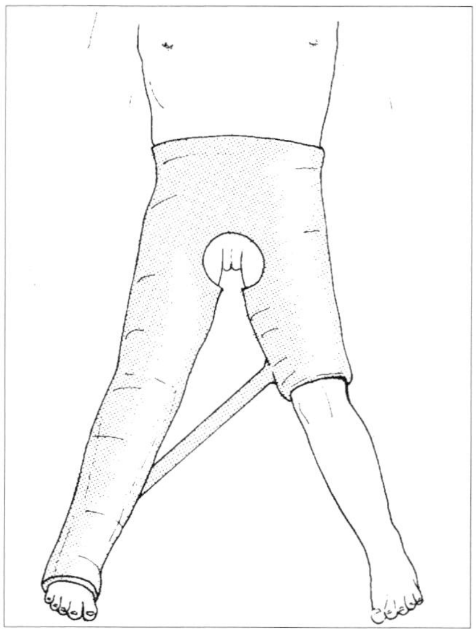

Figure 17.37

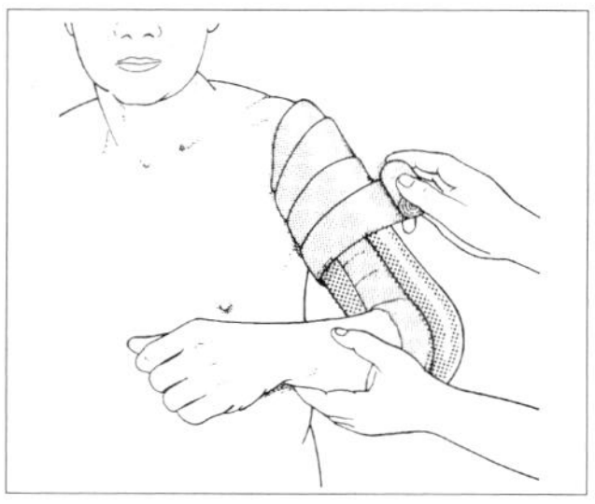

Figure 17.39

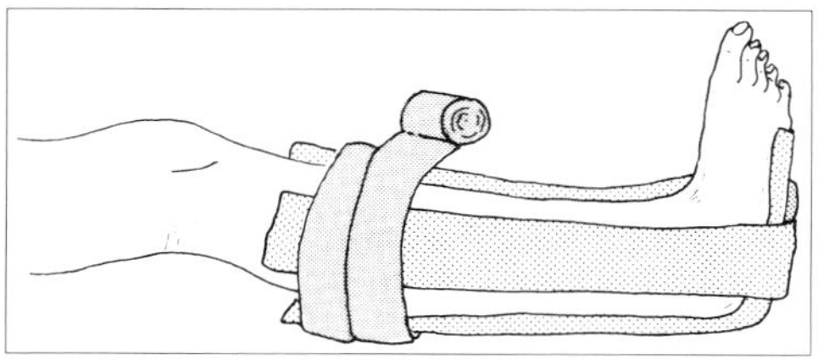

Figure 17.40

KEY POINTS

- External fixation is a technique for immobilizing fractures by placing pins into the bone above and below the fracture and connecting the pins to an external device
- The fracture position is adjusted by making changes to the external components in an outpatient setting
- Wounds are accessible for dressing changes, debridement and secondary closure or skin grafting.

17.3 APPLICATION OF EXTERNAL FIXATION

MATERIALS

- Arrange the fixation frame to best accommodate the fracture pattern and the stability needed (Figures 17.41 and 17.42).
- Partially threaded pins, 3–6 mm diameter, work best but smooth pins will work if threaded ones are not available. Half pins are threaded on the end (Figure 17.41) and transfixation pins are threaded in the middle (Figure 17.42).

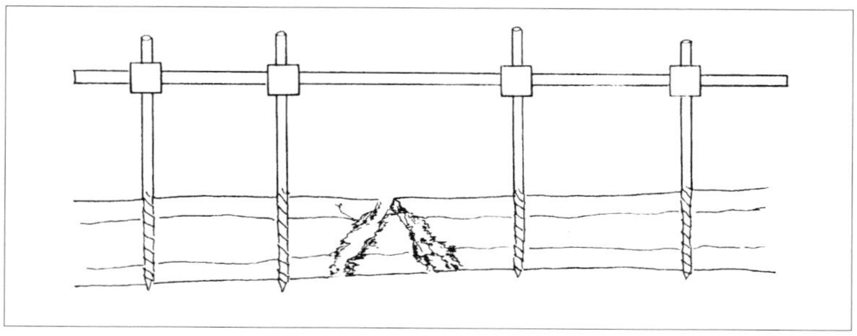

Figure 17.41

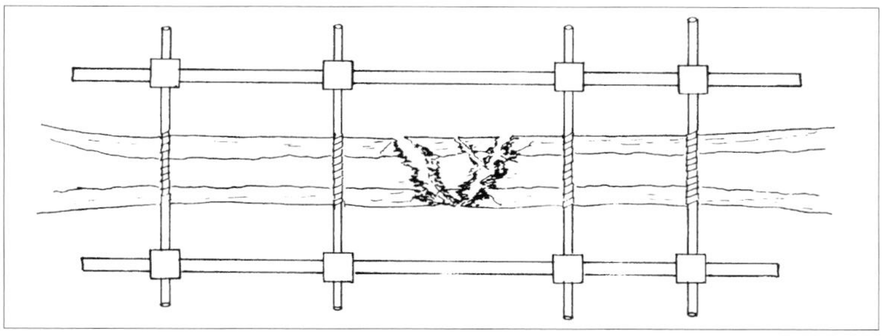

Figure 17.42

- The connector frame consists of clamps to hold the pins to a rod or bar that spans the distance between pin sets. Frames can be purchased or locally made. The simplest frame is constructed of a metal or wooden rod fastened to the pins with plaster of Paris. More complex devices will provide greater stabilization or manoeuvrability.

Application technique

1 Prepare and drape the extremity in a sterile manner. Pin placement is comfortable using local injection anaesthesia at the pin site, but manipulation of the fracture may require a general anaesthetic. Place the pins in safe zones to avoid damage to the vessels and nerves. These areas include:
   - Percutaneous borders of the tibia
   - Calcaneus
   - Radius
   - Ulna.

   Use only half pins in the radius and ulna. Approach the humerus and femur from the lateral side, following the intermuscular septum; use only half pins for these bones also.

2 Make a small incision over the insertion site in the sterile area. Sharp pins should be advanced to the bone and drilled through both cortices. In areas where half pins are used, be careful not to advance the pins beyond the second cortex. When using transfixation pins, advance the pin through the skin on the opposite side, leaving enough protruding to attach the frame on both sides (Figure 17.42).

3 Apply sterile gauze dressings around the pins and attach the frame. For increased stability, place the frame close to the skin allowing adequate clearance for dressings.

4 Place at least two pins in each major bone fragment to provide rotational stability. A third pin will give more stability, but more than three pins per fragment are of no benefit. Align the pins with the long axis of the bone to allow proper alignment of the connecting frame. A wide separation between the pins in each fragment will provide a more stable total system.

Complications

- Injury to nerves and vessels by the pins
- Infection about the pins is common. This can be lessened by careful daily skin cleansing at the pin sites. Most infections are superficial and are controlled by local cleansing and antibiotics. If the infection persists, the pin should be removed and a new pin placed at a different site.

17.4 DIAGNOSTIC IMAGING

Conventional X-ray images (radiographs) are produced by passing high-energy electromagnetic rays ("X-rays") through the body before inducing an image on a photographic plate/film ("analogue" image) or an electronic detector ("digital" image). The denser the tissue, the less residual energy or rays will pass through, so the resulting image will have:

- Bright areas: small amounts let through: i.e. bone and metallic implants
- Dark areas: large amounts let through: i.e. air and fluid, including blood
- Large number of grey tones: i.e. various soft tissues and parenchymatous organs.

Computerized scans (CT scans) use similar technology, but the rays are captured in a computer and a cross sectional body image is produced.

Magnetic Resonance Imaging (MRI) is accomplished using very strong magnetic fields and radio waves. Final images are generated by computers and are displayed on computer screens or TV monitors.

Nuclear medicine imaging ("scintigraphy") is produced by recording ionizing radiation emitted after a substance marked with a radioactive isotope is (mostly intravenously) injected. Various substances and isotopes are used; they will accumulate more in certain pathologic processes, such as a fracture or tumour formation, than in surrounding, normal tissue.

Ultrasound imaging is based on the differential reflection of high frequency sound waves as they pass from one tissue surface to the next. The returning wave pattern is recorded as an image. Ultrasound is less expensive than the other techniques and is especially useful for examination of the abdomen.

Conventional X-ray imaging is the most readily available technique at the district hospital. It is important to decide what information is needed before ordering or asking for an X-ray. If the outcome would not change your treatment, do not waste resources taking the X-ray.

In many locations the equipment is not available to take reliable X-ray images. You must be able to initiate treatment with or without X-ray studies. Do not wait for X-rays or refer patients long distances to obtain them in acute or emergency situations. This handbook explains methods of diagnosis and treatment of most injuries, with and without the use of X-ray imaging.

KEY POINTS

- Diagnostic imaging refers to a variety of graphic techniques: routine X-ray images, ultrasound, nuclear bone scans, MRI scans, CT scans
- X-ray is the most common imaging technique available at the district hospital
- X-ray images are a useful additional aid for diagnosis and treatment, but practitioners must be able to provide care without them
- The most useful and common X-ray examinations include the chest, spine, pelvis and the extremities; skull radiographs are often of limited value as they neither exclude nor confirm possible life-threatening intracranial damage
- In patients with acute abdominal disorders, including trauma injuries, ultrasound examination is the first method of choice, where available
- When performed by well-trained operators, the sensitivity of ultrasound for detecting intraperitoneal bleeding is about 90% and the specificity is close to 100%.

Techniques

X-ray imaging requires a generator powered by electricity to produce the X-ray, a film to capture the image and a method to develop the film. This equipment can be stationary in an X-ray department or mobile for use in the hospital ward, operating theatre or emergency room. Mobile units usually do not produce an image of such high quality, but are useful for patients with fractures treated in traction, or for those with severe injuries who cannot be moved safely to a remote X-ray department.

The following are basic examinations and projections for commonly ordered studies. Since all diagnostic imaging procedures should be "tailor-made" to the specific patient, try to inform the radiological technologist or radiologist about the diagnostic information you need and what you would like to prove or exclude.

Head

- Anterior posterior (AP) and lateral views of the skull.

Chest

- Standing upright film with full inspiration
- AP minimum
- Lateral and additional projections according to clinical situation
- When standing upright is not possible: supine AP.

Abdomen: acute abdominal pain

- AP standing
- AP supine, lateral decubitus views.

Abdomen: abdominal trauma

- Supine AP and lateral views.

Spine

- Unconscious patient: cervical spine, lateral view most important
- AP and lateral views of area involved
- Include an open mouth odontoid view with cervical spine films
- Oblique views of the cervical and lumbar spine will show the facet joints.

Pelvis

- AP view will show the pelvic bones and hip joints
- For fractures, take oblique and inlet/outlet views.

Extremities

- AP and lateral views to include the joint above and below the involved bone
- Oblique and special views are useful in certain areas.

Shoulder

- Axillary lateral.

Ankle

- 15 degree internal rotation (mortise) view.

Knee

- Patella sunrise view.

17.5 PHYSICAL THERAPY

WHY, WHO, WHAT AND HOW

Why?

Immobilized extremities quickly lose their functional abilities through disuse of muscle, bone and joints. The muscle mass decreases and strength decreases. Without weight-bearing stresses, bone loses mineral content and becomes more vulnerable to fracture. Joint motion is necessary for nutrition of the articular cartilage; if joints are immobilized for long periods, fibrous tissue bridges will begin to develop across the joint surfaces.

KEY POINTS

- Physical therapy keeps the musculoskeletal system functional while the injured bone, muscle or ligament heals
- Restoring movement early in the healing process helps to prevent venous thrombosis and pressure sores and enhances pulmonary function.

The goal of physical therapy is to prevent these changes and to keep the musculoskeletal system functional while waiting for the injured bone, muscle or ligaments to heal. Other organ systems also clearly benefit from early functional return: maintaining normal mobility helps to prevent venous thrombosis and pressure sores and enhances pulmonary function.

Who should provide this care?

All care providers should be familiar with the concepts and basic techniques of physical therapy. If a trained physical therapist is available, that person should direct the therapy, but often there will be a need for other providers to participate. If there is no therapist available, other care givers should assume the responsibility. These might include:

- Physical therapy aide
- Nurse
- Physician
- Medical assistant
- Patient's family.

The patient and family members should be taught how to perform the necessary functions and be provided with clear written instructions. Ultimately, it is the motivation of the patient that will determine the outcome.

What materials are necessary?

Expensive equipment is not essential. Most materials can be gathered locally or be made by a carpenter from available supplies.

Basic equipment includes:

- Overhead bed frame: needed on some beds, especially if using traction
- Crutches and walkers: a ready supply is required
- Foam, inner tube or other padding: for use with patients in traction to prevent pressure sores
- Weights: free weights for extremity strengthening.

How should therapy be performed?

Techniques vary with the injury and with the ability of the patient to perform certain tasks. Begin a range of motion and strengthening on the affected extremity as the injury permits. This will change as healing progresses, and is described for specific injuries in Unit 18: *Orthopaedic Trauma*. Begin motion and strengthening of uninjured extremities as soon as possible.

Techniques

Techniques are classified as:

- Active: the patient moves the extremity with or without resistance
- Active assisted: the patient moves the joint with help from the therapist
- Passive: the therapist alone moves the joint.

Active and active assisted therapy are preferable in most cases.

Isometric exercise

Isometric exercise involves muscle contraction without joint motion and is useful across injured joints to keep the muscles functioning.

Motion with gravity

Motion with gravity allows the extremity to be dependent, unweighting the joint and allowing motion with little stress on the bone. It works well for shoulder injuries (see pages 18–2 to 18–3).

Assisted walking

- With a cane, crutches, walker or stick
- The amount of weight placed on the extremity is classified as:
  - Non-weight bearing: the extremity is held off the ground
  - Touch down: the weight of the limb only is rested on the ground, causing less force across the hip area than non-weight bearing
  - Partial weight bearing: placing part of the body weight on the limb, part on an assistive device and varying the proportions of weight as the injury heals
  - Full weight bearing: the assistive device is used for balance and in case of emergency.

17.6 CRANIAL BURR HOLES

INTRACRANIAL TENSION

Increased intracranial tension or pressure will cause secondary injury to the brain. It results from:

- Cerebral swelling from the accumulation of carbon dioxide in the brain
- Hypoxia
- Hypotension
- Epidural, subdural and intracranial haematomas.

The clinical features of increased intracranial pressure include:

- Deteriorating level of consciousness
- Slowing of the pulse
- Dilating pupils
- Focal seizures
- Hemiparesis
- Extensor posturing of the limbs.

Acute extradural and acute subdural haematomas are the only two conditions that may benefit from burr holes. A history of trauma and a clear clinical diagnosis are essential before undertaking the procedure.

KEY POINTS

- Traumatic bleeding within the epidural and subdural spaces increases intracranial pressure and causes neurological impairment
- Clinical features of extremely increased pressure include decreased consciousness, a slow pulse rate, dilated pupils, seizures and hemiparesis
- Release of the pressure with cranial burr holes is an emergency and life-saving procedure.

Acute extradural haematoma

The signs classically consist of:

- Loss of consciousness following an lucid interval, with rapid deterioration

- Middle meningeal artery bleeding with rapid raising of intracranial pressure
- Development of hemiparesis on the opposite side with a dilating pupil on the same side as the impact area, with rapid deterioration.

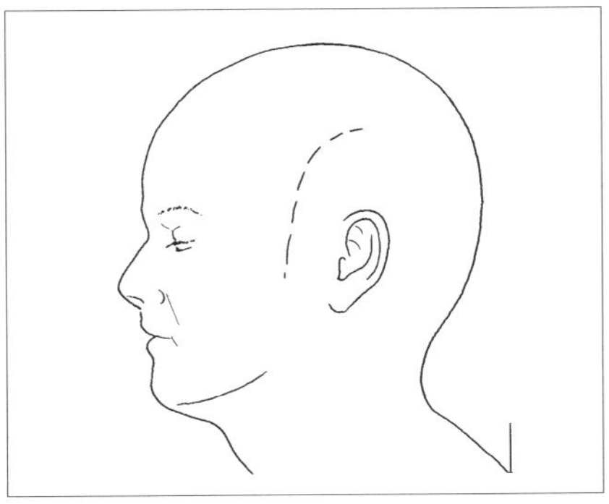
Figure 17.43

Acute subdural haematoma

Acute subdural haematoma, with clotted blood in the subdural space accompanied by severe contusion of the underlying brain, occurs from the tearing of bridging vein between the cortex and the dura.

Management is surgical and every effort should be made to do burr-hole decompressions. The diagnosis can be made on history and examination.

Creating burr holes through the skull to drain the haematoma is often an emergency and life-saving procedure.

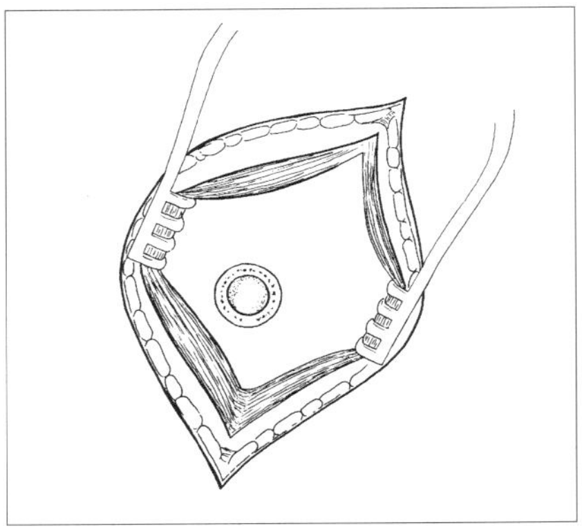
Figure 17.44

Technique

1 Shave and prepare the skull over the temporal region between the ear and the external limit of the orbit on the side of the suspected compression (Figure 17.43).

2 Infiltrate the scalp with a local anaesthetic, and make a 3 cm incision through skin and temporal fascia. Separate the temporalis muscle and incise the periosteum. Control bleeding with retractors or electric cautery. Epinephrine in the local anaesthetic will also help control superficial bleeding (Figure 17.44).

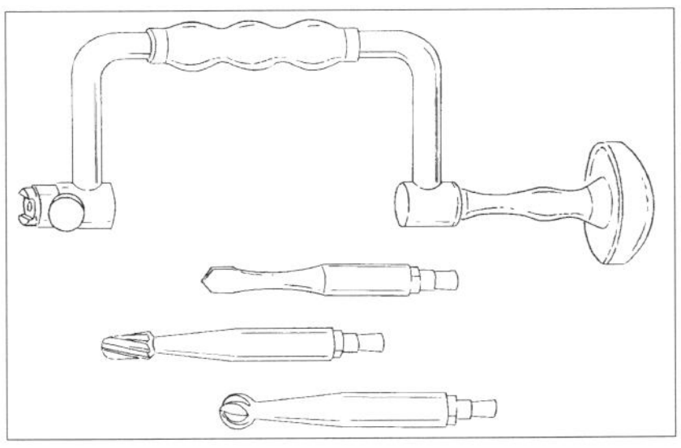
Figure 17.45

3 Make the burr hole 2 cm above and behind the orbital process of the frontal bone. Using a drill cutter, begin to make a hole through the outer and inner tables. Use little pressure when cutting the inner table to avoid plunging through into the brain. Switch to a conical or cylindrical burr to carefully enlarge the opening (Figure 17.45).

4 If necessary, enlarge the opening further with a ronguer (Figure 17.46):
   - Control bleeding from the anterior branch of the middle meningeal artery using cautery or ligature
   - Control venous bleeding with a piece of crushed muscle or a gelatin sponge
   - Control bone bleeding with bone wax.

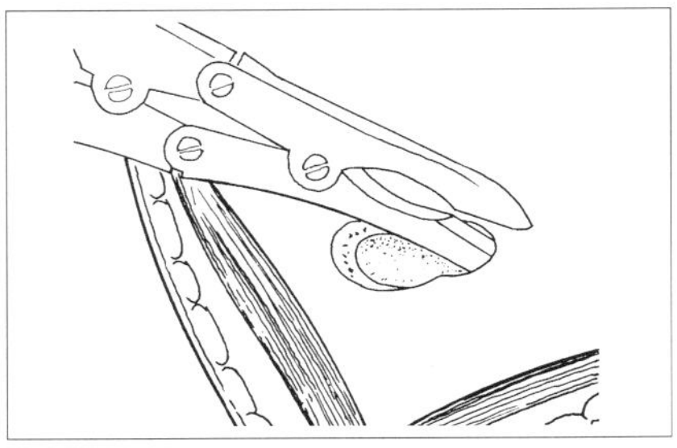
Figure 17.46

5 Wash out the extradural haematoma with a hand syringe. If an extradural haematoma is not found, look for a subdural haematoma. If present, consider opening the dura to release it or arranging for care at a referral hospital. If no haematoma is found, create a burr hole on the opposite side to exclude contra coup bleeding.

6 Close the scalp in two layers. If there is a dural fluid leak, do not use a drain but close the wound tightly to prevent persistent drainage and a secondary infection.

Orthopaedic trauma 18

18.1 UPPER EXTREMITY INJURIES

CLAVICLE FRACTURES

Evaluation

A physical examination shows tenderness over the mid or distal clavicle, with swelling, visible and palpable deformity and, often, crepitus. X-rays confirm diagnosis, but are not essential (Figure 18.1).

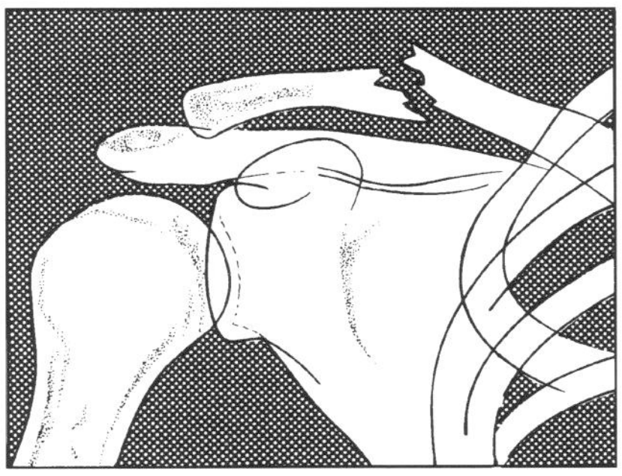

Figure 18.1

Treatment

- Apply a sling as shown in Figure 18.2; a figure-of-8 splint provides some comfort, but is not essential for fracture healing
- Fractures are rarely positioned anatomically, but will heal satisfactorily with little or no functional loss. The patient should continue with the sling until pain free. This will take 4–6 weeks in adults and 3–4 weeks in children.

Rehabilitation

Begin elbow extension and hanging arm exercises in the sling within a few days (Figure 18.3).

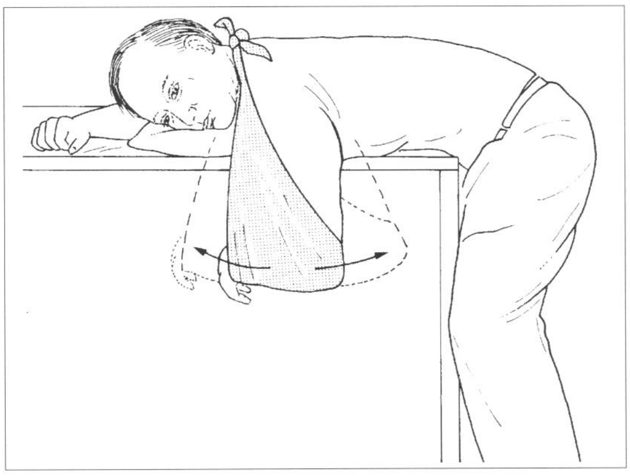

Figure 18.3

KEY POINTS

- Diagnose fractures from the history and by physical examination
- Treat with a sling and early range of motion
- Fracture healing takes 4 weeks in children and 6–8 weeks in adults.

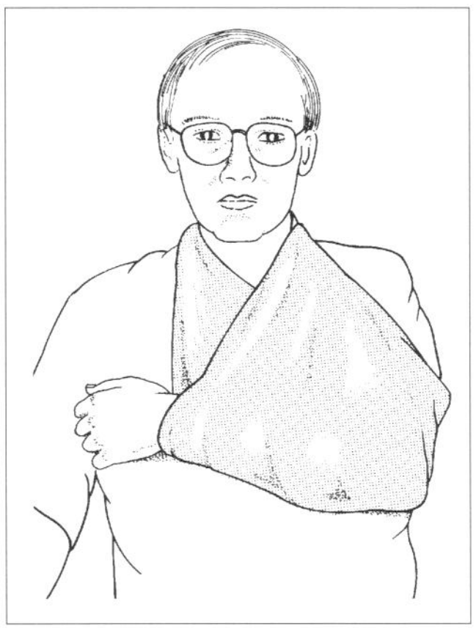

Figure 18.2

> **KEY POINTS**
> - Make the diagnosis based on the history and a physical examination
> - Treat with an arm sling
> - When comfortable, begin a range of motion and active muscle strengthening in the shoulder.

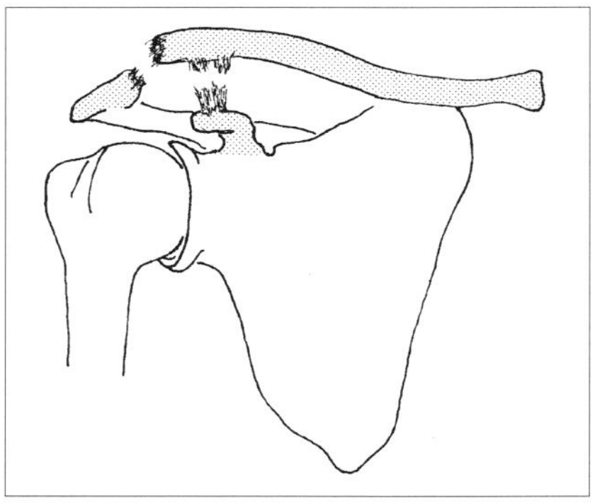

Figure 18.4

ACROMIAL-CLAVICULAR JOINT SEPARATION

Separation of the acromial-clavicular joint results from falls on the tip of the shoulder. Cases are classified by the amount of upward displacement of the clavicle (Figure 18.4).

Evaluation

The acromial-clavicular joint is tender to palpation and the end of the clavicle is prominent. X-rays are not essential but confirm the diagnosis and determine if there is a fracture.

Treatment

- Apply an arm sling to support the weight of the arm and to remove the deforming force from the joint. This will not keep the joint in the anatomical position, but the remaining deformity will cause little functional loss.
- Release the sling daily to allow elbow extension. Begin hanging arm exercises when comfortable and begin active muscle strengthening by the second week.

> **KEY POINTS**
> - Make the diagnosis by physical examination
> - Treat with closed manipulation
> - X-rays help to evaluate the reduction and the presence of fractures
> - Recurrent dislocations are common, especially in younger patients.

SHOULDER DISLOCATION

Anterior dislocations result from injuries that place the arm in abduction, external rotation and extension. Posterior dislocations are less common; the arm position is not important as they follow seizures or electric shocks.

Evaluation

- The contour of the shoulder is changed from the usual curved appearance to one that is much more angular, with a hollow area in place of the humeral head (Figures 18.5 and 18.6)
- Any shoulder movement is painful; X-rays help to determine if there is a fracture
- Perform a careful neurological examination to evaluate for peripheral nerve or brachial plexus injury.

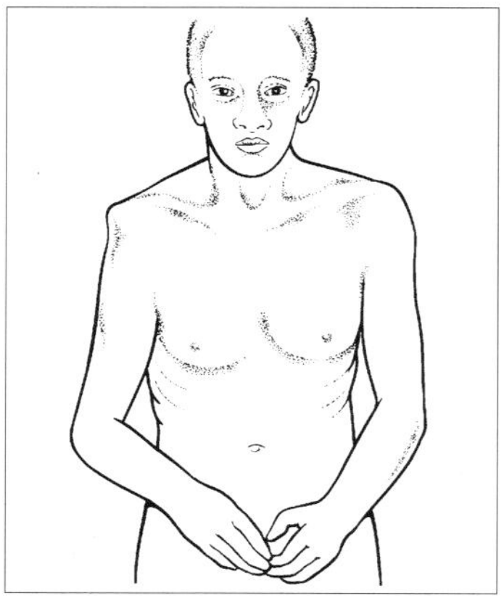

Figure 18.5

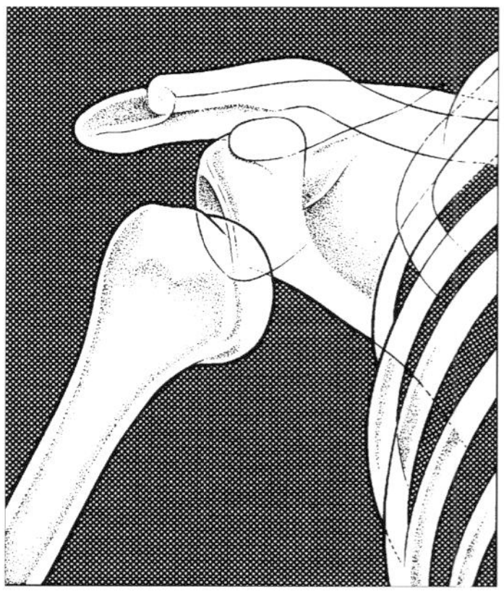

Figure 18.6

Treatment

1 Reduce acute dislocations with the patient supine.

2 If you have an assistant, he/she should place a sheet or other material under the axilla for counter traction. Pull slowly and steadily on the flexed elbow (Figure 18.7). When the patient relaxes the shoulder muscles, you will feel the humeral head move into the joint socket.

If you are alone, place your foot in the axilla for counter traction and gently pull on the arm (Figure 18.8).

3 After reduction, place the arm in a sling and swath to prevent abduction and external rotation (Figure 18.9).

4 Begin strengthening exercises at 6 weeks, with an emphasis on internal rotation strength.

5 Recurrent dislocations are treated similarly. After multiple dislocations, consider surgical shoulder stabilization to prevent further occurrences.

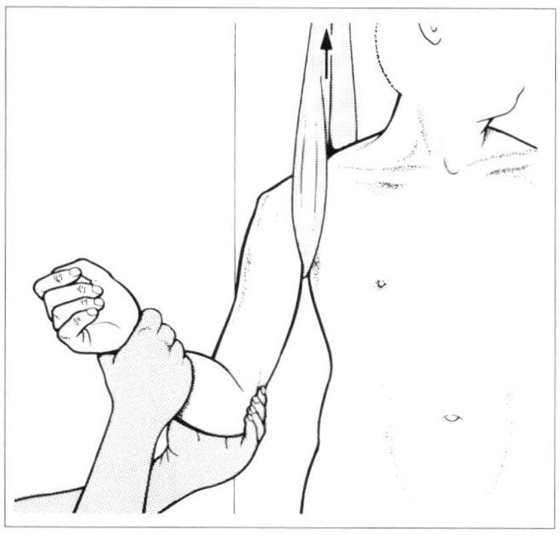

Figure 18.7

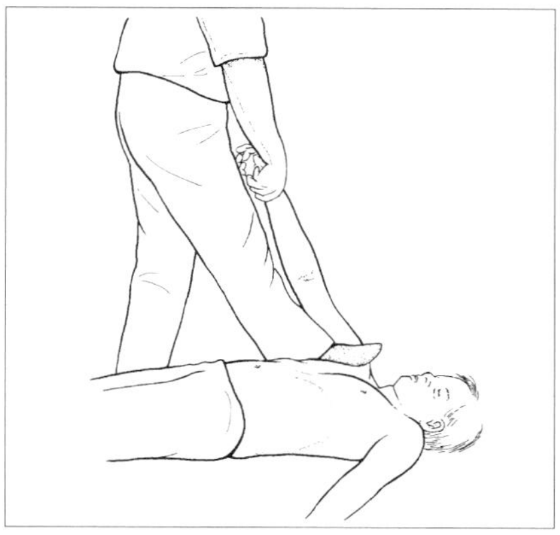

Figure 18.8

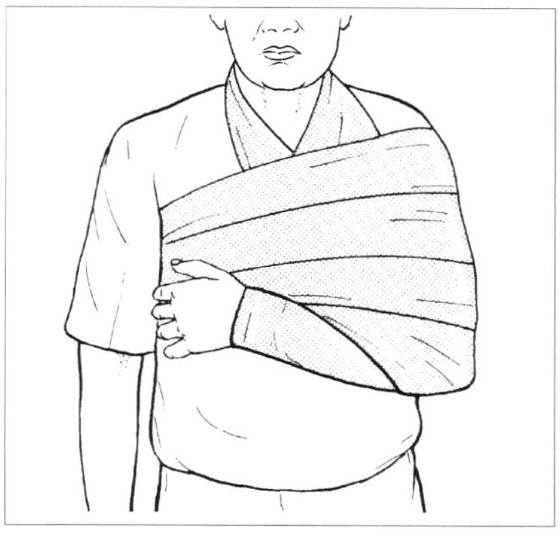

Figure 18.9

PROXIMAL HUMERUS FRACTURES

Fractures of the proximal humerus result from direct or indirect trauma and are classified by the anatomical region injured:

- Greater tuberosity (Figure 18.10)
- Surgical neck (Figure 18.11)
- Anatomic neck
- Humeral head.

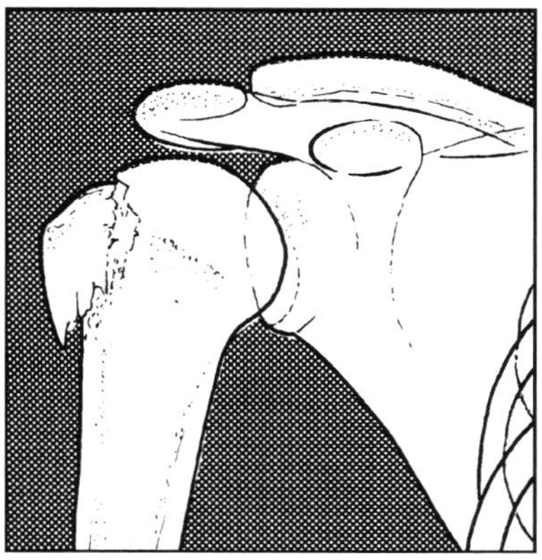

Figure 18.10

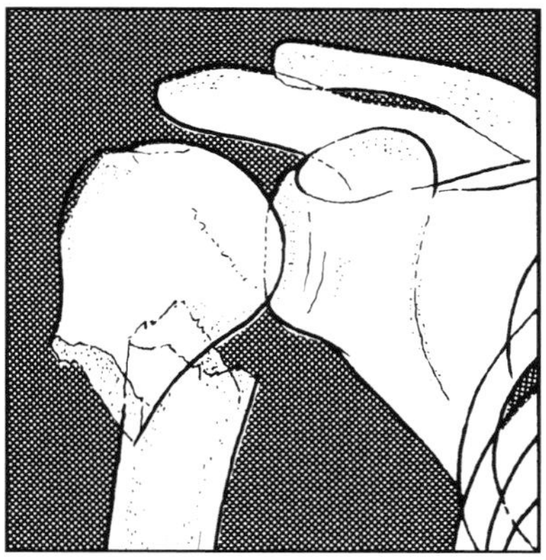

Figure 18.11

KEY POINTS

- The anatomical location of the fracture defines the treatment
- X-rays are needed to evaluate the injury
- Treat displaced fractures with closed manipulation
- The major complication is shoulder stiffness.

18

Evaluation

Suspect the diagnosis from the history and the physical findings of pain, swelling and loss of motion of the shoulder joint. You will need X-rays to confirm the type of fracture and to direct treatment.

Treatment

- Immobilize non-displaced fractures in a sling and swath. Begin mobilization of the shoulder joint within a few days.
- Treat displaced fractures and fracture dislocations by closed manipulation under anaesthesia. If the reduction is not acceptable, consider surgical treatment.
- Begin motion as soon as the patient can tolerate hanging arm exercises (Figure 18.3). Begin active motion against gravity or with weights when the fracture has healed. This is usually at 6–8 weeks.

KEY POINTS

- Humeral shaft fractures result from direct trauma or rotation of the arm
- Treat by closed means in a coaptation splint
- The most significant complications are radial nerve injury and non-union.

HUMERAL SHAFT FRACTURES

Fractures of the shaft of the humerus are the result of direct trauma or rotational injuries (Figure 18.12). The radial nerve wraps around the posterior midshaft of the bone and is injured in about 15 per cent of shaft fractures (Figure 18.13).

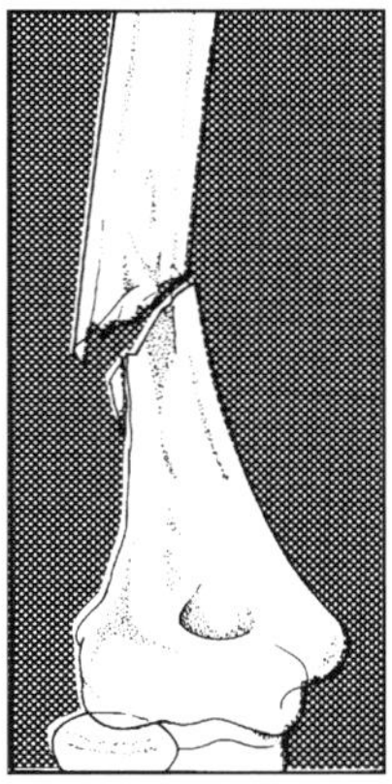
Figure 18.12

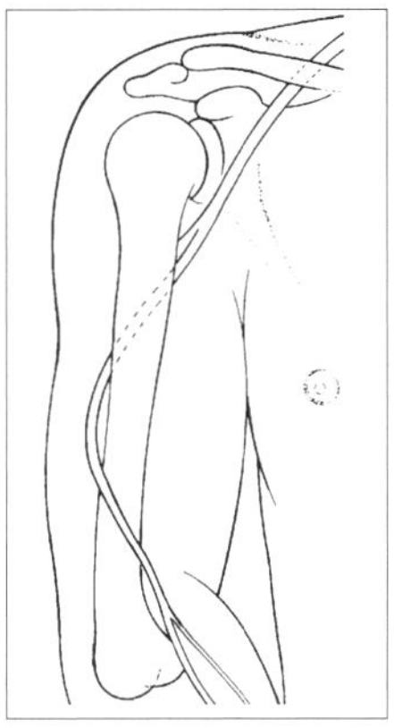
Figure 18.13

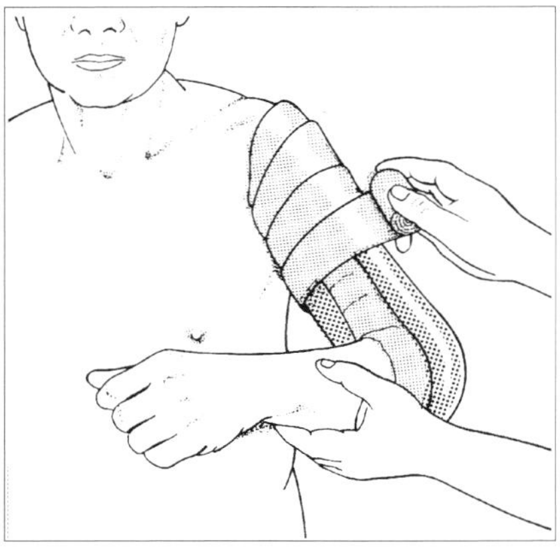
Figure 18.14

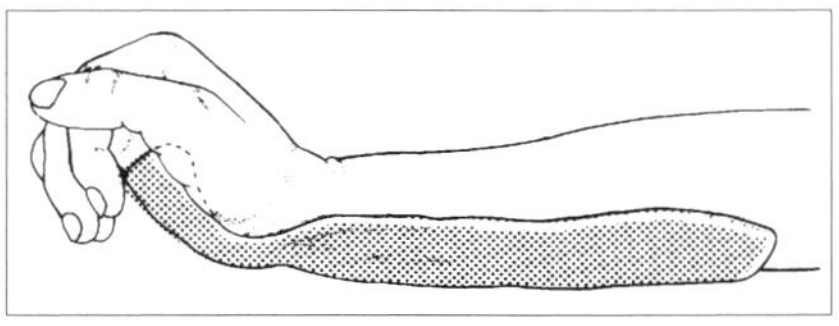
Figure 18.15

Evaluation

Suspect the diagnosis from the clinical findings of tenderness, deformity and instability of the bone. X-rays help to confirm diagnosis, but are most useful in judging the position and healing of the fracture during treatment. Always check the radial nerve function before and after fracture reduction.

Treatment

- Treat with closed reduction and application of a coaptation splint (Figure 18.14). Alignment need not be anatomical; a few degrees of angulation or rotation will not impair function.
- Radial nerve palsy not associated with an open fracture will resolve in most cases. Splint the wrist in extension, and begin passive extension exercise until motor function returns (Figure 18.15).

SUPRACONDYLAR FRACTURES OF THE HUMERUS

Fracture patterns include:

- Supracondylar
- Intercondylar (Figure 18.16)
- Fractures of the medial and lateral epicondyles
- Isolated fractures of the capitellum and trochlea.

KEY POINTS

- Supracondylar fractures of the humerus are complex, unstable fractures
- Treat with closed reduction, followed by a cast or traction
- In cases of incomplete reduction in adults, consider open treatment
- Injury to nerves and arteries leads to significant complications.

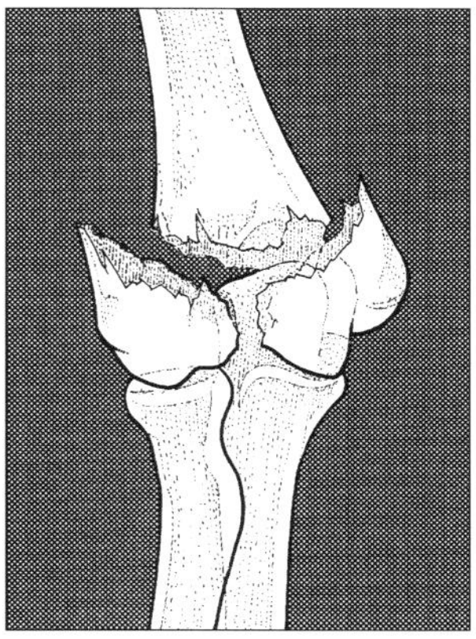

Figure 18.16

Evaluation

The patient has swelling and tenderness about the elbow and pain with attempted motion. Because deformity is often masked by swelling, confirm the type of fracture by X-ray.

Evaluate the neurological and vascular status of the arm. Arterial injuries lead to compartment syndrome (see page 18–33) in the forearm and are associated with:

- Extreme pain
- Decreased sensation
- Pain with passive extension of the digits
- Decreased pulse at the wrist
- Pallor of the hand.

Treatment

1 Perform a closed reduction, using longitudinal traction on the extended arm, followed by flexion at the elbow with anterior pressure on the olecranon (Figures 18.17 and 18.18).

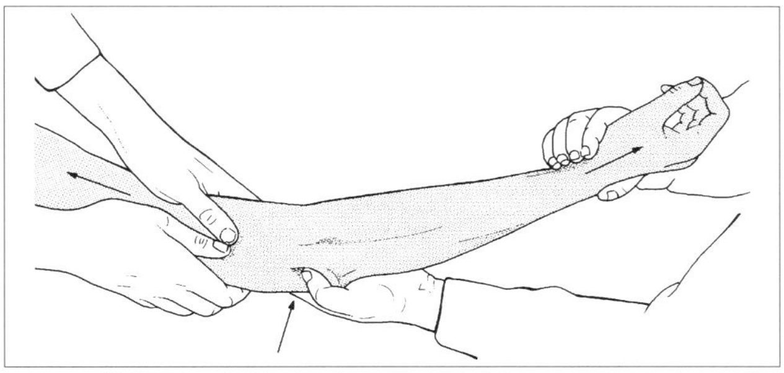

Figure 18.17

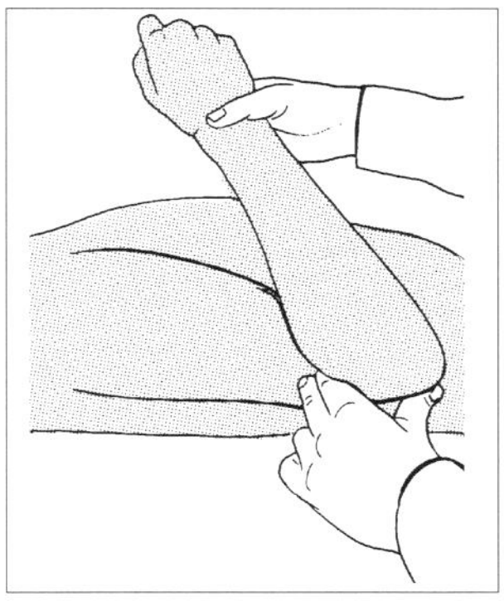

Figure 18.18

2 Monitor the pulse during the reduction. If it decreases, extend the elbow until it returns, and apply a posterior splint in this position. Check the reduction by X-ray.

If a satisfactory reduction cannot be obtained, other options include:

- Overhead traction using an olecranon pin
- A removable splint with early motion
- Open surgical stabilization.

Traction and early motion are useful techniques for severely comminuted fractures and gunshot injuries.

KEY POINTS

- Make the diagnosis by clinical examination and confirm by X-ray
- Treat non-displaced fractures with a long arm splint at 90 degrees
- Splint displaced fractures with the elbow extended or consider surgical stabilization.

OLECRANON FRACTURES

Olecranon fractures result from a fall on the tip of the elbow. The triceps muscle pulls the fracture fragments apart (Figure 18.19).

Evaluation

Physical examination shows swelling about the olecranon and a palpable gap at the fracture site. Examine the ulnar nerve function. X-rays confirm the fracture and associated injuries.

Treatment

- Treat non-displaced fractures in a splint with the elbow at 90 degrees
- Treat displaced fractures with the elbow in full extension; displaced fractures may a have better outcome if treated surgically
- Simple methods include:
  - Suture of the torn triceps tendon (Figure 18.20)
  - Placement of percutaneous pins with rubber bands (Figures 18.21 and 18.22).

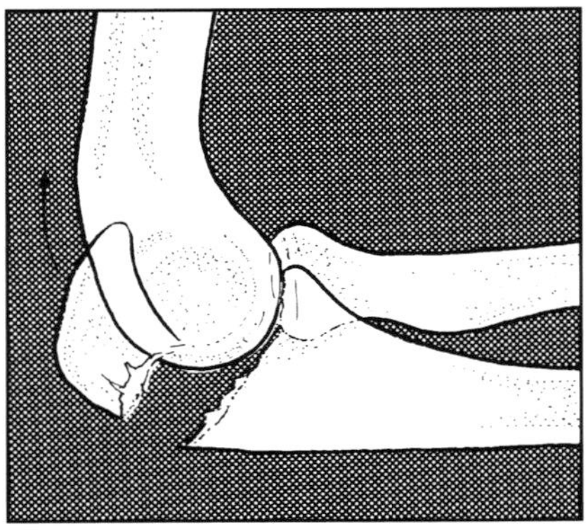

Figure 18.19

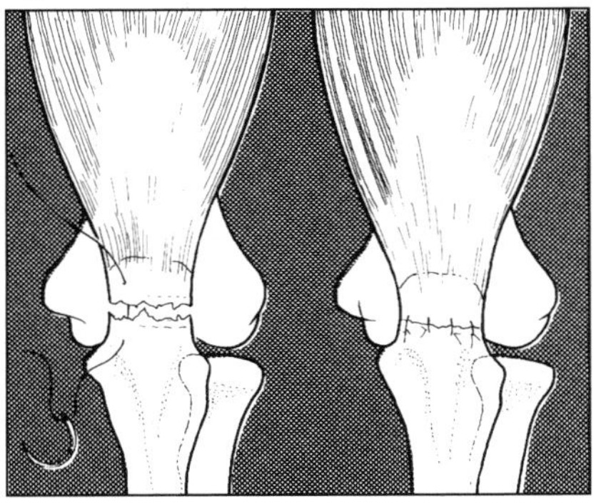

Figure 18.20

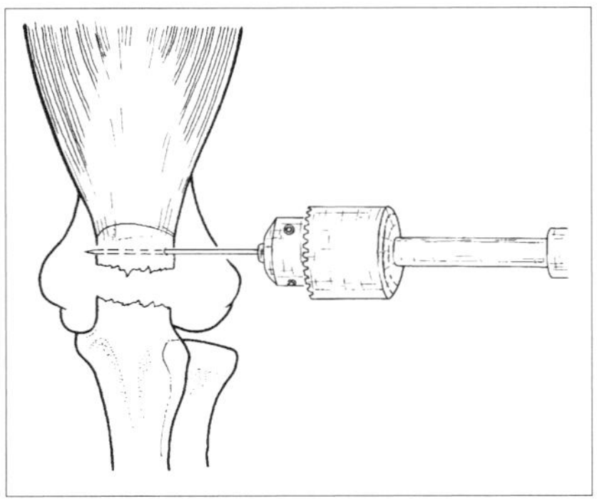

Figure 18.21

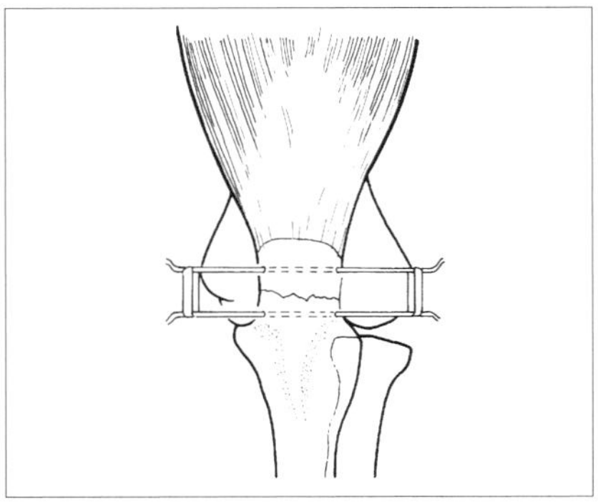

Figure 18.22

KEY POINTS

- In fractures with minimal displacement, treat with closed reduction and a posterior splint and begin motion as soon as comfortable
- Treat displaced intra-articular fractures with early motion and consider surgical treatment, if available.

FRACTURES OF THE RADIAL HEAD AND NECK

The radial head is important for pronation and supination of the forearm as well as for flexion and extension motions at the elbow. Fractures are classified by the articular involvement (Figure 18.23).

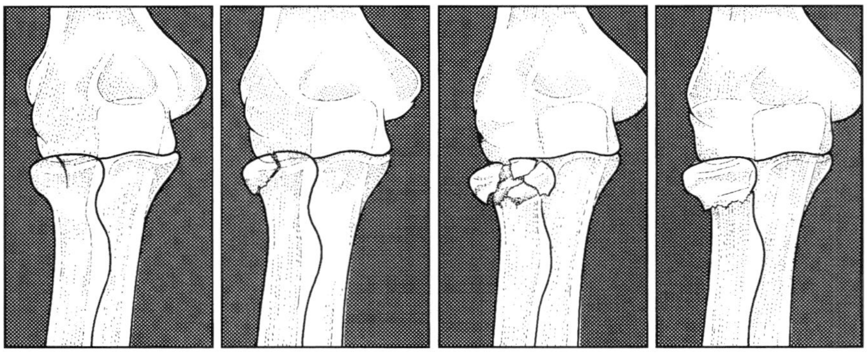

Figure 18.23

Evaluation

Patients have pain and swelling over the lateral aspect of the elbow. Some motion remains in minimally displaced fractures. X-rays confirm the diagnosis.

Treatment

1 Treat fractures with minimal displacement in an arm sling and begin motion when comfortable.
2 To reduce displaced fractures of the radial neck:
   - Place your thumb over the radial head and apply longitudinal traction with a varus stress to the arm
   - Gently rotate the forearm while applying medial pressure with your thumb to the radial head
   - Place the arm in a long arm splint
   - Begin motion out of the splint at 3 weeks.
3 Treat comminuted or displaced intra-articular fractures with early motion. If available, alternatives are surgical stabilization or radial head excision.

ELBOW DISLOCATION

Dislocations of the elbow occur with a fall on the outstretched arm. They may be in the posterior or posterior lateral direction (Figure 18.24).

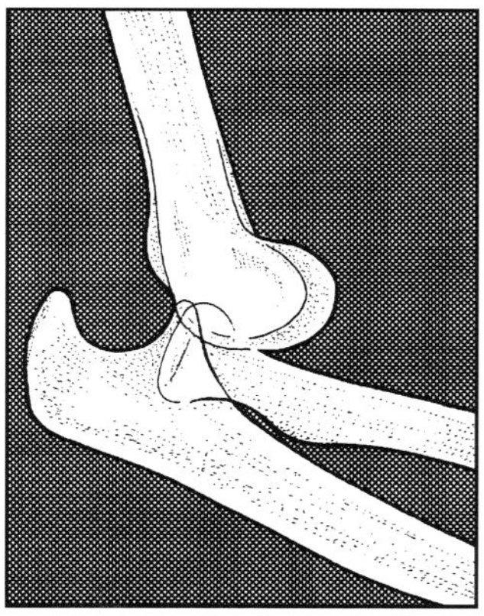

Figure 18.24

KEY POINTS

- Injury occurs with a fall on the outstretched arm
- Treat with immediate closed reduction
- In children, the medial epicondyle may become entrapped in the joint and may require surgical removal.

In children, the medial epicondyle of the humerus is often pulled off as the radius and ulna move posteriorly and laterally. With reduction, this fragment may become lodged in the joint and require surgical removal.

Evaluation

Clinically examine the triangular relationship of the ulna and the two epicondyles to ascertain if it is disturbed. The olecranon is felt protruding in a posterior direction and any elbow motion is painful. Assess and record ulnar nerve function.

Treatment

1 Treat with immediate closed reduction: apply traction to the arm with the elbow in slight flexion and direct pressure on the tip of the olecranon to push it distally and anteriorly.

18

2 When reduced, the elbow will have a free range of motion. After reduction, confirm the position of the epicondyle by X-ray.

3 Place the arm in a posterior splint at 90 degrees of flexion.

4 Begin a range of motion at the elbow after 10 days, or as soon as the pain and swelling permit, removing the splint for short periods. Discontinue the splint at 4–6 weeks.

KEY POINTS

- Forearm fractures are complex fractures which, in adults, usually require surgical stabilization
- They occur as three major types:
  - Midshaft fractures
  - Proximal (Monteggia) dislocations
  - Distal (Galeazzi) fracture dislocations
- The most common complication is loss of forearm rotation.

FOREARM FRACTURES

Forearm fractures are caused by direct trauma or by a fall on the outstretched arm with an accompanying rotatory or twisting force.

Evaluation

The forearm is swollen and tender, with limited motion. Evaluate vascular function by checking pulse, capillary refill and skin temperature of the hand. Check sensory and motor function of the radial, median and ulnar nerves. X-rays confirm the nature of the fracture.

Monteggia fractures involve the proximal ulna with dislocation of the radial head, usually in the anterior direction (Figure 18.25).

Galeazzi fractures are the reverse of the above, with a fracture of the distal radius and a dislocation of the radial-ulnar joint at the wrist. The radius fracture is usually oblique, causing the bone to shorten (Figure 18.26).

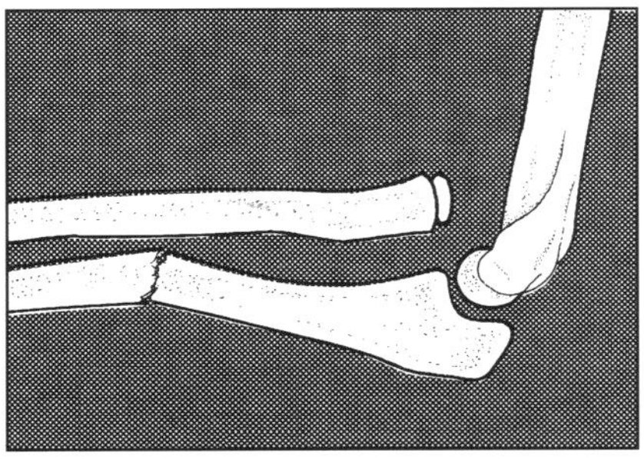

Figure 18.25

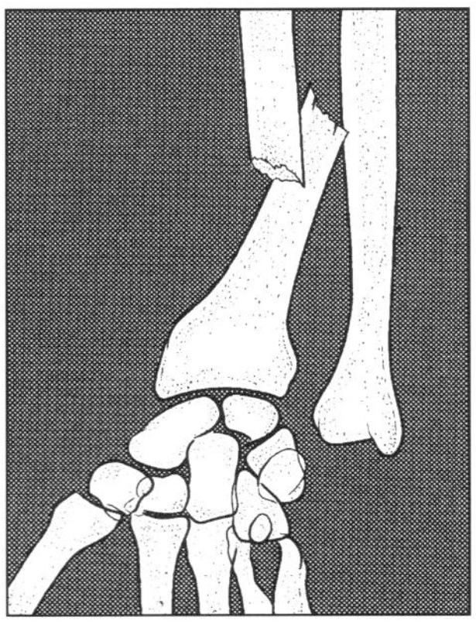

Figure 18.26

Treatment

- Midshaft fractures may involve one or both bones; treat single bone fractures with minimal displacement in a long arm cast, with the elbow at 90 degrees and the forearm in neutral rotation
- Treat displaced fractures by closed reduction and application of a long arm splint; perform the reduction by applying traction to the fingers and manipulating the forearm with the elbow bent to 90 degrees. Apply counter-traction above the bent elbow (Figure 18.27)
- Reduce Monteggia fractures as described for displaced fractures (Figure 18.28). Apply a long arm cast in supination. It is possible to obtain a satisfactory reduction in children, but adults often require surgical treatment.

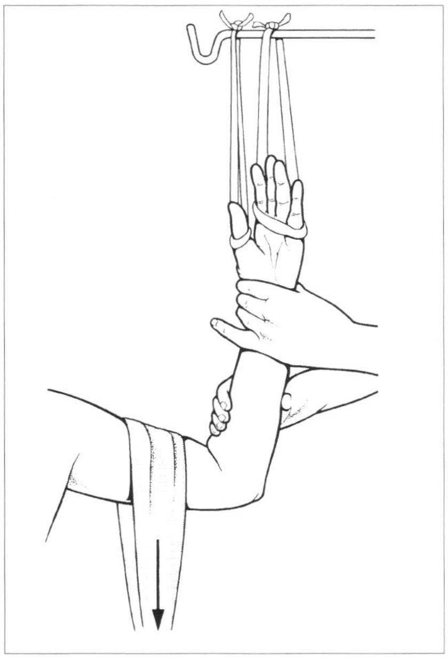

Figure 18.27

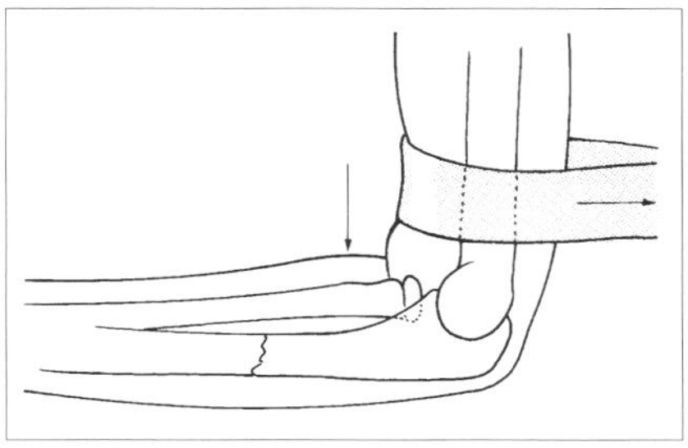

Figure 18.28

- Treat Galeazzi fractures as described for midshaft fractures. They are unstable and often need surgical stabilization.

Rehabilitation

Begin motion out of the cast at 6–8 weeks.

DISTAL RADIUS FRACTURES

Fractures of the distal radius occur with a fall on the outstretched hand. The direction of the deformity depends on the position of the wrist at the time of impact (Figure 18.28).

The goal of fracture treatment is to restore the normal anatomy of the following deformities:

- Shortening of the radius relative to the ulna (Figure 18.29)
- Loss of the volar tilt of the radial articular surface, seen in the lateral X-ray (Figure 18.30)
- Disruption of the articular surface.

KEY POINTS

- The distal radius is one of the most common upper extremity fractures
- Treatment is usually by closed reduction and application of a U-shaped splint coaptation
- The adequacy of the reduction can be judged by specific parameters visible on the post-reduction X-ray
- The most common complication is malposition and loss of motion.

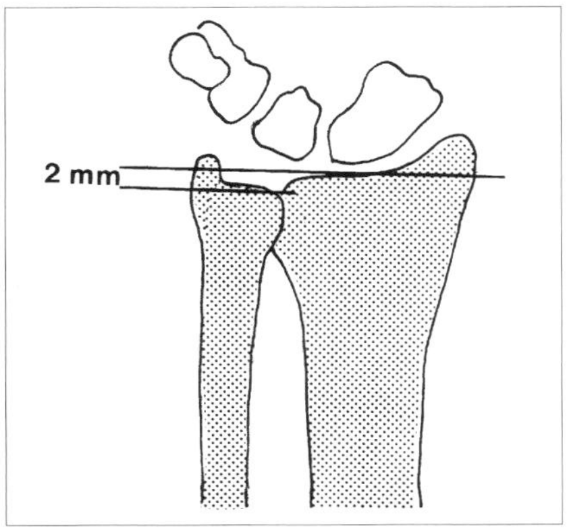

Figure 18.29

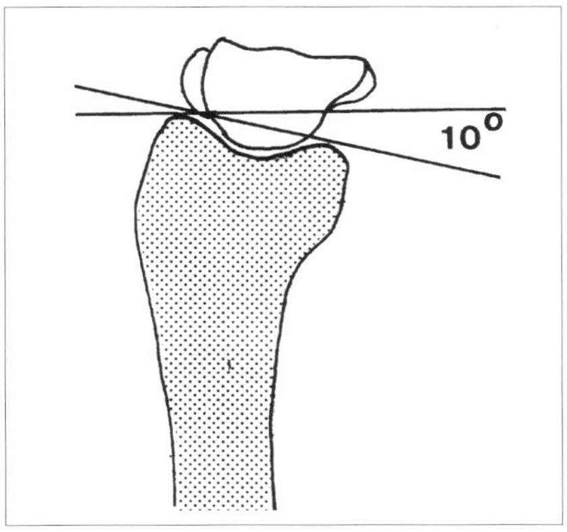

Figure 18.30

Evaluation

- Make the diagnosis based on the history of a fall on the outstretched hand, swelling and tenderness about the wrist and the presence of deformity
- Evaluate tendon function, vascular supply and sensation in the hand
- X-rays distinguish radius fractures from carpal injuries and determine if the fracture is adequately reduced.

Treatment

1 Anaesthetize for closed reduction, using general anaesthesia (ketamine), an intravenous lidocaine block or a haematoma block. A haematoma block involves placing 5–10 ml of 2% lidocaine directly into the fracture haematoma, using a strict aseptic technique (Figure 18.31).

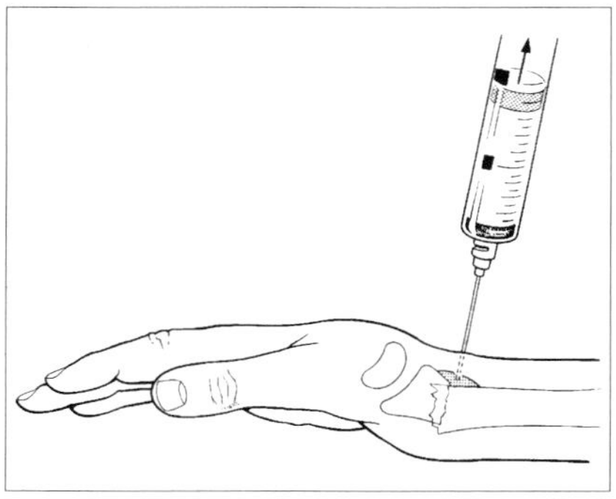

Figure 18.31

2 Reduce the fracture by placing longitudinal traction across the wrist and applying pressure to the distal radial fragment to correct the angular deformity (Figure 18.32). For fractures that are dorsally angulated (Colle's fractures), this is accomplished by wrist flexion and slight ulnar deviation.

3 Next, apply a sugar tong splint, moulded to maintain the fracture position. Three point moulding involves application of pressure above and below the fracture and counter pressure on the opposite side of the bone near the fracture apex.

4 Between 10 days and 2 weeks, change the sugar tong splint to a short arm cast and check the fracture position by X-ray. Healing takes about 6 weeks.

5 If a satisfactory position of the fracture fragments cannot be obtained or maintained, consider open reduction and internal fixation, placement of an external fixator or closed reduction with percutaneous pin fixation.

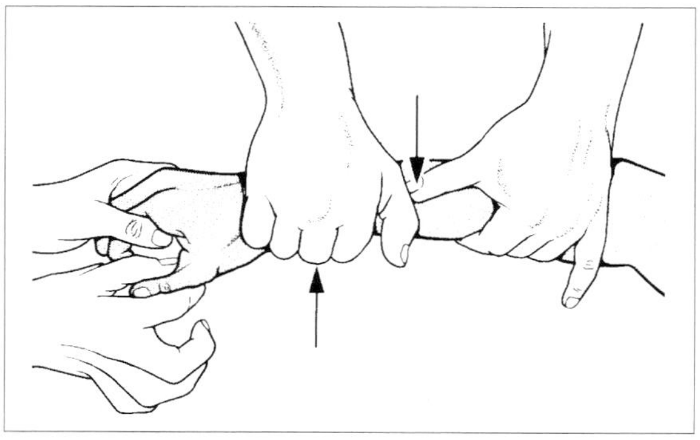

Figure 18.32

KEY POINTS

- The injury results from a fall on the outstretched hand in hyperextension
- Diagnosis is difficult and is often overlooked
- Adequate X-rays are necessary for accurate diagnosis
- Closed reduction is the initial treatment, but surgical stabilization may be necessary.

CARPAL FRACTURES AND FRACTURE DISLOCATIONS

Injuries to the carpal bones fall into three major categories:

- Scaphoid fractures
- Trans-scaphoid perilunate fracture/dislocations
- Perilunate dislocations.

The scaphoid bone (S) bridges the proximal and distal rows of carpal bones, making it especially vulnerable to injury. Most commonly, fractures occur at the waist but may also involve the proximal or distal pole (Figure 18.33).

Perilunate dislocations occur with or without an accompanying scaphoid fracture. The lunate (L) stays in a volar position while the remaining carpal bones dislocate posteriorly (Figure 18.34).

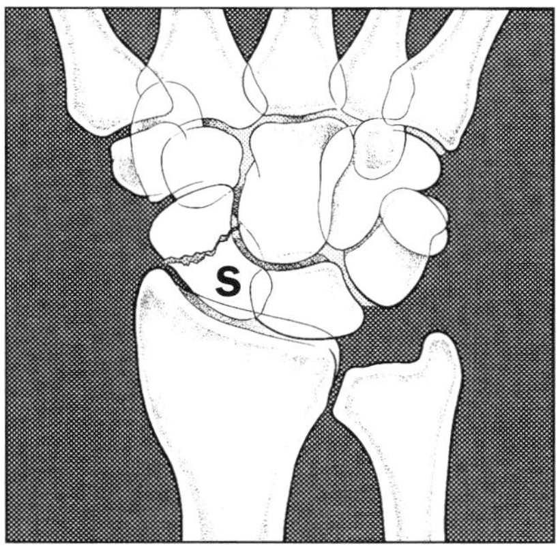

Figure 18.33

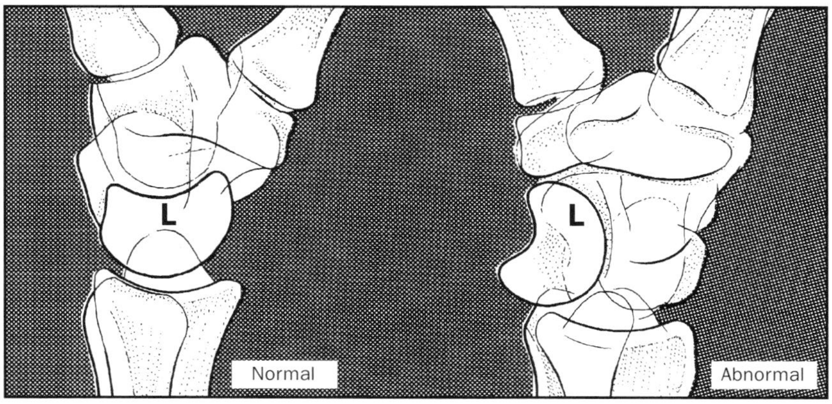

Figure 18.34

Evaluation

The wrist appears swollen and painful to move.

- Scaphoid fractures are tender in the anatomic snuff box and over the scaphoid tubercle on the volar aspect of the wrist. If a perilunate dislocation has occurred, these findings are diffuse about the wrist. X-rays are necessary to make a definitive diagnosis.
- In perilunate dislocations, the lateral X-ray shows an anteriorly displaced lunate bone, with its concavity facing forward (Figure 18.34). The carpus is shortened and the proximal margin of the capitate does not articulate with the concavity of the lunate.

Treatment

- Treat scaphoid fractures with minimal displacement in a thumb spica splint or cast. Healing time is between 6 and 20 weeks.
- Perilunate dislocations require reduction followed by placement in a long arm thumb spica splint. The reduction is usually unstable over time and most patients will need surgical stabilization.

18.2 THE HAND

LACERATIONS

Evaluation

- Treat open injuries of the hand promptly. Perform a local examination to check circulation, sensation and motor function.
- Gently examine the wound using aseptic technique to determine if it is clean or contaminated. A contaminated wound contains foreign material and crushed or dead tissue.

Treatment

1 Debride and lavage all wounds in the operating room or emergency area. If a local anaesthetic is needed, use 1% lidocaine *without epinephrine.*

KEY POINTS

- Treat lacerations promptly with careful evaluation, debridement and lavage
- Close wounds only when clean, using suture, spontaneous healing or skin grafts
- After injury, elevate the hand to control swelling and begin motion early
- Nail bed injuries require special treatment.

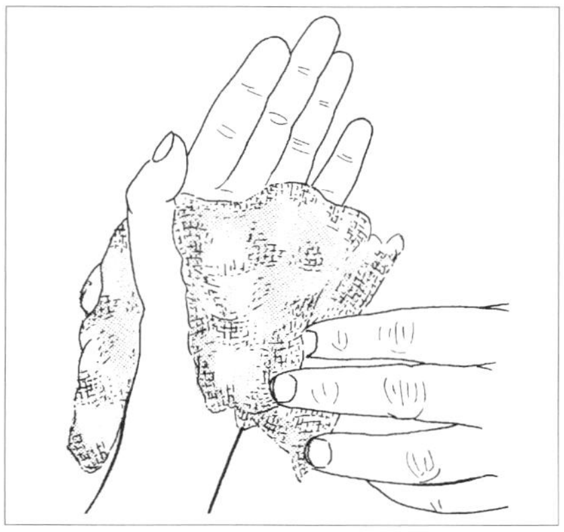

Figure 18.35

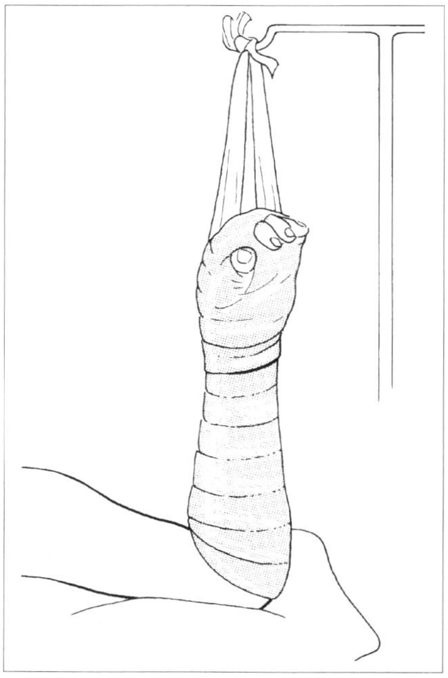

Figure 18.36

2 Administer tetanus toxoid and antibiotics. Obtain X-rays to check underlying bones and joints.

3 Stop bleeding by compression with sterile gauze. If necessary, extend the wound, being careful not to cross skin creases in the palm or digits. Remove all foreign material and devitalized tissue, but *do not excise any skin unless it is dead.*

4 If the wound is clean, repair extensor tendons but not flexor tendons or nerves.

5 Close a clean wound over a drain using interrupted sutures if there is no tension on the skin. If the wound is contaminated, delay closure until after a second debridement. Wounds less than 1 cm square will granulate spontaneously. Use skin grafts for larger wounds, which will not close without skin tension.

6 Cover the hand with sterile gauze and a compression dressing (Figure 18.35).

7 Apply a plaster splint to hold the wrist in 20 degrees of extension, with the metacarpophalangeal joints in 90 degrees of flexion and the interphalangeal joints in full extension. Keep the fingertips exposed unless they are injured.

8 To control oedema, elevate the limb for the first week, either by attachment to an overhead frame or by the use of a triangular sling (Figure 18.36).

9 Begin active exercises as soon as possible and inspect the wound in 2–3 days to remove drains.

Nail bed injuries

- Subungual haematoma causes severe pain resulting from a collection of blood deep under the nail. This can be seen as a dark red to black collection beneath the nail. To relieve pain, make one or two small holes in the nail with a hot safety pin or the tip of sterile number 11 scalpel blade.
- If not repaired, lacerations of the nail bed may result in lasting nail deformity. Remove the nail and, after debridement and lavage, repair the laceration using fine suture. If possible, replace the nail over the sutured laceration until it heals and a new nail has begun to grow.

FRACTURES AND DISLOCATIONS

Fracture dislocation of the first carpometacarpal joint (Bennett's fracture)

This is an oblique fracture of the base of the thumb metacarpal involving the first carpometacarpal joint (Figure 18.37).

1 Reduce the fracture with longitudinal traction to the thumb held in the abducted position.

2 Apply lateral pressure to the base of the metacarpal to reduce the fracture and the dislocation (Figure 18.38).

3 Maintain the reduction with a thumb spica splint.

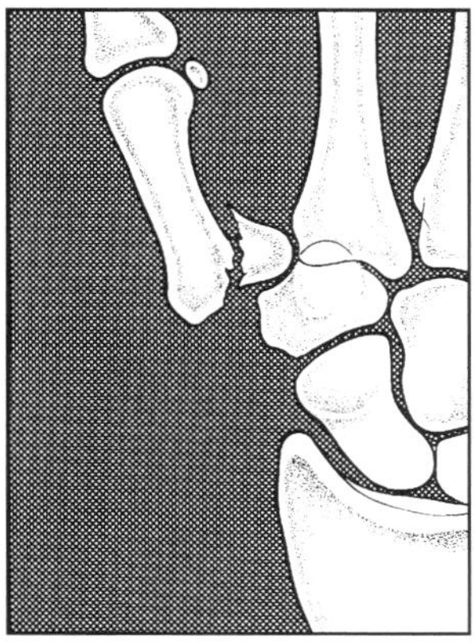

Figure 18.37

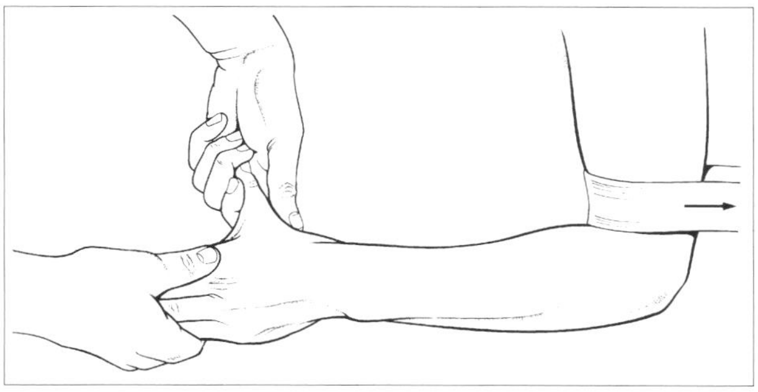

Figure 18.38

Metacarpal fractures

Metacarpal fractures commonly occur at the base, midshaft and neck. Most fractures are stable and can be treated with closed manipulation and plaster immobilization. Rotation is the most important deformity to correct. If it persists, the digits will cross with flexion, impairing general function of the hand.

- Treat with a short arm cast or splint with the wrist in extension and three point moulding about the fracture. When treating unstable fractures, extend the cast to include the involved digit or tape the digit to an adjacent digit to provide rotational stability.
- Healing time is 4–6 weeks.

Phalanges

- Treat non-displaced, stable fractures by taping the fractured digit to the adjacent uninjured digit (buddy tape, Figure 18.39), or with a simple dorsal splint

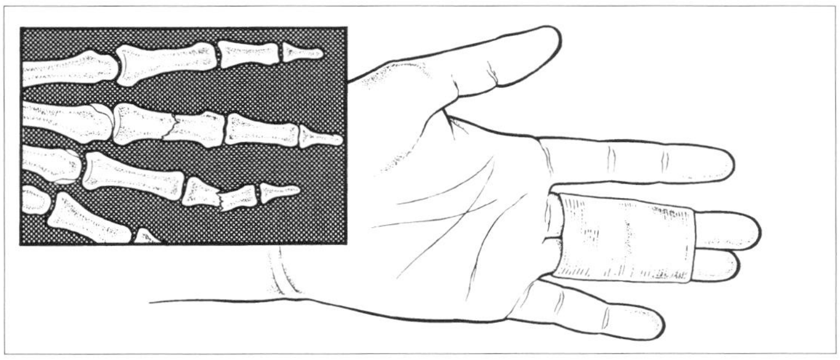

Figure 18.39

- Reduce displaced fractures with traction and direct pressure to correct the deformity. Apply a short arm cast with an attached metal splint extending under or over the digit.

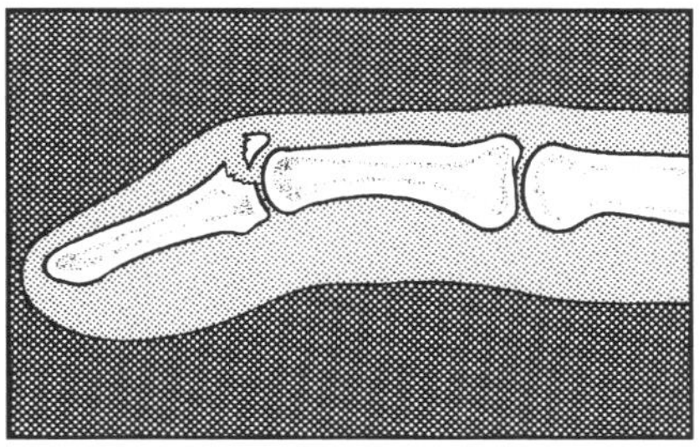

Figure 18.40

Mallet finger

Mallet finger results from a tear of the long extensor tendon at its insertion into the distal phalanx. It may be associated with an avulsion fracture of the dorsal lip of the distal phalanx (Figure 18.40).

Treat by splinting the distal phalanx in slight hyperextension (Figure 18.41). Maintain continuous extension for 6–8 weeks.

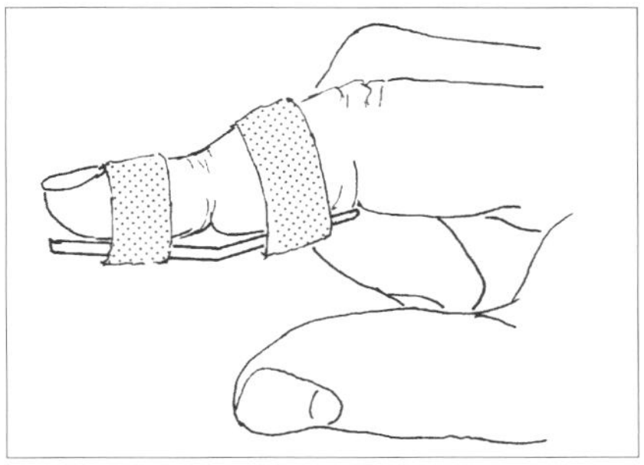

Figure 18.41

KEY POINTS

- Pelvic ring fractures result from high-energy trauma and are classified as stable or unstable
- Unstable fractures are associated with significant blood loss and multiple system injury
- Treat initially with systemic resuscitation and temporary pelvic compression
- Complications include deep vein thrombosis, sciatic nerve injury and death from bleeding or internal organ damage.

18.3 FRACTURES OF THE PELVIS AND HIP

PELVIC RING FRACTURES

Pelvic fractures occur as a result of high-energy trauma and are frequently accompanied by injuries to the genitourinary system and abdominal organs. Internal blood loss caused by fracture of the pelvis and soft organ damage causes hypovolaemic shock (see page 13–8).

Stable fractures are those with a single fracture component (Figure 18.42). Unstable patterns result from fractures at two or more sites, or those associated with disruption of the symphysis pubis or sacroiliac articulation (Figure 18.43).

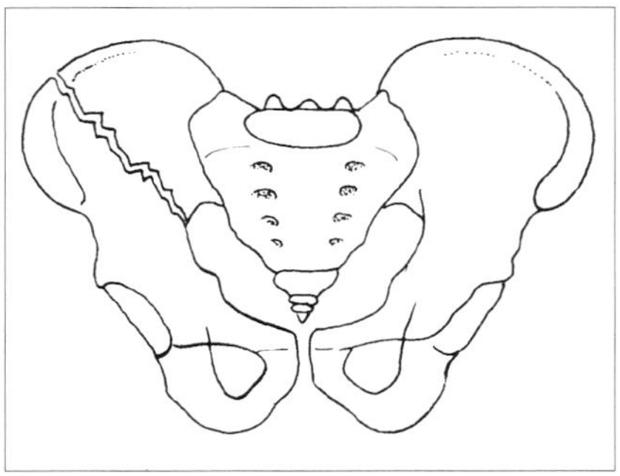

Figure 18.42

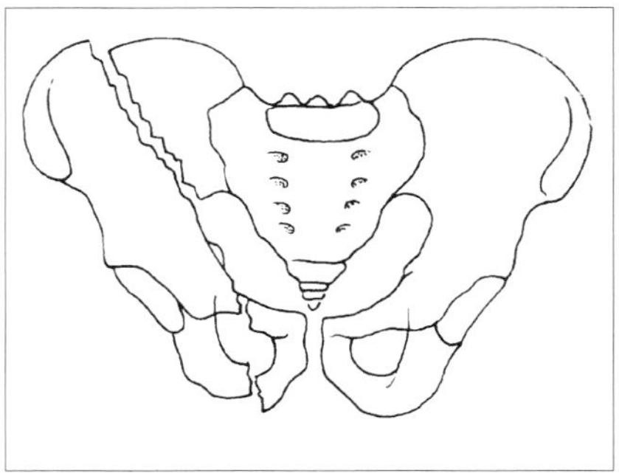

Figure 18.43

Evaluation

Physical examination findings include:

- Flank ecchymosis
- Labial or scrotal swelling
- Abnormal position of the lower extremities
- Pain with pelvic rim compression.

If the fracture is unstable, you will feel differential motion of the pelvic components when gently manipulating them. Place your hands on the iliac wings and gently rock the pelvis. Confirm the diagnosis with an anterior-posterior X-ray of the pelvis. Additional inlet and outlet views help determine the extent of the fractures.

> Remember to focus on a systematic examination of the whole patient (see page 16–2).

Treatment

- Focus the initial management on general resuscitation efforts (see page 13–1 to 13–9).
- Manage stable pelvic fractures with bed rest and analgesics. Stable fractures are rarely associated with significant blood loss.

Unstable fractures

Unstable fractures are associated with visceral damage and there is often significant bleeding. As an emergency procedure:

1 Place compression on the iliac wings, using a sheet or sling to close the pelvic space and tamponade active bleeding (Figure 18.44).
2 Treat with a pelvic sling and/or traction on the leg to reduce the vertical shear component of the fracture (Figure 18.45).
3 Maintain the traction until the fracture has consolidated. This usually takes 8–12 weeks.

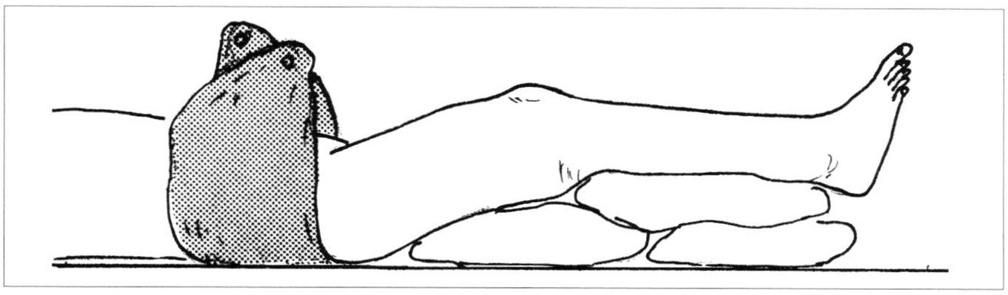

Figure 18.44

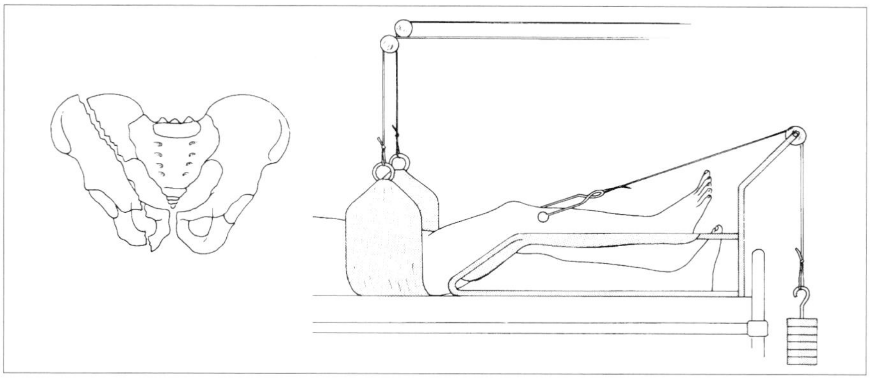

Figure 18.45

ACETABULAR FRACTURES

The fracture disrupts the congruence of the femoral head with the acetabulum and causes damage to the articular surface. A small number of fractures will be combined acetabular and pelvic ring injuries.

KEY POINTS

- Acetabular fractures result from high-energy pelvic injuries
- Treatment aims to restore the congruence of the femoral head with the acetabulum by traction or by surgery if available
- Complications include deep venous thrombosis, sciatic nerve injury and late degenerative arthritis of the hip.

Evaluation

History and physical findings are similar to those in pelvic ring fractures.

- Evaluate and treat hypovolaemic shock and visceral organ damage as an emergency (see page 13–8).
- Evaluate sciatic nerve function and look for an associated femoral shaft fracture.
- Obtain an initial anterior-posterior pelvic X-ray. If a fracture is evident, oblique views show the articular surfaces more clearly. X-ray the femoral shaft.

Treatment

Minimally displaced fractures

Treat minimally displaced fractures with bed rest and gradual mobilization. When comfortable, begin partial weight bearing until fracture healing has occurred. This usually takes about 12 weeks.

Displaced and unstable fractures

Treat displaced and unstable fractures with traction to maintain the congruence of the femoral head with the weight-bearing portion of the acetabulum. If a satisfactory position cannot be maintained, or if there are bone chips within the hip joint, surgical stabilization is indicated.

> Do not send the patient to another hospital unless you are certain that this complicated surgery is available there.

FRACTURES OF THE PROXIMAL FEMUR (HIP FRACTURES)

KEY POINTS

- Hip fractures are classified as intra-capsular (femoral neck fractures) or extra-capsular (inter-trochanteric and sub-trochanteric fractures)
- Treat displaced intra-capsular fractures with internal fixation, prosthetic replacement or early ambulation
- Treat extra-capsular fractures with traction or internal fixation
- Perkin's traction works well and avoids the immobilization necessary with other techniques.

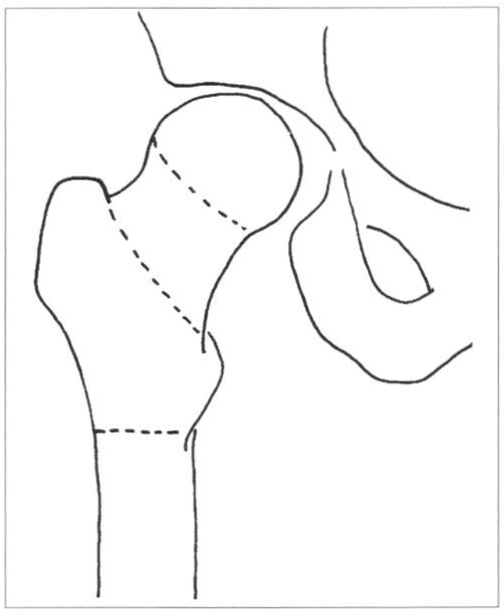

Figure 18.46

Hip fractures in elderly people with osteoporotic (weak) bone frequently occur following simple falls. In younger people, a moderately severe trauma is required to produce a fracture in this region.

Classify fractures by their anatomic location (Figure 18.46):

- Intra-capsular (femoral neck fractures)
- Extra-capsular: intertrochanteric
- Extra-capsular: subtrochanteric.

In intra-capsular fractures, the blood supply to the femoral head is disrupted. This may lead to the secondary complication of avascular necrosis of the femoral head.

Evaluation

Make the diagnosis from a history of a fall, pain about the hip and inability to bear weight on the extremity.

The physical examination reveals a leg that is shortened and externally rotated. The pain is made worse by attempted motion of the hip, especially with rotation. Confirm diagnosis by X-ray.

Treatment

Intra-capsular fractures

Treat with internal fixation or prosthetic replacement of the femoral head. If this cannot be done:

- Treat non-displaced or impacted fractures with light skin traction and a gentle range of motion until the fracture has healed; this will be in about 8–12 weeks
- Treat displaced fractures initially in light traction for a few weeks to control pain, then begin sitting and walking with crutches.

Extra-capsular fractures

Treat with Perkin's traction (see page 17–5) or surgical fixation. Perkin's traction will maintain the fracture position while permitting the patient to sit up to move the knee and hip joint, preventing pressure sores and pneumonia.

HIP DISLOCATIONS

Dislocations of the hip joint result from high-energy trauma and are associated with injuries of the acetabulum, femoral shaft and patella. Posterior dislocations are most common.

Evaluation

Make the diagnosis from the history of the injury and the physical findings of a flexed, adducted, internally rotated hip that is painful to move. The clinical examination is sufficient to make the diagnosis, but X-rays are necessary to identify associated fractures.

Examine the sciatic nerve function by testing foot and ankle strength and sensation.

Treatment

1 Reduce the dislocation as soon as possible:
   - With the patient supine, apply traction to the flexed hip while an assistant holds the pelvis down for counter traction (Figure 18.47); muscle relaxation is usually necessary
   - If you have no assistant, use an alternative method with the patient prone:
     - Apply traction downward with the leg flexed over the edge of the table
     - Gently rotate the hip while applying pressure on the femoral head in the gluteal region (Figure 18.48).

2 Place the patient in post-reduction skin traction for a few days and then begin non-weight bearing ambulation with crutches. Allow weight bearing after 12 weeks. If there is a large posterior rim fracture, treat the patient in traction for 8–12 weeks while the fracture unites.

KEY POINTS

- Make the diagnosis from the history and from clinical findings; use X-rays to confirm associated fractures
- To avoid the complications of vascular necrosis and loss of joint motion, reduce the dislocation as soon as possible
- Closed reduction is usually successful if carried out promptly.

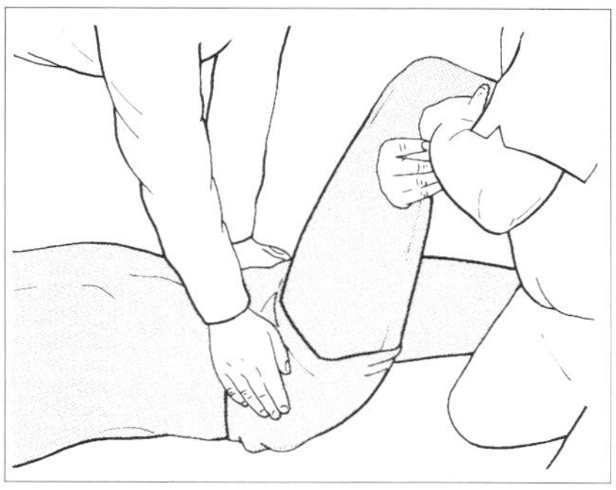

Figure 18.47

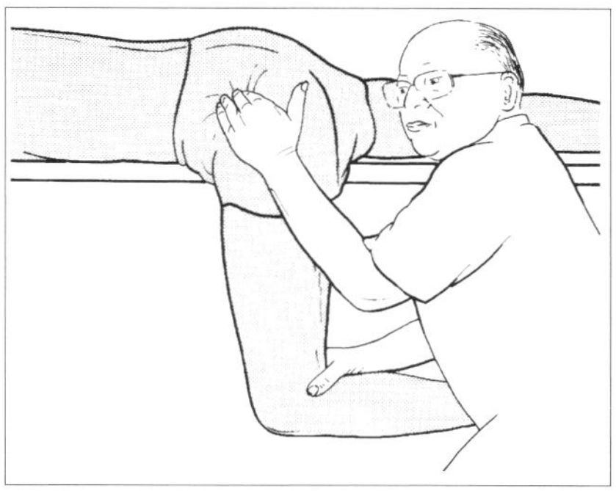

Figure 18.48

18.4 INJURIES OF THE LOWER EXTREMITY

FEMORAL SHAFT FRACTURES

Evaluation

Make the diagnosis based on a history of major trauma and the clinical findings of swelling, pain, angular or rotational deformity or abnormal motion at the fracture site. Examine the skin and soft tissue on all sides of the limb to check for possible open fractures.

Evaluate the neurological and vascular status for injury to the sciatic nerve and the femoral artery. Confirm the diagnosis with X-rays of the entire femur, including the femoral neck.

KEY POINTS

- Femoral shaft fractures result from high-energy trauma and are often associated with other significant injuries
- Debride and lavage open fractures under sterile conditions as soon as possible
- Treat in traction and monitor the fracture position with or without X-rays
- Fracture of the femoral neck is the most common associated skeletal injury and is frequently overlooked.

18

Treatment

1 Immediately debride and lavage open fractures in the operating room. Expose the bone ends and clean of all foreign material.

2 Apply traction to control alignment, length and discomfort:
- For children below the age of six years, use Russell's skin traction (see page 17–5)
- Older children and adults require skeletal traction to accommodate the weight needed to control the fracture position; balanced suspension and Perkin's traction (see page 17–5) work well
- In fractures of the upper third of the femur, the proximal fragment will be pulled into flexion and abduction
  - Adjust the traction to maintain alignment with the proximal fragment
  - Use 90/90 traction in older children (see page 17–5)
- Use portable X-rays for monitoring fracture position and healing in traction; if not available, measure the leg lengths and visually estimate angulation and rotation as a guide to traction adjustment
- Perkin's traction allows the patient to flex his/her knees and hips to 90 degrees. In this position, the rotation of the limb through the fracture will be maintained in an acceptable position.

Fracture healing in adults takes about 10–12 weeks. By 6–8 weeks, the fracture will show early signs of consolidation and it may be possible to place the patient in a hip spica cast and begin non-weight bearing ambulation. Treat fractures in the middle and distal third of the femur with a brace cast and hinged knee instead of a spica.

External fixation is not sufficient to control the fracture position in large muscular patients or in patients with unstable fracture patterns. It is a useful method for temporary stabilization of femoral fractures in multiple trauma patients. Place the frame on the lateral side of the thigh.

If the fracture position cannot be obtained or maintained, consider internal fixation.

DISTAL FEMORAL FRACTURES

Supracondylar fractures occur just above the knee joint. The distal fragment angulates posteriorly because of the pull of the gastrocnemius muscle at its attachment on the posterior aspect of the distal femur (Figure 18.49).

Intra-articular fractures occur as either a single femoral condyle fracture (Figure 18.50) or as a supracondylar fracture with extension distally into the joint (Figure 18.51).

KEY POINTS

- Distal femoral fractures occur as supracondylar fractures or extend into the knee joint as intercondylar fractures
- Treat non-displaced fractures in a cast
- Treat displaced fractures in traction.

Evaluation

There is a history of a high-energy injury and swelling and deformity just above the knee. X-rays are necessary to confirm the diagnosis and to evaluate articular surface injury. Carefully check sensation, motor power and the vascular status of the leg and foot.

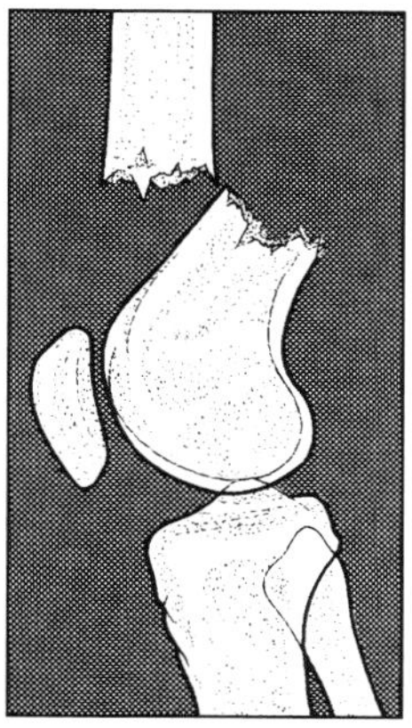

Figure 18.49

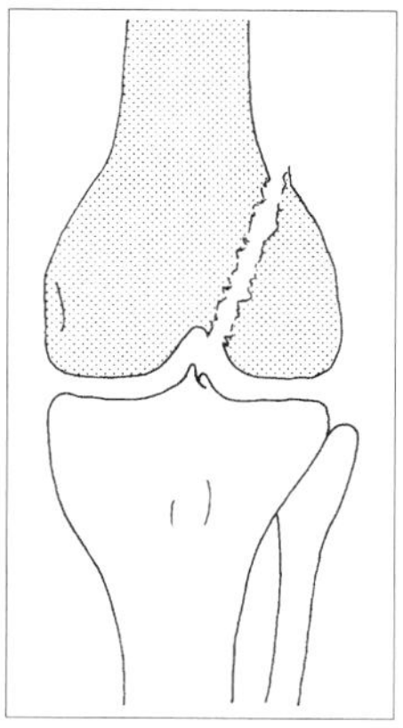

Figure 18.50

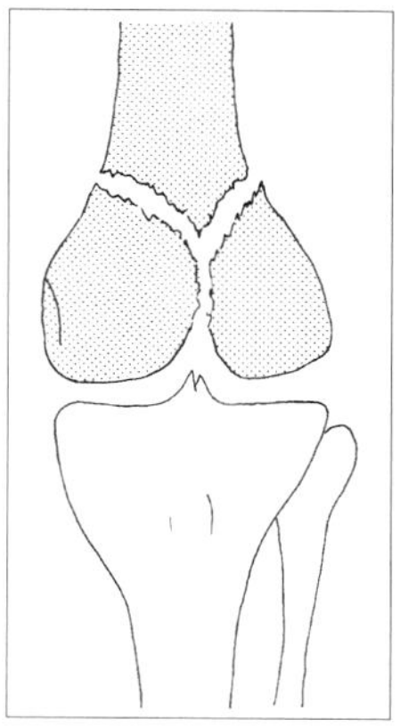

Figure 18.51

Treatment

Non-displaced fractures

Treat non-displaced fractures in a long leg cast without weight bearing.

Displaced fractures

1. Treat displaced fractures in skeletal traction using a tibial pin. Flexing the knee will help to reduce the angular deformity of the distal femur. This is done with pillows under the knee, balanced suspension or using Perkin's traction.
2. Align the articular surfaces to within a few millimetres using traction, closed manipulation or open surgical reduction.
3. Begin quadraceps muscle strengthening in traction when pain permits.
4. When the fracture is united (at 4–6 weeks), transfer the patient to a long leg cast or cast brace with knee hinges.
5. Begin weight bearing at 3 months when the fracture is solidly healed.

Popliteal artery injuries require immediate surgical correction if the limb is to be saved.

PATELLA INJURIES

The fracture will displace if the quadriceps tendon is torn and the quadriceps muscle pulls the fragments apart.

Lateral patella dislocations follow a direct force to the medial side of the bone or from a twisting injury in a developmentally unstable patella. To reduce the dislocation, place the knee in extension and push the patella medially.

KEY POINTS

- Patella injuries are caused by direct trauma to the anterior knee
- Displaced fractures are associated with rupture of the quadriceps tendon complex; they need surgical repair to restore knee extensor function.

Evaluation

Suspect a fracture from the history of the injury and from swelling and pain directly over the anterior knee. If the fracture is displaced, the patient is unable to extend the leg and a gap is often palpable between the displaced fragments.

A rupture of the quadriceps tendon proximal to the patella, or to the patella tendon distal to it, has similar physical findings. X-rays confirm diagnosis.

18

Treatment

Non-displaced fractures

Treat non-displaced fractures in a splint or cylinder cast for 4–6 weeks. Permit full weight bearing in the cast.

Displaced fractures

Treat displaced fractures by surgical repair of the fracture, or by suture of the quadriceps tendon mechanism (Figure 18.52). Remove comminuted fragments and, if necessary, remove a portion of the patella. Place in a splint or cast as for non-displaced fractures.

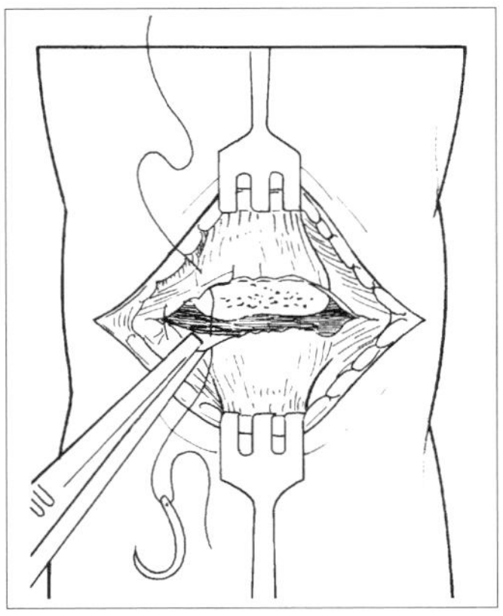

Figure 18.52

TIBIAL PLATEAU FRACTURES

KEY POINTS

- Tibial plateau fractures are intra-articular injuries of the weight-bearing portion of the knee joint
- Treat non-displaced fractures with a splint or cast
- Treat displaced or unstable fractures with traction or surgical stabilization
- Evaluate for injury to the popliteal vessels.

Tibial plateau fractures result from a vertical or lateral force driving the femoral condyles into the tibial articular surface of the knee.

The most unstable fractures involve both plateaux and cross the tibial shaft (Figure 18.53).

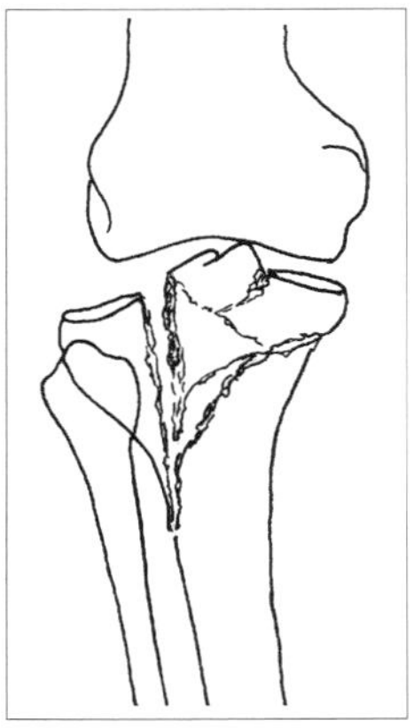

Figure 18.53

Evaluation

The knee is swollen, painful and shows deformity at the location of the injury. X-rays determine the location of the fracture and indicate the treatment.

Perform a careful examination of the neurological and vascular functions at the foot and ankle. Injury to the popliteal artery requires immediate repair if the leg is to be saved.

Treatment

Non-displaced fractures

Treat non-displaced fractures, and fractures with less than 5 mm of articular surface depression, in a splint initially. In 1–2 weeks, begin a range of motion out of the splint. Keep the patient non-weight bearing for 6 weeks and partial weight bearing with crutches or a stick for an additional 6 weeks.

Displaced fractures

Treat displaced or unstable fractures by closed reduction followed by a cast, calcaneal traction or surgical reduction and internal fixation.

TIBIAL SHAFT FRACTURES

Fractures in this region are often open because of the proximity of the anterior tibia to the skin surface.

Fracture patterns include: (Figure 18.54)

- Spiral fractures, from low energy injuries (A)
- Short oblique fractures (B)
- Transverse fractures (C).

The amount of soft tissue (skin, muscle, nerve, artery) damage influences the rate of healing and the chance of subsequent infection.

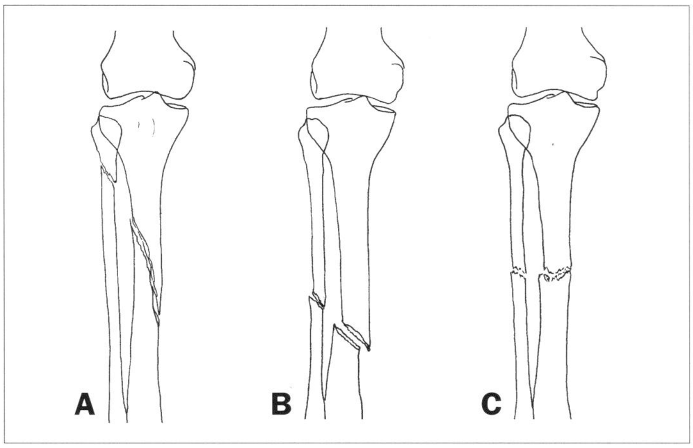

Figure 18.54

KEY POINTS

- Healing response and complication rate are related to the extent of soft tissue injury
- Open fractures are common and require immediate debridement
- Closed reduction and cast application is appropriate for most fractures
- External fixation is useful for fractures associated with open wounds or severe comminution and instability
- Complications include compartment syndrome, non-union and infection.

Evaluation

Inspect the skin closely for any wounds. Full thickness breaks in the skin indicate an open fracture and you should prepare for debridement and lavage of the fracture.

During the initial examination, check the neurological and vascular function to the foot. Signs of a developing compartment syndrome include:

- Increasing pain
- Coolness and pallor of the foot and toes
- Pain with passive extension or flexion of the toes or ankle
- Increasing tight feeling in the compartments in the calf.

Treat with surgical release of the four leg compartments as soon as possible (see pages 18–34 to 18–35).

Treatment

1 Immediately debride open fractures.

2 Reduce tibial fractures by hanging the leg over the end of the examination table and apply longitudinal traction.

3 Place the limb in a long leg three way splint with the knee in 10–20 degrees of flexion.

4 In 2–3 weeks, remove the splint and apply a long leg cast.

18

5 Recheck the patient about every three weeks. X-rays are useful to check the position of the fracture and the extent of healing.

6 When the fracture position feels stable, place the patient in a patella tendon bearing cast (see page 17–9) and begin knee motion and weight bearing. The healing time for uncomplicated tibial fractures is about six months.

Open fractures that require dressing changes or skin grafts and unstable comminuted fractures are best managed using an external fixation frame (see pages 17–10 to 17–11). Use either a unilateral or a bilateral frame. When the skin has been closed and the fracture is stable, remove the frame and apply a cast for the remainder of the treatment period.

KEY POINTS

- Ankle fractures result from inversion, eversion/external rotation and vertical forces
- The anatomic structures involved include the tibia, fibula and talus and three sets of ligaments
- Isolated fibula fractures are stable. Most other injuries involve two or more of the above structures and require closed reduction or surgical stabilization. External fixation may be used in vertical load fractures.

ANKLE FRACTURES

Isolated fractures of the distal fibula are caused by an eversion/external rotation force through the ankle. With only one component of the articular ring disrupted, these are stable injuries (Figure 18.55).

A similar injury combined with a fracture of the medial malleolus or tear of the deltoid ligament (Figure 18.56) is not stable and causes subluxation of the ankle joint.

Inversion injuries result in medial subluxation of the joint and fractures of both malleoli (Figure 18.57).

A vertical load causes the distal tibial articular surface to fracture (Figure 18.58), resulting in a compression injury to the cancellous bone and significant disruption of the articular cartilage of the ankle.

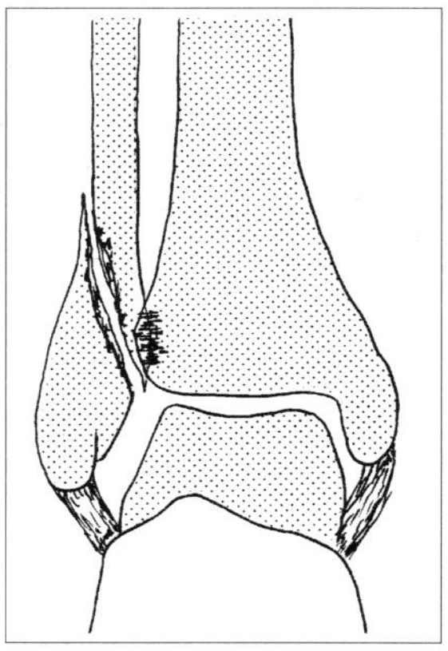

Figure 18.55

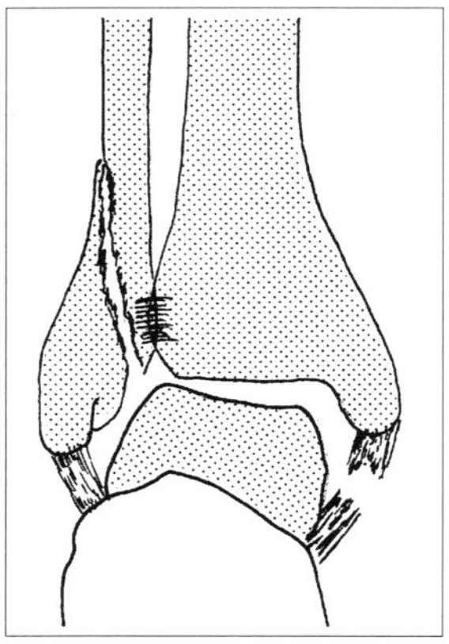

Figure 18.56

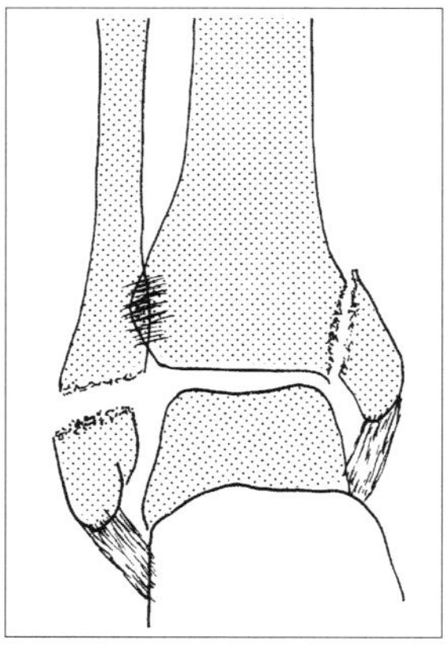

Figure 18.57

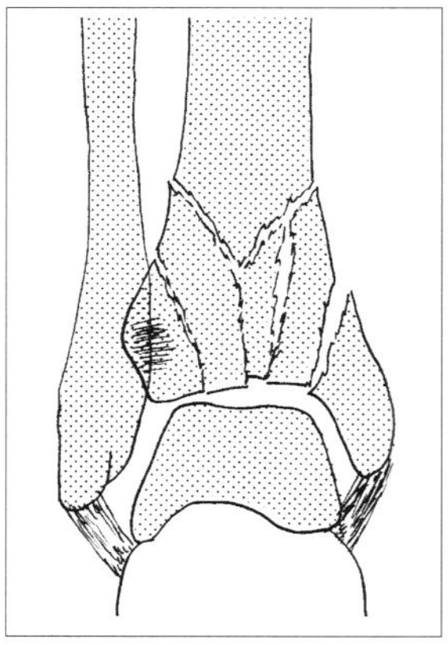

Figure 18.58

Evaluation

Ankle fractures result from low-energy injuries such as a fall from a low step. Inspection for deformity and palpation of the area of maximum tenderness will enable you to make an accurate diagnosis. X-rays are most useful to evaluate the position of the ankle joint after closed reduction.

The reduction is satisfactory if X-rays show the cartilage clear space has a uniform thickness on all three sides of the joint when viewed in the mortise view (anterior-posterior view with the ankle in 15 degrees of internal rotation) and there is a normal relationship of the distal tibial surface to the talus.

Treatment

Treat isolated fibula fractures in a 3-way splint (see page 17–10), followed after 7–10 days by a weight bearing short leg cast.

Unstable fractures

Reduce unstable fractures with gentle longitudinal traction followed by manipulation in the opposite direction to the deformity:

- Position eversion/external rotation fractures with the heel in inversion, the foot internally rotated and the ankle at 90 degrees of flexion; maintain this position by holding the big toe to support the weight of the leg, while an assistant applies the splint
- Position inversion type fractures with the heel everted slightly, the foot in neutral and the ankle at 90 degrees of flexion.

Vertical load fractures (Figure 18.58), are difficult to treat by closed reduction. If gentle traction and manipulation of the fragments does not result in a satisfactory reduction, consider calcaneal traction or an external fixation frame.

FOOT INJURIES

Talus fractures

Talar neck fractures result from an axial load which forces the foot into dorsiflexion. The neck of the talus is pushed against the anterior tibia, fracturing the neck (Figure 18.59). Continuation of this force produces a dislocation of the subtalar joint as the body of the talus extrudes posterior medially from the ankle joint.

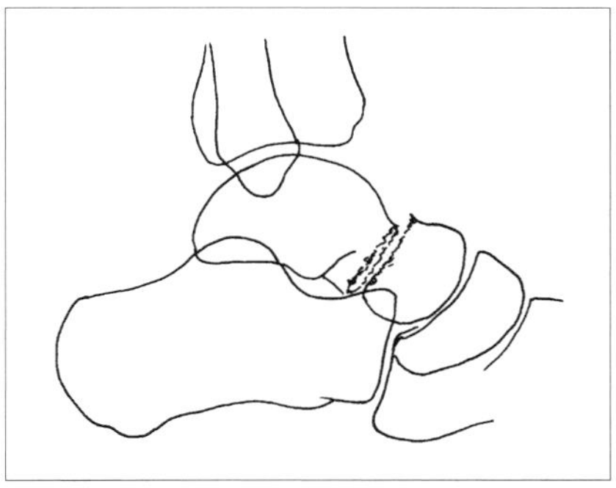

Figure 18.59

KEY POINTS

- Clinical examination suggests this fracture, but X-rays are needed to confirm the diagnosis and to guide treatment
- Treat with closed reduction and immobilization
- Fracture dislocations may require open reduction.

Evaluation

Diagnosis is based on a history of a dorsiflexion injury, with swelling and pain about the ankle and hind foot. Obtain ankle and foot X-rays to confirm the location and extent of the fracture.

Treatment

Treat minimally displaced fractures in a splint followed by a short leg non-weight bearing cast for 6–8 weeks.

18

Reduce displaced fractures with gentle longitudinal traction, pulling the heel forward and dorsiflexing the foot. Next, evert the foot and bring it into plantar flexion to align the major fragments. Apply a short leg cast.

If the talus is dislocated, apply direct pressure over the extruded fragment during the reduction manoeuvre.

KEY POINTS

- Calcaneal fractures occur either through the body of the calcanous and into the subtalar joint, or as avulsion fractures of the posterior portion of the tuberosity
- The mechanism of the injury is a vertical load which may also cause vertebral body compression fractures
- Treat with compression, elevation, splinting and gradual resumption of weight bearing.

Calcaneus fractures

Calcaneous fractures result from a vertical load force driving the talus downward into the subtalar joint and the body of the calcaneus (Figure 18.60).

Avulsion fractures of the calcaneal tuberosity are produced by the contracting Achilles tendon (Figure 18.61). These fractures usually do not enter the subtalar joint and have a better prognosis.

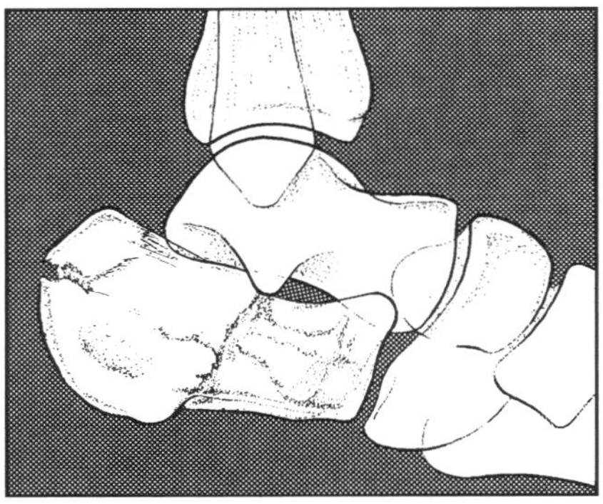

Figure 18.60

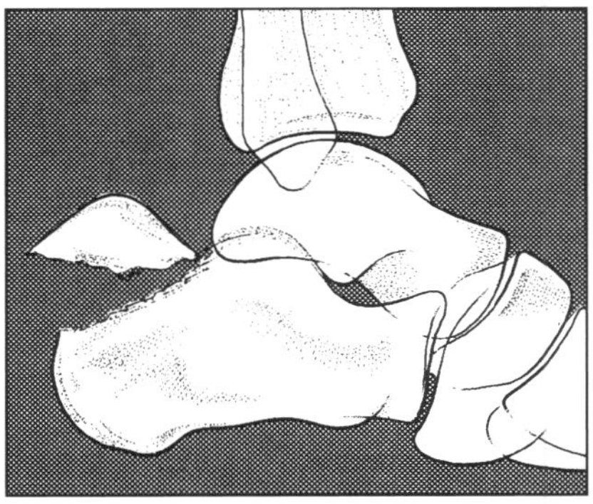

Figure 18.61

Evaluation

The physical examination reveals swelling and tenderness about the hind foot. X-rays will confirm diagnosis. Ask about low or mid-back pain and palpate the spine to evaluate for a vertebral fracture.

Treatment

Treat calcaneal fractures with a compression dressing, short leg splint and elevation.

Keep the patient from bearing weight on the affected limb. Encourage toe and knee motion while the limb is elevated. Begin partial weight bearing 6–8 weeks after the injury and full weight bearing, as tolerated, by 3 months.

KEY POINTS

- The injury results from forced plantar flexion of the forefoot
- Diagnosis is by X-ray showing fractures of the base of the metatarsal bones with subluxation or dislocation of the tarsal-metatarsal joints
- Treat with closed reduction and immobilization
- Pin fixation may be necessary to secure the position
- Long-term mid-foot pain is common.

Fracture dislocation of the tarsal-metatarsal joint (Lisfranc injuries)

The injury causes dislocation of the tarsal-metatarsal joints and fractures of the metatarsals and tarsal bones (Figure 18.62).

Evaluation

Deformity is often not evident because of the large amount of swelling present. On the X-ray, the medial borders of the second and fourth metatarsals should be aligned with the medial borders of the second cuneiform and the cuboid respectively.

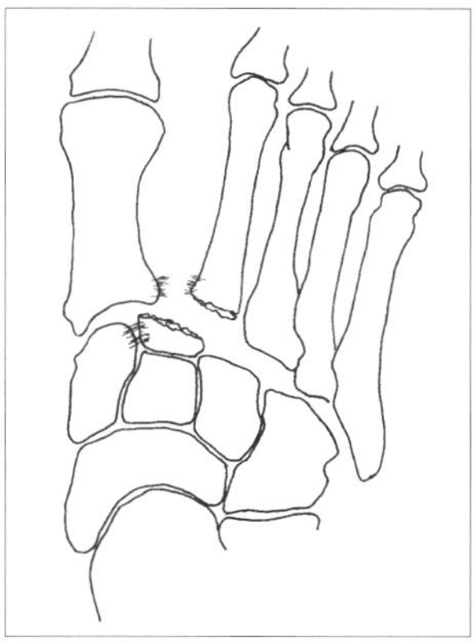

Figure 18.62

Treatment

Perform a closed reduction to return the mid-foot to the anatomic position. Apply a short leg splint and ask the patient to keep the limb elevated. If reduction cannot be attained or maintained, consider stabilization with pins or screws.

Fractures of the metatarsals and toes

Evaluation

Clinical findings are tenderness and swelling. Deformity is not always evident. X-rays confirm diagnosis.

Overuse fractures (stress fractures) occur in the metatarsal bones. The patient has pain and tenderness but no history of acute trauma.

Treatment

- Treat dislocations and angulated fractures with closed reduction. Immobilize metatarsal fractures in a firm bottom shoe or a short leg cast.
- Treat toe fractures and dislocations by taping the toe to a normal adjacent toe (Figure 18.63).
- Treat stress fractures by limiting the amount of time the patient spends on his/her feet. If necessary, use a firm shoe or cast until pain free.

KEY POINTS

- Fractures of the metatarsals and toes are common injuries resulting from minor trauma
- Treat fractures and dislocations in this area by closed reduction and immobilization.

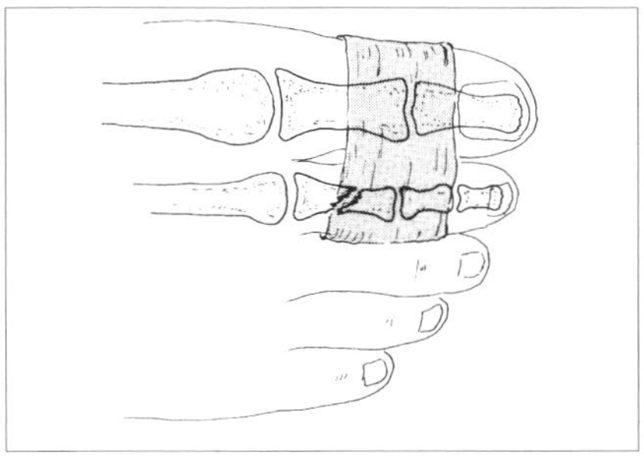

Figure 18.63

18.5 SPINE INJURIES

Fractures are stable if further deformity is unlikely. They are unstable if a change in the fracture position is expected with mobilization.

Spinal cord injury is complete if there is no nerve function below the level of injury and if improvement or return of function is unlikely. Incomplete injuries have some nerve function below the injury level and may show improvement with treatment.

Evaluation

1 Ask the patient if he/she has neck or back pain or has lost feeling in the arms or legs. Assume that an unconscious patient has a spine injury until he/she wakes up enough to answer these questions or until adequate X-rays show the spine to be normal.

KEY POINTS

- Evaluate the spine based on a history of injury, physical examination, a complete neurological examination and X-rays
- Spinal column injuries are stable or unstable, based on bone and ligament damage
- Neurological function may be normal, show incomplete injury or complete spinal cord disruption
- Base your treatment on the extent of injury.

2 Inspect the entire spine by log rolling the patient gently on to his/her side. Look for swelling and bruising. Palpate the spine for areas of tenderness and check for gaps or changes in the alignment of the spinous processes.

3 Perform a careful and complete neurological examination as outlined in Table 18.1 and record your findings. If there is a neurological deficit, determine the level from a motor and sensory examination. The injury is complete if there is no neurological function below that spinal cord level. In incomplete injuries, the sacral nerve roots will often function.

During the period of spinal shock (usually the first 48 hours after injury) there may be no spinal cord function. As shock wears off, some neurological recovery may occur with incomplete injuries. The ultimate prognosis cannot be accurately determined during the first several days.

Neurological examination in the spinal injury patient

Sensation
- Test sensation to pinprick in the extremities and trunk
- Test perianal sensation to evaluate the sacral roots

Motor function
- Evaluate motion and strength of the major muscle groups
- Determine if rectal sphincter tone is normal

Reflexes
- Deep tendon reflexes in the upper and lower extremities
- Bulbocavernosus reflex: squeeze the glans penis – the bulbocavernosus muscle contracts in a positive test
- Anal wink: scratch the skin next to the anus – the anus contracts in a positive test
- Babinsky reflex: stroke the bottom of the foot – the toes flex normally and extend with an upper motor nerve injury

X-ray examination

X-ray the entire spine in patients not mentally responsive enough to cooperate with the clinical examination. In patients who are awake:
- X-ray the symptomatic areas of the cervical, thoracic and lumbar spine
- X-ray the cervical spine in all patients involved in high-energy multiple trauma.

Evaluate the cervical spine:
- With lateral and AP films
- Make sure to include all seven cervical vertebrae
- Obtain an open mouth odontoid view.

Take AP and lateral views of the thoracic and lumbar spine.

The most common areas of injury are C2, C5–6 and T12–L1. In patients with pain but normal X-rays, take flexion and extension lateral X-rays of the cervical spine.

X-ray interpretation

The bony spine is anatomically divided into three sections or columns (Figure 18.64).

Injuries are unstable if there is:

- Injury to two or more columns
- Rotational mal-alignment
- Subluxation or dislocation of one vertebra on another
- Fracture of the odontoid
- Up to 50% vertebral body compression in the thoracolumbar spine
- Increased width between the pedicles on the AP view.

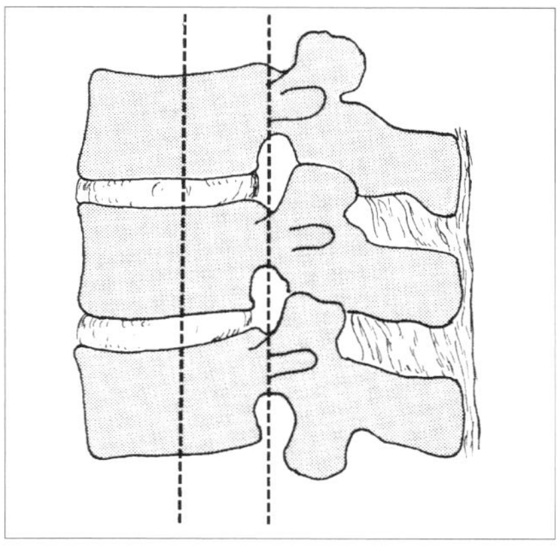

Figure 18.64

Treatment

Cervical spine

- C1: The first cervical vertebra has ample room for the spinal cord and neurological injury is unusual:
  - Initially, place patients in skull traction (see page 17–4) to maintain the fracture position and to control discomfort
  - When stable, change to a Minerva cast or a rigid cervical collar Healing takes about 3 months
- C2: Odontoid fractures at the junction of the vertebral body are unstable (Figure 18.65):
  - To reduce the fracture, place the patient in skull traction with slight hyperextension of the head
  - At 4–6 weeks, change to a Minerva cast or a halo vest
- C2: Vertebral body:
  - Reduce the fracture by placing the neck in the neutral position and apply a Minerva cast or rigid collar
  - Avoid traction because it will distract this fracture
- C3–7: Treat fractures, dislocations and fracture-dislocations (Figure 18.66) in skull traction followed, after 4–6 weeks, by a Minerva cast or halo vest. Healing time is 3–4 months, usually with a spontaneous fusion.

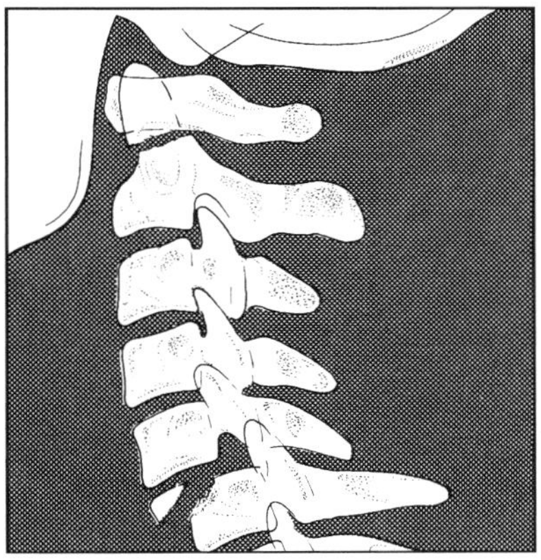

Figure 18.65

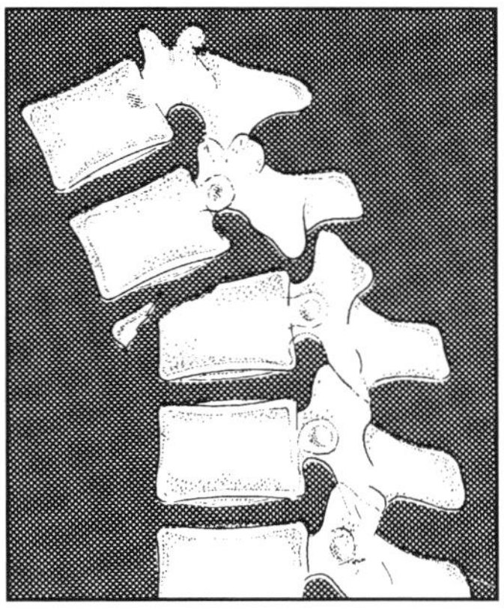

Figure 18.66

Facet dislocations or subluxations

Gradually increase the traction weight (5 kg/hour up to 20 kg) while monitoring neurological signs and taking frequent lateral X-rays. When the facet joints are unlocked, attempt to reduce the dislocation by gently rotating and extending the neck. If this is unsuccessful, allow it to remain dislocated and treat as above.

18

Neurological damage

Spinal cord injury above C5 causes paralysis of the respiratory muscles and patients usually die before reaching a medical care facility. At or below this level, treat similarly to patients without neurological deficit. However, begin care of the skin, bowel and bladder immediately.

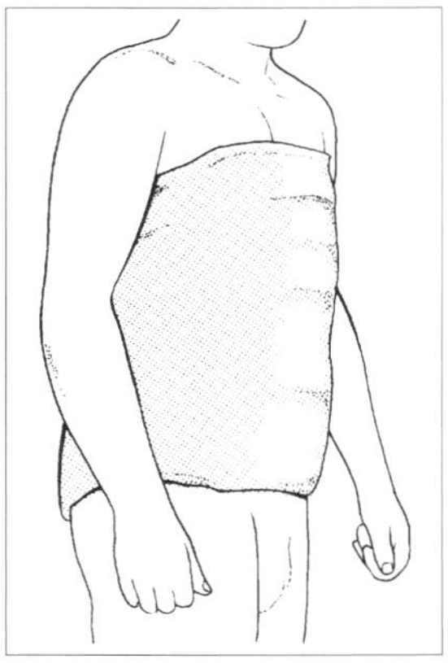

Figure 18.67

Thoracolumbar spine

1 Place the patient at bed rest on a soft pad and move only by log roll. A paralytic ileus is common following lumbar fractures. Give the patient nothing by mouth until bowel sounds return. Regularly monitor and record the neurological status.
2 If there is no neurological damage, begin ambulation, when comfortable, using a brace or body cast (Figure 18.67). A sitting lateral X-ray will confirm fracture stability. The patient should not bend or lift for at least 3 months.

For incomplete neurological injury, treat as above but monitor the neurological status closely until recovery has stabilized.

With complete neurological disruption, begin the rehabilitation programme immediately to prevent potential complications.

KEY POINTS

- Open growth plates and the thick periosteal membrane make fractures in children different from those in adults
- Treat fractures by closed reduction; certain displaced epiphyseal fractures may need surgical reduction
- Future growth will remodel some residual deformity in length, angulation and displacement but not in rotation.

18.6 FRACTURES IN CHILDREN

Growth in length occurs through the cartilaginous epiphyseal plates and growth in width through the periosteal membrane. The latter is a thick fibrous layer that covers the bone and provides stability to torus (Figure 18.68) and greenstick fractures (Figure 18.69).

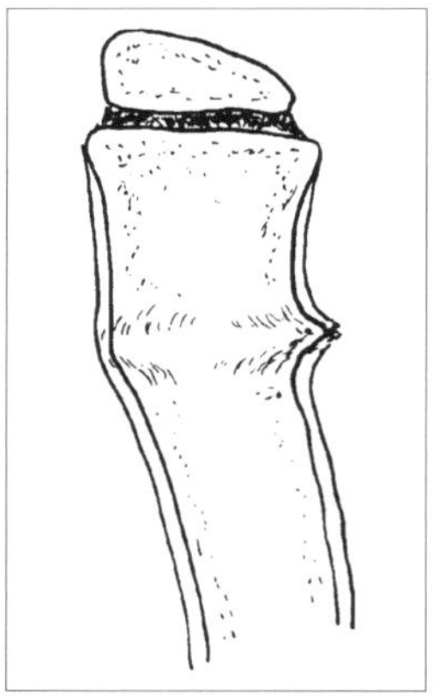

Figure 18.68

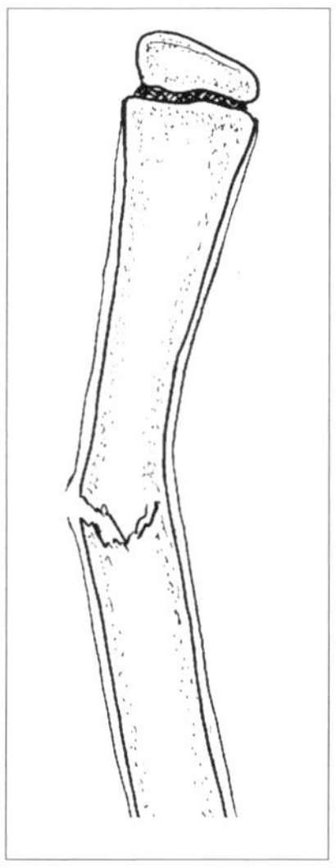

Figure 18.69

Epiphyseal plate fractures are classified by location and by the path of the fracture line across the epiphyseal plate (Figure 18.70).

If the growth potential of the epiphyseal cartilage is damaged, the growth pattern will be altered and deformity of the extremity is likely.

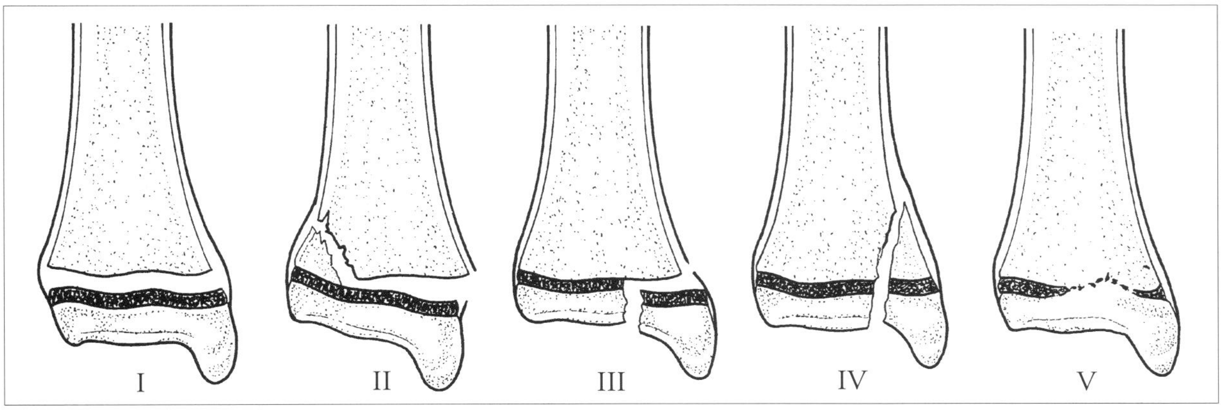

Figure 18.70

Evaluation

Identify the fracture by findings of tenderness, swelling, bruising and deformity. Obtain X-rays, if available. If you cannot identify a fracture, consider the possibility of infection.

Joint instability in children occurs because of torn ligaments and epiphyseal fractures. Take an X-ray while applying stress across the joint to show the location of the instability.

Treatment

- Treat epiphyseal fractures with gentle closed reduction. Make one or two attempts only, as repeated manipulation will further injure growth potential.
- Minor residual deformity in fractures of type I and II will remodel. Type III and IV fractures involve the joint cartilage as well as the epiphyseal plate. If displacement of more than a few millimetres remains in these structures after closed reduction, consider open reduction.
- In general, fractures not involving the growth plate will heal in an acceptable position as long as the general alignment of the limb is maintained. The remodelling potential declines with age, and younger children are able to correct greater deformities.

Expected correction following long bone fractures in children

Length	1.5–2 cm
Angulation	30 degrees
Rotation	None
Displacement	100 %

18

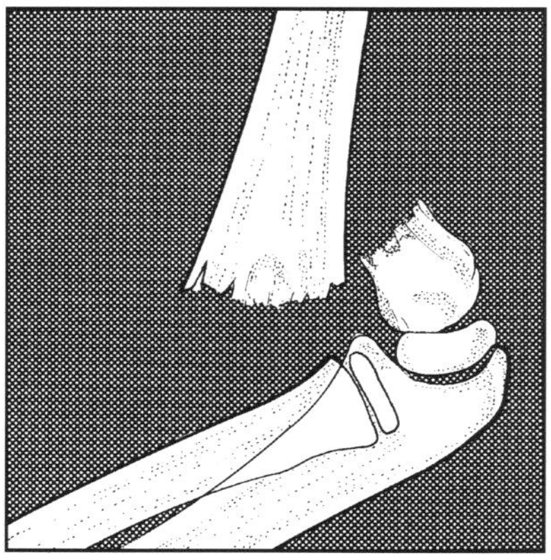

Figure 18.71

Specific fracture types

Supracondylar fractures of the humerus

Age	Most common from 18 months to 5 years
Mechanism	Fall on extended arm
Evaluation	Pain, swelling and deformity just above elbow
	Examine the vascular and nerve function in the forearm and hand
X-ray	Helpful but not essential. Do not delay treatment if X-ray is unavailable (Figure 18.71).

Treatment

1 With the patient lying face up, apply traction on the forearm with the elbow near full extension.

2 While maintaining traction, grasp the distal fragment of the humerus and correct medial and lateral displacement and rotation (Figure 18.72).

3 Next, flex the elbow slowly while pushing the distal fragment forward into the reduced position (Figure 18.73).

4 Check the radial pulse before and after the reduction. If it diminishes as the elbow is flexed, extend the forearm until the pulse returns. Immobilize the arm in a posterior splint at 120 degrees of flexion or in the position where the pulse remains intact.

5 If the circulation is in question, or if it is not possible to obtain a satisfactory reduction, treat the patient in olecranon or Dunlap's traction (see page 7–5).

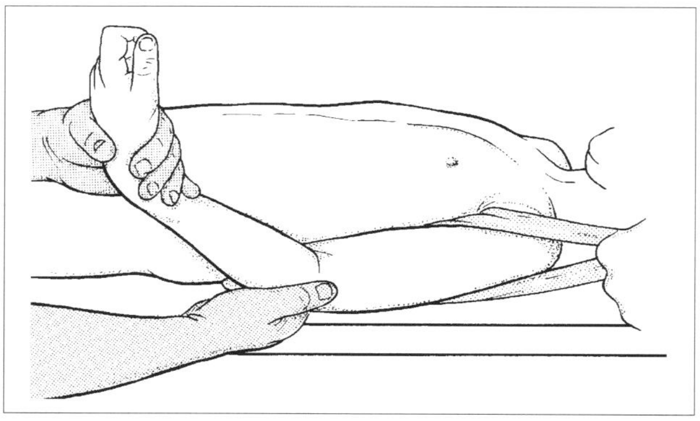

Figure 18.72

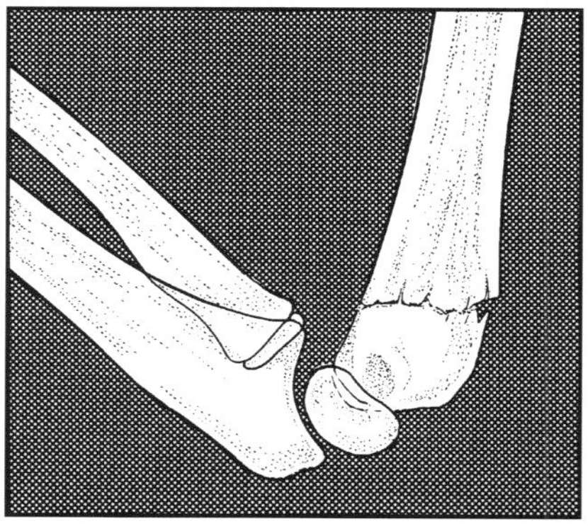

Figure 18.73

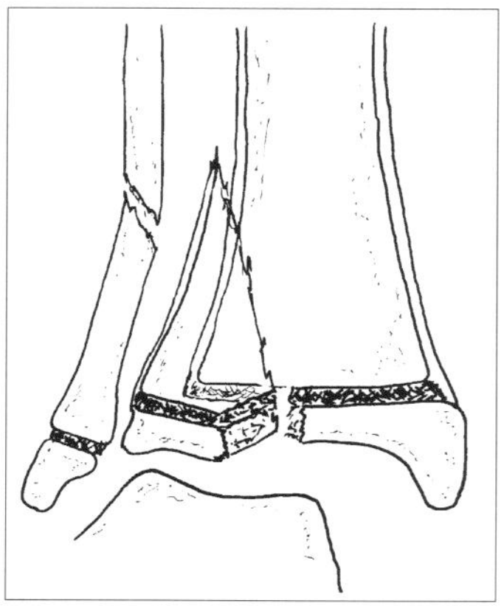

Figure 18.74

Triplane fractures of the distal tibia (Figure 18.74)

Age	12–15 years, at the time of closure of the distal tibial epiphysis
Mechanism	Abduction, external rotation force to the ankle joint
Evaluation	Painful, swollen ankle with or without other deformity
	X-ray is needed to make the diagnosis but, if unavailable, begin treatment

Treatment

1 Apply longitudinal traction to the foot by holding the mid-foot and heel.

2 Invert the heel, bring the ankle from plantar flexion to neutral (90 degrees) and internally rotate the foot.

3 Maintain the reduction by grasping the great toe, allowing the foot to hang, while a three-way splint is applied.
4 Mould the plaster as it dries.
5 Obtain post-reduction X-rays when possible.

18.7 AMPUTATIONS

Amputation refers to the surgical or traumatic removal of the terminal portion of the upper or lower extremity.

Perform surgical amputations to:

- Remove a malignant tumour
- Treat severe infections
- Treat end stage arterial disease
- Remove a limb following irreparable trauma to the extremity.

Determine the amputation level by the quality of tissue and by the requirements for prosthetic fitting. The standard levels for lower extremity amputations are shown in Figure 18.75. In the upper extremity, preserve as much limb length as possible.

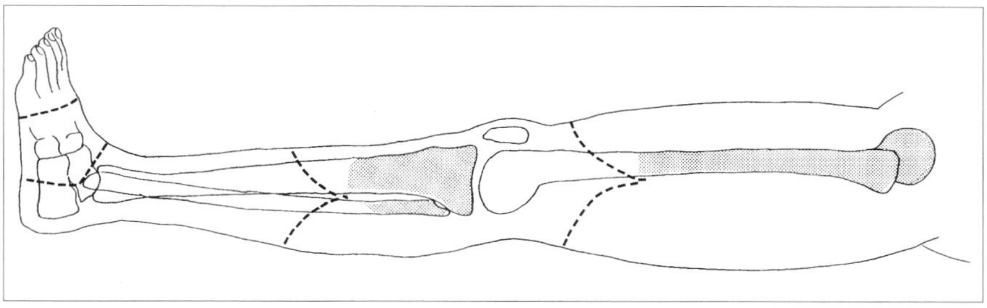

Figure 18.75

KEY POINTS

- Limb amputation is a definitive procedure, which requires careful preoperative thought and consultation
- Amputations are performed in emergency situations for severe limb trauma and in elective situations for infection or tumours
- Amputations in children should, when possible, preserve the growth plates
- Rehabilitation efforts are focused on the substitution of lost function.

Evaluation

- Evaluate skin, muscle, vascular supply, nerve function and bone integrity. Wound healing requires normal blood flow. It is possible to substitute for loss of muscle function, but protective skin sensation is necessary at the amputation site.
- The mangled but intact extremity following trauma requires careful evaluation, and consultation with a colleague and the patient, before amputation is carried out.
- If the vascular supply and the sensation are lost, amputation is indicated. Severe damage to three of the five major tissues (artery, nerve, skin, muscle and bone) is an indication for early amputation.

Techniques

Guillotine amputation

Use a guillotine amputation in emergency situations for contaminated wounds or infection as a quick means of removing diseased or damaged tissue.

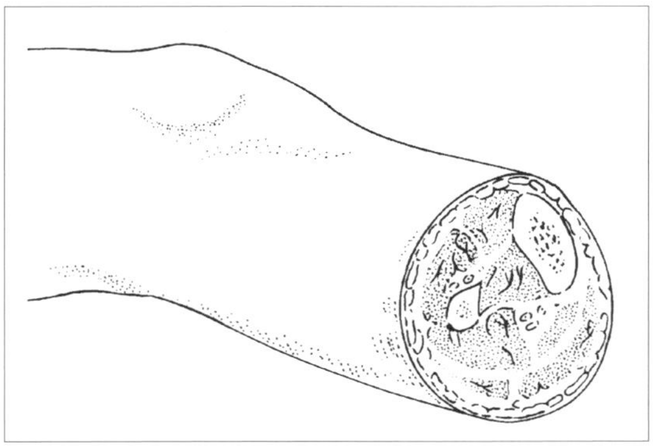

Figure 18.76

1 Divide the skin, muscle and bone at or near the same level, without attempting to fashion flaps or close the wound (Figure 18.76).

2 Tie all bleeding vessels and cut the nerves sharply while under gentle tension, allowing them to retract into the wound. Tack skin flaps loosely with a few stitches to prevent further retraction. Apply a sterile dressing and, if possible, an elastic stump wrap.

3 Debride and lavage the wound every 2–5 days until it is free of dead tissue and infection. At that point, perform a definitive amputation and closure.

Definitive amputation

Perform a definitive amputation as an elective procedure when the extremity is clean and non-infected or following a guillotine amputation.

In the upper limb, preserve as much of the limb as possible. The ideal levels for a lower extremity amputation are 12 cm proximal to the knee joint (transfemoral) and 8–14 cm distal to the knee joint (transtibial). When possible, save the knee joint to improve function with a prosthesis. Amputations through the knee are acceptable in children.

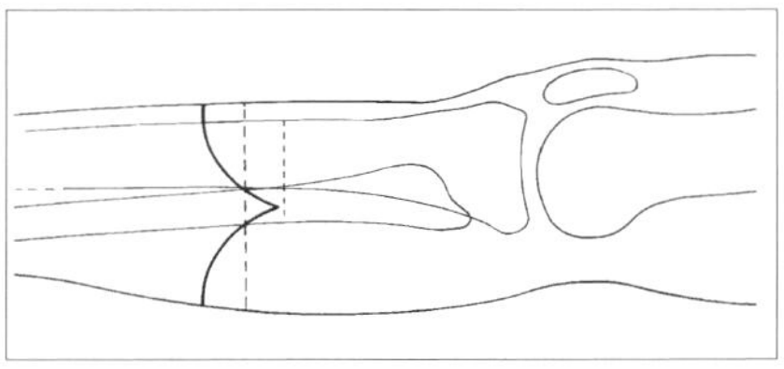

Figure 18.77

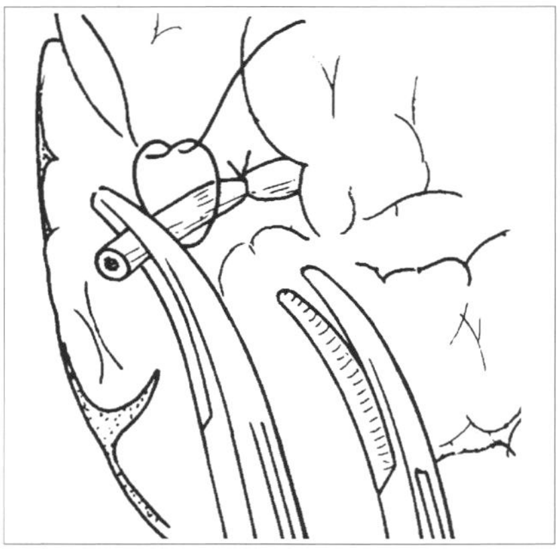

Figure 18.78

1 Cut the skin flaps 5–6 cm, and the muscles 2–4 cm, distal to the proposed level of bone section (Figure 18.77).

2 Fashion the skin flaps so that the sum of the lengths of the flaps is one and a half times the diameter of the limb. Local conditions may necessitate unequal or irregular flaps.

3 Taper the anterior end of the bone and cut the fibula 3 cm proximal to the tibial cut.

4 Doubly ligate all major vessels (Figure 18.78).

5 Cut the nerves sharply while under gentle tension and allow them to retract into the wound. Stitch opposing muscles over the end of the bone and attach the muscle flaps to the bone through the periosteum or a drill hole.

6 Release the tourniquet and stop all bleeding before closing further.

7 Suture the skin and fascia loosely in two layers, using interrupted stitches. If skin closure is a problem, use split thick skin grafts on non-weight bearing portions of the stump. Do not close the skin under tension.

8 In most cases, use a drain and plan to remove it in 1–2 days. Apply a firm bandage and place the remaining limb in a plaster splint.

9 Make the stump cylindrical with even muscle distribution. A conical or bulbous stump will be painful and difficult to fit to the prosthetic socket.

Foot amputations

Perform amputations within the foot at the base of the toes or through the metatarsals, depending on the level of viable tissue. Amputations more proximal on the foot (tarsometatarsal joint or midtarsal joint) are acceptable, but may lead to muscle imbalance. They may require splinting and tendon transfers in order to maintain a plantagrade foot for walking.

Upper extremity amputations

- Save as much of the extremity as possible. A prosthesis will often not be available for upper extremities and any preserved function will be useful.
- Split thickness skin grafts work satisfactorily for most stumps.
- At the wrist level, preserve carpal joints to allow terminal flexion and extension movements.
- Saving the radial-ulnar joint allows pronation and supination of the forearm.
- Patients with bilateral upper extremity amputations may benefit from a Krukenberg operation. This is an elective procedure that splits the radius and ulna and provides muscle power to each. The resulting forearm has simple grasp and sensation.

Amputations in children

Children adapt more easily than adults to amputations and prosthetic use. When possible, preserve the growth plate and the epiphysis to allow normal growth of the extremity. Trans-articular amputations are well tolerated, as is the use of split thickness skin grafts on the weight-bearing surface of the limb.

18.8 COMPLICATIONS

COMPARTMENT SYNDROME

Increased compartment pressure is commonly caused by:

- Tight casts or dressings
- External limb compression
- Burn eschar
- Fractures
- Soft tissue crush injuries
- Arterial injury.

The most common areas involved are the anterior and deep posterior compartment of the leg and the volar forearm compartment. Other areas include the thigh, the dorsal forearm, the foot, the dorsal hand and, rarely, the buttocks.

Diagnostic physical findings include:

- Pain out of proportion to the injury
- Tense muscle compartments to palpation

KEY POINTS

- Compartment syndrome is caused by swelling within closed fascial spaces; as the intra-compartmental pressure increases, blood supply to the muscles is lost
- Treat with immediate surgical release of the skin and fascia over the involved compartment.

18

- Pain with passive stretch of the involved muscle
- Decreased sensation
- Weakness of the involved muscle groups
- Pallor and decreased capillary refill (late finding)
- Elevated compartment pressure (if measurement is possible).

Treatment

Split the cast and dressings, if present. Do not elevate the limb, but observe carefully for improvement. If signs and symptoms persist, treat the acute compartment syndrome with immediate surgical decompression.

Even short delays will increase the extent of irreversible muscle necrosis so, if you suspect a compartment syndrome, proceed with the decompression immediately.

Techniques

Leg

1 Use two full length incisions to decompress the four leg compartments (Figures 18.79 and 18.80).

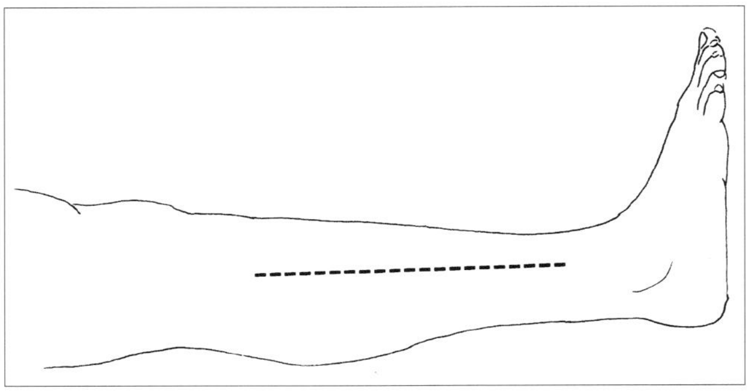

Figure 18.79

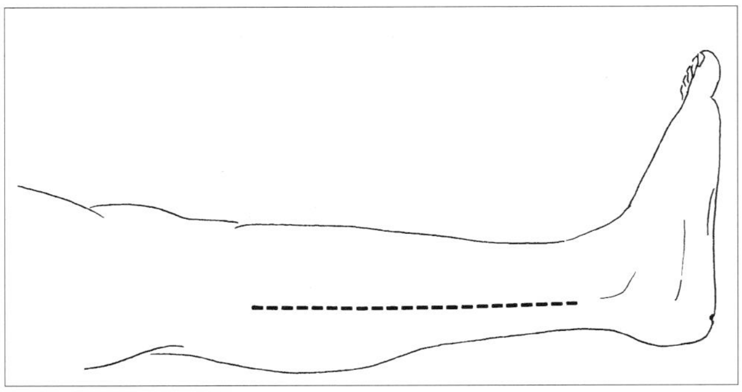

Figure 18.80

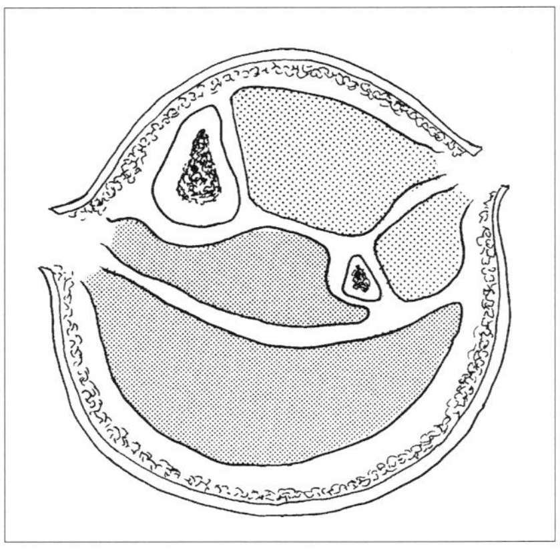

Figure 18.81

2 Place one incision on the anterior lateral aspect of the leg just anterior to the fibula. Divide skin and the fascia surrounding the anterior and lateral compartments.

3 Place the second incision 1–2 cm posterior to the medial border of the tibia to access the superficial and deep posterior compartments (Figure 18.81).

Forearm

1 Decompress the superficial and deep volar compartments through a single incision beginning proximal to the elbow and extending across the carpal canal (Figure 18.82).

2 Divide the superficial fascia for this entire length, being sure to open the carpal canal to decompress the median nerve. Expose the deep compartment muscles and incise the fascia surrounding the pronator teres, the pronator quadratus, the flexor digitorum and the flexor pollicis longus muscles (Figure 18.83).

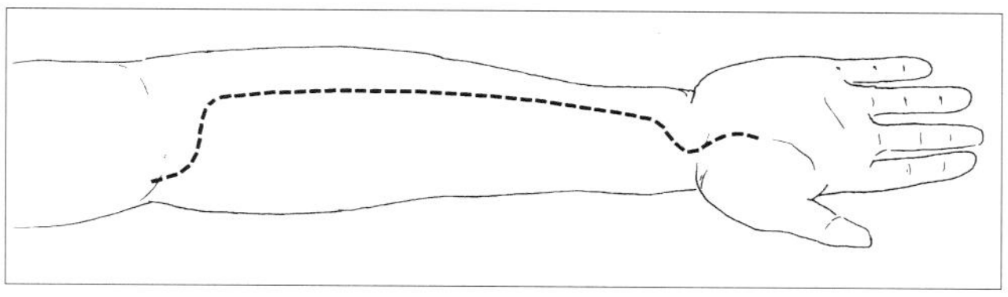

Figure 18.82

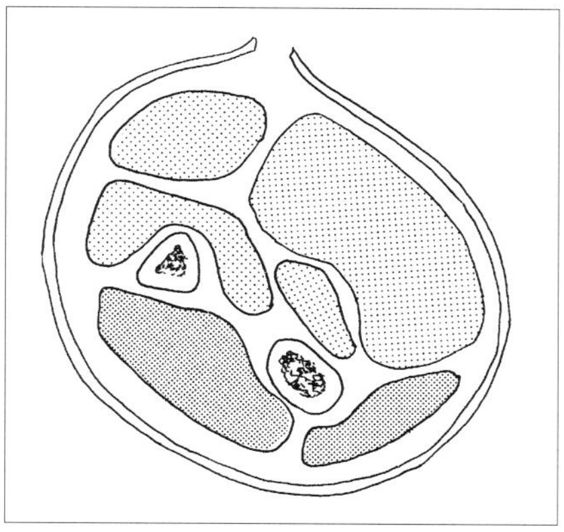

Figure 18.83

3 Inspect the muscles for signs of necrosis. Dead muscle has a dark purple colour, does not bleed if cut, does not twitch if pinched and has a flabby consistency. Remove obviously dead muscle but, if in doubt, leave it and re-evaluate in 1–2 days. Do not close the wound.

4 Apply sterile dressings and splint the extremity. If there is an associated fracture, apply an external fixation apparatus, traction or a cast. Return the patient to the operating theatre for re-debridement in 1–2 days. When the wound is clean and the swelling has decreased sufficiently, close the wound or apply a split thickness skin graft.

FAT EMBOLISM SYNDROME

Fat embolism syndrome follows major long bone trauma. The etiology remains elusive, but seems to involve a showering of bone marrow contents into the bloodstream. These lodge in the lungs, brain and other organs. The syndrome becomes clinically evident on the second or third day post injury. The lung involvement causes respiratory distress, which is fatal in a small percentage of patients.

Signs include:

- Confusion and anxiety
- Increased pulse and respiratory rate
- Petechiae located in the axilla, conjunctiva, palate and neck
- A chest X-ray showing fluffy infiltrates
- Low arterial oxygen content (if test available).

Treatment

1 Stabilize long bone fractures. *Early stabilization may prevent the syndrome.*

18

KEY POINTS

- The severity of the gunshot wound is related to bullet size, shape and velocity
- Low velocity injuries cause minor wounds and are treated with superficial debridement, antibiotics and tetanus prophylaxis
- High velocity injuries cause extensive soft tissue and bone damage and are treated with careful debridement and lavage, as are all open fractures; do not close the wound initially
- Treat associated fractures with plaster, traction or external fixation.

2 Administer oxygen and support respiration if breathing effort becomes great.

The syndrome is self-limited, lasting usually just a few days. Permanent effects are rare, but include impaired vision, kidney abnormalities and mental changes.

18.9 WAR RELATED TRAUMA

GUNSHOT WOUNDS

Tissue damage from missile wounds is related to the mass and shape of the missile (bullet) and the square of the speed at which it travels. Heavier bullets have more momentum and release more energy when they hit an object. The external shape of the bullet determines whether it will penetrate smoothly, splatter into multiple fragments or tumble. Mine fragments (see pages 18–37 to 18–38) are irregular in shape and tear their way through tissue.

Tissue damage occurs from direct injury from the missile, a shock wave resulting from the dissipation of energy as the missile slows down and from a cavitation effect produced by the vacuum behind the advancing missile. Small entrance and exit wounds may coexist with extensive muscle and bone injury.

Evaluation and diagnosis

Since multiple sites are common, inspect the entire body of the patient to identify all wounds. Injuries to the head, chest and abdomen may be life threatening and the patient should be evaluated as outlined on pages 16–4 to 16–7 and the Annex: *Primary Trauma Care Manual*.

Carefully check the sensation, muscle power and circulation of the injured extremities and record your findings. X-rays are not essential, but will help you to evaluate the type of fracture and ascertain if any missile fragments are retained within a joint. If present, these must be removed.

Treatment

Your treatment should be guided by the type of weapon that caused the injury and by the extent of soft tissue injury.

Low velocity injuries

For minor wounds caused by a missile speed less than 1500 feet/second:

1 Debride the wounds superficially. This is usually done in the outpatient department.
2 Lavage the wound with fluid.
3 Do *not* close the skin.
4 Administer intravenous antibiotics for 1–3 days.
5 Give tetanus prophylaxis.
6 Treat fractures by closed means with a cast, traction or external fixation.
7 If bullet fragments remain in a joint cavity, arrange to have them removed within a few weeks.

High velocity injuries

For major wounds caused by missile speeds greater than 1500 feet/second:

1 Debride the wounds in the operating theatre, using adequate anaesthesia.

2 Lavage each wound after removing all dead tissue and foreign material as outlined in the section on open fractures (see pages 5–10 to 5–11).

3 Lavage between the entrance and exit wounds, passing gauze through the tract if necessary.

4 Do *not* close the wound. Re-debride in 2–5 days and close or skin graft when clean.

5 Administer antibiotics and tetanus prophylaxis as above.

6 Treat fractures with a cast or, preferably, external fixation or traction.

LANDMINE INJURIES

Landmines are classified as either blast or fragmentation types. Blast mines are pressure sensitive and are detonated by stepping on them or by gripping them with the hand. They produce damage from the concussion effect of the blast. Clothing, grass and injured body parts become secondary missiles.

Fragmentation mines are positioned above the ground and detonate with a trip-wire. Injuries are caused by metal or plastic fragments propelled by the explosion.

KEY POINTS

- Injury patterns are related to the type of landmine encountered
- Blast injuries occur from pressure sensitive mines, while trip-wire mines produce injury from multiple flying fragments
- Evaluate the entire patient for injury to multiple systems
- Treat extremity injuries with debridement and skin coverage
- Amputation is often necessary.

Patterns of injury

Step on blast mine:

- Lose foot and part of leg
- Tears and shreds skin, muscle and bone
- Bone becomes a secondary missile which can injure the abdomen and perineum.

Pick up blast mine:

- Lose hand and arm
- Injures eyes and face.

Fragmentation mine:

- Puncture wounds all over body
- Injuries common to head, chest and abdomen
- Fragments are missiles of both high and low velocity (see gunshot injuries).

Evaluation and diagnosis

Perform basic resuscitation as outlined in Unit 16: *Acute Trauma Management* and the Annex: *Primary Trauma Care Manual.* Inspect the patient's entire body to determine the location of all wounds and to evaluate injuries to the head, chest, abdomen and perineum.

Extremity injuries commonly follow blast injuries and a terminal portion of the extremity may be missing. Examine the remaining extremity to determine the tissues with blood and nerve supply which will be used to reconstruct the limb.

Treatment

1 Cover the wounds with sterile dressings.

2 Splint fractures temporarily until the patient is transported to the operating room.

3 Administer intravenous antibiotics and tetanus prophylaxis, as with open fractures.

4 Debride the wounds, removing all dead and foreign material. During this initial debridement, it is difficult to determine which tissues have an adequate blood supply. If in doubt, save the tissue and re-evaluate it on the next debridement. Muscle is judged on colour, bleeding and ability to contract.

5 Remove bone fragments with no soft tissue attachment.

6 Save all bleeding skin for coverage of the stump. Save skin from amputated parts as split thickness skin graft for later use.

7 Re-debride the wounds in the operating theatre every 2–5 days until ready to close or skin graft.

8 Treat fractures with splints, traction or external fixation. It is not always necessary to amputate the limb at the most proximal fracture. Try to save as much limb as practical. External fixation is especially useful in injuries with extensive soft tissue wounds.

Rehabilitation

- Begin a range of motion exercise of the remaining joints as soon as possible. The extensive scarring from mine injuries leads to severe contractures.
- Coverage of the weight-bearing portion of amputation stumps with full thickness skin will provide a better prosthetic fit but, if necessary, a prosthesis will work with split thickness skin only.
- Arrange for lower extremity prosthetic fitting, if available, when the skin has matured. For bilateral upper extremity amputations, consider a Krukenberg procedure (see page 18–33). This provides a grasp with some sensation and is especially useful for bilateral amputees and for patients with impaired vision.

General orthopaedics

19

19.1 CONGENITAL AND DEVELOPMENTAL PROBLEMS

HIP DISORDERS IN CHILDREN

Each of the hip disorders that affect children has a different etiology, but all cause damage to the proximal femoral epiphysis and lead to impaired hip function by altering normal growth.

Developmental dysplasia, or congenital dislocation of the hip, is caused by instability of the hip in the socket. The altered pressure causes the socket to grow with a shallow rim (Figure 19.1). As the hip slides laterally out of the socket, the leg shortens and the articular cartilage eventually degenerates.

Septic arthritis destroys the articular and growth cartilage through bacterial enzyme release into the infected joint.

Impairment of the blood supply to the hip causes necrosis of the bone with collapse of the round contour of the femoral head. This impairs motion and leads to later degenerative arthritis.

Slipping of the femoral epiphysis changes the contour of the femoral head in the socket, impairs motion and causes degenerative arthritis (Figure 19.2).

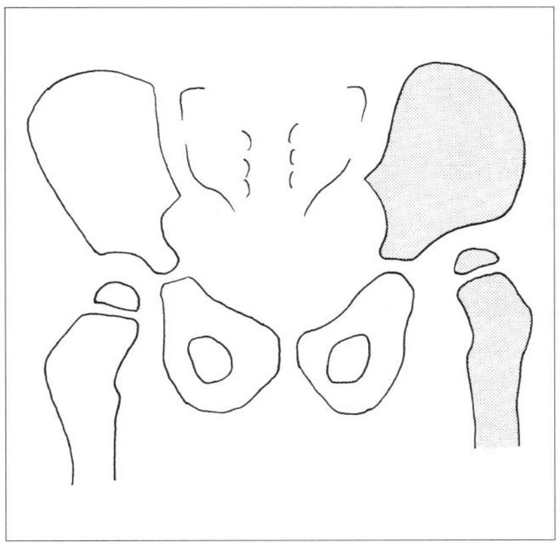

Figure 19.1

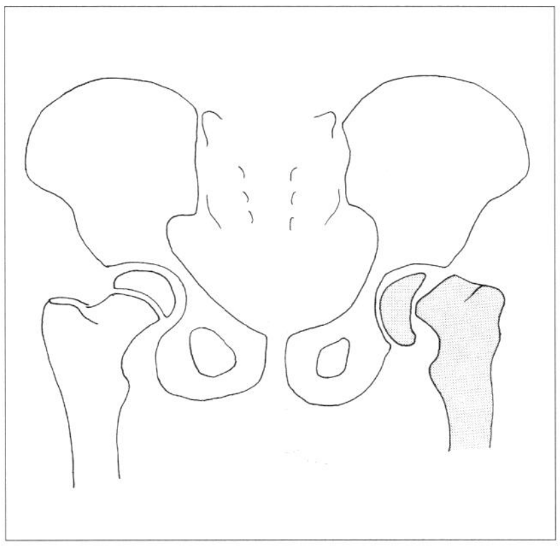

Figure 19.2

Evaluation and diagnosis

Age is a useful indicator of the diagnosis. All of these disorders are associated with decreased motion, but loss of internal rotation is seen earliest. In the older child, knee pain and limp are common presentations. Infection is associated with the systemic signs of fever and malaise. X-rays are helpful but not essential initially. If available, they help to determine the long term prognosis during the follow-up period.

KEY POINTS

- There are four major hip disorders in children; each occurs within a specific age range and may cause severe hip deformity if not treated early
- They include:
  - Developmental dysplasia of the hip
  - Septic arthritis
  - Avascular necrosis (Legg-Calve-Perthe's Disease)
  - Slipped capital femoral epiphysis
- Diagnosis is made by clinical examination. X-rays are useful for follow-up care, but are not essential.

19

Age at presentation	
• Developmental dysplasia	Present at birth
• Septic arthritis	Throughout childhood
• Avascular necrosis	4–8 years
• Slipped epiphysis	7–15 years

Presenting findings

- **Developmental dysplasia**
  - First born child
  - Breech delivery
  - Unstable hip at birth
  - Short leg
  - Asymmetric thigh skin folds
- **Septic arthritis**
  - Systemic signs
  - Pain with any hip motion
  - Hip held in flexed and abducted position
- **Avascular necrosis**
  - Limp without known injury
  - Knee pain with normal knee examination
  - Loss of internal rotation
- **Slipped epiphysis**
  - Limp
  - Knee pain with normal knee examination
  - Loss of internal rotation.

Treatment

- Treat patients with developmental dysplasia at birth with gentle closed reduction and application of a Pavlick harness (if available) or a double hip spica cast with the hips in abduction and flexion. Position the hips so that the reduction feels stable, but do not flex them greater than 90 degrees.
- Septic arthritis requires immediate surgical drainage (see pages 19–5 to 19–6). Aspiration will confirm infection by finding a cloudy or purulent joint fluid. In this case, perform surgical drainage immediately without waiting for culture results.
- If Perthe's disease is suspected, place the child at bed rest with straight leg skin traction and a few kilos of weight. As the pain subsides, begin active and active assisted motion. When full painless motion is regained, begin ambulation, partial weight bearing with crutches, and progress to full weight bearing as tolerated. Check the child frequently to be certain that a painless range of motion persists. If not, repeat the above process. The course of revascularization of the epiphysis takes 1–2 years.
- Slipping of the proximal femoral epiphysis requires pin fixation to prevent further displacement. This is a complex procedure requiring special pins and X-ray equipment. While arranging for this treatment, place the child in straight leg traction. If the child must travel for surgical treatment, keep him/her non-weight bearing with crutches or apply a hip spica cast.

TALPES EQUINOVARUS (CLUB FOOT)

This condition is present at birth and is distinguished by rigid inversion of the heel and forefoot and a plantar flexed ankle (Figure 19.3). Other less severe deformities are correctable with gentle stretching and involve either the forefoot or the ankle but not both. Other causes of deformity with a similar appearance, include arthrogryposis, poliomyelitis and myelomeningocele. These are associated with multiple abnormalities and are treated differently.

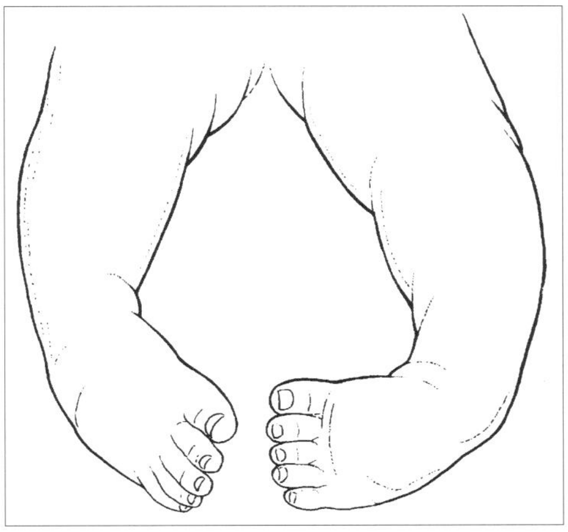

Figure 19.3

KEY POINTS

- The heel and forefoot are inverted, with the ankle in plantar flexion; the deformity is not correctable with manipulation
- Begin treatment as early as possible with manipulation and repetitive casts
- Patients presenting after 6–12 months of age will need surgical correction.

Treatment

Begin treatment as soon as possible with gentle manipulation and cast application. Change the cast weekly until correction is achieved.

Technique

1 Place the child in a comfortable supine position on an examination table or in the mother's lap.

2 Gently manipulate the foot by pushing the forefoot from the varus to a valgus position. Place your thumb on the base of the fifth metatarsal to serve as a fulcrum while pushing the forefoot laterally (Figure 19.4).

3 Next, evert the inverted heel, gently stretching the tight medial structures. Grasp the heel in your hand and rotate the whole foot outward.

4 When these deformities correct to 'normal', begin to bring the foot upward out of the plantar flexed position. Place your hand around the heel and rotate the foot upward pushing on the midfoot. Do not push up on the metatarsal heads as this will cause the foot to bend in the middle, creating a curved or rocker bottom.

5 Hold the corrected position in a padded long leg plaster cast, with the knee flexed or use an elastic or plaster splint (Figure 19.5).

6 Change the cast or splint weekly, slowly bringing the foot to a normal plantigrade position. Once corrected, hold the position with a cast or brace until the child is of walking age. Severely deformed feet may not correct completely with cast or splint treatment and surgery may be required.

19

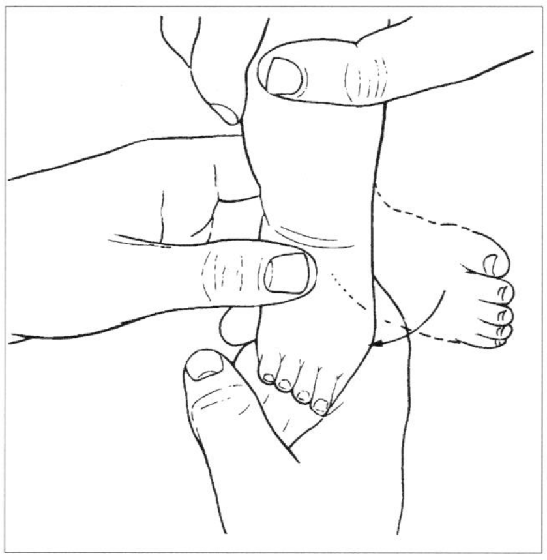

Figure 19.4

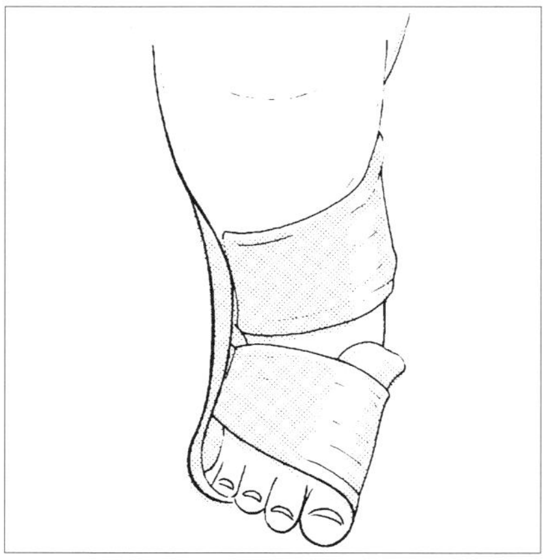

Figure 19.5

KEY POINTS

- Tumours in bone are either primary (originating in the bone) or metastatic (originating elsewhere and spreading to bone)
- Differentiating between benign and malignant tumours requires X-rays and, usually, biopsy
- Treatment of malignant bone tumours requires special facilities, including chemotherapy, radiation therapy and surgery.

19.2 BONE TUMOURS

Tumours metastatic to bone are found most commonly in the pelvis, spine, ribs, proximal femur and proximal humerus. They come from the breast, prostrate, lungs, kidney and thyroid gland. Check these areas if metastatic disease is suspected.

Primary bone tumours arise from bone tissue, cartilage, synovium, collagen and bone marrow cells. Malignant tumours have a high mortality rate and most commonly metastasize to the lungs.

Evaluation and diagnosis

Presenting signs and symptoms include:

- Deep pain which may not be not related to activities
- Swelling and tenderness
- Pathological fracture.

X-ray and biopsy are necessary to determine the diagnosis. Obtain a chest X-ray if metastatic lesions are suspected. The major differential diagnosis is infection. If in doubt, aspirate the lesion to look for pus.

X-ray characteristics

- **Benign tumours**
  - Lucent area surrounded by dense bone which contains the lesion
  - Cortex intact
  - No soft tissue mass
- **Malignant tumours**
  - Lucent area diffuse, without surrounding dense bone
  - Often has a patchy type of bone destruction with perforation of the cortex
  - May have periosteal new bone at the tumour margins
  - May have soft tissue mass
- **Metastatic tumours**
  - Similar to malignant tumours
  - May have sclerotic bone in lesions from the prostrate or breast.

Treatment

Arrange for treatment where the facilities are adequate. Benign tumours may be watched or have bone graft inserted to prevent a fracture through the lesion. If such fractures occur, treat them using the usual closed methods. When healed, arrange for definitive treatment of the tumour. Malignant tumours need special facilities, including chemotherapy, radiation therapy and surgery.

19.3 INFECTION

SEPTIC ARTHRITIS

Infection in a joint is caused by an open wound or puncture directly into the joint, from spread through the bloodstream from an infection elsewhere or from adjacent osteomyelitis. Pyogenic infections result most frequently from staphylococcus species. Other organisms responsible for joint infections include mycobacterium tuberculosis, brucellosis, salmonella and various types of fungus.

Enzymes released by organisms within the joint destroy the articular cartilage, leading to loss of motion, degenerative arthritis and spread of the infection to surrounding tissues. Prompt drainage of the purulent fluid and administration of antibiotics is necessary to preserve joint function.

KEY POINTS

- Joint infections arise from infections elsewhere in the body or from a direct wound into the joint
- Suspect infection when there is swelling, pain and loss of joint motion
- Confirm diagnosis by aspiration of purulent fluid from the joint
- Treat with needle or open joint drainage and antibiotics.

Evaluation and diagnosis

Patients have pain and tense swelling of the joint. The area around the joint is warm, red and tender and any joint motion is painful. A fever is usually present and, if laboratory studies are available, they will show an elevated white blood cell count and sedimentation rate. A history of a wound near the joint, or of an infection elsewhere in the body, should increase suspicion. Confirm the diagnosis by needle aspiration of the joint. Infected fluid is cloudy or overtly purulent. Send it for culture and sensitivity testing, but do not wait for the results before beginning treatment.

Aspiration technique

Perform a surgical scrub, and drape a sterile field about the joint. Use 1% lidocaine anaesthesia for the skin and tissue down to the joint capsule. Sedation may be necessary for aspiration of the hip joint. Insert a large bore needle directly into the joint and withdraw as much fluid as possible. Send the initial aspirate for culture.

Hip

With the patient supine, insert a spinal needle just anterior to the greater trochanter at an angle of 45 degrees (Figure 19.6). Advance the needle while aspirating. You will feel a "pop" when the needle goes through the joint capsule and fluid will fill the syringe.

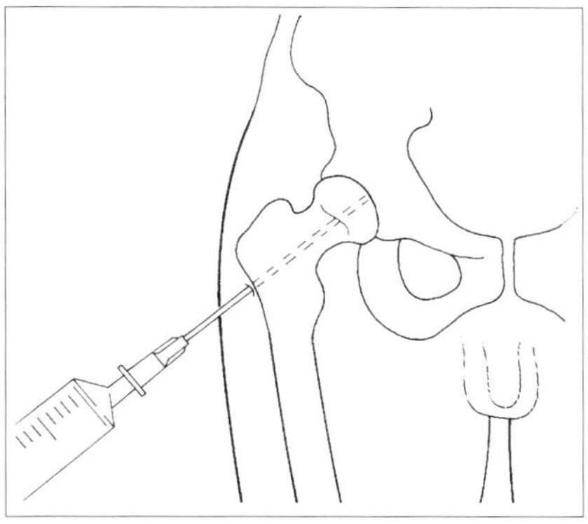

Figure 19.6

Knee

Aspirate the knee through a medial or lateral approach at the superior margin of the patella (Figure 19.7).

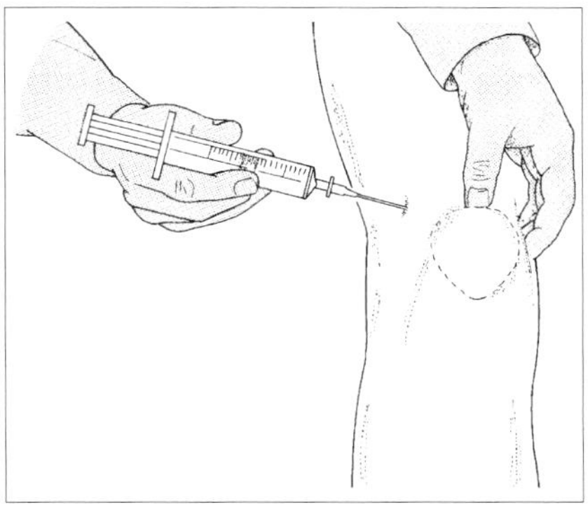

Figure 19.7

19

Ankle

Aspirate the ankle through an anterior lateral or anterior medial approach at the level of the distal tibia, and just lateral or medial to the extensor tendons.

Treatment

Treat septic joints with prompt drainage and systemic antibiotics. Drain the joint by open lavage, if it is possible at your hospital. If it is not, perform repeated daily aspirations until the fluid becomes clear and free of infection. Apply a splint to rest the joint during the initial treatment phase. Do not allow the patient to bear weight on the affected joint. Continue antibiotics for a total of at least 6 weeks. Switch to oral doses when joint swelling subsides and motion is no longer painful. This is usually after about 10–14 days.

KEY POINTS

- Bone infections come from haematogenous spread from a distant site, from penetrating wounds and after surgery
- Acute infections are treated with antibiotics; once an abscess forms, surgical drainage is necessary
- Chronic osteomyelitis is the most common type; a draining sinus and sequestrum (dead bone fragment) are usually present
- Removing the sequestrum is necessary to control the infection, but it should not be performed until the involucrum (new reactive bone) has fully formed.

PYOGENIC OSTEOMYELITIS

Infection of bone, osteomyelitis, occurs by direct inoculation from an overlying wound or from haematogenous spread from another infected site. It occurs as an acute form or, if untreated, as a chronic form.

In many areas of the world, osteomyelitis is endemic, existing as a chronic quiescent disease. The most common organism is staphylococcus and the most common sites of infection are the femur and tibia.

Haematogenous infections begin with the lodging of bacteria in the postcapillary sinusoids on the metaphyseal side of the epiphyseal plate. The organisms proliferate in this area of sluggish circulation, forming an intramedullary infection. This is the acute phase. If the infection is not treated, it forms an abscess cavity within the bone. Pressure within the abscess causes purulent material to penetrate the cortical bone. The periosteum is elevated and a subperiosteal abscess forms (Figure 19.8).

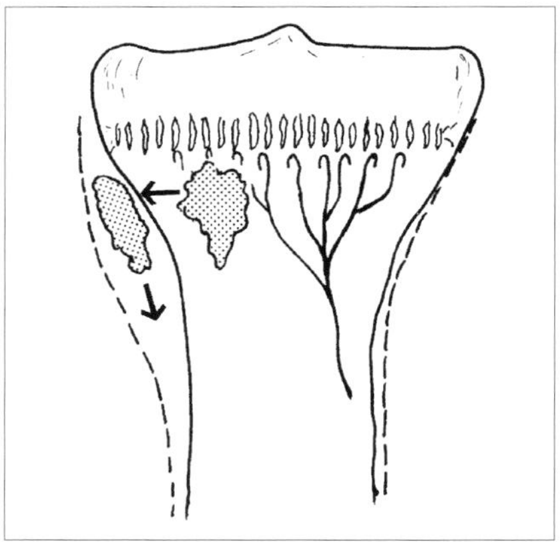

Figure 19.8

This marks the physiological beginning of the chronic form of the disease. There is usually clinical evidence of soft tissue involvement at this point, with swelling, redness and tenderness. If left untreated, the infection will either drain through the skin to decompress the abscess and/or dissect under the periosteum, encompassing much of the diaphysis. When the latter occurs, the original diaphysis becomes engulfed in the abscess, is devoid of a blood supply and becomes a sequestrum.

The most important aspect of this process now occurs: the elevated periosteal sleeve begins to form new bone which becomes the involucrum (Figure 19.9).

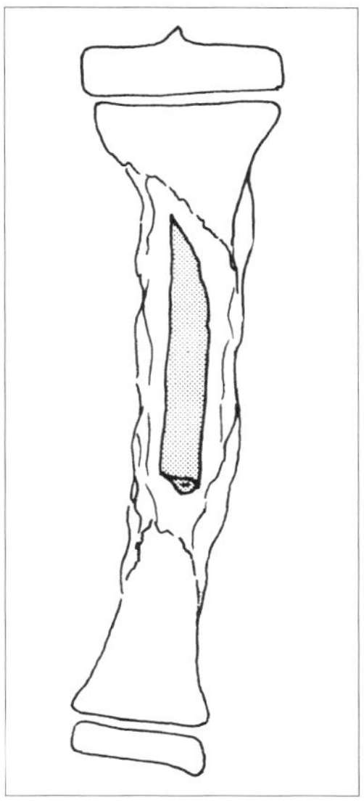

Figure 19.9

The integrity of the involucrum determines the final form and function of the limb. Injury to the periosteum, either from overwhelming infection or from premature surgical debridement, results in incomplete involucrum formation and impaired limb morphology. The epiphyseal plate might also be injured if the infection is severe.

Evaluation and diagnosis

Patients with acute osteomyelitis have pain, fever, malaise, local swelling and limited use of the limb. There may be a history of trauma, sore throat or other intercurrent infection.

Tenderness is greatest in the metaphyseal region of the involved bone. Movement of neighbouring joints is limited, but some painless motion is usually possible. X-rays of the bone are usually normal during this phase but may show soft tissue swelling.

In the quiescent phase, chronic osteomyelitis may be without signs or symptoms other than minimal persistent swelling of the limb. When the infection reactivates, the limb becomes swollen and painful, as it would with an acute infection. As the infection pushes to the surface, a draining sinus forms. This often relieves some of the swelling and pain. X-rays taken during this phase show a deformed bone, usually with a cavity containing a dense piece of dead bone – the sequestrum.

Treatment

When the patient is seen less than 48 hours from the beginning of symptoms, treat acute osteomyelitis with intravenous antibiotics. Switch to oral antibiotics at 4–6 weeks if the infection is controlled. This will be evident by absence of fever, decreased pain, swelling and tenderness, and an increased use of the limb.

X-rays taken after 2–3 weeks of treatment may show decreased bone density and minimal periosteal new bone formation. These are typical findings and do not mean that the infection is out of control. X-rays should be repeated in 2–4 weeks. If the infection is controlled, the X-rays will return towards normal. If an abscess forms, the infection is beyond the acute phase and surgical drainage is necessary.

Technique for draining the abscess

1 Using anaesthesia, perform a surgical preparation of the affected region. Make an incision directly over the metaphyseal region of the affected bone in the area of the most swelling.

2 Carry the incision through the skin, subcutaneous tissue, muscle and periosteum. If pus is not evident, make multiple drill holes through the cortex of the bone into the medullary canal to allow the trapped pus to escape.

3 Irrigate the cavity to remove all purulent material. Close the skin loosely over a drain and send a sample of the infected material for bacteriological examination.

19

4 For infections after the acute phase, treatment is aimed at drainage of the abscess cavity while allowing involucrum formation to proceed.

5 Delay removal of the sequestrum until the involucrum has matured, a process which takes between 6 and 12 months. Antibiotic use at this stage should be limited to treatment of active soft tissue infection, systemic illness, locally aggressive infection, or before and after surgical sequestrectomy.

6 When the involucrum has formed adequately, the sequestrum can be removed to control the residual infection. Sequestrectomy may be difficult if the sequestrum is large, and care should be taken to avoid fracture of the remaining involucrum. The sequestrum may become trapped within the involucrum and might need to be fragmented for removal. After surgery, protect the limb with a cast to prevent a fracture. Close the wound over drains or leave it open for later split thickness skin grafting.

7 Patients with an acute flare of a chronic osteomyelitis are common. It is not unusual for the infection to have been silent for many years, then to flare, accompanied by an acute soft tissue infection, with or without a draining sinus. Usually a sequestrum can be found as the source of the residual infection. Treat with antibiotics, drainage of the soft tissue abscess and removal of the sequestrum.

8 If the involucrum has not formed or is insufficient to maintain a functional extremity, reconstructive procedures are usually necessary once the infection is controlled. These are elective procedures which may not be appropriate in the district hospital.

19.4 DEGENERATIVE CONDITIONS

KEY POINTS

- Arthritis is an abnormality of joints arising from overuse or injury (degenerative arthritis) or inflammation (rheumatoid arthritis)
- Diagnosis is made from the history, physical examination and distinctive X-ray changes
- Non-surgical treatment consists of anti-inflammatory medication, injections, muscle strengthening and rest.

ARTHRITIS

Arthritis is a process of irritation or inflammation of the joints. The articular cartilage is primarily affected, at first becoming rough and irregular and eventually being destroyed completely. This results in pain, swelling and loss of motion. Degenerative arthritis occurs from wear and tear of the cartilage. This is associated with ageing, joint injury or following a joint infection. Inflammatory or rheumatoid arthritis is secondary to an immune reaction that destroys the articular cartilage. It usually involves multiple joints and leads to progressive joint deformities.

Evaluation and diagnosis

Degenerative arthritis

Degenerative arthritis is characterized by:

- History
  - Slow onset of pain with use
  - Decreased motion and stiffness
  - Mild swelling
- Examination
  - Tenderness about the joint
  - Palpable spurs at the joint margins
  - Loss of motion

- X-ray
  - Decreased cartilage space
  - Sclerosis of bone about the weight bearing surfaces
  - Spur formation
  - Subchondral cysts.

Rheumatoid arthritis

Rheumatoid arthritis is characterized by:

- History
  - Joints painful and swollen with morning stiffness
  - Multiple joints frequently affected
  - Possible family history of similar problems
- Examination
  - Joints swollen and tender with decreased range of motion
  - Hands and feet frequently involved
  - Deformity common
  - 75 per cent of patients have dangerous laxity of the C1–C2 vertebral bodies
- X-ray
  - Decrease in cartilage space along with bone density
  - Erosions at the joint margins are common
  - Bone spurs are rare.

Treatment

Rest

Decrease activities to protect the joint from further injury. During acute episodes of rheumatoid arthritis, splint the joint with a removable plaster dressing. Begin a range of motion as soon as pain allows.

Medication

Give oral anti-inflammatory medication, such as aspirin or ibuprofen. Patients with rheumatoid arthritis may benefit from oral corticosteroid medication or other special drugs.

Injections

For degenerative arthritis, use intra-articular injections of cortisone with caution, as it often speeds up the cartilage deterioration.

In patients with rheumatoid arthritis, cortisone helps to control the inflammation and periodic injections may be helpful.

Muscle strengthening

For both types of arthritis, try to preserve joint motion and extremity muscle strength. Strong muscles will protect the joint and delay deterioration.

Surgery

Surgery may be needed for end stage joint destruction or for lack of response to medical treatment in patients with rheumatoid arthritis.

KEY POINTS

- Bursitis and tendinitis result from an inflammatory response to overuse
- Common locations for bursitis are the shoulder, elbow, hip and knee
- Tendinitis is most common at the lateral elbow, radial side of the wrist, knee, Achilles tendon at the ankle, plantar surface of the foot
- Treat with rest and anti-inflammatory medication. Corticosteroid injections into bursa are helpful, but they should not be used around large tendons.

BURSITIS AND TENDINITIS

Bursa are sacs lined by synovial tissue containing a small amount of fluid. They are positioned between structures that move over each other and act to reduce friction. When subjected to increased pressure or excessive motion, they become inflamed, fill with fluid and are painful.

Tendons are most vulnerable to inflammatory overuse symptoms in places where they attach to bone (the lateral epicondyle of the humerus) or travel within a surrounding sheath (the flexor tendons of the digits or the Achilles tendon at the ankle).

Evaluation and diagnosis

Make the diagnosis based on a history of overuse and the physical findings of tenderness, swelling and pain with use.

Common sites of bursitis and tendinitis

Bursitis

- Subcromial bursa (Figure 19.10)
  Located between the acromion process and the rotator cuff tendon. Causes painful abduction or flexion of the shoulder joint (impingement syndrome).
- Olecranon bursa (Figure 19.11)
  A common problem caused by resting the elbow on hard surfaces. Infectious bursitis is common at this location, so aspirate the bursa fluid and examine it for infection before treating as an inflammatory bursitis. Infected fluid will be cloudy and will contain bacteria on Gram stain. Treat the infection with surgical drainage and antibiotics.

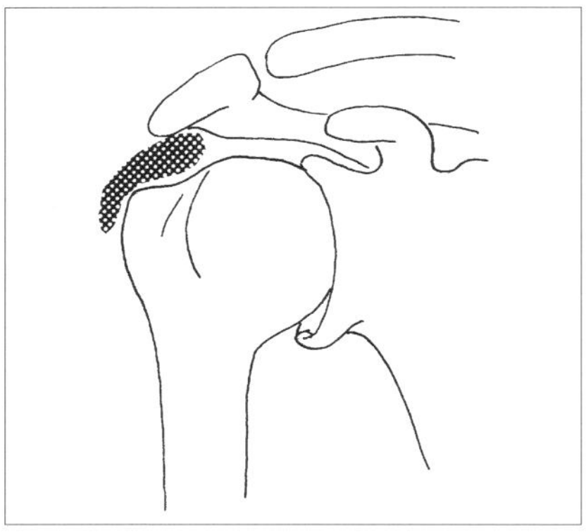

Figure 19.10

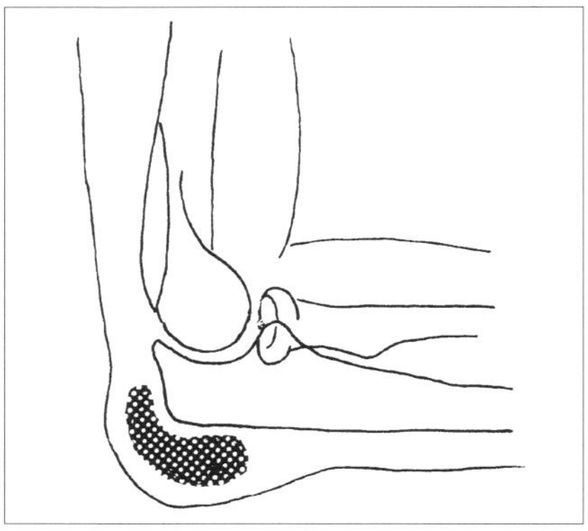

Figure 19.11

- Trochanteric bursa (Figure 19.12)
  A common cause of lateral hip pain. Diagnose by history of pain with walking, pain while lying on the affected side and tenderness to palpation directly over and slightly posterior to the greater trochanter of the femur.
- Prepatella bursa (Figure 19.13)
  Each of the four bursa about the knee may, at times, become inflamed and painful. Prepatella bursitis is the most common of these conditions. It is caused by direct pressure on the anterior aspect of the knee from activities such as kneeling. The other bursa (pes anserine, infrapatella, fibular collateral) are irritated by excessive use associated with walking or climbing.

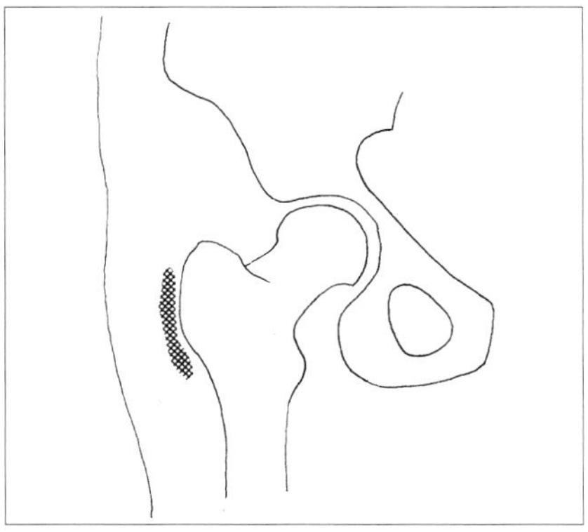

Figure 19.12

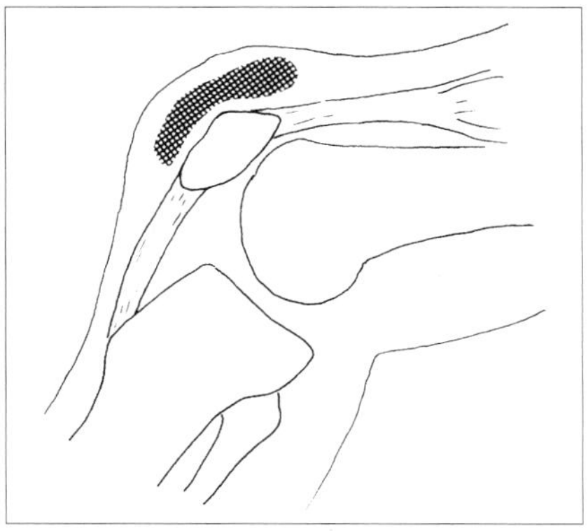

Figure 19.13

Tendinitis

- Lateral epicondylitis (tennis elbow) (Figure 19.14)
  There is pain with use of the hand for gripping activities and tenderness at the insertion of the extensor muscles of the forearm into the lateral epicondyle of the humerus.
- De Quervain's tenosynovitis (Figure 19.15)
  Occurs from motion of the abductor pollicis longus and extensor pollicis brevis tendons within their tendon sheaths on the radial side of the wrist joint.
- Trigger finger (Figure 19.16)
  Tenosynovitis of the flexor tendons within the tendon sheaths leads to nodule formation on the tendons at the level of the distal palm. As the tendons move in and out of the sheath, the nodule catches at the edge, causing the finger to "trigger" (snap into flexion or extension).

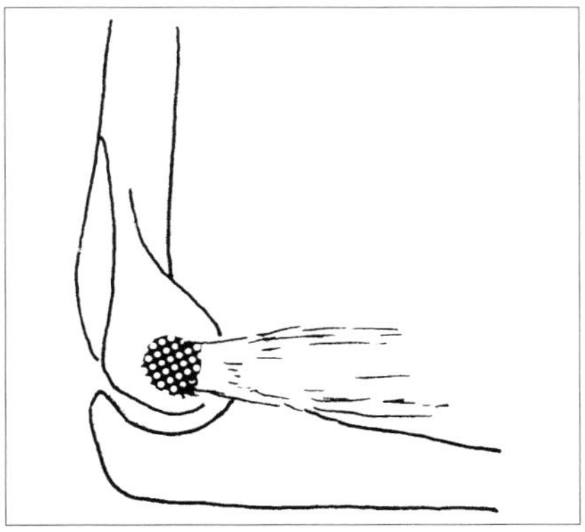

Figure 19.14

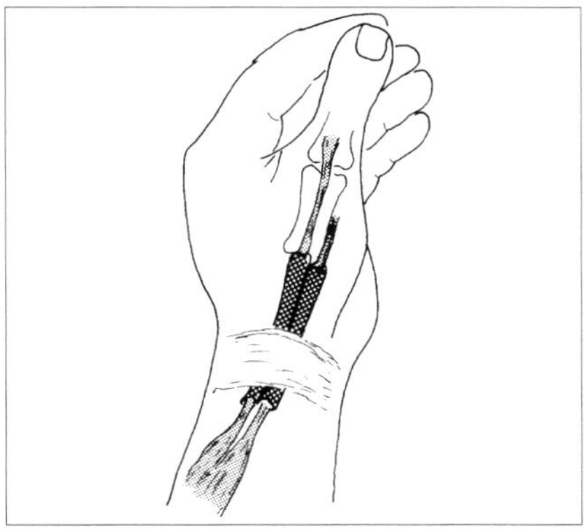

Figure 19.15

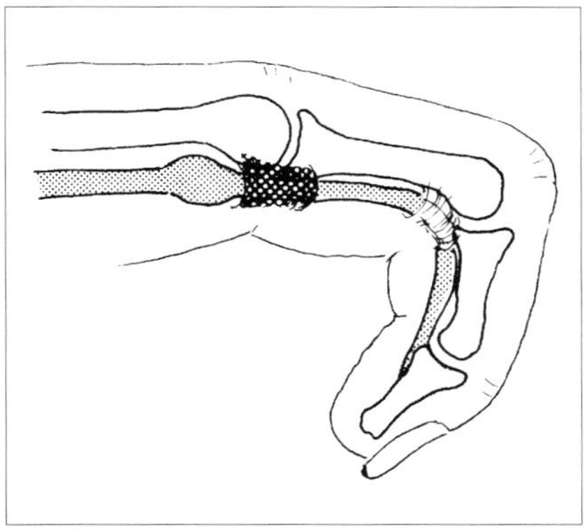

Figure 19.16

- Achilles tendinitis (Figure 19.17)
  There is pain in the tendinous portion of the gastrosoleus muscle complex, at or above the insertion into the posterior calcaneus. The tendon is contained within a sheath and nodule formation or calcification of the tendon is common.
- Plantar fasciitis (Figure 19.18)
  Causes pain with weight bearing at the insertion of the plantar fascia into the calcaneus.

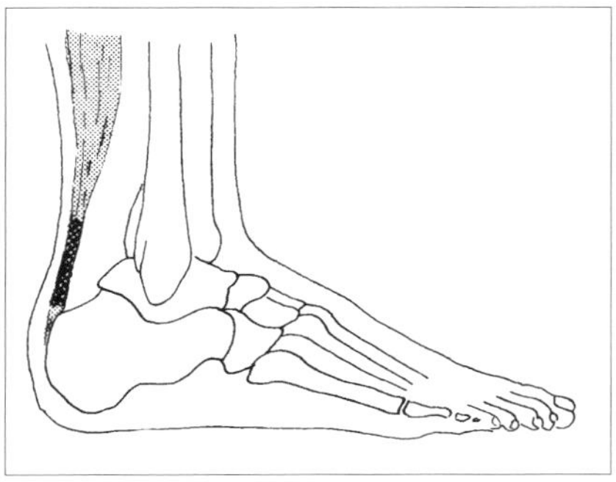

Figure 19.17

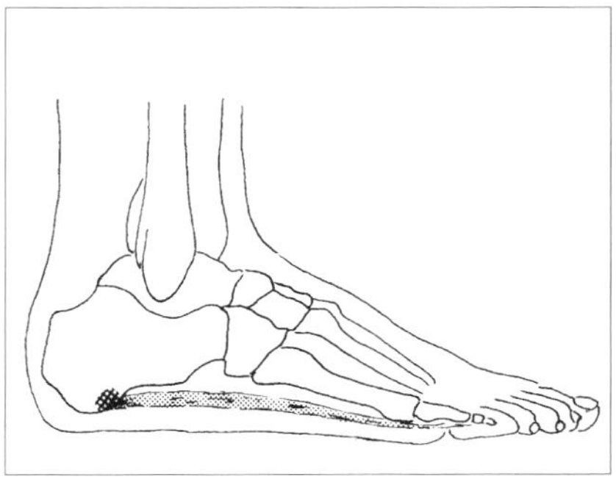

Figure 19.18

Treatment

Rest

The patient should decrease activities or use a plaster splint for a short time and gradually resume activities when they do not cause pain. Heat or cold treatments may help to decrease the inflammation.

Medication

Give oral anti-inflammatory drugs (aspirin or ibuprofen). Corticosteroid injections into bursa and tendon sheaths may help if other methods fail.

Do not inject steroids directly into tendons. They decrease tendon strength and lead to ruptures.

Surgery

Occasionally, surgical release of the tendon sheath is necessary to prevent continuing irritation of the tendon. This is especially helpful for trigger fingers and De Quervain's tenosynovitis.

Annex

The Primary Trauma Care Manual

A Manual for Trauma Management in District and Remote Locations

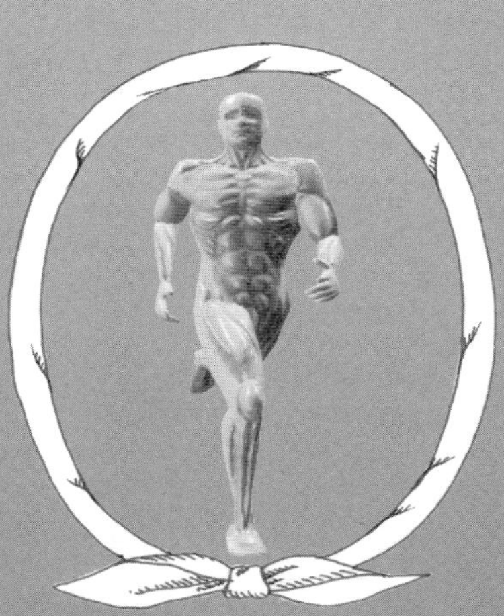

Douglas A. Wilkinson
Marcus F. Skinner

Contents

ABCDE of trauma

The management of severe multiple injury requires clear recognition of management priorities and the goal of the initial assessment is to determine those injuries that threaten the patient's life. If performed correctly, this first survey (the "primary survey") should identify such life-threatening injuries such as:

- Airway obstruction
- Chest injuries with breathing difficulties
- Severe external or internal haemorrhage
- Abdominal injuries.

If there is more than one injured patient, treat patients in order of priority (triage). Successful triage requires rapid assessment and clear thinking.

THE PRIMARY SURVEY

First, carry out the ABCDE survey:

- Airway
- Breathing
- Circulation
- Disability
- Exposure.

The ABCDE survey is sometimes referred to as the "primary survey". Its primary function is to diagnose and treat life threatening injuries which, if left undiagnosed and untreated, could lead to death:

- Airway obstruction
- Chest injuries with breathing difficulties
- Severe external or internal haemorrhage
- Abdominal injuries.

When more than one life threatening state exists, simultaneous treatment of injuries is essential and requires effective teamwork.

Airway

Assess the airway. Can the patient talk and breathe freely? If obstructed, consider the following steps.

- Chin lift/jaw thrust (tongue is attached to the jaw)
- Suction (if available)
- Guedel airway/nasopharyngeal airway
- Intubation; keep the neck immobilized in neutral position.

Breathing

Assess airway patency and breathing adequacy by clinical observation. If inadequate, consider:

- Artificial ventilation
- Decompression and drainage of tension pneumothorax/haemothorax
- Closure of open chest injury.

Reassess the ABCs if the patient is unstable.

Circulation

Assess the patient's circulation as you recheck the oxygen supply, airway patency and breathing adequacy. If inadequate, you may need to:

- Stop external haemorrhage
- Establish 2 large-bore IV lines (14 or 16 G) if possible
- Administer fluids, if available.

Give oxygen, if available.

Disability

Make a rapid neurological assessment (is the patient awake, vocally responsive to pain or unconscious?) There is no time to do the Glasgow Coma Scale (page PCTM –23) so use the following clear, quick system at this stage:

A Awake
V Verbal response
P Painful response
U Unresponsive

Exposure

Undress the patient and look for injury. If you suspect a neck or spinal injury, in-line immobilization is important.

Take care when moving the patient, especially if he or she is unconscious.

Notes . . .

Airway management

The first priority is establishment or maintenance of airway patency.

1 Talk to the patient

A patient who can speak clearly must have a clear airway. Airway obstruction by the tongue in the unconscious patient is often a problem. The unconscious patient may require assistance with airway and/or ventilation. If you suspect a head, neck or chest injury, protect the cervical spine during endotracheal intubation.

2 Give oxygen

Give oxygen, if available, via self-inflating bag or mask.

3 Assess the airway

Signs of airway obstruction include:

- Snoring or gurgling
- Stridor or abnormal breath sounds
- Agitation (hypoxia)
- Using the accessory muscles of ventilation/paradoxical chest movements
- Cyanosis.

Be alert for foreign bodies. Intravenous sedation is absolutely contraindicated in this situation.

4 Consider the need for advanced airway management

Indications for advanced airway management techniques include:

- Persisting airway obstruction
- Penetrating neck trauma with haematoma (expanding)
- Apnoea
- Hypoxia
- Severe head injury
- Chest trauma
- Maxillofacial injury.

Airway obstruction requires *urgent* treatment.

Airway management techniques

BASIC TECHNIQUES

Chin lift and jaw thrust

To perform a *chin lift*, place two fingers under the mandible and gently lift upward to bring the chin anterior. During this manoeuvre, be careful not to hyperextend the neck. Care should be given to neck stabilization, if appropriate.

The *jaw thrust* is performed by manually elevating the angles of the mandible to obtain the same effect.

Remember these are not definitive procedures and obstruction may occur at any time.

Oropharyngeal airway

Insert the oral airway into the mouth behind the tongue; it is usually inserted upside down until the palate is encountered and is then rotated 180 degrees. Take particular care in children because of the possibility of soft tissue damage.

Nasopharyngeal airway

Insert a nasopharyngeal airway (well lubricated) via a nostril and pass it into the posterior oropharynx. It is well tolerated.

ADVANCED TECHNIQUES

Orotracheal intubation

Uncontrolled laryngoscopy may produce cervical hyperextension. It is essential that in line neck immobilization is maintained by an assistant. Cricoid pressure may be necessary if a full stomach is suspected. Inflate the cuff and check the correct placement of the tube by checking for normal bilateral breath sounds.

Consider tracheal intubation when there is a need to:

- Establish a patent airway and prevent aspiration
- Deliver oxygen while not being able to use mask and airway
- Provide ventilation and prevent hypercarbia.

Tracheal intubation should be performed in no more than 30 seconds. If you are unable to intubate, continue ventilation of the patient via mask.

> Remember: patients die from lack of oxygen, not lack of an endotracheal tube (ETT).

Surgical cricothyroidotomy

Surgical cricothyroidotomy should be conducted in any patient where intubation has been attempted twice and failed and/or the patient cannot be ventilated.

Technique

1 Hyperextend the neck, making the patient comfortable.

2 Identify the groove between the cricoid and thyroid cartilages just below the "Adam's apple" (the protruding thyroid).

3 Clean the area and infiltrate with local anaesthetic.

4 Incise through the skin vertically with a 1.5 cm cut and use blunt dissection to ensure that you can see the membrane between the thyroid and cricoid (Figure 1).

5 With a #22 or #23 scalpel blade, stab through the membrane into the hollow trachea.

6 Rotate the blade 90° (Figure 2), insert a curved artery forceps alongside the blade, remove the blade and open the forceps side to side, widening the space between the thyroid and cricoid cartilages (Figure 3).

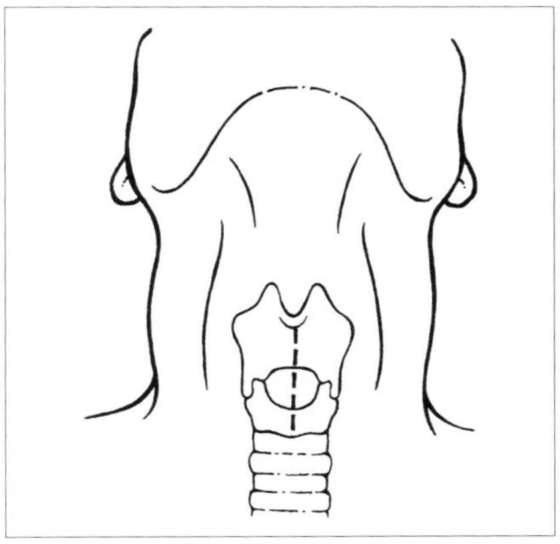

Figure 1

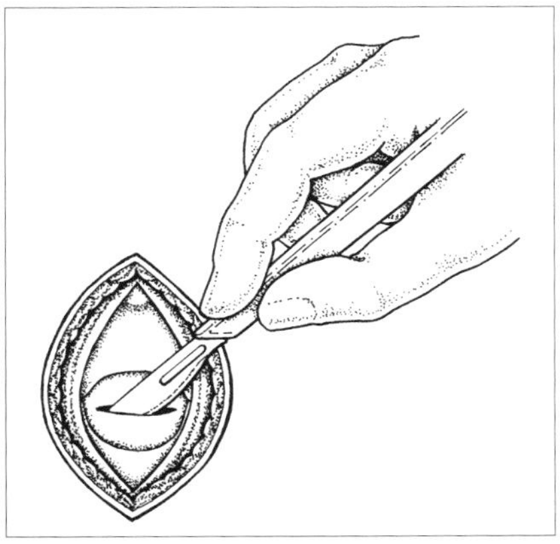

Figure 2

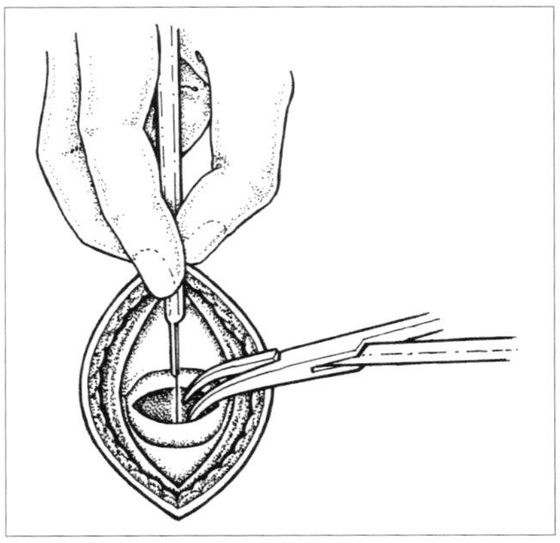

Figure 3

7 Pass a thin introducer or a nasogastric tube into the trachea if very small access (Figure 4) or proceed to 9.

8 Run a 4–6 endotracheal tube over the introducer and pass it into the trachea (Figure 5).

9 Remove the introducer, if used.

This tube can stay in place for up to 3 days. Do not attempt this procedure in a child under the age of 10 years; passing several needles through the membrane will give enough air entry.

This procedure should be performed by an experienced person, with prior knowledge of the anatomy and medical condition of the patient.

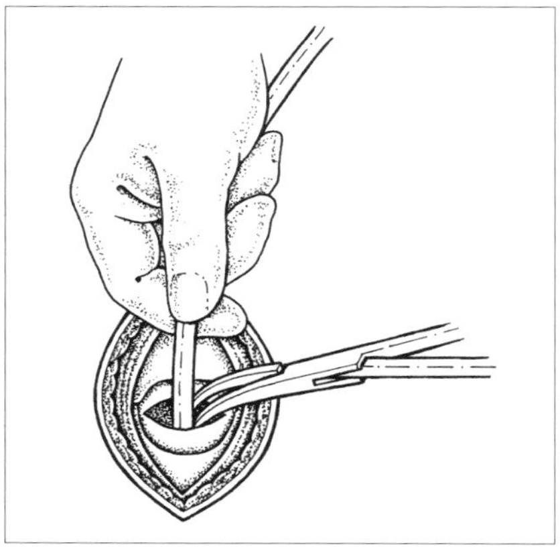

Figure 4

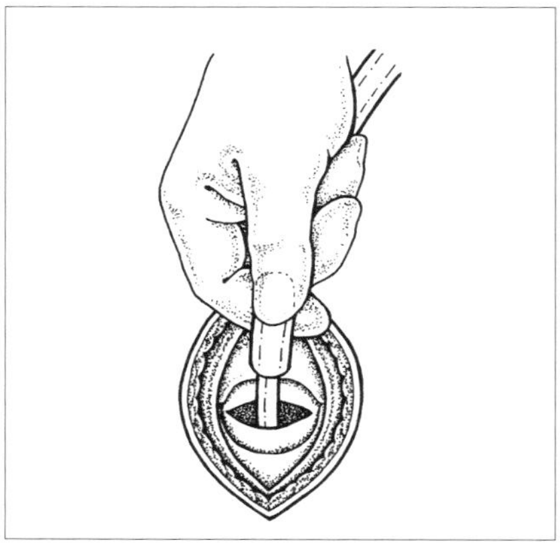

Figure 5

This procedure should not be undertaken lightly, as wrong placement, bleeding and delay can cause death.

Notes . . .

Ventilation (breathing) management

The second priority is the establishment of adequate ventilation.

1 Inspect (LOOK)

Inspection of respiratory rate is essential. Are any of the following present?

- Cyanosis
- Penetrating injury
- Presence of flail chest
- Sucking chest wounds
- Use of accessory muscles.

2 Palpate (FEEL)

Palpate for:

- Tracheal shift
- Broken ribs
- Subcutaneous emphysema.

Percussion is useful for diagnosis of haemothorax and pneumothorax.

3 Auscultate (LISTEN)

Auscultate for:

- Pneumothorax (decreased breath sounds on site of injury)
- Detection of abnormal sounds in the chest.

4 Resuscitation action

- Insert an intercostal drainage tube as a matter of priority, and before chest X-ray if respiratory distress exists, to drain the chest pleura of air and blood
- When indications for intubation exist but the trachea cannot be intubated, consider using a laryngeal mask airway or direct access via a cricothyroidotomy.

SPECIAL NOTES

- If available, maintain the patient on oxygen until complete stabilization is achieved

- If a you suspect a tension pneumothorax, introduce a large-bore needle into the pleural cavity through the second intercostal space, mid clavicular line, to decompress the tension and allow time for the placement of an intercostal tube
- If intubation in one or two attempts is not possible, a cricothyroidotomy should be considered a priority. This depends on experienced medical personnel being available, with appropriate equipment, and may not be possible in many places.

Do *not* persist with intubation attempts without ventilating the patient.

Notes . . .

Circulatory management

The third priority is establishment of adequate circulation.

"Shock" is defined as inadequate organ perfusion and tissue oxygenation. In the trauma patient, it is most often due to haemorrhage and hypovolaemia.

The diagnosis of shock is based on clinical findings: hypotension, tachycardia and tachypnoea, as well as hypothermia, pallor, cool extremities, decreased capillary refill and decreased urine production.

HAEMORRHAGIC (HYPOVOLAEMIC) SHOCK

Haemorrhagic (hypovolaemic) shock is due to acute loss of blood or fluids. The amount of blood loss after trauma is often poorly assessed and in blunt trauma is usually underestimated. Remember:

- Large volumes of blood may be hidden in the abdominal and pleural cavity
- Femoral shaft fracture may lose up to 2 litres of blood
- Pelvic fracture often loses in excess of 2 litres of blood.

CARDIOGENIC SHOCK

Cardiogenic shock is due to inadequate heart function. This may result from

- Myocardial contusion (bruising)
- Cardiac tamponade
- Tension pneumothorax (preventing blood returning to heart)
- Penetrating wound of the heart
- Myocardial infarction.

Assessment of the jugular venous pressure is essential in these circumstances and an ECG should be recorded, if available.

NEUROGENIC SHOCK

Neurogenic shock is due to the loss of sympathetic tone, usually resulting from spinal cord injury. The classical presentation is hypotension without reflex tachycardia or skin vasoconstriction.

SEPTIC SHOCK

Septic shock is rare in the early phase of trauma, but is a common cause of late death (via multi-organ failure) in the weeks following injury. It is most commonly seen in penetrating abdominal injury and burns patients.

Hypovolaemia is a life-threatening emergency and must be recognized and treated aggressively.

Circulatory resuscitation measures

The goal is to stop bleeding and restore oxygen delivery to the tissues. As the usual problem is loss of blood, fluid resuscitation must be a priority.

1 Obtain adequate vascular access

This requires the insertion of at least two large-bore cannulas (14–16 G), if available. Peripheral cut down may be necessary.

2 Give fluids

Infusion fluids (crystalloids, such as normal saline, as the first line) should be warmed to body temperature, if possible (prewarm in a bucket of warmed water).

Remember:

- Hypothermia can lead to abnormal blood clotting
- Avoid solutions containing glucose.

3 Take specimens

Take any specimens you need for laboratory tests and crossmatching.

FIRST PRIORITY: STOP THE BLEEDING

Injuries to the limbs

Tourniquets do not work and, besides, cause reperfusion syndromes and add to the primary injury.

The recommended procedure of "pressure dressing" is an ill-defined entity. Severe bleeding from high-energy penetrating injuries and amputation wounds can be controlled by:

- Subfascial gauze pack placement

Plus

- Manual compression on the proximal artery

Plus

- Carefully applied compressive dressing of the entire injured limb.

Injuries to the chest

The most common source of bleeding is chest wall arteries. Immediate in-field placement of a chest tube drain plus efficient analgesia (IV ketamine is the drug of choice) expands the lung and seals off the bleeding.

CARDIAC LIFE SUPPORT

Ensure the safety of your patient and yourself

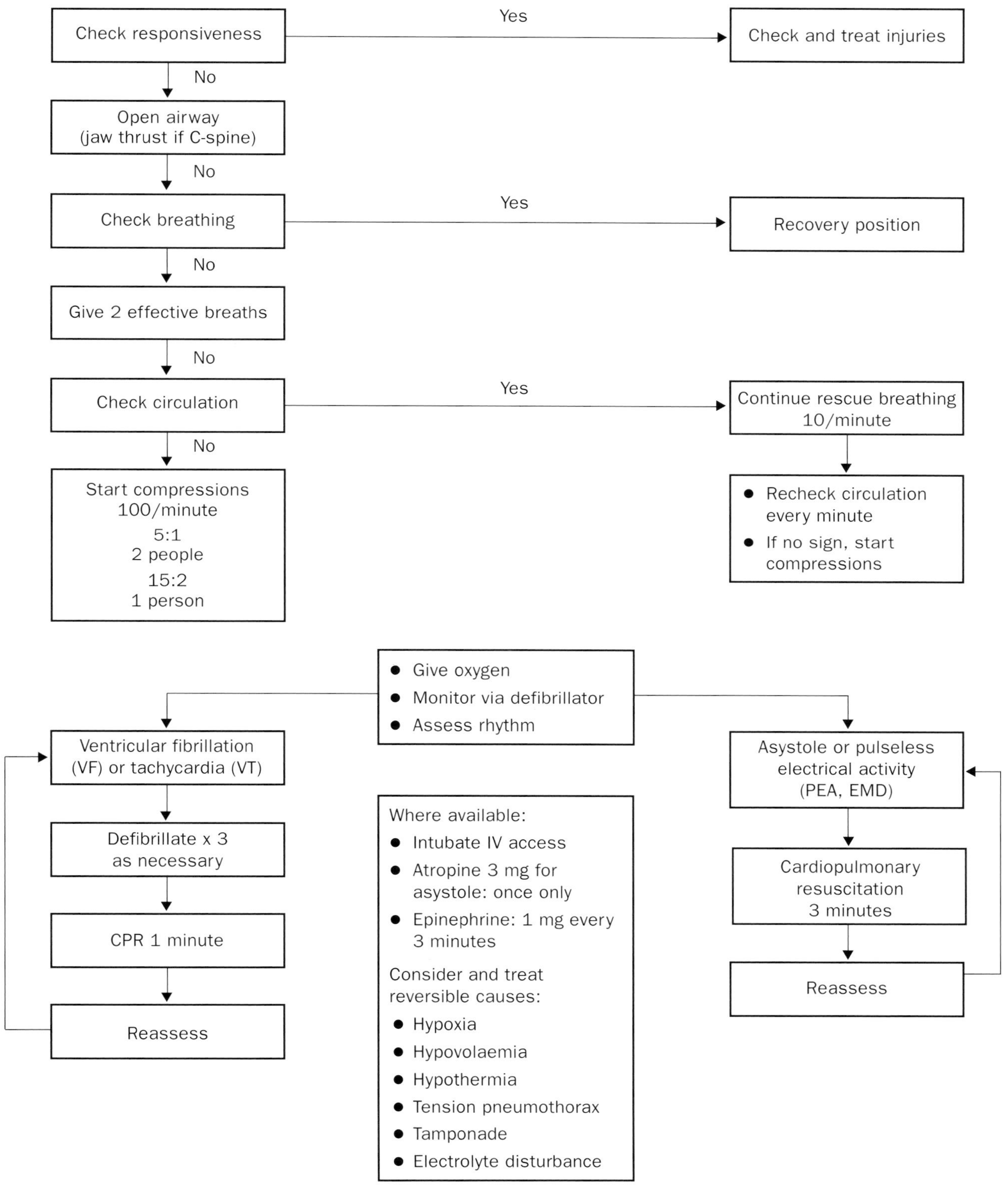

Injuries to the abdomen

"Damage control (DC) laparotomy" should be performed as soon as possible on cases where fluid resuscitation cannot maintain a systolic BP at 80–90 mmHg. The sole objective of DC laparotomy is to gauze pack the bleeding abdominal quadrants, after which the midline incision is temporarily closed within 30 minutes with towel clamps.

DC laparotomy is not surgery, but a resuscitative procedure that any trained doctor or nurse at district level should be able to do under ketamine anaesthesia. The technique needs to be observed before performing it but, done correctly, it can save lives.

> Loss of blood is the main cause of shock in trauma patients.

Bleeding from massive pelvic fractures

Bleeding from massive pelvic fractures may be controlled by tying a sheet around the pelvis.

SECOND PRIORITY: VOLUME REPLACEMENT, WARMING AND KETAMINE ANALGESIA

Replacement fluids

Replacement fluids should be warm. Physiological coagulation works best at 38.5 °C and haemostasis is difficult at core temperatures below 35 °C. Hypothermia in trauma patients is common during protracted improvised outdoor evacuations – even in the tropics. It is easy to cool a patient but difficult to re-warm, hence prevention of hypothermia is essential.

Oral and IV fluids should have a temperature of 40 °C – 42 °C; using IV fluids at "room temperature" means cooling!

Hypotensive fluid resuscitation

In cases where the haemostasis is insecure or not definitive, control the fluid volume to maintain systolic BP at 80–90 mmHg during the transfer of a critically-ill, bleeding patient.

Oral resuscitation

Per-oral resuscitation is safe and efficient in patients without abdominal injury who have a positive gag reflex:

- Oral fluids should be low in sugar and salts; concentrated solutions can cause an osmotic pull over the intestinal mucosa and the effect will be negative
- Diluted cereal porridges, based on local foodstuffs, are recommended.

Analgesia

Ketamine is the analgesic choice in repeated IV doses of 0.2 mg/kg during evacuation of all severe trauma cases because of the positive inotropic effects and the fact that it does not affect the gag reflex.

Cardiovascular parameters

Blood loss	Heart rate	Blood pressure	Capillary refill	Respir. rate	Urine volume	Mental state
Up to 750 ml	< 100	Normal	Normal	Normal	> 30 ml/hour	Normal
750–1500 ml	> 100	Systolic normal	Positive	20–30	20–30	Mild concern
1500–2000 ml	> 120	Decreased	Positive	30–40	5–15	Anxious/ confused
More than 2000 ml	> 140	Decreased	Positive	> 40	< 10	Confused/ coma

Urine

Measure urine output as an indicator of circulation reserve. Output should be more than 0.5 ml/kg/hour. Unconscious patients may need a urinary catheter if they are persistently shocked.

Blood transfusion

There may be considerable difficulty in getting blood. Remember possible incompatibility and the risks of transfusion-transmissible infection (including HIV, malaria, syphilis), even among the patient's own family.

Blood transfusion must be considered when the patient has persistent haemodynamic instability despite fluid (colloid/crystalloid) infusion. If type-specific or crossmatched blood is not available, use group O negative packed red blood cells. Transfusion should, however, be seriously considered if the haemoglobin level is less than 7 g/dl and the patient is still bleeding.

Notes . . .

Secondary survey

Undertake the secondary survey only when the patient's ABCs are stable.

If any deterioration occurs during this phase, it must be interrupted by another **primary survey**. Documentation is required for all procedures undertaken.

Undertake a head-to-toe examination, noting particularly the following.

HEAD EXAMINATION

- Scalp and ocular abnormalities
- External ear and tympanic membrane
- Periorbital soft tissue injuries.

NECK EXAMINATION

- Penetrating wounds
- Subcutaneous emphysema
- Tracheal deviation
- Neck vein appearance.

NEUROLOGICAL EXAMINATION

- Brain function assessment: use the Glasgow Coma Scale (page PTCM–23)
- Spinal cord motor activity
- Sensation and reflex.

CHEST EXAMINATION

- Clavicles and all ribs
- Breath sounds and heart tones
- ECG monitoring (if available).

ABDOMINAL EXAMINATION

- Penetrating abdominal wound requiring surgical exploration
- Blunt trauma: insert a nasogastric tube is inserted (not in the presence of facial trauma)
- Rectal examination
- Insert urinary catheter (check for meatal blood before insertion).

Suspect cervical spine injury in head injury patients until proven otherwise.

PELVIS AND LIMBS

- Fractures
- Peripheral pulses
- Cuts, bruises and other minor injuries.

X-RAYS (if possible and where indicated)

- Chest, lateral neck and pelvis X-rays may be needed during primary survey
- Cervical spine films (it is important to see all 7 vertebrae)
- Pelvic and long bone X-rays
- Skull X-rays may be useful to search for fractures when head injury is present without focal neurological deficit, but are seldom indicated.

Notes . . .

Chest trauma

Approximately a quarter of deaths due to trauma are attributed to thoracic injury. Immediate deaths are essentially due to major disruption of the heart or of great vessels. Early deaths due to thoracic trauma include airway obstruction, cardiac tamponade or aspiration.

The majority of patients with thoracic trauma can be managed by simple manoeuvres and do not require surgical treatment.

RESPIRATORY DISTRESS

Respiratory distress may be caused by:

- Rib fractures/flail chest
- Pneumothorax
- Tension pneumothorax
- Haemothorax
- Pulmonary contusion (bruising)
- Open pneumothorax
- Aspiration.

HAEMORRHAGIC SHOCK

Haemorrhagic shock may be due to:

- Haemothorax
- Haemomediastinum.

RIB FRACTURES

Fractured ribs may occur at the point of impact and damage to the underlying lung may produce lung bruising or puncture. In the elderly patient, fractured ribs may result from simple trauma. The ribs usually become fairly stable within 10 days to two weeks. Firm healing with callus formation is seen after about six weeks.

FLAIL CHEST

The unstable segment moves separately and in an opposite direction from the rest of the thoracic cage during the respiration cycle. Severe respiratory distress may ensue. This is a medical emergency and can be treated with positive pressure ventilation and analgesia.

TENSION PNEUMOTHORAX

Tension pneumothorax develops when air enters the pleural space but cannot leave. The consequence is progressively increasing intrathoracic pressure in the affected side resulting in mediastinal shift. The patient will become short of breath and hypoxic.

Urgent needle decompression is required prior to the insertion of an intercostal drain. The trachea may be displaced (late sign) and is pushed away from the midline by the air under tension. Immediate decompression can be achieved by needle decompression, as described above, but a definitive chest drain should be inserted as soon as possible.

The extent of internal injuries cannot be judged by the appearance of a skin wound.

HAEMOTHORAX

Haemothorax is more common in penetrating than in non-penetrating injures to the chest. If the haemorrhage is severe hypovolaemic shock will occur as well as respiratory distress due to compression of the lung on the involved side.

Optimal therapy consists of the placement of a large chest tube.

- A haemothorax of 500–1500 ml that stops bleeding after insertion of an intercostal catheter can generally be treated by closed drainage alone
- A haemothorax of greater than 1500–2000 ml or with continued bleeding of more than 200–300 ml per hour may be an indication for further investigation, such as thoracotomy.

PULMONARY CONTUSION

Pulmonary contusion (bruising) is common after chest trauma. It is a potentially life-threatening condition. The onset of symptoms may be slow and may progress over 24 hours post injury. It is likely to occur in cases of high-speed accidents and falls from great heights.

Symptoms and signs include:

- Dyspnoea (shortness of breath)
- Hypoxaemia
- Tachycardia
- Rare or absent breath sounds
- Rib fractures
- Cyanosis.

OPEN CHEST WOUNDS

In open or "sucking" wounds of the chest wall, the lung on the affected side is exposed to atmospheric pressure with lung collapse and a shift of the mediastinum to the uninvolved side. This must be treated rapidly. A seal, such as a plastic packet, is sufficient to stop the sucking, and can be applied until reaching hospital. In compromised patients intercostal drains, intubation and positive pressure ventilation is often required.

OTHER INJURIES

The injuries listed below are also possible in trauma, but carry a high mortality risk even in regional centres. They are mentioned for educational purposes.

MYOCARDIAL CONTUSION

Myocardial contusion is associated, in chest blunt trauma, with fractures of the sternum or ribs. The diagnosis is supported by abnormalities on ECG and elevation of serial cardiac enzymes, if these are available. Cardiac contusion can simulate a myocardial infarction. The patient must be submitted to observation with cardiac monitoring, if available. This type of injury is more common than generally realized and may be a cause of sudden death well after the accident.

> Beware pulmonary contusion and delay in deterioration of respiratory state

PERICARDIAL TAMPONADE

Penetrating cardiac injuries (for example, following stab wounds) are a leading cause of death in urban areas. It is rare to have pericardial tamponade with blunt trauma. Pericardiocentesis must be undertaken early if this injury is considered likely. Look for it in patients with:

- Shock
- Distended neck veins
- Cool extremities and no pneumothorax
- Muffled heart sounds

Treatment is pericardiocentesis which is potentially hazardous and should only be undertaken by experienced clinicians.

THORACIC GREAT VESSEL INJURIES

Injury to the pulmonary veins and arteries is often fatal, and is one of the major causes of on-site death.

RUPTURE OF TRACHEA OR MAJOR BRONCHI

Rupture of the trachea or major bronchi is a serious injury with an overall estimated mortality of at least 50%. The majority (80%) of ruptures of bronchi are within 2.5 cm of the carina. The usual signs of tracheobronchial disruption are the following:

- Haemoptysis
- Dyspnoea
- Subcutaneous and mediastinal emphysema
- Occasionally cyanosis.

TRAUMA TO THE OESOPHAGUS

Trauma to the oesophagus is rare in patients following blunt trauma injury. Perforation of the oesophagus is more frequently caused by penetrating injury. It is lethal if unrecognized because of mediastinitis. Patients often complain of sudden sharp pain in the epigastrium and chest with radiation to the back. Dyspnoea, cyanosis and shock occur, but these may be late symptoms.

DIAPHRAGMATIC INJURIES

Diaphragmatic injuries occur more frequently in blunt chest trauma, paralleling the rise in frequency of car accidents. The diagnosis is often missed. Diaphragmatic injuries should be suspected in any penetrating thoracic wound.

- Below 4th intercostal space anteriorly
- 6th interspace laterally
- 8th interspace posteriorly
- Usually the left side.

THORACIC AORTA RUPTURE

Thoracic aorta rupture occurs following severe decelerating forces such as high speed car accidents or falls from great heights. Patients have high mortality as the cardiac output is 5 litres/minute and the total blood volume in an adult is 5 litres.

Beware pericardial tamponade in penetrating chest trauma.

Notes . . .

Abdominal trauma

The abdomen is commonly injured in multiple trauma. The liver is the commonest organ injured in penetrating trauma. In blunt trauma, the spleen is often torn and ruptured.

The initial evaluation of the abdominal trauma patient must include:

A Airway and cervical spine
B Breathing
C Circulation
D Disability and neurological assessment
E Exposure.

Any patient involved in any serious accident should be considered to have an abdominal injury until proved otherwise. Unrecognized abdominal injury remains a frequent cause of preventable death after trauma.

There are two basic categories of abdominal trauma.

1 Penetrating trauma where surgical consultation is important: e.g.
   - Gunshot
   - Stabbing
2 Non-penetrating trauma: e.g.
   - Compression
   - Crush
   - Seat belt
   - Acceleration/deceleration injuries.

About 20% of trauma patients with acute haemoperitoneum (blood in abdomen) have no signs of peritoneal irritation at the first examination and the value of a *repeated primary survey* cannot be overstated.

Blunt trauma can be very difficult to evaluate, especially in the unconscious patient. These patients may need a peritoneal lavage. An exploratory laparotomy may be the best definitive procedure if abdominal injury needs to be excluded.

Complete physical examination of the abdomen includes rectal examination, assessing:

- Sphincter tone
- Integrity of rectal wall
- Blood in the rectum
- Prostate position.

Remember to check for blood at the external urethral meatus.

Deep penetrating foreign bodies should remain in situ until theatre exploration.

Women of childbearing age should be considered pregnant until proven otherwise. A shocked pregnant mother at term can usually be resuscitated properly only after delivery of the baby. The fetus may be salvageable and the best treatment of the fetus is resuscitation of the mother.

DIAGNOSTIC PERITONEAL LAVAGE (DPL)

Diagnostic peritoneal lavage (DPL) may help in determining the presence of blood or enteric fluid due to intra-abdominal injury. The results can be highly suggestive, but a negative result does not rule out intra-abdominal injury. If there is any doubt, a laparotomy is still necessary.

Indications for diagnostic peritoneal lavage include:

- Unexplained abdominal pain
- Trauma of the lower part of the chest
- Hypotension, systolic 90 mmHg, haematocrit fall with no obvious explanation
- Any patient suffering abdominal trauma and who has an altered mental state (drugs, alcohol, brain injury)
- Patient with abdominal trauma and spinal cord injuries
- Pelvic fractures.

The relative contraindications for lavage are:

- Pregnancy
- Previous abdominal surgery
- Operator inexperience
- If the result does not change your management.

OTHER SPECIFIC ISSUES WITH ABDOMINAL TRAUMA

Pelvic fractures are often complicated by massive haemorrhage and urology injury.

- Examining the rectum for the position of the prostate and for the presence of blood or rectal or perineal laceration is essential
- X-ray of the pelvis, if clinical diagnosis is difficult.

The management of pelvic fractures includes:

- Resuscitation (ABC)
- Transfusion
- Immobilization and assessment for surgery
- Analgesia.

Pelvic fractures often cause massive blood loss.

Head trauma

Delay in the early assessment of head-injured patients can have devastating consequence in terms of survival and patient outcome. Hypoxia and hypotension double the mortality of head-injured patients.

The following conditions are potentially life-threatening, but difficult to treat in district hospitals. It is important to treat what you can, within your expertise and resources, and to triage casualties carefully.

ACUTE EXTRADURAL

Classically, the signs consist of:

- Loss of consciousness following a lucid interval, with rapid deterioration
- Middle meningeal artery bleeding with rapid raising of intracranial pressure
- Development of hemiparesis on the opposite side of the impact area with a dilating pupil on the same side, with rapid deterioration.

ACUTE SUBDURAL HAEMATOMA

Acute subdural haematoma (clotted blood in the subdural space accompanied by severe contusion of the underlying brain) occurs from the tearing of bridging veins between the cortex and the dura.

Management is surgical and every effort should be made to do burr hole decompressions. The diagnosis can be made on history and examination.

The conditions below should be treated with more conservative medical management, as neurosurgery usually does not improve the outcome.

BASE-OF-SKULL FRACTURES

Bruising of the eyelids (Racoon eyes) or over the mastoid process (Battle's sign); cerebrospinal fluid (CSF) leak from ears and/or nose.

CEREBRAL CONCUSSION

Cerebral concussion with temporary altered consciousness.

DEPRESSED SKULL FRACTURE

A depressed skull fracture is an impaction of fragmented skull that may result in penetration of the underlying dura and brain.

INTRACEREBRAL HAEMATOMA

Intracerebral haematoma may result from acute injury or progressive damage secondary to contusion.

Alteration of consciousness is the hallmark of brain injury.

COMMON ERRORS

The most common errors in head injury evaluation and resuscitation are:

- Failure to perform ABC and prioritize management
- Failure to look beyond the obvious head injury
- Failure to assess the baseline neurological examination
- Failure to re-evaluate a patient who deteriorates.

MANAGEMENT

Stabilize the Airway, Breathing and Circulation and immobilize the cervical spine, if possible. Vital signs of important indicators in the patient's neurological status must be monitored and recorded frequently. Undertake a Glasgow Coma Scale (GCS) evaluation.

Glasgow Coma Scale

Function	Response	Score
Eyes (4)	Open spontaneously	4
	Open to command	3
	Open to pain	2
	None	1
Verbal (5)	Normal	5
	Confused talk	4
	Inappropriate words	3
	Inappropriate sounds	2
	None	1
Motor (6)	Obeys command	6
	Localizes pain	5
	Flexes limbs normally to pain	4
	Flexes limbs abnormally to pain	3
	Extends limbs to pain	2
	None	1

Never assume that alcohol is the cause of drowsiness in a confused patient.

Remember:

- Severe head injury: GCS of 8 or less
- Moderate head injury: GCS between 9 and 12
- Minor head injury: GCS between 13 and 15.

Deterioration may occur due to bleeding:

- Unequal or dilated pupils may indicate an increase in intracranial pressure
- Head or brain injury is never the cause of hypotension in the adult trauma patient
- Sedation should be avoided as it not only interferes with the state of consciousness, but will promote hypercarbia (slow breathing with retention of CO_2)
- The Cushing response is a specific response to a lethal rise in intracranial pressure. This is a late and poor prognostic sign. The hallmarks are:
  - Bradycardia
  - Hypertension
  - Decreased respiratory rate.

Basic medical management

Basic medical management for severe head injuries includes:

- Intubation and moderate hyperventilation, producing moderate hypocapnia (PCO_2 to 4.5–5 Kpa)
  - This will temporarily reduce both intracranial blood volume and intracranial pressure
  - Hypoxia and hypoventilation may kill patients
- Sedation with possible paralysis
- Moderate IV fluid input with diuresis: i.e. do not overload
- Nurse head up 20%
- Prevent hyperthermia.

Caution: Never transport a patient with a suspected cervical spine injury in the sitting or prone position; always make sure the patient is stabilized before transferring.

Notes . . .

Spinal trauma

The incidence of nerve injury in multiple trauma is high. Injury to the cervical spine and the thoraco-lumbar junction T12–L1 are common. Other common injuries include brachial plexus injury and nerve damage to legs and fingers.

The first priority is to undertake the primary survey with evaluation of ABCDE.

A Airway maintenance with care and control of a possible injury to the cervical spine

B Breathing control or support

C Circulation control and blood pressure monitoring

D Disability: the observation of neurological damage and state of consciousness

E Exposure of the patient to assess skin injuries and peripheral limb damage.

Examination of spine-injured patients must be carried out with the patient in the neutral position (i.e. without flexion, extension or rotation) and without any movement of the spine. The patient should be:

- Log-rolled i.e. moved by several people, working together to keep neck and spine immobilized
- Properly immobilized: in-line immobilization, stiff neck cervical collar or sandbags
- Transported in a neutral position: i.e. supine.

With vertebral injury (which may cause spinal cord injury), look for:

- Local tenderness
- Deformities as well as for a posterior "step-off" injury
- Oedema (swelling).

Clinical findings indicating injury of the cervical spine include:

- Difficulties in respiration (diaphragmatic breathing – check for paradoxical breathing)
- Flaccid and no reflexes (check rectal sphincter)
- Hypotension with bradycardia (without hypovolaemia).

Cervical spine

In addition to the initial X-rays, all patients with a suspicion of cervical spine injury should have an anterior–posterior (AP) and a lateral X-ray with a view of the atlas-axis joint. All seven cervical vertebrae must be seen on both views.

Neurological assessment

Assessment of the level of injury must be undertaken. If the patient is conscious, ask questions relevant to his or her sensation. Check the motor function of the upper and lower extremities by asking the patient to do minor movements.

The following summarizes key reflex assessment to determine the level of lesion.

MOTOR RESPONSE

• Diaphragm intact level	C3, C4, C5
• Shrug shoulders	Accessory nerve, cranial nerve 11
• Shoulder abduction	C5
• Biceps (flex elbows)	C6
• Extension of wrist	C6
• Extension of elbow	C7
• Flexion of wrist	C7
• Abduction of fingers	C8–T1
• Active chest expansion	Tl–T12
• Hip flexion	L2
• Knee extension	L3–L4
• Ankle dorsiflexion	L5–S1
• Ankle plantarflexion	S1–S2

SENSORY RESPONSE

• Antero-medial thigh	L2
• Anterior knee	L3
• Anterolateral ankle	L4
• Dorsum great and 2nd toe	L5
• Lateral side of foot	Sl
• Posterior calf	S2
• Perianal sensation (perineum)	S2–S5

If no sensory or motor function is exhibited with a complete spinal cord lesion, the chance of recovery is small.

Loss of autonomic function with spinal cord injury may occur rapidly and resolve slowly.

Limb trauma

Examination must include:

- Skin colour and temperature
- Distal pulse assessment
- Grazes and bleeding sites
- Limb alignment and deformities
- Active and passive movements
- Unusual movements and crepitation
- Level of pain caused by the injury.

MANAGEMENT OF EXTREMITY INJURIES

Management of extremity injuries should aim to:

- Keep blood flowing to peripheral tissues
- Prevent infection and skin necrosis
- Prevent damage to peripheral nerves.

SPECIAL ISSUES RELATING TO LIMB TRAUMA

1 Stop active bleeding by direct pressure, rather than by tourniquet. Tourniquets can be left on by mistake which can result in ischaemic damage.

2 Compartment syndrome is caused by an increase in the internal pressure of fascial compartments; this pressure results in a compression of vessels and peripheral nerves situated in these regions. Tissue perfusion is limited; the final result is ischaemic or even necrotic muscles with restricted function.

3 Body parts, traumatically amputated, should be covered with moistened sterile gauze towels and put into a sterile plastic bag. A non-cooled amputated part may be used within 6 hours after the injury, a cooled one as late as 18 to 20 hours.

Bladder catheterization (with caution in pelvic injury) is important.

LIMB SUPPORT: EARLY FASCIOTOMY

The problem of compartment syndrome is often underestimated.

TISSUE DAMAGE DUE TO HYPOXAEMIA

Compartment syndromes with increased intramuscular (IM) pressures and local circulatory collapse are common in injuries with intramuscular haematomas, crush injuries, fractures or amputations. If the perfusion pressure (systolic BP) is low, even a slight rise in IM pressure causes local hypoperfusion. With normal body temperature, peripheral limb circulation starts to decrease at a systolic BP around 80 mmHg.

REPERFUSION

The damage caused by reperfusion is often serious. If there is local hypoxaemia (high IM pressure, low blood pressure) for more than two hours, the reperfusion can cause extensive vascular damage. For this reason, decompression should be performed early.

In particular, the forearm and lower leg compartments are at risk.

Notes . . .

Special trauma cases

PAEDIATRICS

Trauma is a leading cause of death for all children, with a higher incidence in boys. The survival of children who sustain major trauma depends on pre-hospital care and early resuscitation.

The initial assessment of the paediatric trauma patient is identical to that for an adult. The first priorities are:

- Airway
- Breathing
- Circulation
- Early neurological assessment
- Exposure of the child, without losing heat.

The normal blood volume is proportionately greater in children and is calculated at 80 ml/kg in a child and 85–90 ml/kg in the neonate. Using a height/weight chart is often the easiest method of finding the approximate weight of a seriously-ill child.

Age	Pulse rate beats/min	Blood pressure systolic mmHg	Respiratory rate breaths/min	Blood volume ml/kg
<1 year	120–160	70–90	30–40	85–90
1–5 years	100–120	80–90	25–30	80
6–12 years	80–100	90–110	20–25	80
>12 years	60–100	100–120	15–20	70

Venous access in children who are hypovolaemic can be difficult. Useful sites for cannulation include the long saphenous vein over the ankle, the external jugular vein and femoral veins.

The intraosseous route can provide the quickest access to the circulation in a shocked child in whom venous cannulation is impossible. Fluids, blood and many drugs can be administered by this route. The intraosseous needle is normally sited in the anterior tibial plateau, 2–3 cm below the tibial tuberosity, thereby avoiding the epiphysial growth plate.

Once the needle has been located in the marrow cavity, fluids may need to be administered under pressure or via a syringe when rapid replacement is required. If purpose-designed intraosseous needles are unavailable, use a spinal, epidural or bone marrow biopsy needle as an alternative. The intraosseous route has been used in all age groups, but is generally most successful in children below about six years of age.

Hypovolaemia

Recognition of hypovolaemia can be more difficult than in the adult. The increased physiological reserves of the child may result in the vital signs being only slightly abnormal, even when up to 25% of blood volume is lost (Class I and II hypovolaemia).

Tachycardia is often the earliest response to hypovolaemia, but this can also be caused by fear or pain.

Classification of hypovolaemia in children

	Class I	Class II	Class III	Class IV
Blood volume lost	<15%	15–25%	25–40%	>40%
Pulse rate	Increased	>150	>150	Increased or bradycardia
Pulse pressure	Normal	Reduced	Very reduced	Absent
Systolic blood	Normal	Reduced	Very reduced	Unrecordable pressure
Capillary refill time	Normal	Prolonged	Very prolonged	Absent
Respiratory rate	Normal	Increased	Increased	Slow sighing respiration
Mental state	Normal	Irritable	Lethargic	Comatosed
Urine output	<1 ml/kg/hr	<1 ml/kg/hr	<1ml/kg/hr	<1 ml/kg/hr

Because the signs of hypovolaemia may only become apparent after 25% of the blood volume is lost, the initial fluid challenge in a child should represent this amount. Therefore, 20 ml/kg of crystalloid fluid should be given initially to the child showing signs of Class II hypovolaemia or greater. Depending on the response, this may need to be repeated up to three times (up to 60 ml/kg).

Children who have a transient or no response to the initial fluid challenge clearly require further crystalloid fluids and blood transfusion. 20 ml/kg of whole blood or 10 ml/kg of packed red cells should be initially transfused in these circumstances.

Due to the high surface-to-mass ratio in a child, heat loss occurs rapidly. A child who is hypothermic may become refractory to treatment. It is therefore vital to maintain the body temperature.

Acute gastric dilatation is commonly seen in the seriously ill or injured child. Gastric decompression, usually via a nasogastric tube, is therefore an essential component of their management.

After initial fluid resuscitation, and in the absence of a head injury, do not withhold analgesia. A recommended regime is:

- 50 microgm/kg intravenous bolus of morphine, followed by 10–20 microgm/kg increments at 10 minute intervals until an adequate response is achieved.

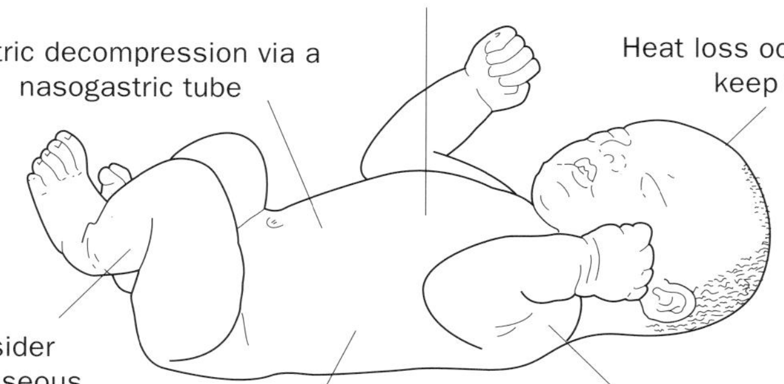

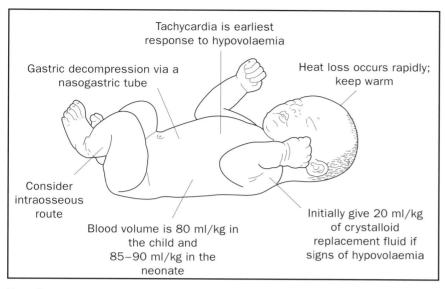

Figure 6

The principles in managing paediatric trauma patients are the same as for the adult.

Specific resuscitation and intubation issues in the young

- Relatively larger head and larger nasal airway and tongue
- Nose breathing in small babies
- Angle of the jaw is greater, larynx is higher and epiglottis is proportionally bigger and more "U"-shaped
- Cricoid is the narrowest part of the larynx which limits the size of the ETT; by adult life, the larynx has grown and the narrowest part is at the cords
- Trachea in the full-term newborn is about 4 cm long and will admit a 2.5 or 3.0 mm diameter ETT (the adult trachea is about 12 cm long)
- Gastric distension is common following resuscitation, and a nasogastric tube is useful to decompress the stomach.

If tracheal intubation is required, avoid cuffed tubes in children less than 10 years old so as to minimize subglottic swelling and ulceration. Oral intubation is easier than nasal for infants and young children.

Shock in the paediatric patient

The femoral artery in the groin and the brachial artery in the antecubital fossa are the best sites to palpate pulses in the child. If the child is pulseless, cardiopulmonary resuscitation should be commenced.

Signs of shock in paediatric patients include:

- Tachycardia
- Weak or absent peripheral pulses
- Capillary refill >2 seconds

- Tachypnoea
- Agitation
- Drowsiness
- Poor urine output.

Hypotension may be a late sign, even in the presence of severe shock.

Vascular access should be obtained. Two large bore intravenous cannulae should be inserted. Attempt peripheral veins first and avoid central venous catheters. Good sites are the long saphenous vein at the ankle and the femoral vein in the groin.

Hypothermia is a potentially major problem in a child. Because of the child's relatively large surface area to volume ratio, they lose proportionally more heat through the head. All fluids should be warmed. Exposure of the child is necessary for assessment, but consider covering as soon as possible.

The child should be kept warm and close to family, if at all possible.

Respiratory parameters and endotracheal tube size and placement

Age	Weight (kg)	Respiratory rate (breaths/min)	ETT size	ETT at lip (cm)	ETT at nose (cm)
Newborn	1.0–3.0	40–50	3.0	5.5–8.5	7–10.5
Newborn	3.5	40–50	3.5	9	11
3 months	6.0	30–50	3.5	10	12
1 year	10	20–30	4.0	11	14
2 years	12	20–30	4.5	12	15
3 years	14	20–30	4.5	13	16
4 years	16	15–25	5.0	14	17
6 years	20	15–25	5.5	15	19
8 years	24	10–20	6.0	16	20
10 years	30	10–20	6.5	17	21
12 years	38	10–20	7.0	18	22

Notes . . .

PREGNANCY

The ABCDE priorities of trauma management in pregnant patients is the same as those in non-pregnant patients.

Anatomical and physiological changes occur in pregnancy which are extremely important in the assessment of the pregnant trauma patient.

Anatomical changes

- The size of the uterus gradually increases and becomes more vulnerable to damage both by blunt and penetrating injury
  - At 12 weeks of gestation the fundus is at the symphysis pubis
  - At 20 weeks it is at the umbilicus
  - At 36 weeks it is at the xiphoid
- The fetus at first is well protected by the thick walled uterus and large amounts of amniotic fluid.

Physiological changes

- Increased tidal volume and respiratory alkalosis
- Increased heart rate
- 30% increased cardiac output
- Blood pressure is usually 15 mmHg lower
- Aortocaval compression in the third trimester with hypotension.

Special issues in the traumatized pregnant female

Blunt trauma may lead to:

- Uterine irritability and premature labour
- Partial or complete rupture of the uterus
- Partial or complete placental separation (up to 48 hours after trauma)
- With pelvic fracture, be aware of severe blood loss potential.

Priorities

- Assessment of the mother according to ABCDE
- Resuscitate in left lateral position to avoid aortocaval compression
- Vaginal examination (speculum) for vaginal bleeding and cervical dilatation
- Mark fundal height and tenderness and foetal heart rate, monitoring as appropriate.

Resuscitation of the mother may save the baby. There are times when the mother's life is at risk and the fetus may need to be sacrificed in order to save the mother.

> Aortocaval compression must be prevented in resuscitation of the traumatized pregnant woman. Remember left lateral tilt.

BURNS

The burns patient has the same priorities as all other trauma patients.

Assess:

- Airway
- Breathing: beware of inhalation and rapid airway compromise
- Circulation: fluid replacement
- Disability: compartment syndrome
- Exposure: percentage area of burn.

The source of the burn is important: e.g. fire, hot water, paraffin, kerosene. Electrical burns are often more serious than they appear. Remember damaged skin and muscle can results in acute renal failure.

Essential management points:

- Stop the burning
- ABCDE
- Determine the percentage area of burn (Rule of 9's)
- Good IV access and early fluid replacement.

The severity of the burn is determined by:

- Burned surface area
- Depth of burn
- Other considerations.

The burned surface area

Morbidity and mortality rises with increasing burned surface area. It also rises with increasing age so that even small burns may be fatal in elderly people.

Burns greater than 15% in an adult, greater than 10% in a child, or any burn occurring in the very young or elderly are considered serious.

Adults

The "Rule of 9's" is commonly used to estimate the burned surface area in adults. The body is divided into anatomical regions that represent 9% (or multiples of 9%) of the total body surface (Figure 7). The outstretched palm and fingers approximates to 1% of the body surface area. If the burned area is small, assess how many times your hand covers the area.

Children

The 'Rule of 9's' method is too imprecise for estimating the burned surface area in children because the infant or young child's head and lower extremities represent different proportions of surface area than in an adult (see Figure 8 on page PTCM–36).

Clinical manifestations of inhalation injury may not appear for the first 24 hours.

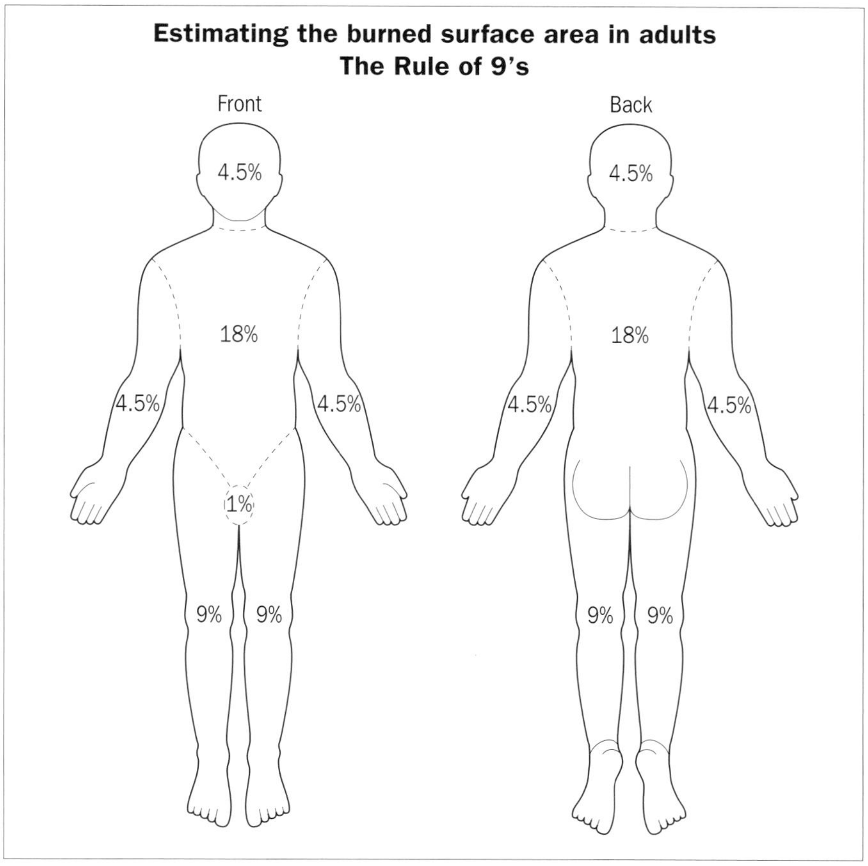

Figure 7

Depth of burn

It is important to estimate the depth of the burn to assess its severity and to plan future wound care. Burns can be divided into three types, as shown below.

Depth of burn	Characteristics	Cause
First degree burn	• Erythema • Pain • Absence of blisters	• Sunburn
Second degree (partial thickness)	• Red or mottled • Flash burns	• Contact with hot liquids
Third degree (full thickness)	• Dark and leathery • Dry	• Fire • Electricity or lightning • Prolonged exposure to hot liquids/objects

It is common to find all three types within the same burn wound and the depth may change with time, especially if infection occurs. Any full thickness burn is considered serious.

Estimating the burned surface area in children

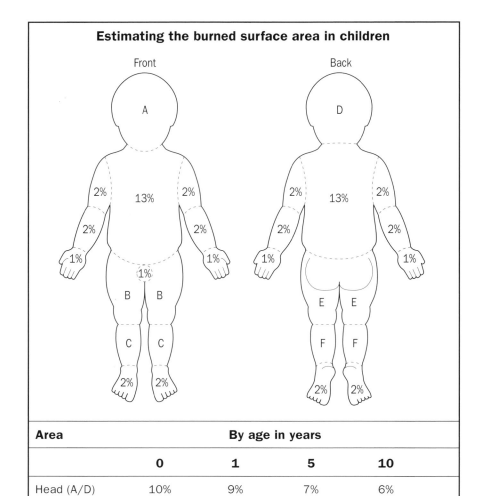

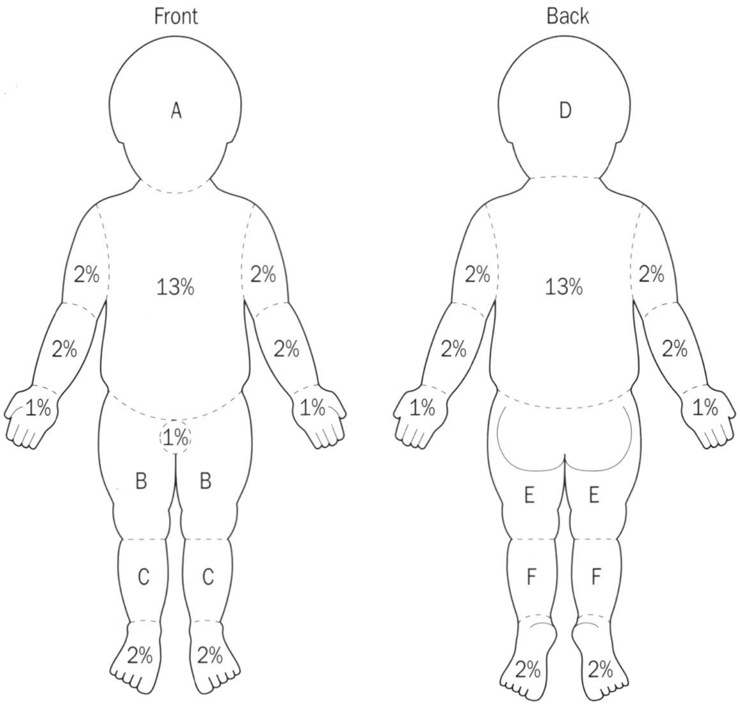

Area	By age in years			
	0	**1**	**5**	**10**
Head (A/D)	10%	9%	7%	6%
Thigh (B/E)	3%	3%	4%	5%
Leg (C/F)	2%	3%	3%	3%

Figure 8

Other considerations

In addition to the area and depth of burn, the site of burn also determines its severity. Burns to the face, neck, hands, feet, perineum and circumferential burns (those encircling a limb, neck, etc.) are classified as serious.

Serious burn requiring hospitalization

- Greater than 15% burns in an adult
- Greater than 10% burns in a child
- Any burn in the very young, the elderly or the infirm
- Any full thickness burn
- Burns of special regions: face, hands, feet, perineum
- Circumferential burns
- Inhalation injury
- Associated trauma or significant pre-burn illness: e.g. diabetes

Remember: patients with trauma of the face and neck are at risk for airway obstruction.

Specific issues for burns patients

The following principles can be used as a guide to detect and manage respiratory injury in the burn patient:

- Burns around the mouth
- Facial burns or singed facial or nasal hair
- Hoarseness, rasping cough
- Evidence of glottic oedema
- Circumferential, full-thickness burns of chest or neck.

Nasotracheal or endotracheal intubation is indicated especially if patient has severe increasing hoarseness, difficulty swallowing secretions, or increased respiratory rate with history of inhalation injury.

The burn patient requires at least 2–4 ml of crystalloid solution per kg body weight per percent body surface burn in the first 24 hours, starting from the time of the burn, to maintain an adequate circulating blood volume and provide adequate renal output. The estimated fluid volume is then proportioned in the following manner:

- One half of the total estimated fluid is provided in the first 8 hours post-burn
- The remaining one half is administered in the next 24 hours, to maintain an average urinary output of 0.5–1.0 ml/kg/hour.

Assessment of the size and extent of the burn is difficult. This formula is only a rough guide and it is essential to reassess the fluid state of the patient regularly.

Undertake the following, if possible:

- Pain relief
- Bladder catheterization if burn > 20%
- Nasogastric drainage
- Tetanus prophylaxis.

Notes . . .

Transport of critically ill patients

Transporting patients is risky. It requires good communication, planning and appropriate staffing. Any patient who requires transportation must be effectively stabilized before departure. As a general principle, patients should be transported only if they are going to a facility that can provide a higher level of care.

Planning and preparation include consideration of:

- Type of transport (car, landrover, boat, etc.)
- Personnel to accompany the patient
- Equipment and supplies required en route for routine and emergency treatment
- Potential complications
- Monitoring and final packaging of the patient.

Effective communication is essential with:

- The receiving centre
- The transport service
- Escorting personnel
- The patient and relatives.

Effective stabilization necessitates:

- Prompt initial resuscitation
- Control of haemorrhage and maintenance of the circulation
- Immobilization of fractures
- Analgesia.

Remember, if the patient deteriorates

- Re-evaluate the patient by using the primary survey
- Check and treat life threatening conditions
- Make a careful assessment focusing on the affected system.

> Be prepared: if anything can go wrong, it will – and at the worst possible time!

Notes . . .

Trauma response

Long before any trauma patient arrives in your medical care, roles must be identified and allocated to each member of the trauma team.

TEAM MEMBERS

The membership of the trauma team will depend on the availability of staff. Ideally, it should comprise:

- On-duty emergency doctor or experienced health worker (team leader)
- On-duty emergency nurse
- 1 or 2 additional helpers.

Trauma team roles

Team leader (doctor)	Nurse
• Coordinate ABCs • Take patient history from the patient or family • Request X-rays (if possible) • Perform the secondary survey • Consider tetanus prophylaxis and antibiotics • Reassess the patient • Prepare the patient for transfer • Complete the documentation	• Help co-ordinate early resuscitation • Liaise with relatives • Check documentation including: – Allergies – Medications – Past history – Last meal – Events leading to injury • Notify nursing staff in other areas

When the patient actually arrives, a rapid overview is necessary. This is known as *triage*. Triage means to prioritize patient management according to:

- Medical need
- Personnel available
- Resources available.

Notes . . .

Activation plan for trauma team

CRITERIA

The following patients should undergo full trauma assessment:

History

- Fall >3 metres
- Motor vehicle accident: net speed >30 km/hour
- Thrown from vehicle/trapped in vehicle
- Death of a person in accident
- Pedestrian *vs* car/cyclist *vs* car/ unrestrained occupant.

Examination

- Airway or respiratory distress
- BP >100 mmHg
- Glasgow Coma Scale <13/15 (see page PTCM–23)
- >1 area injured
- Penetrating injury.

DISASTER MANAGEMENT

Disasters do occur and disaster planning is an essential part to any trauma service. A disaster is any event that exceeds the ability of local resources to cope with the situation.

A simple disaster plan must include:

- Disaster scenarios practice
- Disaster management protocols including:
  - On-scene management
  - Key personnel identification
  - Trauma triage
- Medical team allocations from your hospital
- Agreement in advance on who will be involved in the event of a disaster:
  - Ambulance
  - Police/army
  - National/international authorities
  - Aid and relief agencies.
- Evacuation priorities
- Modes of transport: road/air (helicopter/fixed wing)/sea
- Communications strategies.

Index

D

I

M

N

O

P

T

U

V

W

X